The Maudsley

The South London and Maudsley NHS Foundation Trust
&
Oxleas NHS Foundation Trust

PRESCRIBING GUIDELINES

10th Edition

David Taylor
Carol Paton
Shitij Kapur

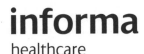

informa
healthcare

Reprinted 2010

First published in the United Kingdom in 2009 by Informa Healthcare, Telephone House,
69-77 Paul Street, London EC2A 4LQ. Informa Healthcare is a trading division of Informa
UK Ltd. Registered Office: 37/41 Mortimer Street, London W1T 3JH. Registered in England
and Wales number 1072954.

www.informahealthcare.com

A CIP record for this book is available from the British Library.
Library of Congress Cataloging-in-Publication Data

Data available on application

ISBN-13: 978 1 84184 699 6

Distributed in North and South America by
Taylor & Francis
6000 Broken Sound Parkway, NW, (Suite 300)
Boca Raton, FL 33487, USA

Within Continental USA
Tel: 1 (800) 272 7737; Fax: 1 (800) 374 3401
Outside Continental USA
Tel: (561) 994 0555; Fax: (561) 361 6018
Email: orders@crcpress.com

Book orders in the rest of the world
Telephone: +44 (0)20 7017 5540
Email: CSDhealthcarebooks@informa.com

Composition by Exeter Premedia Services Pvt Ltd, Chennai, India
Printed and bound in Great Britain by the MPG Books Group, Bodmin, Cornwall, UK

Authors and editors

David Taylor
Chief Pharmacist, South London and Maudsley NHS Foundation Trust
Professor of Psychopharmacology, King's College, London

Carol Paton
Chief Pharmacist, Oxleas NHS Foundation Trust
Honorary Research Fellow, Imperial College, London

Shitij Kapur
Vice Dean and Professor, Institute of Psychiatry, London

Preface

The 10th edition of the *Maudsley Prescribing Guidelines* fully updates the 9th edition and includes new sections offering guidance on, for example, the use of psychotropics in atrial fibrillation, alternative routes for antidepressant administration, the treatment of velo-cardio-facial syndrome and the covert administration of medicines. Where possible guidance has been aligned with the most recently issued guidelines from UK NICE and the latest Cochrane reviews. There has also been an attempt to make the text 'future-proof' (at least for a year or two) by anticipating new drug introductions and changes in Product Licences.

Following the tragic loss of Rob Kerwin in 2007, we now welcome Shitij Kapur as a co-author of the Prescribing Guidelines. Shitij is one of the world's foremost researchers in the field of schizophrenia and is widely recognised for his innovative and cogently argued theories on the causes and treatment of psychosis. We are honoured to have Shitij as part of our team and it serves as an honour to Rob Kerwin that only an illustrious clinician as Shitij could be considered a suitable replacement.

As before, we are indebted to a great many people who have contributed their time and expertise to the Prescribing Guidelines in expectation of no more than being mentioned on the following page. The Guidelines would be nothing without their invaluable contributions. Thanks are also due to those who have written to me making suggestions about the Guidelines and to both formal and internet reviewers who have provided precious feedback on previous editions. Particular thanks are due to Maria O'Hagan who has managed the production of this and several previous editions of the *Maudsley Prescribing Guidelines*.

David Taylor
June 2009

vi

Acknowledgements

We are deeply indebted to previous contributors and to the following contributors to the present edition of the *Maudsley Prescribing Guidelines*.

Ayesha Ali
Azizah Attard
Sube Banerjee
Elizabeth Bevan
Delia Bishara
Steve Bleakley
Anthony Cleare
Anne Connolly
Richard Corrigall
Sarah Curran
Anthony David
Sarah Elliott
Emily Finch
Russell Foster
Deborah Green
Lucinda Green
Paul Gringras
Isobel Heyman
Louise Howard
Bimpe Idowu
Sally Jones
Theresa Joyce
Jenny Keech
Mike Kelleher
Shubhra Mace
Jane Marshall
Gordana Milavic
Quynh-Anh Nguyen
Ifeoma Okonkwo
Carmine Pariente
Mike Philpot
Sally Porter
Kylie Reed
Eli Silber
Emily Simonoff
Anna Sparshatt
Argyris Stringaris
Gay Sutherland
Eric Taylor
Rochelle Tsang

Special thanks to

Jo Taylor

Notes on using *The Maudsley Prescribing Guidelines*

The main aim of *The Guidelines* is to provide clinicians with practically useful advice on the prescribing of psychotropic agents in commonly encountered clinical situations. The advice contained in this handbook is based on a combination of literature review, clinical experience and expert contribution. We do not claim that this advice is necessarily 'correct' or that it deserves greater prominence than guidance provided by other professional bodies or special interest groups. We hope, however, to have provided guidance that helps to assure the safe, effective and economic use of medicines in mental health. We hope also to have made clear the sources of information used to inform the guidance given.

Please note that many of the recommendations provided here go beyond the licensed or labelled indications of many drugs, both in the UK and elsewhere. Note also that, while we have endeavoured to make sure all quoted doses are correct, clinicians should always consult statutory texts before prescribing. Users of *The Guidelines* should also bear in mind that the contents of this handbook are based on information available to us up to June 2009. Much of the advice contained here will become outdated as more research is conducted and published.

No liability is accepted for any injury, loss or damage, however caused.

Notes on inclusion of drugs

The Guidelines are used in many other countries outside the UK. With this in mind, we have included in this edition those drugs in widespread use throughout the western world in June 2009. Thus, we have included, for example, ziprasidone and iloperidone, even though these drugs are not marketed in the UK at this time. Their inclusion gives *The Guidelines* relevance in those countries where ziprasidone and iloperidone are marketed and may also be of benefit to UK readers, since many unlicensed drugs can be obtained through formal pharmaceutical importers. We have also tried to include information on drugs likely to be introduced into practice in the next two years. Many older drugs (methotrimeprazine, pericyazine, maprotiline, etc.) are either only briefly mentioned or not included on the basis that these drugs are not in widespread use at the time of writing.

Notes on commonly used abbreviations

Throughout this text we have abbreviated *British National Formulary* to BNF and extrapyramidal side-effects to EPS. We have also used FGA for first generation antipsychotics and SGA for second generation antipsychotics (broadly speaking, those antipsychotics marketed in the UK since 1990). SPC refers to the UK Summary of Product Characteristics for the drug in question.

All other abbreviations are explained in the text itself.

Contents

Plasma level monitoring of psychotropics and anticonvulsants

Introduction

Plasma drug concentration or 'plasma level' monitoring is a process surrounded by some confusion and misunderstanding. Drug level monitoring, when appropriately used, is of considerable help in optimising treatment and assuring adherence. However, in psychiatry, as in other areas of medicine, plasma level determinations are frequently undertaken without good cause and results acted upon inappropriately[1]. Conversely, in other instances, plasma levels are underused.

Before taking a blood sample for plasma level assay, make sure that the following criteria are satisfied:

- **Is there a clinically useful assay method available?**
  Only a minority of drugs have available assays. The assay must be clinically validated and results available within a clinically useful timescale.

- **Is the drug at 'steady state'?**
  Plasma levels are usually meaningful only when samples are taken after steady-state levels have been achieved. This takes 4–5 drug half-lives.

- **Is the timing of the sample correct?**
  Sampling time is vitally important for many but not all drugs. If the recommended sampling time is 12 hours post-dose, then the sample should be taken 11–13 hours post-dose if possible; 10–14 hours post-dose, if absolutely necessary. For trough or 'pre-dose' samples, take the blood sample immediately before the next dose is due. Do not, under any circumstances, withhold the next dose for more than 1 or (possibly) 2 hours until a sample is taken. Withholding for longer than this will inevitably give a misleading result (it will give a lower result than that ever seen in the usual, regular dosing), and this may lead to an inappropriate dose increase. Sampling

time is less critical with drugs with a long half-life (e.g. olanzapine) but, as an absolute minimum, prescribers should always record the time of sampling and time of last dose.

If a sample is not taken within 1–2 hours of the required time, it has the potential to mislead rather than inform. The only exception to this is if toxicity is suspected – sampling at the time of suspected toxicity is obviously appropriate.

- **Will the level have any inherent meaning?**
Is there a target range of plasma levels? If so, then plasma levels (from samples taken at the right time) will usefully guide dosing. If there is not an accepted target range, plasma levels can only indicate adherence or potential toxicity. However, if the sample is being used to check compliance, then bear in mind that a plasma level of zero indicates only that the drug has not been taken in the past several days. Plasma levels above zero may indicate erratic compliance, full compliance or even long-standing non-compliance disguised by recent taking of prescribed doses. Note also that target ranges have their limitations: patients may respond to lower levels than the quoted range and tolerate levels above the range; also, ranges quoted by different laboratories vary sometimes widely without explanation.

- **Is there a clear reason for plasma level determination?**
Only the following reasons are valid:
  - to confirm compliance (but see above)
  - if toxicity is suspected
  - if drug interaction is suspected
  - if clinical response is difficult to assess directly (and where a target range of plasma levels has been established)
  - if the drug has a narrow therapeutic index and toxicity concerns are considerable.

Interpreting sample results

The basic rule for sample level interpretation is to act upon assay results in conjunction with reliable clinical observation (*'treat the patient, not the level'*). For example, if a patient is responding adequately to a drug but has a plasma level below the accepted target range, then the dose should not normally be increased. If a patient has intolerable adverse effects but a plasma level within the target range, then a dose decrease may be appropriate.

Where a plasma level result is substantially different from previous results, a repeat sample is usually advised. Check dose, timing of dose and recent compliance but ensure, in particular, the correct timing of the sample. Many anomalous results are the consequence of changes in sample timing.

Table Interpreting sample results

Drug	Target range	Sample timing	Time to steady state	Comments
Amisulpride	200–320 µg/L	Trough	3 days	Refer to text
Aripiprazole	150–210 µg/L	Trough	15–16 days	Refer to text
Carbamazepine[2,3]	>7 mg/L bipolar disorder	Trough	2 weeks	Carbamazepine induces its own metabolism. Time to steady state dependent on auto-induction
Clozapine	350–500 µg/L Upper limit of target range is ill-defined	Trough	2–3 days	Refer to text
Lamotrigine[4–7]	Not established but suggest 2.5–15 mg/L	Trough	5 days Auto-induction is thought to occur, so time to steady state may be longer	Some debate over utility of lamotrigine levels, especially in bipolar disorder. Toxicity may be increased above 15 mg/L
Lithium[8–11]	0.6–1.0 mmol/L (may be >1.0 mmol/L in mania)	12 hours	5 days post-dose	Well-established target range
Olanzapine	20–40 µg/L	12 hours	1 week	Refer to text
Phenytoin[3]	10–20 mg/L	Trough	Variable	Follows zero-order kinetics. Free levels may be useful
Quetiapine	Around 50–100 µg/L?	Trough?	2–3 days oral	Target range not defined. Plasma level monitoring not recommended. Refer to text
Risperidone	20–60 µg/L (active moiety)	Trough	2–3 days oral 6–8 weeks injection	Plasma level monitoring is not recommended Refer to text
Tricyclics[12]	Nortriptyline 50–150 µg/L Amitriptyline 100–200 µg/L	Trough	2–3 days	Rarely used and of dubious benefit. Use ECG to assess toxicity
Valproate[2,3,13–16]	50–100 mg/L Epilepsy and bipolar	Trough	2–3 days	Some doubt over value of levels in epilepsy and bipolar disorder. Some evidence that levels up to 125 mg/L are tolerated and more effective than lower levels (in mania)

Amisulpride

Amisulpride plasma levels are closely related to dose with insufficient variation to recommend routine plasma level monitoring. Higher levels observed in women[17–19] and older age[17,19] seem to have little significant clinical implication for either therapeutic response or adverse effects. A (trough) threshold for clinical response has been suggested to be approximately 100 µg/L[20] and mean levels of 367 µg/L[19] noted in responders in individual studies. Adverse effects (notably EPS) have been observed at mean levels of 336 µg/L[17], 377 µg/L[20] and 395 µg/L[18]. A plasma level threshold of below 320 µg/L has been found to predict avoidance of EPS[20]. A review of the current literature[21] has suggested an approximate range of **200 µg/L to 320 µg/L** for optimal clinical response and avoidance of adverse effects.

In practice, amisulpride plasma level monitoring is rarely undertaken and few laboratories offer amisulpride assays. The dose–response relationship is sufficiently robust to obviate the need for plasma sampling within the licensed dose range; adverse effects are well managed by dose adjustment alone. Plasma level monitoring is best reserved for those in whom clinical response is poor, adherence is questioned and in whom drug interactions or physical illness may make adverse effect more likely.

Aripiprazole

Plasma level monitoring of aripiprazole is rarely carried out in practice. The dose–response relationship of aripiprazole is well established with a plateau in clinical response and D_2 dopamine occupancy seen in doses above approximately 10 mg/day[22]. Plasma levels of aripiprazole, its metabolite, and the total moiety (parent plus metabolite) strongly relate linearly to dose, making it possible to predict, with some certainty, an approximate plasma level for a given dose[23]. Target plasma level ranges for optimal clinical response have been suggested as 146–254 µg/L[24] and 150–300 µg/L[25], with adverse effects observed above 210 µg/L[25]. Inter-individual variation in aripiprazole plasma levels has been observed but not fully investigated, although gender appears to have little influence[26,27]. Age, metabolic enzyme genotype and interacting medications seem likely causes of variation[25–28], however there are too few reports regarding their clinical implication to recommend specific monitoring in light of these factors. A putative range of between **150 µg/L and 210 µg/L**[23] has been suggested as a target for patients taking aripiprazole who are showing little or no clinical response or intolerable EPS. However, for reasons described here, plasma level monitoring is not advised in routine practice.

Clozapine

Clozapine plasma levels are broadly related to daily dose[29], but there is sufficient variation to make impossible any precise prediction of plasma level. Plasma levels are generally lower in younger patients, males[30] and smokers[31] and higher in Asians[32]. A series of algorithms has been developed for the approximate prediction of clozapine levels according to patient factors and are recommended[33]. Algorithms cannot, however, account for other influences on clozapine plasma levels such as changes in adherence, inflammation[34] and infection[35].

The plasma level threshold for acute response to clozapine has been suggested to be 200 µg/L[36], 350 µg/L[37–39], 370 µg/L[40], 420 µg/L[41], 504 µg/L[42] and 550 µg/L[43]. Limited data suggest a level of at least 200 µg/L is required to prevent relapse[44].

Despite these varied estimates of response threshold, plasma levels can be useful in optimising treatment. In those not responding to clozapine, dose should be adjusted to give plasma levels in the range **350–500 μg/L**. Those not tolerating clozapine may benefit from a reduction to a dose giving plasma levels in this range. An upper limit to the clozapine target range has not been defined. Plasma levels do seem to predict EEG changes[45] and seizures occur more frequently in patients with levels above 1000 μg/L[46], so levels should probably be kept well below this. Other non-neurological clozapine-related adverse effects also seem to be plasma level related[47] as might be expected. Note also that clozapine metabolism may become saturated at higher doses: the ratio of clozapine to norclozapine rises with increasing plasma levels, suggesting saturation[48–50]. The effect of fluvoxamine also suggests that metabolism via CYP1A2 to norclozapine can be overwhelmed[51].

A further consideration is that placing an upper limit on the target range for clozapine levels may discourage potentially worthwhile dose increases within the licensed dose range. Before plasma levels were widely used, clozapine was fairly often dosed to 900 mg/day, with valproate being added when the dose reached 600 mg/day. It remains unclear whether using these high doses can benefit patients with plasma levels already above the accepted threshold. Nonetheless, it is prudent to use valproate as prophylaxis against seizures and myoclonus when plasma levels are above 500–600 μg/L and certainly when levels approach 1000 μg/L.

Olanzapine

Plasma levels of olanzapine are linearly related to daily dose, but there is substantial variation[52], with higher levels seen in women[42], non-smokers[53] and those on enzyme-inhibiting drugs[53,54]. With once-daily dosing, the threshold level for response in schizophrenia has been suggested to be 9.3 μg/L (trough sample)[55], 23.2 μg/L (12-hour post-dose sample)[42] and 23 μg/L at a mean of 13.5 hours postdose[56]. There is evidence to suggest that levels greater than around 40 μg/L (12-hour sampling) produce no further therapeutic benefit than lower levels[57]. Severe toxicity is uncommon but may be associated with levels above 100 μg/L, and death is occasionally seen at levels above 160 μg/L[58] (albeit when other drugs or physical factors are relevant). A target range for therapeutic use of **20–40 μg/L** (12-hour post-dose sample) has been proposed[59] for schizophrenia (the range for mania is probably similar[60]). Notably, significant weight gain seems most likely to occur in those with plasma levels above 20 μg/L[61]. Constipation, dry mouth and tachycardia also seem to be plasma level related[62].

In practice, the dose of olanzapine should be governed by response and tolerability. Plasma level determinations should be reserved for those suspected of non-adherence or those not responding to the maximum licensed dose. In the latter case, dose may then be adjusted to give 12-hour plasma levels of **20–40 μg/L**.

Quetiapine

The dose of quetiapine is weakly related to trough plasma levels[63–66]. Mean levels reported within the dose range 150 mg/day to 800 mg/day range from 27 μg/L to 387 μg/L[66–73], although the highest and lowest levels are not necessarily found at the lowest and highest doses. Age, gender and co-medication may contribute to the significant inter-individual variance observed in TDM studies, with female gender[72,74], older age[71,72] and CYP3A4-inhibiting drugs[66,71,72] likely to increase quetiapine concentration. Reports of these effects are conflicting[63,64,68,73] and not sufficient to support the routine use of plasma level monitoring based on these factors alone. Thresholds for clinical response have been proposed as **77 µg/L**[63,64] and **50–100 µg/L**[73]; EPS has been observed in females with levels in excess of 210 µg/L[63,64]. Despite the substantial variation in plasma levels at each dose, there is insufficient evidence to suggest a target therapeutic range, thus plasma level monitoring has little value. Most current reports of quetiapine concentrations are from trough samples. Because of the short half life of quetiapine, plasma levels tend to drop to within a relatively small range regardless of dose and previous peak level. Thus peak plasma levels may be more closely related to dose and clinical response, although monitoring of such is not currently justified in the absence of an established peak plasma target range. Quetiapine has an established dose–response relationship, and appears to be well tolerated at doses well beyond the licensed dose range[75]. In practice, dose adjustment should be based on patient response and tolerability.

Risperidone

Risperidone plasma levels are rarely measured in the UK and very few laboratories have developed assay methods for its determination. In any case, plasma level monitoring is probably unproductive (dose–response is well described) except where compliance is in doubt and in such cases measurement of prolactin will give some idea of compliance.

The therapeutic range for risperidone is said to be **20–60 µg/L** of the active moiety (risperidone + 9-OH-risperidone)[76,77]. Plasma levels of this magnitude are usually provided by oral doses of between 3 mg and 6 mg a day[76,78–80]. Occupancy of striatal dopamine D_2 receptors has been shown to be around 65% (the minimum required for therapeutic effect) at plasma levels of approximately 20 µg/L[77].

Risperidone long-acting injection (25 mg/2 weeks) appears to afford plasma levels averaging between 4.4 and 22.7 µg/L[79]. Dopamine D_2 occupancies at this dose have been variously estimated at between 25% and 71%[77,81,82]. There is considerable inter-individual variation around these mean values with a substantial minority of patients with plasma levels above those shown. Nonetheless, these data do cast doubt on the efficacy of a dose of 25 mg/2 weeks[79], although it is noteworthy that there is some evidence that long-acting preparations are effective despite apparently sub-therapeutic plasma levels and dopamine occupancies[83].

References

1. Mann K et al. Appropriateness of therapeutic drug monitoring for antidepressants in routine psychiatric inpatient care. Ther Drug Monit 2006; 28:83–8.
2. Taylor D et al. Doses of carbamazepine and valproate in bipolar affective disorder. Psychiatr Bull 1997; 21:221–3.
3. Eadie MJ. Anticonvulsant drugs. Drugs 1984; 27:328–63.
4. Cohen AF et al. Lamotrigine, a new anticonvulsant: pharmacokinetics in normal humans. Clin Pharmacol Ther 1987; 42:535–41.
5. Kilpatrick ES et al. Concentration–effect and concentration–toxicity relations with lamotrigine: a prospective study. Epilepsia 1996; 37:534–8.
6. Johannessen SI et al. Therapeutic drug monitoring of the newer antiepileptic drugs. Ther Drug Monit 2003; 25:347–63.
7. Lardizabal DV et al. Tolerability and pharmacokinetics of oral loading with lamotrigine in epilepsy monitoring units. Epilepsia 2003; 44:536–9.
8. Schou M. Forty years of lithium treatment. Arch Gen Psychiatry 1997; 54:9–13.
9. Anon. Using lithium safely. Drug Ther Bull 1999; 37:22–4.
10. Nicholson J et al. Monitoring patients on lithium – a good practice guideline. Psychiatr Bull 2002; 26:348–51.
11. National Institute for Health and Clinical Excellence. Bipolar disorder. The management of bipolar disorder in adults, children and adolescents, in primary and secondary care. Clinical Guidance 38. http://www.nice.org.uk. 2006.
12. Taylor D et al. Plasma levels of tricyclics and related antidepressants: are they necessary or useful? Psychiatr Bull 1995; 19:548–50.
13. Davis R et al. Valproic acid – a reappraisal of its pharmacological properties and clinical efficacy in epilepsy. Drugs 1994; 47:332–72.
14. Perucca E. Pharmacological and therapeutic properties of valproate. CNS Drugs 2002; 16:695–714.
15. Allen MH et al. Linear relationship of valproate serum concentration to response and optimal serum levels for acute mania. Am J Psychiatry 2006; 163:272–5.
16. Bowden CL et al. Relation of serum valproate concentration to response in mania. Am J Psychiatry 1996; 153:765–70.
17. Muller MJ et al. Amisulpride doses and plasma levels in different age groups of patients with schizophrenia or schizoaffective disorder. J Psychopharmacol 2008; 23:278–86.
18. Muller MJ et al. Gender aspects in the clinical treatment of schizophrenic inpatients with amisulpride: a therapeutic drug monitoring study. Pharmacopsychiatry 2006; 39:41–6.
19. Bergemann N et al. Plasma amisulpride levels in schizophrenia or schizoaffective disorder. Eur Neuropsychopharmacol 2004; 14:245–50.
20. Muller MJ et al. Therapeutic drug monitoring for optimizing amisulpride therapy in patients with schizophrenia. J Psychiatr Res 2007; 41:673–9.

21. Sparshatt A et al. Amisulpride - dose, plasma concentration, occupancy and response: implications for therapeutic drug monitoring. Acta Psychiatr Scand 2009; Epub ahead of print. DOI: 10.1111/j.1600–0447.2009.01429.x.
22. Mace S et al. Aripiprazole: dose–response relationship in schizophrenia and schizoaffective disorder. CNS Drugs 2008; In Press.
23. Sparshatt A et al. Aripiprazole – dose, plasma concentration, receptor occupancy and response: implications for therapeutic drug monitoring. J Clin Psychiatry 2009; In Press.
24. Kirschbaum KM et al. Therapeutic monitoring of aripiprazole by HPLC with column-switching and spectrophotometric detection. Clin Chem 2005; 51:1718–21.
25. Kirschbaum KM et al. Serum levels of aripiprazole and dehydroaripiprazole, clinical response and side effects. World J Biol Psychiatry 2008; 9:212–18.
26. Molden E et al. Pharmacokinetic variability of aripiprazole and the active metabolite dehydroaripiprazole in psychiatric patients. Ther Drug Monit 2006; 28:744–9.
27. Bachmann CJ et al. Large variability of aripiprazole and dehydroaripiprazole serum concentrations in adolescent patients with schizophrenia. Ther Drug Monit 2008; 30:462–6.
28. Hendset M et al. Impact of the CYP2D6 genotype on steady-state serum concentrations of aripiprazole and dehydroaripiprazole. Eur J Clin Pharmacol 2007; 63:1147–51.
29. Haring C et al. Influence of patient-related variables on clozapine plasma levels. Am J Psychiatry 1990; 147:1471–5.
30. Haring C et al. Dose-related plasma levels of clozapine: influence of smoking behaviour, sex and age. Psychopharmacology 1989; 99 Suppl:S38–40.
31. Taylor D. Pharmacokinetic interactions involving clozapine. Br J Psychiatry 1997; 171:109–12.
32. Ng CH et al. An inter-ethnic comparison study of clozapine dosage, clinical response and plasma levels. Int Clin Psychopharmacol 2005; 20:163–8.
33. Rostami-Hodjegan A et al. Influence of dose, cigarette smoking, age, sex, and metabolic activity on plasma clozapine concentrations: a predictive model and nomograms to aid clozapine dose adjustment and to assess compliance in individual patients. J Clin Psychopharmacol 2004; 24:70–8.
34. Haack MJ et al. Toxic rise of clozapine plasma concentrations in relation to inflammation. Eur Neuropsychopharmacol 2003; 13:381–5.
35. de Leon J et al. Serious respiratory infections can increase clozapine levels and contribute to side effects: a case report. Prog Neuropsychopharmacol Biol Psychiatry 2003; 27:1059–63.
36. VanderZwaag C et al. Response of patients with treatment-refractory schizophrenia to clozapine within three serum level ranges. Am J Psychiatry 1996; 153:1579–84.
37. Perry PJ et al. Clozapine and norclozapine plasma concentrations and clinical response of treatment refractory schizophrenic patients. Am J Psychiatry 1991; 148:231–5.
38. Miller DD. Effect of phenytoin on plasma clozapine concentrations in two patients. J Clin Psychiatry 1991; 52:23–5.
39. Spina E et al. Relationship between plasma concentrations of clozapine and norclozapine and therapeutic response in patients with schizophrenia resistant to conventional neuroleptics. Psychopharmacology 2000; 148:83–9.
40. Hasegawa M et al. Relationship between clinical efficacy and clozapine concentrations in plasma in schizophrenia: effect of smoking. J Clin Psychopharmacol 1993; 13:383–90.
41. Potkin SG et al. Plasma clozapine concentrations predict clinical response in treatment-resistant schizophrenia. J Clin Psychiatry 1994; 55 Suppl B:133–6.
42. Perry PJ. Therapeutic drug monitoring of antipsychotics. Psychopharmacol Bull 2001; 35:19–29.
43. Llorca PM et al. Effectiveness of clozapine in neuroleptic-resistant schizophrenia: clinical response and plasma concentrations. J Psychiatry Neurosci 2002; 27:30–7.
44. Xiang YQ et al. Serum concentrations of clozapine and norclozapine in the prediction of relapse of patients with schizophrenia. Schizophr Res 2006; 83:201–10.
45. Khan AY et al. Examining concentration-dependent toxicity of clozapine: role of therapeutic drug monitoring. J Psychiatr Pract 2005; 11:289–301.
46. Greenwood-Smith C et al. Serum clozapine levels: a review of their clinical utility. J Psychopharmacol 2003; 17:234–8.
47. Yusufi B et al. Prevalence and nature of side effects during clozapine maintenance treatment and the relationship with clozapine dose and plasma concentration. Int Clin Psychopharmacol 2007; 22:238–43.
48. Volpicelli SA et al. Determination of clozapine, norclozapine, and clozapine-N-oxide in serum by liquid chromatography. Clin Chem 1993; 39:1656–9.
49. Guitton C et al. Clozapine and metabolite concentrations during treatment of patients with chronic schizophrenia. J Clin Pharmacol 1999; 39:721–8.
50. Palego L et al. Clozapine, norclozapine plasma levels, their sum and ratio in 50 psychotic patients: influence of patient-related variables. Prog Neuropsychopharmacol Biol Psychiatry 2002; 26:473–80.
51. Wang CY et al. The differential effects of steady-state fluvoxamine on the pharmacokinetics of olanzapine and clozapine in healthy volunteers. J Clin Pharmacol 2004; 44:785–92.
52. Aravagiri M et al. Plasma level monitoring of olanzapine in patients with schizophrenia: determination by high-performance liquid chromatography with electrochemical detection. Ther Drug Monit 1997; 19:307–13.
53. Gex-Fabry M et al. Therapeutic drug monitoring of olanzapine: the combined effect of age, gender, smoking, and comedication. Ther Drug Monit 2003; 25:46–53.
54. Bergemann N et al. Olanzapine plasma concentration, average daily dose, and interaction with co-medication in schizophrenic patients. Pharmacopsychiatry 2004; 37:63–8.
55. Perry PJ et al. Olanzapine plasma concentrations and clinical response in acutely ill schizophrenic patients. J Clin Psychopharmacol 1997; 6:472–7.
56. Fellows L et al. Investigation of target plasma concentration–effect relationships for olanzapine in schizophrenia. Ther Drug Monit 2003; 25:682–9.
57. Mauri MC et al. Clinical outcome and olanzapine plasma levels in acute schizophrenia. Eur Psychiatry 2005; 20:55–60.
58. Rao ML et al. [Olanzapine: pharmacology, pharmacokinetics and therapeutic drug monitoring]. Fortschr Neurol Psychiatr 2001; 69:510–17.
59. Robertson MD et al. Olanzapine concentrations in clinical serum and postmortem blood specimens – when does therapeutic become toxic? J Forensic Sci 2000; 45:418–21.
60. Bech P et al. Olanzapine plasma level in relation to antimanic effect in the acute therapy of manic states. Nord J Psychiatry 2006; 60:181–2.
61. Perry PJ et al. The association of weight gain and olanzapine plasma concentrations. J Clin Psychopharmacol 2005; 25:250–4.
62. Kelly DL et al. Plasma concentrations of high-dose olanzapine in a double-blind crossover study. Hum Psychopharmacol 2006; 21:393–8.
63. Dragicevic A, Muller MJ, Sachse J, Hartter S, Hiemke C. Therapeutic drug monitoring (TDM) of quetiapine. 2003. Lecture presented at the Symposium of the AGNP, October 8–10, Munich.
64. Hiemke C et al. Therapeutic monitoring of new antipsychotic drugs. Ther Drug Monit 2004; 26:156–60.
65. Gerlach M et al. Therapeutic drug monitoring of quetiapine in adolescents with psychotic disorders. Pharmacopsychiatry 2007; 40:72–6.
66. Hasselstrom J et al. Quetiapine serum concentrations in psychiatric patients: the influence of comedication. Ther Drug Monit 2004; 26:486–91.
67. Winter HR et al. Steady-state pharmacokinetic, safety, and tolerability profiles of quetiapine, norquetiapine, and other quetiapine metabolites in pediatric and adult patients with psychotic disorders. J Child Adolesc Psychopharmacol 2008; 18:81–98.
68. Mauri MC et al. Two weeks' quetiapine treatment for schizophrenia, drug-induced psychosis and borderline personality disorder: a naturalistic study with drug plasma levels. Expert Opin Pharmacother 2007; 8:2207–13.
69. Li KY et al. Multiple dose pharmacokinetics of quetiapine and some of its metabolites in Chinese suffering from schizophrenia. Acta Pharmacol Sin 2004; 25:390–4.
70. McConville BJ et al. Pharmacokinetics, tolerability, and clinical effectiveness of quetiapine fumarate: an open-label trial in adolescents with psychotic disorders. J Clin Psychiatry 2000; 61:252–60.
71. Castberg I et al. Quetiapine and drug interactions: evidence from a routine therapeutic drug monitoring service. J Clin Psychiatry 2007; 68:1540–5.
72. Aichhorn W et al. Influence of age, gender, body weight and valproate comedication on quetiapine plasma concentrations. Int Clin Psychopharmacol 2006; 21:81–5.

73. Dragicevic A, Trotzauer D, Hiemke C, Muller MJ. Gender and age effects on quetiapine serum concentrations in patients with schizophrenia or schizoaffective disorders. 2005. Lecture presented at the 24th Symposium of the AGNP, 5–8 October, Munich.

74. Mauri MC et al. Two weeks' quetiapine treatment for schizophrenia, drug-induced psychosis and borderline personality disorder: a naturalistic study with drug plasma levels. Expert Opin Pharmacother 2007; 8:2207–13.

75. Sparshatt A et al. Quetiapine: dose–response relationship in schizophrenia. CNS Drugs 2008; 22:49–68.

76. Olesen OV et al. Serum concentrations and side effects in psychiatric patients during risperidone therapy. Ther Drug Monit 1998; 20:380–4.

77. Remington G et al. A PET study evaluating dopamine D2 receptor occupancy for long-acting injectable risperidone. Am J Psychiatry 2006; 163: 396–401.

78. Lane HY et al. Risperidone in acutely exacerbated schizophrenia: dosing strategies and plasma levels. J Clin Psychiatry 2000; 61:209–14.

79. Taylor D. Risperidone long-acting injection in practice – more questions than answers? Acta Psychiatr Scand 2006; 114:1–2.

80. Nyberg S et al. Suggested minimal effective dose of risperidone based on PET-measured D2 and 5-HT2A receptor occupancy in schizophrenic patients. Am J Psychiatry 1999; 156:869–75.

81. Medori R et al. Plasma antipsychotic concentration and receptor occupancy, with special focus on risperidone long-acting injectable. Eur Neuropsychopharmacol 2006; 16:233–40.

82. Gefvert O et al. Pharmacokinetics and D2 receptor occupancy of long-acting injectable risperidone (Risperdal Consta™) in patients with schizophrenia. Int J Neuropsychopharmacol 2005; 8:27–36.

83. Nyberg S et al. D2 dopamine receptor occupancy during low-dose treatment with haloperidol decanoate. Am J Psychiatry 1995; 152:173–8.

chapter 2

Schizophrenia

Antipsychotics – general introduction

The NICE guideline for medicines adherence[1] recommends that patients should be as involved as possible in decisions about the choice of medicines that are prescribed for them, and that clinicians should be aware that illness beliefs and beliefs about medicines influence adherence. Consistent with this general advice that covers all of healthcare, the NICE guideline for schizophrenia emphasises the importance of patient choice rather than specifically recommending a class or individual antipsychotic as first-line treatment[2].

Antipsychotics are effective in both the acute and maintenance treatment of schizophrenia and other psychotic disorders. They differ in their pharmacology, kinetics, overall efficacy/effectiveness and tolerability, but perhaps more importantly, response and tolerability differs between patients. This individual response means that there is no clear first-line antipsychotic suitable for all.

Relative efficacy

Further to the publication of CATIE[3] and CUtLASS[4], the World Psychiatric Association reviewed the evidence relating to the relative efficacy of 51 FGAs and 11 SGAs and concluded that, if differences in EPS could be minimised (by careful dosing) and anticholinergic use avoided, there is no convincing evidence to support any advantage for SGAs over FGAs[5]. As a class, SGAs may have a lower propensity for EPS but this is offset by a higher propensity for metabolic side-effects.

When individual non-clozapine SGAs are compared with each other, it would appear that olanzapine is more effective than aripiprazole, risperidone, quetiapine and ziprasidone, and that risperidone has the edge over quetiapine and ziprasidone[6]. FGA-controlled trials also suggest an advantage for olanzapine, risperidone and amisulpride[7,8]. The magnitude of these differences is small and must be weighed against the very different side-effect profiles associated with individual antipsychotics.

Both FGAs and SGAs are associated with a number of adverse effects. These include weight gain, dyslipidaemia, hyperprolactinaemia, sexual dysfunction, EPS, anticholinergic effects, sedation and postural hypotension. The exact profile is drug-specific (see individual sections on adverse effects). Side effects are a common reason for treatment discontinuation[9]. Patients do not always spontaneously report side effects however[10] and psychiatrists' views of the prevalence and importance of adverse effects differs markedly from patient experience[11]. Systematic enquiry along with a physical examination and appropriate biochemical tests is the only way accurately to assess their presence and severity or perceived severity. Patient-completed checklists, such as the Glasgow Antipsychotic Side-Effect Scale (GASS)[12] or the Liverpool University Neuroleptic Side-Effect Ratings Scale (LUNSERS)[13], can be a useful first step in this process.

Non-adherence to antipsychotic treatment is common and here the guaranteed medication delivery associated with depot preparations is potentially advantageous[14]. In comparison with oral antipsychotics, there is a suggestion that depots may be associated with better global outcome[15] and a reduced risk of rehospitalisation[16,17].

In patients whose symptoms have not responded adequately to sequential trials of two or more antipsychotic drugs, clozapine is the most effective treatment[18-20] and its use in these circumstances is recommended by NICE[2].

This section covers the treatment of schizophrenia with antipsychotic drugs, the relative adverse effect profile of these drugs and how adverse effects can be managed.

References

1. National Institute for Health and Clinical Excellence. Medicines adherence: involving patients in decisions about prescribed medicines and supporting adherence. Clinical Guidance CG76. http://www.nice.org.uk/. 2009.
2. National Institute for Health and Clinical Excellence. Schizophrenia: core interventions in the treatment and management of schizophrenia in adults in primary and secondary care (update). http://www.nice.org.uk/
3. Lieberman JA et al. Effectiveness of antipsychotic drugs in patients with chronic schizophrenia. N Engl J Med 2005; 353:1209–1223.
4. Jones PB et al. Randomized controlled trial of the effect on Quality of Life of second- vs first-generation antipsychotic drugs in schizophrenia: Cost Utility of the Latest Antipsychotic Drugs in Schizophrenia Study (CUtLASS 1). Arch Gen Psychiatry 2006; 63:1079–1087.
5. Tandon R et al. World Psychiatric Association Pharmacopsychiatry Section statement on comparative effectiveness of antipsychotics in the treatment of schizophrenia. Schizophr Res 2008; 100:20–38.
6. Leucht S et al. A meta-analysis of head-to-head comparisons of second-generation antipsychotics in the treatment of schizophrenia. Am J Psychiatry 2009; 166:152–163.
7. Davis JM et al. A meta-analysis of the efficacy of second-generation antipsychotics. Arch Gen Psychiatry 2003; 60:553–564.
8. Leucht S et al. Second-generation versus first-generation antipsychotic drugs for schizophrenia: a meta-analysis. Lancet 2009; 373:31–41.
9. Falkai P. Limitations of current therapies: why do patients switch therapies? Eur Neuropsychopharmacol 2008;18 Suppl 3:S135–S139.
10. Yusufi B et al. Prevalence and nature of side effects during clozapine maintenance treatment and the relationship with clozapine dose and plasma concentration. Int Clin Psychopharmacol 2007; 22:238–243.
11. Day JC et al. A comparison of patients' and prescribers' beliefs about neuroleptic side-effects: prevalence, distress and causation. Acta Psychiatr Scand 1998; 97:93–97.
12. Waddell L et al. A new self-rating scale for detecting atypical or second-generation antipsychotic side effects. J Psychopharmacol 2008; 22:238–243.
13. Day JC et al. A self-rating scale for measuring neuroleptic side-effects. Validation in a group of schizophrenic patients. Br J Psychiatry 1995; 166: 650–653.
14. Zhu B et al. Time to discontinuation of depot and oral first-generation antipsychotics in the usual care of schizophrenia. Psychiatr Serv 2008; 59: 315–317.
15. Adams CE et al. Systematic meta-review of depot antipsychotic drugs for people with schizophrenia. Br J Psychiatry 2001; 179:290–299.
16. Schooler NR. Relapse and rehospitalization: comparing oral and depot antipsychotics. J Clin Psychiatry 2003;64 Suppl 16:14–17.
17. Tiihonen J et al. Effectiveness of antipsychotic treatments in a nationwide cohort of patients in community care after first hospitalisation due to schizophrenia and schizoaffective disorder: observational follow-up study. BMJ 2006; 333:224.
18. Kane J et al. Clozapine for the treatment-resistant schizophrenic. A double-blind comparison with chlorpromazine. Arch Gen Psychiatry 1988; 45: 789–796.
19. McEvoy JP et al. Effectiveness of clozapine versus olanzapine, quetiapine, and risperidone in patients with chronic schizophrenia who did not respond to prior atypical antipsychotic treatment. Am J Psychiatry 2006; 163:600–610.
20. Lewis SW et al. Randomized controlled trial of effect of prescription of clozapine versus other second-generation antipsychotic drugs in resistant schizophrenia. Schizophr Bull 2006; 32:715–723.

Antipsychotics – equivalent doses

Antipsychotic drugs vary greatly in potency (not the same as efficacy) and this is usually expressed as differences in 'neuroleptic' or 'chlorpromazine' 'equivalents'. Some of the estimates relating to neuroleptic equivalents are based on early dopamine binding studies and some largely on clinical experience or even inspired guesswork. BNF maximum doses for antipsychotic drugs bear little relationship to their 'neuroleptic equivalents'. The following table gives some approximate equivalent doses for conventional drugs[1,2]. Values given should be seen as a rough guide when transferring from one conventional drug to another. An early review of progress is essential.

Schizophrenia

Table	Equivalent doses	
Drug	*Equivalent dose (consensus)*	*Range of values in literature*
Chlorpromazine	100 mg/day	–
Fluphenazine	2 mg/day	2–5 mg/day
Trifluoperazine	5 mg/day	2.5–5 mg/day
Flupentixol	3 mg/day	2–3 mg/day
Zuclopenthixol	25 mg/day	25–60 mg/day
Haloperidol	3 mg/day	1.5–5 mg/day
Sulpiride	200 mg/day	200–270 mg/day
Pimozide	2 mg/day	2 mg/day
Loxapine	10 mg/day	10–25 mg/day
Fluphenazine depot	5 mg/week	1–12.5 mg/week
Pipotiazine depot	10 mg/week	10–12.5 mg/week
Flupentixol depot	10 mg/week	10–20 mg/week
Zuclopenthixol depot	100 mg/week	40–100 mg/week
Haloperidol depot	15 mg/week	5–25 mg/week

It is inappropriate to convert SGA doses into 'equivalents' since the dose–response relationship is usually well-defined for these drugs. Dosage guidelines are discussed under each individual drug. Those readers eager to find chlorpromazine equivalents for the newer drugs are directed to the only published paper listing such data[3].

References

1. Foster P. Neuroleptic equivalence. Pharm J 1989; 243:431–432.
2. Atkins M et al. Chlorpromazine equivalents: a consensus of opinion for both clinical and research implications. Psychiatr Bull 1997; 21:224–226.
3. Woods SW. Chlorpromazine equivalent doses for the newer atypical antipsychotics. J Clin Psychiatry 2003; 64:663–667.

Antipsychotics – minimum effective doses

The table below suggests the minimum dose of antipsychotic likely to be effective in schizophrenia (first episode or relapse). At least some patients will respond to the dose suggested, although others may require higher doses. Given the variation in individual response, all doses should be considered approximate. Primary references are provided where available, but consensus opinion has also been used (as have standard texts such as the BNF and SPC). Only oral treatment with commonly used drugs is covered.

Table Minimum effective dose/day – antipsychotics

Drug	First episode	Relapse
FGAs		
Chlorpromazine	200 mg*	300 mg
Haloperidol[1–5]	2 mg	>4 mg
Sulpiride[6]	400 mg*	800 mg
Trifluoperazine[7]	10 mg*	15 mg
SGAs		
Amisulpride[8–10]	400 mg*	800 mg
Aripiprazole[11,12]	10 mg*	10 mg
Asenapine[13]	Not known	10 mg*
Bifeprunox[13]	Not known	20 mg*
Iloperidone[14,15]	4 mg*	8 mg*
Olanzapine[5,16,17]	5 mg	10 mg
Paliperidone[18]	3 mg*	3 mg
Quetiapine[19–22]	150 mg*	300 mg
Risperidone[4,23–25]	1–2 mg	3–4 mg
Sertindole[26]	Not appropriate	12 mg
Ziprasidone[27–29]	80 mg*	80 mg
Zotepine[30,31]	75 mg*	150 mg

*Estimate – too few data available.

References

1. Oosthuizen P et al. Determining the optimal dose of haloperidol in first-episode psychosis. J Psychopharmacol 2001; 15:251–255.
2. McGorry PD. Recommended haloperidol and risperidone doses in first-episode psychosis. J Clin Psychiatry 1999; 60:794–795.
3. Waraich PS et al. Haloperidol dose for the acute phase of schizophrenia. Cochrane Database Syst Rev 2002; CD001951.
4. Schooler N et al. Risperidone and haloperidol in first-episode psychosis: a long-term randomized trial. Am J Psychiatry 2005; 162:947–953.
5. Keefe RS et al. Long-term neurocognitive effects of olanzapine or low-dose haloperidol in first-episode psychosis. Biol Psychiatry 2006; 59:97–105.
6. Soares BG et al. Sulpiride for schizophrenia. Cochrane Database Syst Rev 2000; CD001162.
7. Armenteros JL et al. Antipsychotics in early onset Schizophrenia: Systematic review and meta-analysis. Eur Child Adolesc Psychiatry 2006; 15:141–148.
8. Mota NE et al. Amisulpride for schizophrenia. Cochrane Database Syst Rev 2002; CD001357.
9. Puech A et al. Amisulpride, and atypical antipsychotic, in the treatment of acute episodes of schizophrenia: a dose-ranging study vs. haloperidol. The Amisulpride Study Group. Acta Psychiatr Scand 1998; 98:65–72.
10. Moller HJ et al. Improvement of acute exacerbations of schizophrenia with amisulpride: a comparison with haloperidol. PROD-ASLP Study Group. Psychopharmacology 1997; 132:396–401.
11. Taylor D. Aripiprazole: a review of its pharmacology and clinical utility. Int J Clin Pract 2003; 57:49–54.
12. Cutler AJ et al. The efficacy and safety of lower doses of aripiprazole for the treatment of patients with acute exacerbation of schizophrenia. CNS Spectr 2006; 11:691–702.
13. Bishara D et al. Upcoming agents for the treatment of schizophrenia. Mechanism of action, efficacy and tolerability. Drugs 2008; 68:2269–2296.
14. Kane JM et al. Long-term efficacy and safety of iloperidone: results from 3 clinical trials for the treatment of schizophrenia. J Clin Psychopharmacol 2008; 28:S29–S35.
15. Potkin SG et al. Efficacy of iloperidone in the treatment of schizophrenia: initial phase 3 studies. J Clin Psychopharmacol 2008; 28:S4–11.
16. Sanger TM et al. Olanzapine versus haloperidol treatment in first-episode psychosis. Am J Psychiatry 1999; 156:79–87.

17.   Kasper S. Risperidone and olanzapine: optimal dosing for efficacy and tolerability in patients with schizophrenia. Int Clin Psychopharmacol 1998; 13:253–262.
18.   Meltzer HY et al. Efficacy and tolerability of oral paliperidone extended-release tablets in the treatment of acute schizophrenia: pooled data from three 6-week, placebo-controlled studies. J Clin Psychiatry 2008; 69:817–829.
19.   Small JG et al. Quetiapine in patients with schizophrenia. A high- and low-dose double-blind comparison with placebo. Seroquel Study Group. Arch Gen Psychiatry 1997; 54:549–557.
20.   Peuskens J et al. A comparison of quetiapine and chlorpromazine in the treatment of schizophrenia. Acta Psychiatr Scand 1997; 96:265–273.
21.   Arvanitis LA et al. Multiple fixed doses of "Seroquel" (quetiapine) in patients with acute exacerbation of schizophrenia: a comparison with haloperidol and placebo. Biol Psychiatry 1997; 42:233–246.
22.   Kopala LC et al. Treatment of a first episode of psychotic illness with quetiapine: an analysis of 2 year outcomes. Schizophr Res 2006; 81:29–39.
23.   Lane HY et al. Risperidone in acutely exacerbated schizophrenia: dosing strategies and plasma levels. J Clin Psychiatry 2000; 61:209–214.
24.   Williams R. Optimal dosing with risperidone: updated recommendations. J Clin Psychiatry 2001; 62:282–289.
25.   Ezewuzie N et al. Establishing a dose–response relationship for oral risperidone in relapsed schizophrenia. J Psychopharmacol 2006; 20:86–90.
26.   Lindstrom E et al. Sertindole: efficacy and safety in schizophrenia. Expert Opin Pharmacother 2006; 7:1825–1834.
27.   Bagnall A et al. Ziprasidone for schizophrenia and severe mental illness. Cochrane Database Syst Rev 2000; CD001945.
28.   Taylor D. Ziprasidone – an atypical antipsychotic. Pharm J 2001; 266:396–401.
29.   Joyce AT et al. Effect of initial ziprasidone dose on length of therapy in schizophrenia. Schizophr Res 2006; 83:285–292.
30.   Petit M et al. A comparison of an atypical and typical antipsychotic, zotepine versus haloperidol in patients with acute exacerbation of schizophrenia: a parallel-group double-blind trial. Psychopharmacol Bull 1996; 32:81–87.
31.   Palmgren K et al. The safety and efficacy of zotepine in the treatment of schizophrenia: results of a one-year naturalistic clinical trial. Int J Psychiatry Clin Pract 2000; 4:299–306.

Further reading

Davis JM et al. Dose response and dose equivalence of antipsychotics. J Clin Psychopharmacol 2004; 24:192–208.

Antipsychotics – licensed maximum doses

The table below lists the UK licensed maximum doses of antipsychotics.

Drug	Maximum dose
FGAs – oral	
Chlorpromazine	1000 mg/day
Flupentixol	18 mg/day
Haloperidol	30 mg/day (See BNF)
Levomepromazine	1000 mg/day
Pericyazine	300 mg/day
Perphenazine	24 mg/day
Pimozide	20 mg/day
Sulpiride	2400 mg/day
Trifluoperazine	None (suggest 30 mg/day)
Zuclopenthixol	150 mg/day
SGAs – oral	
Amisulpride	1200 mg/day
Aripiprazole	30 mg/day
Clozapine	900 mg/day
Olanzapine	20 mg/day
Paliperidone	12 mg/day
Quetiapine	750/800 mg/day (see BNF)
Risperidone	16 mg/day (see BNF)
Sertindole	24 mg/day
Ziprasidone*	160 mg/day
Zotepine	300 mg/day
Depots	
Flupentixol depot	400 mg/week
Fluphenazine depot	50 mg/week
Haloperidol depot	300 mg every 4 weeks (see BNF)
Pipotiazine depot	50 mg/week
Risperidone**	25 mg/week
Zuclopenthixol depot	600 mg/week

Note: Doses above these maxima should only be used in extreme circumstances: there is no evidence for improved efficacy.
*Not available in the UK at time of publication, European labelling used.
**May only be given two weekly.

New antipsychotics

Asenapine

Asenapine has affinity for D_2, $5HT_{2A}$, $5HT_{2C}$ and α_1/α_2 adrenergic receptors along with relatively low affinity for H_1 and ACh receptors[1]. At a dose of 5 mg twice daily, asenapine has been demonstrated to be more effective than placebo in acute treatment of schizophrenia and more effective than risperidone in the treatment of negative symptoms[2]; perhaps through selective affinity for different dopamine pathways, most notably in the pre-frontal cortex[3]. Asenapine has less potential to raise prolactin than risperidone and may also be associated with a lower risk of weight gain[4].

Bifeprunox

Bifeprunox is a D_2 partial agonist and $5HT_{1A}$ agonist with minimal propensity to increase serum prolactin[5] or cause weight gain or EPS[6]. Bifeprunox 20 mg/day has broadly equivalent therapeutic effects to risperidone 6 mg/day[7]. There are some negative studies[6].

Iloperidone

Iloperidone is a $D_2/5HT_{2A}$ antagonist with little activity at H_1 and muscarinic receptors[8]. In short-term trials, iloperidone 4–24 mg/day was more effective than placebo and doses of 20–24 mg/day showed similar efficacy to haloperidol and risperidone[9,10]. Motor-related adverse effects were rare. Iloperidone 24 mg/day showed similar efficacy and tolerability to ziprasidone 160 mg/day in a 4-week trial with each drug producing similar changes in QTc (around 11 ms increase)[11]. In long-term treatment, iloperidone 4–16 mg/day was equivalent to haloperidol 5–20 mg/day in terms of relapse and QT changes (around 10 ms increase)[12]. Insomnia is the most commonly experienced adverse effect of iloperidone. Mean weight gain in 6-week trials was 2.6 kg; prolactin levels appear not to be affected[8].

Olanzapine pamoate

Olanzapine pamoate is a poorly soluble salt of olanzapine formulated as an aqueous suspension for 2- or 4-weekly IM administration. Doses of 210 mg/2 weeks, 300 mg/2 weeks and 405 mg/4 weeks have been shown to be more effective than placebo with activity seen as early as 3 days after starting treatment[13]. Adverse effects are similar to those seen with oral olanzapine. Treatment is complicated by the risk of sedation syndrome or post injection syndrome (occurring in 0.07% injections)[14] and by a complex dosing regimen[15].

Paliperidone

Paliperidone (9-OH risperidone) is the major active metabolite of risperidone now marketed in most countries. In-vitro data demonstrate rapid dissociation from D_2 receptors, predicting a low propensity to cause EPS[16]. It is a D_2 and $5HT_{2A}$ antagonist[17] formulated as an osmotic controlled-release oral delivery system (OROS) to reduce fluctuations in plasma levels and remove the need for dosage titration[18]. Paliperidone undergoes limited hepatic metabolism and this may reduce the potential for drug interactions[19].

A pooled analysis of three 6-week placebo-controlled studies found paliperidone 3–15 mg to be more effective than placebo and relatively well tolerated[20]. In common with risperidone, paliperidone can cause headache. With respect to weight gain, 9% of paliperidone-treated patients gained >7% of their baseline bodyweight compared with 5% of patients treated with placebo[21]. Extra-pyramidal side effects are fairly common in people receiving 9 mg and 12 mg daily[22]. Doses of 6 mg and 12 mg have been shown to be more effective than placebo and to have equivalent efficacy to olanzapine 10 mg in a 6-week study in adults with schizophrenia[23]. Paliperidone 9 mg or 12 mg a day was more efficacious than quetiapine 600 mg or 800 mg[24]. Doses of 6–9 mg are effective and well tolerated in patients with schizophrenia who are >65 years old[25]. There are some long-term data[26,27] suggesting efficacy in preventing relapse. Paliperidone palmitate is a long-acting formulation which may be given in the deltoid muscle[28].

References

1. Shahid M et al. Asenapine: a novel psychopharmacologic agent with a unique human receptor signature. J Psychopharmacol 2009; 23:65–73.
2. Potkin SG et al. Efficacy and tolerability of asenapine in acute schizophrenia: a placebo- and risperidone-controlled trial. J Clin Psychiatry 2007; 68:1492–1500.
3. Tarazi FI et al. Differential regional and dose-related effects of asenapine on dopamine receptor subtypes. Psychopharmacology (Berl) 2008; 198: 103–111.
4. Potkin SG et al. Efficacy and tolerability of asenapine in acute schizophrenia: a placebo- and risperidone-controlled trial. J Clin Psychiatry 2007; 68:1492–1500.
5. Cosi C et al. Partial agonist properties of the antipsychotics SSR181507, aripiprazole and bifeprunox at dopamine D2 receptors: G protein activation and prolactin release. Eur J Pharmacol 2006; 535:135–144.
6. Bishara D et al. Upcoming agents for the treatment of schizophrenia. Mechanism of action, efficacy and tolerability. Drugs 2008; 68:2269–2296.
7. Casey DE et al. Efficacy and safety of bifeprunox in patients with an acute exacerbation of schizophrenia: results from a randomized, double-blind, placebo-controlled, multicenter, dose-finding study. Psychopharmacology (Berl) 2008; 200:317–331.
8. Citrome L et al. Iloperidone for schizophrenia: a review of the efficacy and safety profile for this newly-commercialised second-generation antipsychotic. Int J Clin Pract 2009; In Press.
9. Weiden PJ et al. Safety profile of iloperidone: a pooled analysis of 6-week acute-phase pivotal trials. J Clin Psychopharmacol 2008; 28:S12–S19.
10. Potkin SG et al. Efficacy of iloperidone in the treatment of schizophrenia: initial phase 3 studies. J Clin Psychopharmacol 2008; 28:S4–11.
11. Cutler AJ et al. Four-week, double-blind, placebo- and ziprasidone-controlled trial of iloperidone in patients with acute exacerbations of schizophrenia. J Clin Psychopharmacol 2008; 28:S20–S28.
12. Kane JM et al. Long-term efficacy and safety of iloperidone: results from 3 clinical trials for the treatment of schizophrenia. J Clin Psychopharmacol 2008; 28:S29–S35.
13. Lauriello J et al. An 8-week, double-blind, randomized, placebo-controlled study of olanzapine long-acting injection in acutely ill patients with schizophrenia. J Clin Psychiatry 2008; 69:790–799.
14. Citrome L. Olanzapine pamoate: a stick in time? Int J Clin Pract 2009; 63:140–150.
15. Taylor DM. Olanzapine pamoate – blockbuster or damp squib? Int J Clin Pract 2009; 63:540–541.
16. Seeman P. An update of fast-off dopamine D2 atypical antipsychotics. Am J Psychiatry 2005; 162:1984–1985.
17. Karlsson P, Dencker E, Nyberg S, Mannaert E, Boom S, Talluri K et al. Pharmacokinetics, dopamine D2 and serotonin 5-HT2A receptor occupancy and safety profile of paliperidone in healthy subjects: two open-label, single-dose studies. 2006. Poster presented at ASCPT 8–11 March 2006, Baltimore.
18. Conley R et al. Clinical spectrum of the osmotic-controlled release oral delivery system (OROS), an advanced oral delivery form. Curr Med Res Opin 2006; 22:1879–1892.
19. Vermeir M et al. Absorption, metabolism and excretion of a single oral dose of 14C-paliperidone 1mg in healthy subjects. Clin Pharmacol Ther 2006; 79:80.
20. Meltzer H et al. Efficacy and tolerability of oral paliperidone extended-release tablets in the treatment of acute schizophrenia: pooled data from three 6-week placebo-controlled studies. J Clin Psychiatry 2006; 69:817–829.
21. Meyer J, Kramer M, Kostic D, Lane R, Lim P, Eerdekens M. Metabolic outcomes in patients with schizophrenia treated with oral paliperidone extended-release tablets: pooled analysis of three 6-week placebo-controlled studies. 2006. Poster presented at CINP 9–13 July 2006, Chicago, IL, USA.
22. Citrome L. Paliperidone: quo vadis? Int J Clin Pract 2007; 61:653–662.
23. Marder SR et al. Efficacy and safety of paliperidone extended-release tablets: results of a 6-week, randomized, placebo-controlled study. Biol Psychiatry 2007; 62:1363–1370.
24. Canuso CM et al. Randomized, double-blind, placebo-controlled study of paliperidone extended-release and quetiapine in inpatients with recently exacerbated schizophrenia. Am J Psychiatry 2009; 166:691–701.
25. Tzimos A et al. Safety and tolerability of oral paliperidone extended-release tablets in elderly patients with schizophrenia: a double-blind, placebo-controlled study with six-month open-label extension. Am J Geriatr Psychiatry 2008; 16:31–43.
26. Kramer M et al. Paliperidone extended-release tablets for prevention of symptom recurrence in patients with schizophrenia: a randomized, double-blind, placebo-controlled study. J Clin Psychopharmacol 2007; 27:6–14.
27. Emsley R et al. Efficacy and safety of oral paliperidone extended-release tablets in the treatment of acute schizophrenia: pooled data from three 52-week open-label studies. Int Clin Psychopharmacol 2008; 23:343–356.
28. Hough D et al. Safety and tolerability of deltoid and gluteal injections of paliperidone palmitate in schizophrenia. Prog Neuropsychopharmacol Biol Psychiatry 2009; In Press.

New antipsychotics – costs

Newer antipsychotics are relatively costly medicines, although their benefits may make them cost-effective in practice. The table below gives the cost (£/patient per 30 days) as of May 2009 of atypicals at their estimated lowest effective dose, their approximate average clinical dose and their licensed maximum dose. The table allows comparison of different doses of the same drug and of different drugs at any of the three doses. It is hoped that the table will encourage the use of lower doses of less expensive drugs, given equality in other respects and allowing for clinical requirements.

Table Monthly costs of new antipsychotics

Drug	Minimum effective dose cost	Approximate average clinical dose cost	Maximum cost
Amisulpride*	400 mg/day £55.68	800 mg/day £111.36	1200 mg/day £167.04
Aripiprazole	10 mg/day £104.65	20 mg/day £209.29	30 mg/day £209.29
Olanzapine	10 mg/day £85.13	15 mg/day £127.69	20 mg/day £170.25
Paliperidone	3 mg/day £104.23	6 mg/day £104.23	12 mg/day £260.57
Quetiapine IR	300 mg/day £85.00	500 mg/day £141.55	750 mg/day £226.55
Quetiapine XL	300 mg/day £85.00	600 mg/day £170.00	800 mg/day £226.20
Risperidone (oral*)	4 mg/day £30.80	6 mg/day £47.72	16 mg/day £126.24
Risperidone (injection)	25 mg/2 weeks £159.38/28 days	37.5 mg/2 weeks £222.64/28 days	50 mg/2 weeks £285.52/28 days
Sertindole	12 mg/day POA	20 mg/day POA	24 mg/day POA
Zotepine	150 mg/day £75.93	300 mg/day £141.84	300 mg/day £141.84

*Generic versions available – costs vary.

Notes:
- costs for UK adults (30 days), MIMS, May 2009
- average clinical doses for inpatients receiving maintenance therapy
- clozapine costs not included because it has different indications.

Antipsychotics – general principles of prescribing

- The lowest possible dose should be used. For each patient, the dose should be titrated to the lowest known to be effective (see section on minimum effective doses); dose increases should then take place only after 2 weeks of assessment during which the patient is clearly showing poor or no response. With depot medication, plasma levels rise for 6–12 weeks after initiation, even without a change in dose. Dose increases during this time are therefore inappropriate.
- For the large majority of patients, the use of a single antipsychotic (with or without additional mood-stabiliser or sedatives) is recommended (see section on antipsychotic polypharmacy). Apart from exceptional circumstances (e.g. clozapine augmentation) antipsychotic polypharmacy should be avoided because of the risks associated with QT prolongation and sudden cardiac death[1].
- Combinations of antipsychotics should only be used where response to a single antipsychotic (including clozapine) has been clearly demonstrated to be inadequate. In such cases, the effect of the combination against target symptoms and the side-effects should be carefully evaluated and documented. Where there is no clear benefit, treatment should revert to single antipsychotic therapy.
- In general, antipsychotics should not be used as 'PRN' sedatives. Short courses of benzodiazepines or general sedatives (e.g. promethazine) are recommended.
- Responses to antipsychotic drug treatment should be assessed by recognised rating scales and be documented in patients' records.
- Those receiving antipsychotics should undergo close monitoring of physical health (including blood pressure, pulse, ECG, plasma glucose and plasma liquids).

Reference

1.   Ray WA et al. Atypical antipsychotic drugs and the risk of sudden cardiac death. N Engl J Med 2009; 360:225–235.

Further reading

Pharmacovigilance Working Party. Public Assessment Report on Neuroleptics and Cardiac safety, in particular QT prolongation, cardiac arrhythmias, ventricular tachycardia and torsades de pointes. http://www.mhra.gov.uk. 2006.

NICE Guidelines – Schizophrenia[1]

The 2009 NICE Guidelines differ importantly from previous guidelines. There is no longer an imperative to prescribe an 'atypical' as first-line treatment and it is now recommended only that clozapine be 'offered' (rather than prescribed) after the prior failure of two antipsychotics. Much emphasis is placed on involving patients and their carers in prescribing decisions. There is some evidence that this is rarely done[2] but that it can be done[3].

NICE Guidelines – a summary

- For people with newly diagnosed schizophrenia, offer oral antipsychotic medication. Provide information and discuss the benefits and side-effect profile of each drug with the service user. The choice of drug should be made by the service user and healthcare professional together, considering:
    - the relative potential of individual antipsychotic drugs to cause extrapyramidal side effects (including akathisia), metabolic side effects (including weight gain) and other side effects (including unpleasant subjective experiences)
    - the views of the carer where the service user agrees.

- Before starting antipsychotic medication, offer the person with schizophrenia an electrocardiogram (ECG) if:
    - specified in the SPC
    - a physical examination has identified specific cardiovascular risk (such as diagnosis of high blood pressure)
    - there is personal history of cardiovascular disease, or
    - the service user is being admitted as an inpatient.

- Treatment with antipsychotic medication should be considered an explicit individual therapeutic trial. Include the following:
    - Record the indications and expected benefits and risks of oral antipsychotic medication, and the expected time for a change in symptoms and appearance of side effects
    - At the start of treatment give a dose at the lower end of the licensed range and slowly titrate upwards within the dose range given in the British National Formulary (BNF) or SPC
    - Justify and record reasons for dosages outside the range given in the BNF or SPC.

- Monitor and record the following regularly and systematically throughout treatment, but especially during titration:
    - efficacy, including changes in symptoms and behaviour
    - side effects of treatment, taking into account overlap between certain side effects and clinical features of schizophrenia, for example the overlap between akathisia and agitation or anxiety
    - adherence
    - physical health
    - record the rationale for continuing, changing or stopping medication, and the effects of such changes
    - carry out a trial of the medication at optimum dosage for 4–6 weeks.

- Do not use a loading dose of antipsychotic medication (often referred to as 'rapid neuroleptisation').

- Do not initiate regular combined antipsychotic medication, except for short periods (for example, when changing medication).

- If prescribing chlorpromazine, warn of its potential to cause skin photosensitivity. Advise using sunscreen if necessary.

- Consider offering depot/long-acting injectable antipsychotic medication to people with schizophrenia:
  - who would prefer such treatment after an acute episode
  - where avoiding covert non-adherence (either intentional or unintentional) to antipsychotic medication is a clinical priority within the treatment plan.

- Offer clozapine to people with schizophrenia whose illness has not responded adequately to treatment despite the sequential use of adequate doses of at least two different antipsychotic drugs. At least one of the drugs should be a non-clozapine SGA.

- For people with schizophrenia whose illness has not responded adequately to clozapine at an optimised dose, healthcare professionals should establish prior compliance with optimised antipsychotic treatment (including measuring therapeutic drug levels) and engagement with psychological treatment before adding a second antipsychotic to augment treatment with clozapine. An adequate trial of such an augmentation may need to be up to 8–10 weeks. Choose a drug that does not compound the common side effects of clozapine.

References

1. National Institute for Health and Clinical Excellence. Schizophrenia: core interventions in the treatment and management of schizophrenia in adults in primary and secondary care (update). 2009. http://www.nice.org.uk/
2. Olofinjana B et al. Antipsychotic drugs – information and choice: a patient survey. Psychiatr Bull 2005; 29:369–371.
3. Whiskey E et al. Evaluation of an antipsychotic information sheet for patients. Int J Psychiatry Clin Pract 2005; 9:264–270.

First-episode schizophrenia

Treatment algorithm

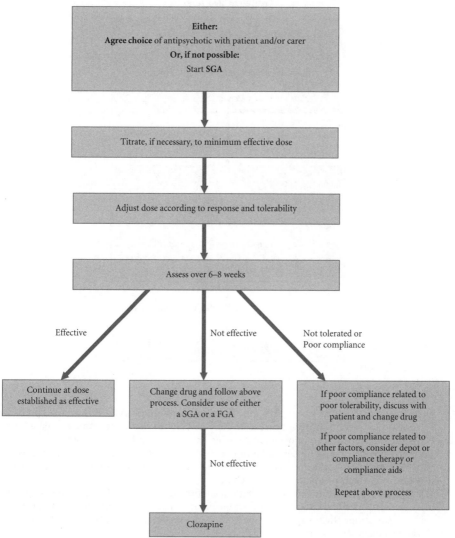

Either:
Agree choice of antipsychotic with patient and/or carer
Or, if not possible:
Start **SGA**

Titrate, if necessary, to minimum effective dose

Adjust dose according to response and tolerability

Assess over 6–8 weeks

Effective

Not effective

Not tolerated or
Poor compliance

Continue at dose
established as effective

Change drug and follow above
process. Consider use of either
a SGA or a FGA

If poor compliance related to
poor tolerability, discuss with
patient and change drug

If poor compliance related to
other factors, consider depot or
compliance therapy or
compliance aids

Repeat above process

Not effective

Clozapine

Relapse or acute exacerbation of schizophrenia

(full adherence to medication confirmed)

Treatment algorithm

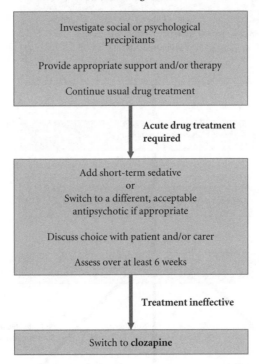

Investigate social or psychological precipitants

Provide appropriate support and/or therapy

Continue usual drug treatment

Acute drug treatment required

Add short-term sedative
or
Switch to a different, acceptable antipsychotic if appropriate

Discuss choice with patient and/or carer

Assess over at least 6 weeks

Treatment ineffective

Switch to **clozapine**

Notes

- First-generation drugs may be slightly less efficacious than some SGAs[1,2]. FGAs should probably be reserved for second-line use because of the possibility of poorer outcome compared with FGAs and the higher risk of movement disorder, particularly tardive dyskinesia[3,4].
- Choice is however based largely on comparative adverse effect profile and relative toxicity. Patients seem able to make informed choices based on these factors[5,6], although in practice they may only very rarely be involved in drug choice[7].
- Where there is prior treatment failure (but not confirmed treatment refractoriness) olanzapine or risperidone may be better options than quetiapine[8]. Olanzapine, because of the wealth of evidence suggesting slight superiority over other antipsychotics, should always be tried before clozapine unless contra-indicated[9-12].
- Where there is confirmed treatment resistance (failure to respond to at least two antipsychotics) evidence supporting the use of clozapine (and only clozapine) is overwhelming[13,14].

Relapse or acute exacerbation of schizophrenia

(adherence doubtful or known to be poor)

Treatment algorithm

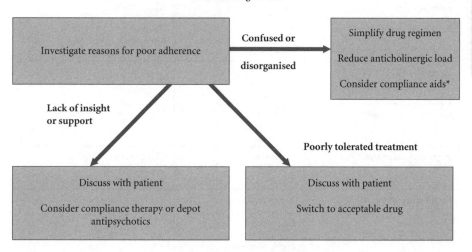

*Compliance aids (e.g. Medidose system) are not a substitute for patient education. The ultimate aim should be to promote independent living, perhaps with patients filling their own compliance aid, having first been given support and training. Note that such compliance aids are of little use unless the patient is clearly motivated to adhere to prescribed treatment. Note also that some medicines are not suitable for storage in compliance aids.

References

1. Davis JM et al. A meta-analysis of the efficacy of second-generation antipsychotics. Arch Gen Psychiatry 2003; 60:553–564.
2. Leucht S et al. Second-generation versus first-generation antipsychotic drugs for schizophrenia: a meta-analysis. Lancet 2009; 373:31–41.
3. Schooler N et al. Risperidone and haloperidol in first-episode psychosis: a long-term randomized trial. Am J Psychiatry 2005; 162:947–953.
4. Oosthuizen PP et al. Incidence of tardive dyskinesia in first-episode psychosis patients treated with low-dose haloperidol. J Clin Psychiatry 2003; 64:1075–1080.
5. Whiskey E et al. Evaluation of an antipsychotic information sheet for patients. Int J Psychiatry Clin Pract 2005; 9:264–270.
6. Stroup TS et al. Results of phase 3 of the CATIE schizophrenia trial. Schizophr Res 2009; 107:1–12.
7. Olofinjana B et al. Antipsychotic drugs – information and choice: a patient survey. Psychiatr Bull 2005; 29:369–371.
8. Stroup TS et al. Effectiveness of olanzapine, quetiapine, risperidone, and ziprasidone in patients with chronic schizophrenia following discontinuation of a previous atypical antipsychotic. Am J Psychiatry 2006; 163:611–622.
9. Haro JM et al. Remission and relapse in the outpatient care of schizophrenia: three-year results from the Schizophrenia Outpatient Health Outcomes study. J Clin Psychopharmacol 2006; 26:571–578.
10. Novick D et al. Recovery in the outpatient setting: 36-month results from the Schizophrenia Outpatients Health Outcomes (SOHO) study. Schizophr Res 2009; 108:223–230.
11. Tiihonen J et al. Effectiveness of antipsychotic treatments in a nationwide cohort of patients in community care after first hospitalisation due to schizophrenia and schizoaffective disorder: observational follow-up study. BMJ 2006; 333:224.
12. Leucht S et al. A meta-analysis of head-to-head comparisons of second-generation antipsychotics in the treatment of schizophrenia. Am J Psychiatry 2009; 166:152–163.
13. McEvoy JP et al. Effectiveness of clozapine versus olanzapine, quetiapine, and risperidone in patients with chronic schizophrenia who did not respond to prior atypical antipsychotic treatment. Am J Psychiatry 2006; 163:600–610.
14. Lewis SW et al. Randomized controlled trial of effect of prescription of clozapine versus other second-generation antipsychotic drugs in resistant schizophrenia. Schizophr Bull 2006; 32:715–723.

Switching antipsychotics because of poor tolerability – recommendations

Schizophrenia

Adverse effect	Suggested drugs	Alternatives
Acute EPS[1-5]	Aripiprazole Olanzapine Quetiapine	Clozapine Risperidone (<6 mg/day) Ziprasidone
Dyslipidaemia[6-9]	Amisulpride Aripiprazole* Ziprasidone	
Impaired glucose tolerance[10-13]	Amisulpride Aripiprazole* Ziprasidone	Risperidone
Hyperprolactinaemia[14-16]	Aripiprazole* Quetiapine	Clozapine Olanzapine Ziprasidone
Postural hypotension	Amisulpride Aripiprazole Haloperidol Sulpiride Trifluoperazine	
QT prolongation[17-20]	Aripiprazole (with ECG monitoring)	Low dose monotherapy of any drug not formally contra-indicated in QT prolongation (with ECG monitoring)
Sedation	Amisulpride Aripiprazole Risperidone Sulpiride	Haloperidol Trifuoperazine Ziprasidone
Sexual dysfuction[21-26]	Aripiprazole Quetiapine	Clozapine
Tardive dyskinesia[27-30]	Clozapine	Aripiprazole Olanzapine Quetiapine
Weight gain[31-35]	Amisulpride Aripiprazole* Haloperidol Trifluoperazine	Quetiapine Risperidone Ziprasidone

*There is evidence that both switching to and co-prescription of aripiprazole are effective in reducing weight, prolactin and dyslipidaemia and in reversing impaired glucose tolerance[36-38].

References

1. Stanniland C et al. Tolerability of atypical antipsychotics. Drug Saf 2000; 22:195–214.
2. Tarsy D et al. Effects of newer antipsychotics on extrapyramidal function. CNS Drugs 2002; 16:23–45.
3. Caroff SN et al. Movement disorders associated with atypical antipsychotic drugs. J Clin Psychiatry 2002;63 Suppl 4:12–19.
4. Lemmens P et al. A combined analysis of double-blind studies with risperidone vs. placebo and other antipsychotic agents: factors associated with extrapyramidal symptoms. Acta Psychiatr Scand 1999; 99:160–170.
5. Taylor DM. Aripiprazole: a review of its pharmacology and clinical use. Int J Clin Pract 2003; 57:49–54.

6. Rettenbacher MA et al. Early changes of plasma lipids during treatment with atypical antipsychotics. Int Clin Psychopharmacol 2006; 21:369–372.
7. Ball MP et al. Clozapine-induced hyperlipidemia resolved after switch to aripiprazole therapy. Ann Pharmacother 2005; 39:1570–1572.
8. Chrzanowski WK et al. Effectiveness of long-term aripiprazole therapy in patients with acutely relapsing or chronic, stable schizophrenia: a 52-week, open-label comparison with olanzapine. Psychopharmacology 2006; 189:259–266.
9. De Hert M et al. A case series: evaluation of the metabolic safety of aripiprazole. Schizophr Bull 2007; 33:823–830.
10. Haddad PM. Antipsychotics and diabetes: review of non-prospective data. Br J Psychiatry Suppl 2004; 47:S80–S86.
11. Berry S et al. Improvement of insulin indices after switch from olanzapine to risperidone. Eur Neuropsychopharmacol 2002; 12:316.
12. Gianfrancesco FD et al. Differential effects of risperidone, olanzapine, clozapine, and conventional antipsychotics on type 2 diabetes: findings from a large health plan database. J Clin Psychiatry 2002; 63:920–930.
13. Mir S et al. Atypical antipsychotics and hyperglycaemia. Int Clin Psychopharmacol 2001; 16:63–74.
14. Turrone P et al. Elevation of prolactin levels by atypical antipsychotics. Am J Psychiatry 2002; 159:133–135.
15. David SR et al. The effects of olanzapine, risperidone, and haloperidol on plasma prolactin levels in patients with schizophrenia. Clin Ther 2000; 22:1085–1096.
16. Hamner MB et al. Hyperprolactinaemia in antipsychotic-treated patients: guidelines for avoidance and management. CNS Drugs 1998; 10:209–222.
17. Glassman AH et al. Antipsychotic drugs: prolonged QTc interval, torsade de pointes, and sudden death. Am J Psychiatry 2001; 158:1774–1782.
18. Taylor D. Antipsychotics and QT prolongation. Acta Psychiatr Scand 2003; 107:85–95.
19. Titier K et al. Atypical antipsychotics: from potassium channels to torsade de pointes and sudden death. Drug Saf 2005; 28:35–51.
20. Ray WA et al. Atypical antipsychotic drugs and the risk of sudden cardiac death. N Engl J Med 2009; 360:225–235.
21. Byerly MJ et al. An open-label trial of quetiapine for antipsychotic-induced sexual dysfunction. J Sex Marital Ther 2004; 30:325–332.
22. Byerly MJ et al. Sexual dysfunction associated with second-generation antipsychotics in outpatients with schizophrenia or schizoaffective disorder: an empirical evaluation of olanzapine, risperidone, and quetiapine. Schizophr Res 2006; 86:244–250.
23. Montejo Gonzalez AL et al. A 6-month prospective observational study on the effects of quetiapine on sexual functioning. J Clin Psychopharmacol 2005; 25:533–538.
24. Dossenbach M et al. Effects of atypical and typical antipsychotic treatments on sexual function in patients with schizophrenia: 12-month results from the Intercontinental Schizophrenia Outpatient Health Outcomes (IC-SOHO) study. Eur Psychiatry 2006; 21:251–258.
25. Kerwin R et al. A multicentre, randomized, naturalistic, open-label study between aripiprazole and standard of care in the management of community-treated schizophrenic patients Schizophrenia Trial of Aripiprazole: (STAR) study. Eur Psychiatry 2007; 22:433–443.
26. Hanssens L et al. The effect of antipsychotic medication on sexual function and serum prolactin levels in community-treated schizophrenic patients: results from the Schizophrenia Trial of Aripiprazole (STAR) study (NCT00237913). BMC Psychiatry 2008; 8:95.
27. Lieberman J et al. Clozapine pharmacology and tardive dyskinesia. Psychopharmacology 1989;99 Suppl 1:S54–S59.
28. O'Brien J et al. Marked improvement in tardive dyskinesia following treatment with olanzapine in an elderly subject. Br J Psychiatry 1998; 172:186.
29. Sacchetti E et al. Quetiapine, clozapine, and olanzapine in the treatment of tardive dyskinesia induced by first-generation antipsychotics: a 124-week case report. Int Clin Psychopharmacol 2003; 18:357–359.
30. Witschy JK et al. Improvement in tardive dyskinesia with aripiprazole use. Can J Psychiatry 2005; 50:188.
31. Taylor DM et al. Atypical antipsychotics and weight gain - a systematic review. Acta Psychiatr Scand 2000; 101:416–432.
32. Allison D et al. Antipsychotic-induced weight gain: A comprehensive research synthesis. Am J Psychiatry 1999; 156:1686–1696.
33. Brecher M et al. The long term effect of quetiapine (Seroquel™) monotherapy on weight in patients with schizophrenia. Int J Psychiatry Clin Pract 2000; 4:287–291.
34. Casey DE et al. Switching patients to aripiprazole from other antipsychotic agents: a multicenter randomized study. Psychopharmacology 2003; 166:3 91–399.
35. Newcomer JW et al. A multicenter, randomized, double-blind study of the effects of aripiprazole in overweight subjects with schizophrenia or schizoaffective disorder switched from olanzapine. J Clin Psychiatry 2008; 69:1046–1056.
36. Shim JC et al. Adjunctive treatment with a dopamine partial agonist, aripiprazole, for antipsychotic-induced hyperprolactinemia: a placebo-controlled trial. Am J Psychiatry 2007; 164:1404–1410.
37. Fleischhacker WW et al. Weight change on aripiprazole-clozapine combination in schizophrenic patients with weight gain and suboptimal response on clozapine: 16-week double-blind study. Eur Psychiatry 2008;23 Suppl 2:S114–S115.
38. Henderson DC et al. Aripiprazole added to overweight and obese olanzapine-treated schizophrenia patients. J Clin Psychopharmacol 2009; 29: 165–169.

Further reading

Devlin MJ et al. Obesity: what mental health professionals need to know. Am J Psychiatry 2000; 157:854–866.
Slovenko R. Update of legal issues associated with tardive dyskinesia. J Clin Psychiatry 1999;61(Suppl. 4):45–57.

Antipsychotic response to increase the dose, to switch, to add or just wait – what is the right move?

For any clinician taking active care of patients with schizophrenia the single most common clinical dilemma is what to do when the current antipsychotic is not optimal for the patient. This may be for two broad reasons; firstly when the symptoms are well controlled but side-effects are problematic, and; secondly where there is inadequate response. Fortunately, given the diversity of antipsychotics available, it is usually possible to find an antipsychotic that has a side-effect profile that is acceptable to the patient. The more difficult question is when there is inadequate symptom response. If the patient has already had 'adequate' trials of two antipsychotics for 'sufficient' duration then clozapine should clearly be considered. However, the majority of the patients in the clinic are those who are either as yet not ready for clozapine or unwilling to choose that option. In those instances the clinician has four main choices: to increase the dose of the current medication; to switch to another antipsychotic; to add an adjunct medication; or just to wait.

When to increase the dose?

While optimal doses of typical antipsychotics were always a matter of debate, the recommended doses of the newer atypical antipsychotics were generally based on careful and extensive clinical trials but even then the consensus on optimal doses has changed with time. For example, when risperidone was first launched it was suggested that optimal titration was from 2 mg to 4 mg to 6 mg or more for all patients, however, the field has tended towards lower doses[1]. On the other hand, when quetiapine was introduced, 300 mg was considered the optimal dose and the overall consensus now is towards higher doses[2], although the evidence does not support this shift[2]. Nonetheless, most clinicians feel comfortable in navigating within the recommended clinical doses. The more critical question is what one should do if one has hit the upper limit of these dose ranges and the patient is tolerating the medication well with limited efficacy benefit.

Dose–response observations

Davis and Chen performed a systematic meta-analysis of the data available up to 2004 and concluded that the average dose that produces maximal benefit was 4 mg for risperidone, 16 mg of olanzapine, 120 mg of ziprasidone and 10–15 mg of aripiprazole (they could not determine such a dose for quetiapine using their method)[3]. More recent trials have tried to compare 'high-dose' versus the standard dose and Kinon et al[4] studied the dose–response relationship of standard and higher doses of olanzapine in a randomized, double-blind, 8-week, fixed-dose study comparing olanzapine 10 mg, 20 mg and 40 mg and found no benefit of the higher doses (i.e. 40 mg was no better than even 10 mg) and clear evidence for increasing side-effects (weight-gain and prolactin) with dose. Similarly, the initial licensing studies of risperidone had compared the usual doses 2–6 mg to the higher doses 8–16 mg/day and had chosen the lower dose ranges and they found little additional benefit at higher doses, but, a clear signal for greater side effects (extrapyramidal side-effects and prolactin). These more recent studies are in accord with older studies involving fixed doses of haloperidol[5]. However, it is important to keep in mind that these doses are extracted from group evidence where patients are assigned to different doses, which is a different question from the clinical one where one considers increasing a dose only in those who have failed an initial dose. To our knowledge only one study has systematically addressed this question in its clinically relevant dimension. Kinon et al.[6] examined patients who failed to respond to the (then) standard dose of fluphenazine (20 mg) and tested three strategies: increasing dose to 80 mg, switching to haloperidol or watchful waiting. All three strategies were equivalent in terms of efficacy. Thus, it seems that at a group level (as opposed to an individual level) there is little evidence to support treatment beyond the recommended doses.

Plasma level variations

However, group-level evidence cannot completely determine individual decisions. There is significant inter-individual variation in plasma levels in patients treated with antipsychotics. One can often encounter a patient who when at the higher end of the dose range (say 6 mg of risperidone or 20 mg of olanzapine) would have plasma levels that are well below the range expected for 2 mg risperidone or 10 mg of olanzapine respectively. In such patients, one can make a rational case for increasing the dose, provided the patient is informed and the side-effects are tolerable, to bring the plasma levels to the median optimal range for the particular medication. More details on plasma levels and their interpretation are provided in Chapter 1. However, one often encounters an unresponsive compliant patient, whose dose has reached the ceiling and plasma levels are also sufficient – what next?

Treatment choices

There are essentially three options here, clozapine, switch to another drug or add another drug. If the patient meets the criteria for clozapine it is undoubtedly the preferred option. However, many patients either do not meet the criteria or do not prefer the idea of regular blood testing and the regular appointments required to receive clozapine. In these patients the choice is to switch to another medication or to add another antipsychotic. The data on switching are sparse. While almost every clinical trial in patients with chronic schizophrenia has entailed the patient switching from one antipsychotic to another – there are no rigorous studies of preferred switch combinations (e.g. if risperidone fails – what next? olanzapine, quetiapine, aripiprazole or ziprasidone). If one looks at only the switching trials which have been sponsored by the drug companies it leads to a rather confusing picture, with the trials' results being very closely linked to the sponsors' interest (see 'Why olanzapine beats risperidone, risperidone beats quetiapine, and quetiapine beats olanzapine: an exploratory analysis of head-to-head comparison studies of SGAs'[7]).

CATIE, a major US-based publicly funded comparative trial, examined patients who had failed their first atypical antipsychotic and were then randomly assigned to a different second one[8] – patients switched to olanzapine and risperidone did better than those switched to quetiapine and ziprasidone. This greater effectiveness is supported by a recent meta-analysis that compared a number of atypicals to first-generation typical antipsychotics and concluded that other than clozapine, only amisulpride, risperidone and olanzapine were superior to first-generation agents in efficacy[9]; and a meta-analysis comparing atypicals amongst themselves which suggests that olanzapine and risperidone (in that order) may be more effective than others[10]. This suggests that if a patient has not tried olanzapine or risperidone as yet, it would be a reasonable decision to switch to these drugs provided the side-effect balance is favourable. But, if patients have already tried olanzapine and risperidone the benefits of switching rather than staying are probably rather marginal[11].

What to choose for someone who fails olanzapine and risperidone (other than clozapine) is not as yet clear. Should one switch (to, say, aripiprazole or ziprasidone or even an older typical agent) or should one add another antipsychotic. It should be borne in mind that after 'switching', adding another antipsychotic is probably the second most common clinical move as 39–43% of patients in routine care are on more than one antipsychotic[12]. Often a second antipsychotic is added to get an additional profile (e.g. sedation with quetiapine, or decrease prolactin with the addition of aripiprazole) – these matters are discussed elsewhere. We concern ourselves solely with the addition of an antipsychotic to another antipsychotic to increase efficacy. From a theoretical point of view since all antipsychotics block D_2 receptors (unlike anti-hypertensives which use different mechanisms) there is limited rationale for addition. Studies of add-ons have often chosen combinations of convenience or based on clinical lore and perhaps the most systematic evidence is available for the addition of antipsychotics to clozapine[13] – perhaps supported by the rationale that since clozapine has low D_2 occupancy, increasing its D_2 occupancy may yield additional benefits[14]. A meta-analysis of all systematic antipsychotic add-on studies seems to suggest at best a modest benefit – more likely when the patient is on clozapine, when a FGA is added, and when both antipsychotics are used at effective doses[15].

When to 'stay'? A review of the above evidence suggests that no one strategy: increasing the dose; switching; or augmenting is a clear winner in all situations. Increase the dose if plasma levels are low; switch if the patient has not tried olanzapine or risperidone; and if failing on clozapine, augmentation may help. Given the limited efficacy of these manoeuvres perhaps an equally important call by the treating doctor is when to just 'stay' with the current pharmacotherapy and focus on non-pharmacological means: engagement in case-management, targeted psychological treatments and vocational rehabilitation as means of enhancing patient well-being. While it may seem a passive option – staying may often do less harm that aimless switching[11].

Summary

When treatment fails

- If dose has been optimised, consider watchful waiting
- Consider increasing antipsychotic dose according to tolerability and plasma levels
- If this fails, consider switching to olanzapine or risperidone (if not already used)
- If this fails, use clozapine (supporting evidence very strong)
- If clozapine fails, use time-limited augmentation strategies (supporting evidence variable)

References

1. Ezewuzie N et al. Establishing a dose–response relationship for oral risperidone in relapsed schizophrenia. J Psychopharmacol 2006; 20:86–90.
2. Sparshatt A et al. Quetiapine: dose–response relationship in schizophrenia. CNS Drugs 2008; 22:49–68.
3. Davis JM et al. Dose response and dose equivalence of antipsychotics. J Clin Psychopharmacol 2004; 24:192–208.
4. Kinon BJ et al. Standard and higher dose of olanzapine in patients with schizophrenia or schizoaffective disorder: a randomized, double-blind, fixed-dose study. J Clin Psychopharmacol 2008; 28:392–400.
5. Van PT et al. A controlled dose comparison of haloperidol in newly admitted schizophrenic patients. Arch Gen Psychiatry 1990; 47:754–758.
6. Kinon BJ et al. Treatment of neuroleptic-resistant schizophrenic relapse. Psychopharmacol Bull 1993; 29:309–314.
7. Heres S et al. Why olanzapine beats risperidone, risperidone beats quetiapine, and quetiapine beats olanzapine: an exploratory analysis of head-to-head comparison studies of second-generation antipsychotics. Am J Psychiatry 2006; 163:185–194.
8. Stroup TS et al. Effectiveness of olanzapine, quetiapine, risperidone, and ziprasidone in patients with chronic schizophrenia following discontinuation of a previous atypical antipsychotic. Am J Psychiatry 2006; 163:611–622.
9. Leucht S et al. Second-generation versus first-generation antipsychotic drugs for schizophrenia: a meta-analysis. Lancet 2009; 373:31–41.
10. Leucht S et al. A meta-analysis of head-to-head comparisons of second-generation antipsychotics in the treatment of schizophrenia. Am J Psychiatry 2009; 166:152–163.
11. Rosenheck RA et al. Does switching to a new antipsychotic improve outcomes? Data from the CATIE Trial. Schizophr Res 2009; 107:22–29.
12. Paton C et al. High-dose and combination antipsychotic prescribing in acute adult wards in the UK: the challenges posed by p.r.n. prescribing. Br J Psychiatry 2008; 192:435–439.
13. Taylor DM et al. Augmentation of clozapine with a second antipsychotic – a meta-analysis of randomized, placebo-controlled studies. Acta Psychiatr Scand 2009; 119:419–425.
14. Kapur S et al. Increased dopamine D2 receptor occupancy and elevated prolactin level associated with addition of haloperidol to clozapine. Am J Psychiatry 2001; 158:311–314.
15. Correll CU et al. Antipsychotic combinations vs monotherapy in schizophrenia: a meta-analysis of randomized controlled trials. Schizophr Bull 2009; 35:443–457.

Speed and onset of antipsychotic action

How quickly a drug acts is of tremendous interest to a clinician as it determines how long one should wait before initiating a change in dose or medication. The question of the speed of onset of antipsychotic action has been clouded. While the very initial observations of antipsychotic action in the 1950s suggested a quick onset (days), over time the field came to accept that the onset of antipsychotic action was delayed – with the standard teaching being that the 'onset' of antipsychotic action may take anywhere from two to three weeks[1]. This position has two major implications:

- For those designing clinical algorithms it suggests that one must wait a long period (four to six weeks) before making medication changes.
- For those attempting to understand antipsychotic action as it suggested that the early changes were non-specific and perhaps not relevant.

Over the last few years this dogma regarding a 'delayed onset' has been questioned and alternative evidence provided. Agid et al.[2] undertook a systematic meta-analysis that involved nearly 7,500 patients with schizophrenia, drawn from nearly 100 studies, using typicals (haloperidol, chlorpromazine) and atypicals (risperidone, olanzapine) and convincingly demonstrated that:

- there is a distinct onset of an antipsychotic effect within this first week – nearly 22% improvement in the first two weeks and only 9% improvement in weeks three or four
- this 'early onset' is evident regardless of measurement scale or antipsychotic or patient characteristics
- the effect is clearly greater than that of placebo even with the very first week; and
- there is a specific effect on psychotic symptoms within the first week – not just a non-specific effect on agitation and hostility.

These data reject the long-held 'delayed-onset' hypothesis and instead demonstrate that the antipsychotics have a quick and specific effect.

This effect has now been confirmed in a number of settings.

- First, it has been shown that the 'early onset' can be observed with even specific D_2/D_3 blockers (i.e. lacking sedative effects) such as amisulpride[3].
- Second, the effect is not just restricted to the four drugs tested in the original meta-analysis – similar findings have now been reported for ziprasidone and quetiapine, and are likely to be true for all antipsychotics provided they can be titrated to their effective dose quickly[4,5].
- Third, imaging studies have shown that early D_2 blockade is a predictor of this antipsychotic effect – thus suggesting that early response is likely to be directly linked to D_2 blockade[6].
- Finally, and perhaps most important clinically, the newer studies also show that if a patient does not show a certain amount of clinical response (currently thought to be about 20% in the first two weeks) the patient has a rather low chance of response on that drug and dose in the future[7,8].

These new findings raise two interesting questions. How could such a simple clinical observation have been hidden for so long and what are its clinical implications?

The main reason why the 'early onset' was obscured is because the field was driven by the 'delayed onset' theory and no group systematically investigated the early stages until the work of Agid et al[2]. The other relevant factor is that while controlled clinical studies measure changes using sensitive measurement scales (e.g. PANSS) most clinical treatment uses simple clinical observation (as expressed in the CGI scale). It is now understood that one requires a 15–20-point change in PANSS before an average clinician can identify 'minimal improvement' by subjective impression[9]. Thus, one can see how even though the onset of improvement is rather early, it does not reach the threshold of 15–20% change till the end of the second week on average, giving an impression of a later onset.

The findings have three important clinical implications.

- First, they emphasise the critical role of the first few days after initiating antipsychotics. The first two weeks on a new antipsychotic or dose are not dormant periods but likely the period of maximum change[1]. This should be communicated to patients and it also emphasises that clinicians need to be particularly attentive to changes early on.
- Secondly, the data highlight the value of using structured scales in daily clinical practice.
- Finally, the data cause one to revisit the question of how long one should wait if a medication is not effective. Should one switch after two, four or six weeks? While most algorithms currently would suggest waiting between four and six weeks on a given drug and dose, the early onset idea, the empirical evidence and clinical imperative suggest that it may be appropriate to switch earlier, say after two weeks, in patients in whom a combination of drug and dose has had *no* clinical improvement at all and where viable other alternatives exist.

Controlled clinical trials comparing clinical strategies which rely on early onset (i.e. use an early cut-off point to determine switching) versus more conservative strategies (wait four to six weeks) are urgently required. Until then, clinicians should make their decisions based on the evidence provided above and their clinical judgement in individual cases.

References

1. Agid O et al. The "delayed onset" of antipsychotic action – an idea whose time has come and gone. J Psychiatry Neurosci 2006; 31:93–100.
2. Agid O et al. Delayed-onset hypothesis of antipsychotic action: a hypothesis tested and rejected. Arch Gen Psychiatry 2003; 60:1228–1235.
3. Leucht S et al. Early-onset hypothesis of antipsychotic drug action: a hypothesis tested, confirmed and extended. Biol Psychiatry 2005; 57:1543–1549.
4. Agid O et al. Early onset of antipsychotic response in the treatment of acutely agitated patients with psychotic disorders. Schizophr Res 2008; 102: 241–248.
5. Small JG et al. Quetiapine in schizophrenia: onset of action within the first week of treatment. Curr Med Res Opin 2004; 20:1017–1023.
6. Agid O et al. Striatal vs extrastriatal dopamine D2 receptors in antipsychotic response. A double-blind PET study in schizophrenia. Neuropsychopharmacology 2006; 32:1209–1215.
7. Correll CU et al. Early prediction of antipsychotic response in schizophrenia. Am J Psychiatry 2003; 160:2063–2065.
8. Kinon BJ et al. Predicting response to atypical antipsychotics based on early response in the treatment of schizophrenia. Schizophr Res 2008; 102: 230–240.
9. Leucht S et al. Linking the PANSS, BPRS, and CGI: clinical implications. Neuropsychopharmacology 2006; 31:2318–2325.

First-generation antipsychotics – place in therapy

Typical and atypical antipsychotics are not categorically delineated. Typical (first-generation) drugs are those which can be expected to give rise to acute EPS, hyperprolactinaemia and, in the longer term, tardive dyskinesia. Atypicals (SGAs), by any sensible definition, might be expected not to be associated with these adverse effects. However, some atypicals show dose-related EPS, some induce hyperprolactinaemia and some may eventually give rise to tardive dyskinesia. To complicate matters further, it has been suggested that the therapeutic and adverse effects of typical drugs can be separated by careful dosing[1] – thus making typical drugs potentially atypical (although there is much evidence to the contrary[2–4]).

Given these observations, it seems unwise and unhelpful to consider so-called typical and atypical drugs as distinct groups of drugs. The essential difference between the two groups is the size of the therapeutic index in relation to acute EPS; for instance haloperidol has an extremely narrow index (probably less than 0.5 mg/day); olanzapine a wide index (20–40 mg/day).

Typical drugs still play an important role in schizophrenia and offer a valid alternative to atypicals where atypicals are poorly tolerated or where typicals are preferred by patients themselves. Typicals may be less effective than some non-clozapine atypicals (amisulpride, olanzapine and risperidone may be more efficacious[5,6]). CATIE[7] and CUtLASS[8], however, found few important differences between atypicals and typicals (mainly sulpiride and perphenazine). Their main drawbacks are, of course, acute EPS, hyperprolactinaemia and tardive dyskinesia. Hyperprolactinaemia is probably unavoidable in practice and, even when not symptomatic, may grossly affect hypothalamic function[9]. It is also associated with sexual dysfunction[10], but be aware that the autonomic effects of some atypicals may also cause sexual dysfunction[11].

Tardive dyskinesia probably occurs more frequently with typicals than atypicals[12–15] (notwithstanding difficulties in defining what is atypical), although there remains some uncertainty[16–18]. Careful observation of patients and the prescribing of the lowest effective dose are essential to help reduce the risk of this serious adverse event[19,20]. Even with these precautions, the risk of tardive dyskinesia with typical drugs may be unacceptably high[21].

References

1. Oosthuizen P et al. Determining the optimal dose of haloperidol in first-episode psychosis. J Psychopharmacol 2001; 15:251–255.
2. Zimbroff DL et al. Controlled, dose–response study of sertindole and haloperidol in the treatment of schizophrenia. Sertindole Study Group. Am J Psychiatry 1997; 154:782–791.
3. Jeste DV et al. Incidence of tardive dyskinesia in early stages of low-dose treatment with typical neuroleptics in older patients. Am J Psychiatry 1999; 156:309–311.
4. Meltzer HY et al. The effect of neuroleptics on serum prolactin in schizophrenic patients. Arch Gen Psychiatry 1976; 33:279–286.
5. Davis JM et al. A meta-analysis of the efficacy of second-generation antipsychotics. Arch Gen Psychiatry 2003; 60:553–564.
6. Leucht S et al. Second-generation versus first-generation antipsychotic drugs for schizophrenia: a meta-analysis. Lancet 2009; 373:31–41.
7. Lieberman JA et al. Effectiveness of antipsychotic drugs in patients with chronic schizophrenia. N Engl J Med 2005; 353:1209–1223.
8. Jones PB et al. Randomized controlled trial of the effect on Quality of Life of second- vs first-generation antipsychotic drugs in schizophrenia: Cost Utility of the Latest Antipsychotic Drugs in Schizophrenia Study (CUtLASS 1). Arch Gen Psychiatry 2006; 63:1079–1087.
9. Smith S et al. The effects of antipsychotic-induced hyperprolactinaemia on the hypothalamic-pituitary-gonadal axis. J Clin Psychopharmacol 2002; 22:109–114.
10. Smith SM et al. Sexual dysfunction in patients taking conventional antipsychotic medication. Br J Psychiatry 2002; 181:49–55.
11. Aizenberg D et al. Comparison of sexual dysfunction in male schizophrenic patients maintained on treatment with classical antipsychotics versus clozapine. J Clin Psychiatry 2001; 62:541–544.
12. Tollefson GD et al. Blind, controlled, long-term study of the comparative incidence of treatment-emergent tardive dyskinesia with olanzapine or haloperidol. Am J Psychiatry 1997; 154:1248–1254.
13. Beasley C et al. Randomised double-blind comparison of the incidence of tardive dyskinesia in patients with schizophrenia during long-term treatment with olanzapine or haloperidol. Br J Psychiatry 1999; 174:23–30.
14. Correll CU et al. Lower risk for tardive dyskinesia associated with second-generation antipsychotics: a systematic review of 1-year studies. Am J Psychiatry 2004; 161:414–425.
15. Tenback DE et al. Effects of antipsychotic treatment on tardive dyskinesia: a 6-month evaluation of patients from the European Schizophrenia Outpatient Health Outcomes (SOHO) Study. J Clin Psychiatry 2005; 66:1130–1133.
16. Halliday J et al. Nithsdale Schizophrenia Surveys 23: movement disorders. 20-year review. Br J Psychiatry 2002; 181:422–427.
17. Novick D et al. Tolerability of outpatient antipsychotic treatment: 36-month results from the European Schizophrenia Outpatient Health Outcomes (SOHO) study. Eur Neuropsychopharmacol 2009; 19:542–550.
18. Miller DD et al. Extrapyramidal side-effects of antipsychotics in a randomised trial. Br J Psychiatry 2008; 193:279–288.
19. Jeste DV et al. Tardive dyskinesia. Schizophr Bull 1993; 19:303–315.
20. Cavallaro R et al. Recognition, avoidance, and management of antipsychotic-induced tardive dyskinesia. CNS Drugs 1995; 4:278–293.
21. Oosthuizen P et al. A randomized, controlled comparison of the efficacy and tolerability of low and high doses of haloperidol in the treatment of first-episode psychosis. Int J Neuropsychopharmacol 2004; 7:125–131.

Antipsychotics – monitoring

This table summarises suggested monitoring for those receiving antipsychotics. More detail and background is provided in specific sections in this chapter.

Parameter/test	Suggested frequency	Action to be taken if results outside reference range	Drugs with special precautions	Drugs for which monitoring is not required
Urea and electrolytes (including creatinine or estimated GFR)	Baseline and yearly	Investigate all abnormalities detected	Amisulpride and sulpiride renally excreted – consider reducing dose if GFR reduced	None
Full blood count (FBC)[1–6]	Baseline and yearly	Stop suspect drug if neutrophils fall below $1.5 \times 10^9/l$. Refer to specialist medical care if neutrophils below $0.5 \times 10^9/l$. Note high frequency of benign ethnic neutropenia in certain ethnic groups	Clozapine – FBC weekly for 18 weeks, then fortnightly up to one year, then monthly	None
Blood lipids[7,8] (cholesterol; triglycerides) Fasting sample, if possible	Baseline, at 3 months then yearly	Offer lifestyle advice. Consider changing antipsychotic and/or initiating statin therapy	Clozapine, olanzapine, quetiapine, phenothiazines – 3 monthly for first year, then yearly	Some antipsychotics (e.g. aripiprazole) not clearly associated with dyslipidaemia but prevalence is high in this patient group[9–11] so all patients should be monitored
Weight[7,8,11] (include waist size and BMI, if possible)	Baseline, frequently for three months then yearly	Offer lifestyle advice. Consider changing antipsychotic and/or dietary/pharmacological intervention	Clozapine, olanzapine – 3 monthly for first year, then yearly	Aripiprazole and ziprasidone not clearly associated with weight gain but monitoring recommended nonetheless – obesity prevalence high in this patient group

Test	Monitoring frequency	Action	Drugs most likely associated	Comments / other drugs
Plasma glucose (fasting sample, if possible)	Baseline, at 4–6 months, then yearly	Offer lifestyle advice. Obtain fasting sample or non-fasting and HbA$_{1C}$; Refer to GP or specialist	Clozapine, olanzapine – test at baseline, one month, then 4–6 monthly	Some antipsychotics not clearly associated with IFG but prevalence is high in this patient group[12,13] so all patients should be monitored
ECG	Baseline and after dose increases (ECG changes rare in practice[14]) on admission to hospital and before discharge if drug regimen changed	Refer to cardiologist if abnormality detected	Haloperidol, pimozide, sertindole – ECG mandatory. Ziprasidone, zotepine – ECG mandatory in some situations	Risk of sudden cardiac death increased with most antipsychotics[15]. Ideally, all patients should be offered an ECG at least yearly
Blood pressure	Baseline; frequently during dose titration	If severe hypotension or hypertension (clozapine) observed, slow rate of titration	Clozapine, chlorpromazine and quetiapine most likely to be associated with postural hypotension	Amisulpride, aripiprazole, trifluoperazine, sulpiride
Prolactin	Baseline, then at 6 months, then yearly	Switch drugs if hyperprolactinaemia confirmed and symptomatic		Aripiprazole, clozapine, quetiapine, olanzapine (<20mg), ziprasidone usually do not elevate prolactin, but worth measuring if symptoms arise
Liver function tests (LFTs)[16–18]	Baseline, then yearly	Stop suspect drug if LFTs indicate hepatitis (transaminases x 3 normal) or functional damage (PT/albumin change)	Clozapine and chlorpromazine associated with hepatic failure	Amisulpride, sulpiride
Creatinine phosphokinase (CPK)	Baseline, then if NMS suspected	See section on NMS	NMS more likely with first generation antipsychotics	None

Other tests:

Patients on clozapine may benefit from an **EEG**[19,20] as this may help determine the need for valproate (although interpretation is obviously complex). Those on quetiapine should have thyroid function tests yearly although the risk of abnormality is very small[21,22].

Key:

BMI – body mass index; ECG – electrocardiograph; EEG – electrocephalogram; GFR – glomerula filtration rate; IFG – impaired fasting glucose.

References

1. Burckart GJ et al. Neutropenia following acute chlorpromazine ingestion. Clin Toxicol 1981; 18:797–801.
2. Grohmann R et al. Agranulocytosis and significant leucopenia with neuroleptic drugs: results from the AMUP program. Psychopharmacology 1989;99 Suppl:S109–S112.
3. Esposito D et al. Risperidone-induced morning pseudoneutropenia. Am J Psychiatry 2005; 162:397.
4. Montgomery J. Ziprasidone-related agranulocytosis following olanzapine-induced neutropenia. Gen Hosp Psychiatry 2006; 28:83–85.
5. Cowan C et al. Leukopenia and neutropenia induced by quetiapine. Prog Neuropsychopharmacol Biol Psychiatry 2007; 31:292–294.
6. Buchman N et al. Olanzapine-induced leukopenia with human leukocyte antigen profiling. Int Clin Psychopharmacol 2001; 16:55–57.
7. Marder SR et al. Physical health monitoring of patients with schizophrenia. Am J Psychiatry 2004; 161:1334–1349.
8. Fenton WS et al. Medication-induced weight gain and dyslipidemia in patients with schizophrenia. Am J Psychiatry 2006; 163:1697–1704.
9. Weissman EM et al. Lipid monitoring in patients with schizophrenia prescribed second-generation antipsychotics. J Clin Psychiatry 2006; 67:1323–1326.
10. Cohn TA et al. Metabolic monitoring for patients treated with antipsychotic medications. Can J Psychiatry 2006; 51:492–501.
11. Paton C et al. Obesity, dyslipidaemias and smoking in an inpatient population treated with antipsychotic drugs. Acta Psychiatr Scand 2004; 110: 299–305.
12. Taylor D et al. Undiagnosed impaired fasting glucose and diabetes mellitus amongst inpatients receiving antipsychotic drugs. J Psychopharmacol 2005; 19:182–186.
13. Citrome L et al. Incidence, prevalence, and surveillance for diabetes in New York State psychiatric hospitals, 1997–2004. Psychiatr Serv 2006; 57: 1132–1139.
14. Novotny T et al. Monitoring of QT interval in patients treated with psychotropic drugs. Int J Cardiol 2007; 117:329–332.
15. Ray WA et al. Atypical antipsychotic drugs and the risk of sudden cardiac death. N Engl J Med 2009; 360:225–235.
16. Hummer M et al. Hepatotoxicity of clozapine. J Clin Psychopharmacol 1997; 17:314–317.
17. Erdogan A et al. Management of marked liver enzyme increase during clozapine treatment: a case report and review of the literature. Int J Psychiatry Med 2004; 34:83–89.
18. Regal RE et al. Phenothiazine-induced cholestatic jaundice. Clin Pharm 1987; 6:787–794.
19. Centorrino F et al. EEG abnormalities during treatment with typical and atypical antipsychotics. Am J Psychiatry 2002; 159:109–115.
20. Gross A et al. Clozapine-induced QEEG changes correlate with clinical response in schizophrenic patients: a prospective, longitudinal study. Pharmacopsychiatry 2004; 37:119–122.
21. Twaites BR et al. The safety of quetiapine: results of a post-marketing surveillance study on 1728 patients in England. J Psychopharmacol 2007; 21: 392–399.
22. Kelly DL et al. Thyroid function in treatment-resistant schizophrenia patients treated with quetiapine, risperidone, or fluphenazine. J Clin Psychiatry 2005; 66:80–84.

Depot antipsychotics

Depot antipsychotics eliminate covert non-adherence, thus ensuring medication delivery. Depot preparations are widely used; it is estimated that between a quarter and a third of people with schizophrenia are prescribed a depot[1]. Approximately half are also prescribed an oral antipsychotic drug, which often results in high-dose prescribing[1].

Advice on prescribing depot medication

- **Give a test dose**
  Depots are long-acting. Any adverse effects that result from injection are likely to be long-lived. For FGA depots, a test dose consisting of a small dose of active drug in a small volume of oil serves a dual purpose; it is a test of the patient's sensitivity to EPS and to reveal any sensitivity to the base oil. For SGA depots, test doses are not required (less propensity to cause EPS and aqueous base not known to be allergenic).
- **Begin with the lowest therapeutic dose**
  There are few data showing clear dose–response effects for depot preparations. There is some information indicating that low doses are at least as effective as higher ones. Low doses are likely to be better tolerated and are certainly less expensive.
- **Administer at the longest possible licensed interval**
  All depots can be safely administered at their licensed dosing intervals. There is no evidence to suggest that shortening the dose interval improves efficacy. Moreover, injections are painful, so less frequent administration is desirable. The 'observation' that some patients deteriorate in the days before the next depot is due is probably fallacious. For some hours (or even days with some preparations) plasma levels of antipsychotics continue to fall, albeit slowly, after the next injection. Thus patients are most at risk of deterioration immediately after a depot injection and not before it. Moreover, in trials, relapse seems only to occur 3–6 months after withdrawing depot therapy; roughly the time required to clear steady-state depot drug levels from the blood.
- **Adjust doses only after an adequate period of assessment**
  Attainment of peak plasma levels, therapeutic effect and steady-state plasma levels are all delayed with depot injections. Doses may be *reduced* if adverse effects occur, but should only be increased after careful assessment over at least 1 month, and preferably longer. The use of adjunctive oral medication to assess depot requirements may be helpful, but it too is complicated by the slow emergence of antipsychotic effects. Note that at the start of therapy, plasma levels of antipsychotic released from a depot increase over several weeks to months without increasing the given dose. (This is due to accumulation: steady state is only achieved after 6–8 weeks.) Dose increases during this time to steady-state plasma levels are thus illogical and impossible to evaluate properly.

Differences between depots

There are few differences between FGA depots. Pipotiazine may be associated with relatively less EPS, and fluphenazine with relatively more EPS, but perhaps less weight gain[2]. Cochrane reviews have been completed for pipotiazine[3], flupentixol[4], zuclopenthixol[5], haloperidol[6] and fluphenazine[7]. With the exception of zuclopenthixol[5] (see below), these depot preparations are equally effective, both with respect to oral antipsychotics and each other. Standard doses are as effective as high doses for flupentixol[4]. It has been argued that compliance with oral antipsychotics decreases over time and that relapse rates in patients prescribed depots decrease in comparison to oral antipsychotics only in the longer term[8]. That is, depots reveal advantages over oral treatment only after several years.

Risperidone and olanzapine long-acting injections have a relatively lower propensity for EPS. Risperidone however increases prolactin, and because of its pharmacokinetic profile, dosage adjustment can be complex. Olanzapine can cause significant weight gain and is associated with inadvertent intravascular (IAIV) injection[9] (also known as 'post injection syndrome'). Unlike risperidone long-acting injection, it is effective almost immediately.

Two differences that do exist between depot antipsychotics are:

- zuclopenthixol may be more effective in preventing relapses than other depots, although this may be at the expense of an increased burden of side-effects[5], and
- flupentixol decanoate can be given in very much higher 'neuroleptic equivalent' doses than the other depot preparations and still remain 'within *BNF* limits'. It is doubtful that this confers any real therapeutic advantage.

Table Antipsychotic depot injections – suggested doses and frequencies[10]

Drug	Trade name	Test dose (mg)	Dose range (mg/week)	Dosing interval (weeks)	Comments
Flupentixol decanoate	Depixol	20	12.5–400	2–4	Maximum licensed dose is very high relative to other depots
Fluphenazine decanoate	Modecate	12.5	6.25–50	2–5	High EPS
Haloperidol decanoate	Haldol	25*	12.5–75	4	High EPS
Pipothiazine palmitate	Piportil	25	12.5–50	4	? Lower incidence of EPS (unproven)
Zuclopenthixol decanoate	Clopixol	100	100–600	2–4	? Slightly better efficacy
Risperidone microspheres	Risperidal Consta	Not required	12.5–25 mg	2	Drug release delayed for 2–3 weeks
Olanzapine pamoate	Zypadhera	Not required	75–150 mg	2–4	Note risk of IVIA/post injection syndrome

Notes:
* Give a quarter to half dose stated doses in elderly.
* After test dose, wait 4–10 days before starting titration to maintenance therapy (see product information for individual drugs).
* Dose range is given in mg/week for convenience only – avoid using shorter dose intervals than those recommended except in exceptional circumstances (e.g. long interval necessitates high volume (>3–4 ml) injection).
*Test dose not stated by manufacturer.

Intramuscular anticholinergics and depots

Depot antipsychotics do not produce acute movement disorder at the time of administration[11]: this may take hours to days. The administration of intramuscular procyclidine routinely with each depot is illogical, as the effects of the anticholinergic drug will have worn off before plasma antipsychotic levels peak.

References

1. Barnes T. Antipsychotic long acting injections: prescribing practice in the UK. Br J Psychiatry 2009; In press.
2. Taylor D. Psychopharmacology and adverse effects of antipsychotic long acting injections. Br J Psychiatry 2009; In press.
3. Dinesh M et al. Depot pipotiazine palmitate and undecylenate for schizophrenia. Cochrane Database Syst Rev 2006; CD001720.
4. David A et al. Depot flupenthixol decanoate for schizophrenia or other similar psychotic disorders. Cochrane Database Syst Rev 2006; CD001470.
5. da Silva Freire Coutinho E et al. Zuclopenthixol decanoate for schizophrenia and other serious mental illnesses. Cochrane Database Syst Rev 2006; CD001164.
6. Quraishi S et al. Depot haloperidol decanoate for schizophrenia. Cochrane Database Syst Rev 2006; CD001361.
7. David A et al. Depot fluphenazine decanoate and enanthate for schizophrenia. Cochrane Database Syst Rev 2006; CD000307.
8. Schooler NR. Relapse and rehospitalization: comparing oral and depot antipsychotics. J Clin Psychiatry 2003;64 Suppl 16:14–17.
9. Citrome L. Olanzapine pamoate: a stick in time? Int J Clin Pract 2009; 63:140–150.
10. Taylor D et al. Antipsychotic depot injections – suggested doses and frequencies. Psychiatr Bull 1995; 19:357.
11. Kane JM et al. Guidelines for depot antipsychotic treatment in schizophrenia. European Neuropsychopharmacology Consensus Conference in Siena, Italy. Eur Neuropsychopharmacol 1998; 8:55–66.

Further reading

Adams CE et al. Systematic meta-review of depot antipsychotic drugs for people with schizophrenia. Br J Psych 2001; 179:290–299.

Barnes TRE. Why indeed?: Invited commentary on….why aren't depot antipsychotics prescribed more often and what can be done about it? Adv Psychiatr Treat 2005; 11:211–213.

Patel MX et al. Why aren't depot antipsychotics prescribed more often and what can be done about it? Adv Psychiatr Treat 2005; 11:203–211.

Taylor D. Depot antipsychotics revisited. Psychiatr Bull 1999; 23:551–553.

Walburn J et al. Systematic review of patient and nurse attitudes to depot antipsychotic medication. Br J Psych 2001; 179:300–307.

Schizophrenia

Risperidone long-acting injection

Risperidone was the first 'atypical' drug to be made available as a depot, or long-acting, injectable formulation. Doses of 25–50 mg every 2 weeks appear to be as effective as oral doses of 2–6 mg/day[1]. The long-acting injection also seems to be well tolerated – fewer than 10% of patients experience EPSEs and fewer than 6% withdrew from a long-term trial because of adverse effects[2]. Few data are available relating to effects on prolactin but, although problems might be predicted[3], prolactin levels appear to reduce somewhat following a switch from oral to injectable risperidone[4–6]. Rates of tardive dyskinesia are said to be low[7].

Confusion remains over the dose–response relationship for RLAI. Studies randomising subjects to different fixed doses of RLAI show no differences in response according to dose[8]. One randomised, fixed-dose year long study suggested better outcome for 50 mg every two weeks than with 25 mg, although no observed difference reached statistical significance[9]. Naturalistic studies indicate doses higher than 25 mg/2 weeks are frequently used[10,11]. One study suggests higher doses are associated with better outcome[12,13].

Plasma levels afforded by 25 mg/2 weeks seem to be similar to, or even lower than, levels provided by 2 mg/day oral risperidone[14,15]. Striatal dopamine D_2 occupancies are similarly low in people receiving 25 mg/2 weeks[16,17]. So, although fixed-dose studies have not revealed clear advantages for doses above 25 mg/2 weeks other indicators cast doubt on the assumption that 25 mg/2 weeks will be adequate for all or even most patients. While this conundrum remains unresolved the need for careful dose titration becomes of great importance. This is perhaps most efficiently achieved by establishing the required dose of oral risperidone and converting this dose into the equivalent injection dose. Trials have clearly established that switching from 2 mg oral to 25 mg injection and 4 mg oral to 50 mg injection is usually successful[2,18,19] (switching from 4 mg/day to 25 mg/2 weeks increases the risk of relapse[20]). There remains a question over the equivalent dose for 6 mg oral: in theory, patients should be switched to 75 mg injection but this showed no advantage over lower doses in trials and is in any case above the licensed maximum dose.

Risperidone long-acting injection differs importantly from other depots and the following should be noted:

- Risperidone depot is not an esterified form of the parent drug. It contains risperidone coated in polymer to form microspheres. These microspheres have to be suspended in an aqueous base immediately before use.
- The injection must be stored in a fridge (consider the practicalities for CPNs).
- It is available as doses of 25, 37.5 and 50 mg. The whole vial must be used (because of the nature of the suspension). This means that there is limited flexibility in dosing.
- A test dose is not required or sensible. (Testing tolerability with oral risperidone is desirable but not always practical.)
- It takes 3–4 weeks for the first injection to produce therapeutic plasma levels. Patients must be maintained on a full dose of their previous antipsychotic for at least 3 weeks after the administration of the first risperidone injection. Oral antipsychotic cover is sometimes required for longer (6–8 weeks). If the patient is not already receiving an oral antipsychotic, oral risperidone should be prescribed. (See table for advice on switching from depots.) Patients who refuse oral treatment and are acutely ill should not be given RLAI because of the long delay in drug release.
- Risperidone depot must be administered every 2 weeks. The Product Licence does not allow longer intervals between doses. There is little flexibility to negotiate with patients about the frequency of administration although monthly injections may be effective[21].

- The most effective way of predicting response to RLAI is to establish dose and response with oral risperidone.
- Risperidone injection is not suitable for patients with treatment refractory schizophrenia.

For guidance on switching to risperidone long-acting injection see below.

Table Switching to risperidone long-acting injection (RLAI)

Switching from	Recommended method of switching	Comments
No treatment (new patient or recently non-compliant)	Start oral risperidone at 2 mg/day and titrate to effective dose. If tolerated, prescribe equivalent dose of RLAI Continue with oral risperidone for at least 3 weeks then taper over 1–2 weeks. Be prepared to continue oral risperidone for longer	Use oral risperidone before giving injection to assure good tolerability Those stabilised on 2 mg/day start on 25 mg/2 weeks Those on higher doses, start on 37.5 mg/2 weeks and be prepared to use 50 mg/2 weeks
Oral risperidone	Prescribe equivalent dose of RLAI	See above
Oral antipsychotics (not risperidone)	**Either:** (a) Switch to oral risperidone and titrate to effective dose. If tolerated, prescribe equivalent dose of RLAI Continue with oral risperidone for at least 3 weeks then taper over 1–2 weeks. Be prepared to continue oral risperidone for longer Or: (b) Give RLAI and then slowly discontinue oral antipsychotics after 3–4 weeks. Be prepared to continue oral antipsychotics for longer	Dose assessment is difficult in those switching from another antipsychotic. Broadly speaking, those on low oral doses should be switched to 25 mg/2 weeks. 'Low' in this context means towards the lower end of the licensed dose range or around the minimum dose known to be effective Those on higher oral doses should receive 37.5 mg or 50 mg every 2 weeks. The continued need for oral antipsychotics after 3–4 weeks may indicate that higher doses of RLAI are required
Depot antipsychotic	Give RLAI one week **before** the last depot injection is given	Dose of RLAI difficult to predict. For those on low doses (see above) start at 25 mg/2 weeks and then adjust as necessary Start RLAI at 37.5 mg/2 weeks in those previously maintained on doses in the middle or upper range of licensed doses. Be prepared to increase to 50 mg/2 weeks
Antipsychotic polypharmacy with depot	Give RLAI one week before the last depot injection is given Slowly taper oral antipsychotics 3–4 weeks later. Be prepared to continue oral antipsychotics for longer	Aim to treat patient with RLAI as the sole antipsychotic. As before, RLAI dose should be dictated, as far as is possible, by the total dose of oral and injectable antipsychotic

References

1. Chue P et al. Comparative efficacy and safety of long-acting risperidone and risperidone oral tablets. Eur Neuropsychopharmacol 2005; 15:111–117.
2. Fleischhacker WW et al. Treatment of schizophrenia with long-acting injectable risperidone: a 12-month open-label trial of the first long-acting second-generation antipsychotic. J Clin Psychiatry 2003; 64:1250–1257.
3. Kleinberg DL et al. Prolactin levels and adverse events in patients treated with risperidone. J Clin Psychopharmacol 1999; 19:57–61.
4. Bai YM et al. A comparative efficacy and safety study of long-acting risperidone injection and risperidone oral tablets among hospitalized patients: 12-week randomized, single-blind study. Pharmacopsychiatry 2006; 39:135–141.
5. Bai YM et al. Pharmacokinetics study for hyperprolactinemia among schizophrenics switched from risperidone to risperidone long-acting injection. J Clin Psychopharmacol 2007; 27:306–308.
6. Peng PW et al. The disparity of pharmacokinetics and prolactin study for risperidone long-acting injection. J Clin Psychopharmacol 2008; 28:726–727.
7. Gharabawi GM et al. An assessment of emergent tardive dyskinesia and existing dyskinesia in patients receiving long-acting, injectable risperidone: results from a long-term study. Schizophr Res 2005; 77:129–139.
8. Kane JM et al. Long-acting injectable risperidone: efficacy and safety of the first long-acting atypical antipsychotic. Am J Psychiatry 2003; 160: 1125–1132.
9. Simpson GM et al. A 1-year double-blind study of 2 doses of long-acting risperidone in stable patients with schizophrenia or schizoaffective disorder. J Clin Psychiatry 2006; 67:1194–1203.
10. Turner M et al. Long-acting injectable risperidone: safety and efficacy in stable patients switched from conventional depot antipsychotics. Int Clin Psychopharmacol 2004; 19:241–249.
11. Taylor DM et al. Early clinical experience with risperidone long-acting injection: A prospective, 6-month follow-up of 100 patients. J Clin Psychiatry 2004; 65:1076–1083.
12. Taylor DM et al. Prospective 6-month follow-up of patients prescribed risperidone long-acting injection: factors predicting favourable outcome. Int J Neuropsychopharmacol 2005; 23:1–10.
13. Taylor DM et al. Risperidone long-acting injection: a prospective 3-year analysis of its use in clinical practice. J Clin Psychiatry 2009; 70:196–200.
14. Nesvag R et al. Serum concentrations of risperidone and 9-OH risperidone following intramuscular injection of long-acting risperidone compared with oral risperidone medication. Acta Psychiatr Scand 2006; 114:21–26.
15. Castberg I et al. Serum concentrations of risperidone and 9-hydroxyrisperidone after administration of the long-acting injectable form of risperidone: evidence from a routine therapeutic drug monitoring service. Ther Drug Monit 2005; 27:103–106.
16. Gefvert O et al. Pharmacokinetics and D2 receptor occupancy of long-acting injectable risperidone (Risperdal Consta™) in patients with schizophrenia. Int J Neuropsychopharmacol 2005; 8:27–36.
17. Remington G et al. A PET study evaluating dopamine D2 receptor occupancy for long-acting injectable risperidone. Am J Psychiatry 2006; 163: 396–401.
18. Lasser RA et al. Clinical improvement in 336 stable chronically psychotic patients changed from oral to long-acting risperidone: a 12-month open trial. Int J Neuropsychopharmacol 2005; 8:427–438.
19. Lauriello J et al. Long-acting risperidone vs. placebo in the treatment of hospital inpatients with schizophrenia. Schizophr Res 2005; 72:249–258.
20. Bai YM et al. Equivalent switching dose from oral risperidone to risperidone long-acting injection: a 48-week randomized, prospective, single-blind pharmacokinetic study. J Clin Psychiatry 2007; 68:1218–1225.
21. Uchida H et al. Monthly administration of long-acting injectable risperidone and striatal dopamine D2 receptor occupancy for the management of schizophrenia. J Clin Psychiatry 2008; 69:1281–1286.

Management of patients on long-term depots – dose reduction

All patients receiving long-term treatment with antipsychotic medication should be seen by their psychiatrist at least once a year (ideally more frequently) in order to review their progress and treatment. A systematic assessment of side-effects should constitute part of this review. There is no simple formula for deciding when to reduce the dose of maintenance antipsychotic treatment; therefore, a risk/benefit analysis must be done for every patient. The following prompts may be helpful:

- Is the patient symptom-free and if so for how long? Long-standing, non-distressing symptoms which have not previously been responsive to medication may be excluded
- What is the severity of the side-effects (EPS, TD, obesity, etc.)?
- What is the previous pattern of illness? Consider the speed of onset, duration and severity of episodes and any danger posed to self or others.
- Has dosage reduction been attempted before? If so, what was the outcome?
- What are the patient's current social circumstances? Is it a period of relative stability, or are stressful life events anticipated?
- What is the social cost of relapse (e.g. is the patient the sole breadwinner for a family)?
- Is the patient able to monitor his/her own symptoms? If so, will he/she seek help?

If after consideration of the above, the decision is taken to reduce medication dose, the patient's family should be involved and a clear explanation given of what should be done if symptoms return/worsen. It would then be reasonable to proceed in the following manner:

- If it has not already been done, oral antipsychotic medication should be discontinued first.
- The interval between injections should be increased to up to 4 weeks before decreasing the dose given each time. Note: *not* with risperidone.
- The dose should be reduced by no more than a third at any one time. Note: special considerations apply to risperidone.
- Decrements should, if possible, be made no more frequently than every 3 months, preferably every 6 months.
- Discontinuation should be seen as the end point of the above process.

If the patient becomes symptomatic, this should be seen not as a failure, but rather as an important step in determining the minimum effective dose that the patient requires.

Combined antipsychotics

There is no good objective evidence that combined antipsychotics (that do not include clozapine) offer any efficacy advantage over the use of a single antipsychotic. The evidence base supporting such combinations consists for the most part of small open studies and case series[1-6]. A questionnaire survey of US psychiatrists found that, in patients who did not respond to a single antipsychotic, two thirds of psychiatrists switched to another single antipsychotic, while a third added a second antipsychotic. Those who switched were more positive about outcomes than those who augmented[7].

There are a number of published case reports of clinically significant side-effects such as an increased prevalence of EPS[8], severe EPS[9], increased metabolic side-effects[6], paralytic ileus[10], grand mal seizures[11] and prolonged QTc[12] associated with combined antipsychotics. Despite this, such prescriptions are commonly seen[13]. National surveys have repeatedly shown that up to 50% of patients prescribed atypical antipsychotics receive a typical drug as well[14-17]. Anticholinergic medication is then often required[15].

A UK audit of antipsychotic prescribing in hospitalised patients found that 20% of all patients prescribed antipsychotics were prescribed doses above the *BNF* maximum. Very few of these prescriptions were for single antipsychotics[13] (high doses were the result of combined antipsychotics). Monitoring of patients receiving high doses or combinations was very poor. Prescribers would seem not to be aware of the potential for increased side-effects, particularly QTc prolongation[18] resulting from antipsychotic polypharmacy. Clinical factors such as age (young), gender (male) and diagnosis (schizophrenia) were associated with antipsychotic polypharmacy, albeit only a small proportion of the total[19]. A recent national quality improvement programme conducted through the Prescribing Observatory for Mental Health (POMH-UK) found that combined antipsychotics were prescribed for 43% of patients in acute adult wards in the UK at baseline and 39% at re-audit one year later[17]. In the majority of cases, the second antipsychotic was prescribed PRN and the most common reason given for prescribing in this way was to manage behavioural disturbance[17]. Initiatives to reduce the prevalence of combined antipsychotic prescribing appear to have only modest effects[17,20-23].

A study which followed a cohort of patients with schizophrenia prospectively over a 10-year period found that receiving more than one antipsychotic concurrently was associated with substantially increased mortality[24]. There was no association with the total number of antipsychotics given sequentially as monotherapy, the maximum daily antipsychotic dose, duration of exposure, lifetime intake, or any other measure of illness severity. Interestingly, the prescription of anticholinergics was associated with increased survival. Another study followed up 99 patients with schizophrenia over a 25-year period and found that those who were prescribed three antipsychotics simultaneously were twice as likely to die as those who were prescribed only one[25]. Although these data should be interpreted with some important caveats in mind, they should serve to remind us that antipsychotic monotherapy is desirable and should be the norm. This is emphasised by a study which demonstrated longer patient hospital stay and more frequent adverse effects in people receiving combining antipsychotics[26]. It follows that it should be standard practice to document the rationale for combined antipsychotics in individual cases in clinical notes along with a clear account of any benefits and side-effects. Medicolegally, that would seem to be wise although in practice it is rarely done[27].

Note that NICE explicitly demands that antipsychotics be not prescribed together except when switching[28]. On the basis of risk associated with QT prolongation (common to almost all antipsychotics), concomitant use of antipsychotics should be avoided. Note however that clozapine augmentation strategies often involve combining antipsychotics and this is perhaps the sole therapeutic area where such practice is supportable[29-33]. See section on clozapine augmentation.

Summary

* Antipsychotic polypharmacy is a widespread and resilient practice.
* Substantial evidence suggest that polypharmacy is harmful.
* Very limited evidence supports the efficacy of combined antipsychotics.

References

1. Bacher NM et al. Combining risperidone with standard neuroleptics for refractory schizophrenic patients. Am J Psychiatry 1996; 153:137.
2. Waring EW et al. Treatment of schizophrenia with antipsychotics in combination. Can J Psychiatry 1999; 44:189–190.
3. Zink M et al. Combination of amisulpride and olanzapine in treatment-resistant schizophrenic psychoses. Eur Psychiatry 2004; 19:56–58.
4. Chan J et al. Combination therapy with non-clozapine atypical antipsychotic medication: a review of current evidence. J Psychopharmacol 2007; 21:657–664.
5. Correll CU et al. Antipsychotic combinations vs monotherapy in schizophrenia: a meta-analysis of randomized controlled trials. Schizophr Bull 2009; 35:443–457.
6. Suzuki T et al. Effectiveness of antipsychotic polypharmacy for patients with treatment refractory schizophrenia: an open-label trial of olanzapine plus risperidone for those who failed to respond to a sequential treatment with olanzapine, quetiapine and risperidone. Hum Psychopharmacol 2008; 23:455–463.
7. Kreyenbuhl J et al. Adding or switching antipsychotic medications in treatment-refractory schizophrenia. Psychiatr Serv 2007; 58:983–990.
8. Carnahan RM et al. Increased risk of extrapyramidal side-effect treatment associated with atypical antipsychotic polytherapy. Acta Psychiatr Scand 2006; 113:135–141.
9. Gomberg RF. Interaction between olanzapine and haloperidol. J Clin Psychopharmacol 1999; 19:272–273.
10. Dome P et al. Paralytic ileus associated with combined atypical antipsychotic therapy. Prog Neuropsychopharmacol Biol Psychiatry 2007; 31:557–560.
11. Hedges DW et al. New-onset seizure associated with quetiapine and olanzapine. Ann Pharmacother 2002; 36:437–439.
12. Beelen AP et al. Asymptomatic QTc prolongation associated with quetiapine fumarate overdose in a patient being treated with risperidone. Hum Exp Toxicol 2001; 20:215–219.
13. Harrington M et al. The results of a multi-centre audit of the prescribing of antipsychotic drugs for in-patients in the UK. Psychiatr Bull 2002; 26: 414–418.
14. Taylor D et al. A prescription survey of the use of atypical antipsychotics for hospital inpatients in the United Kingdom. Int J Psychiatry Clin Pract 2000; 4:41–46.
15. Paton C et al. Patterns of antipsychotic and anticholinergic prescribing for hospital inpatients. J Psychopharmacol 2003; 17: 223–229.
16. De Hert M et al. Pharmacological treatment of hospitalised schizophrenic patients in Belgium. Int J Psychiatry Clin Pract 2009; 10:285–290.
17. Paton C et al. High-dose and combination antipsychotic prescribing in acute adult wards in the UK: the challenges posed by p.r.n. prescribing. Br J Psychiatry 2008; 192:435–439.
18. Medicines and Healthcare Products Regulatory Agency. Pharmacovigilance Working Party Public Assessment Report on neuroleptics and cardiac safety, in particular QT prolongation, cardiac arrhythmias, ventricular tachycardia and torsades de pointes. 2006. http://www.mhra.gov.uk/.
19. Lelliott P et al. The influence of patient variables on polypharmacy and combined high dose of antipsychotic drugs prescribed for in-patients. Psychiatr Bull 2002; 26:411–414.
20. Patrick V et al. Best practices: An initiative to curtail the use of antipsychotic polypharmacy in a state psychiatric hospital. Psychiatr Serv 2006; 57:21–23.
21. Baker JA et al. The impact of a good practice manual on professional practice associated with psychotropic PRN in acute mental health wards: an exploratory study. Int J Nurs Stud 2008; 45:1403–1410.
22. Thompson A et al. The DEBIT trial: an intervention to reduce antipsychotic polypharmacy prescribing in adult psychiatry wards – a cluster randomized controlled trial. Psychol Med 2008; 38:705–715.
23. Tucker WM. When less is more: reducing the incidence of antipsychotic polypharmacy. J Psychiatr Pract 2007; 13:202–204.
24. Waddington JL et al. Mortality in schizophrenia. Antipsychotic polypharmacy and absence of adjunctive anticholinergics over the course of a 10-year prospective study. Br J Psychiatry 1998; 173:325–329.
25. Joukamaa M et al. Schizophrenia, neuroleptic medication and mortality. Br J Psychiatry 2006; 188:122–127.
26. Centorrino F et al. Multiple versus single antipsychotic agents for hospitalized psychiatric patients: case-control study of risks versus benefits. Am J Psychiatry 2004; 161:700–706.
27. Taylor D et al. Co-prescribing of atypical and typical antipsychotics – prescribing sequence and documented outcome. Psychiatr Bull 2002; 26: 170–172.
28. National Institute of Clinical Excellence. Guidance on the use of newer (atypical) antipsychotic drugs for the treatment of schizophrenia. Health Technology Appraisal No. 43. 2002. http://www.nice.org.uk/
29. Shiloh R et al. Sulpiride augmentation in people with schizophrenia partially responsive to clozapine. A double-blind, placebo-controlled study. Br J Psychiatry 1997; 171:569–573.
30. Josiassen RC et al. Clozapine augmented with risperidone in the treatment of schizophrenia: a randomized, double-blind, placebo-controlled trial. Am J Psychiatry 2005; 162:130–136.
31. Paton C et al. Augmentation with a second antipsychotic in patients with schizophrenia who partially respond to clozapine: a meta-analysis. J Clin Psychopharmacol 2007; 27:198–204.
32. Barbui C et al. Does the addition of a second antipsychotic drug improve clozapine treatment? Schizophr Bull 2009; 35: 458–468.
33. Taylor DM et al. Augmentation of clozapine with a second antipsychotic – a meta-analysis of randomized, placebo-controlled studies. Acta Psychiatr Scand 2009; 119:419–425.

Further reading

Tranulis C et al. Benefits and risks of antipsychotic polypharmacy: an evidence-based review of the literature. Drug Saf 2008; 31:7–20.

Schizophrenia

High-dose antipsychotics: prescribing and monitoring

'High dose' can result from the prescription of either:

- a single antipsychotic in a dose that is above the recommended maximum

  or

- two or more antipsychotics that, when expressed as a percentage of their respective maximum recommended doses and added together, result in a cumulative dose of >100%.

Efficacy

There is no firm evidence that high doses of antipsychotics are any more effective than standard doses. This holds true for the use of antipsychotics in rapid tranquillisation, the management of acute psychotic episodes, chronic aggression and relapse prevention. Approximately a quarter to a third of hospitalised patients are prescribed high-dose antipsychotics, the vast majority through the cumulative effect of combinations[1,2]; the common practice of prescribing antipsychotic drugs on a PRN basis makes a major contribution.

A review of the dose–response effects of a variety of antipsychotics revealed no evidence whatever for increasing doses above accepted licensed ranges[3]. Effect appears to be optimal at low doses: 4 mg/day risperidone[4]; 300 mg/day quetiapine[5], olanzapine 10mg[6], etc. There are a small number of RCTs that examine the efficacy of high versus standard doses in patients with treatment-resistant schizophrenia[7,8]. Some demonstrated benefit[9] but the majority of these studies are old, the number of patients randomised is small and study design is poor by current standards. Some studies used doses equivalent to more than 10 g chlorpromazine. More recently, one small (n = 12) open study of high-dose quetiapine (up to 1400 mg/day) found modest benefits in a third of subjects[10] (other studies of quetiapine have shown no benefit for higher doses[5]). In a further small (n = 40) RCT of high-dose olanzapine (up to 45 mg/day) versus clozapine, high-dose olanzapine showed similar efficacy to clozapine[11]. In both studies, the side-effect burden associated with high-dose treatment was considerable.

Adverse effects

The majority of side-effects associated with antipsychotic treatment are dose-related. These include EPS, sedation, postural hypotension, anticholinergic effects, QTc prolongation and sudden cardiac death[12]. High-dose antipsychotic treatment clearly worsens adverse effect incidence and severity[13,14]. Polypharmacy (with the exception of augmentation strategies for clozapine) also seems to be ineffective[15–17] and to produce more severe adverse effects including increased mortality[12,16,18]. A recent meta-analysis[19] revealed small but significant benefit for polypharmacy over single-drug treatment but this was in the context of poor-quality studies and publication bias. There is some evidence that dose reduction from very high (mean 2253 mg chlorpromazine equivalents per day) to high (mean 1315 mg chlorpromazine equivalents per day) dose leads to improvements in cognition and negative symptoms[20].

Recommendations

The use of high-dose antipsychotics should be an exceptional clinical practice and only ever employed when standard treatments, including clozapine, have failed. Documentation of target symptoms, response and side-effects, ideally using validated rating scales, should be standard practice so that there is ongoing consideration of the risk–benefit ratio for the patient. Close physical monitoring (including ECG) is essential.

References

1. Royal College of Psychiatrists. Consensus statement on high-dose antipsychotic medication (Council Report 138). 2006. London, Royal College of Psychiatrists.
2. Paton C et al. High-dose and combination antipsychotic prescribing in acute adult wards in the UK: the challenges posed by p.r.n. prescribing. Br J Psychiatry 2008; 192:435–439.
3. Davis JM et al. Dose response and dose equivalence of antipsychotics. J Clin Psychopharmacol 2004; 24:192–208.
4. Ezewuzie N et al. Establishing a dose–response relationship for oral risperidone in relapsed schizophrenia. J Psychopharmacol 2006; 20:86–90.
5. Sparshatt A et al. Quetiapine: dose–response relationship in schizophrenia. CNS Drugs 2008; 22:49–68.
6. Kinon BJ et al. Standard and higher dose of olanzapine in patients with schizophrenia or schizoaffective disorder: a randomized, double-blind, fixed-dose study. J Clin Psychopharmacol 2008; 28:392–400.
7. Hirsch SR et al. Clinical use of high-dose neuroleptics. Br J Psychiatry 1994; 164:94–96.
8. Thompson C. The use of high-dose antipsychotic medication. Br J Psychiatry 1994; 164:448–458.
9. Aubree JC et al. High and very high dosage antipsychotics: a critical review. J Clin Psychiatry 1980; 41:341–350.
10. Boggs DL et al. Quetiapine at high doses for the treatment of refractory schizophrenia. Schizophr Res 2008; 101:347–348.
11. Meltzer HY et al. A randomized, double-blind comparison of clozapine and high-dose olanzapine in treatment-resistant patients with schizophrenia. J Clin Psychiatry 2008; 69:274–285.
12. Ray WA et al. Atypical antipsychotic drugs and the risk of sudden cardiac death. N Engl J Med 2009; 360:225–235.
13. Bollini P et al. Antipsychotic drugs: is more worse? A meta-analysis of the published randomized control trials. Psychol Med 1994; 24:307–316.
14. Baldessarini RJ et al. Significance of neuroleptic dose and plasma level in the pharmacological treatment of psychoses. Arch Gen Psychiatry 1988; 45:79–90.
15. Taylor D et al. Co-prescribing of atypical and typical antipsychotics – prescribing sequence and documented outcome. Psychiatr Bull 2002; 26: 170–172.
16. Centorrino F et al. Multiple versus single antipsychotic agents for hospitalized psychiatric patients: case-control study of risks versus benefits. Am J Psychiatry 2004; 161:700–706.
17. Kreyenbuhl J et al. Adding or switching antipsychotic medications in treatment-refractory schizophrenia. Psychiatr Serv 2007; 58:983–990.
18. Waddington JL et al. Mortality in schizophrenia. Antipsychotic polypharmacy and absence of adjunctive anticholinergics over the course of a 10-year prospective study. Br J Psychiatry 1998; 173:325–329.
19. Correll CU et al. Antipsychotic combinations vs monotherapy in schizophrenia: a meta-analysis of randomized controlled trials. Schizophr Bull 2009; 35:443–457.
20. Kawai N et al. High-dose of multiple antipsychotics and cognitive function in schizophrenia: the effect of dose-reduction. Prog Neuropsychopharmacol Biol Psychiatry 2006; 30:1009–1014.

Schizophrenia

Prescribing high-dose antipsychotics

Before using high doses, ensure that:
- Sufficient time has been allowed for response (see section on time to response)
- At least two different antipsychotics have been tried sequentially (one atypical)
- Clozapine has failed or not been tolerated due to agranulocytosis. Most other side-effects can be managed. A very small proportion of patients may also refuse clozapine outright
- Compliance is not in doubt (use of blood tests, liquids/dispersible tablets, depot preparations, etc.)
- Adjunctive medications such as antidepressants or mood stabilisers are not indicated
- Psychological approaches have failed or are not appropriate

The decision to use high doses should:
- Be made by a consultant psychiatrist
- Involve the multidisciplinary team
- Be done if possible, with the patient's informed consent

Process
- Exclude contra-indications (ECG abnormalities, hepatic impairment)
- Consider and minimise any risks posed by concomitant medication (e.g. potential to cause QTc prolongation, electrolyte disturbance or pharmacokinetic interactions via CYP inhibition)
- Document the decision to prescribe high doses in the clinical notes along with a description of target symptoms. The use of an appropriate rating scale is advised
- Adequate time for response should be allowed after each dosage increment before a further increase is made

Monitoring
- Physical monitoring should be carried out as outlined in monitoring section
- All patients on high doses should have regular ECGs (base-line, when steady-state serum levels have been reached after each dosage increment, and then every 6–12 months). Additional biochemical/ECG monitoring is advised if drugs that are known to cause electrolyte disturbances or QTc prolongation are subsequently co-prescribed
- Target symptoms should be assessed after 6 weeks and 3 months. If insufficient improvement in these symptoms has occurred, the dose should be decreased to the normal range

Negative symptoms

The literature pertaining to the pharmacological treatment of negative symptoms largely consists of sub-analyses of acute efficacy studies, correlational analysis and path analyses[1]. Few studies specifically recruit patients with persistent negative symptoms.

The aetiology of negative symptoms is complex and it is important to determine the most likely cause in any individual case before embarking on a treatment regimen. Negative symptoms can be either primary (transient or enduring) or secondary to positive symptoms (e.g. asociality secondary to paranoia), EPS (e.g. bradykinesia, lack of facial expression), depression (e.g. social withdrawal) or institutionalisation[2]. Secondary negative symptoms are obviously best dealt with by treating the relevant cause (EPS, depression, etc.). In general:

- The earlier a psychotic illness is effectively treated, the less likely is the development of negative symptoms over time[3,4]. In first episode patients, response of negative symptoms to antipsychotic treatment may be determined by $5HT_{1A}$ genotype[5].
- Older antipsychotics have only a small effect against primary negative symptoms and can cause secondary negative symptoms (via EPS).
- Some SGAs have been shown to be generally superior to first-generation antipsychotics in the treatment of negative symptoms[6], in the context of overall treatment response in non-selected populations[7]. Data support the effectiveness of amisulpride in primary negative symptoms[8,9], but not clear superiority over low-dose haloperidol[10]. There are many small RCTs in the literature reporting equivalent efficacy for different SGAs, e.g. quetiapine and olanzapine[11]; ziprasidone and amisulpride[12]. A well-conducted study appeared to show superiority for olanzapine (only at 5 mg/day) over amisulpride[13]. A further small study shows superiority of olanzapine over haloperidol but the magnitude of the effect was modest[14].
- Low serum folate[15] and glycine[16] concentrations have been found in patients with predominantly negative symptoms.

A Cochrane review concluded that antidepressants may be effective in the treatment of affective flattening, alogia and avolition[17], while a meta-analysis of SSRI augmentation of an antipsychotic was less positive[18]. Small RCTs have demonstrated some benefit for selegiline[19,20], testosterone (applied topically)[21], ondansetron[22] and ginkgo biloba[23]. Data for rTMS are mixed[24–26]. A small case series suggests that memantine may have some efficacy[27]. A large (n = 250) RCT in adults[28] and a smaller RCT in elderly patients[29] each found no benefit for donepezil. There is also a small negative RCT of modafinil[30]. Patients who misuse psychoactive substances experience fewer negative symptoms than patients who do not[31]. It is not clear if this cause or effect.

References

1. Buckley PF et al. Pharmacological treatment of negative symptoms of schizophrenia: therapeutic opportunity or cul-de-sac? Acta Psychiatr Scand 2007; 115:93–100.
2. Carpenter WT. The treatment of negative symptoms: pharmacological and methodological issues. Br J Psychiatry 1996; 168:17–22.
3. Waddington JL et al. Sequential cross-sectional and 10-year prospective study of severe negative symptoms in relation to duration of initially untreated psychosis in chronic schizophrenia. Psychol Med 1995; 25:849–857.
4. Melle I et al. Prevention of negative symptom psychopathologies in first-episode schizophrenia: two-year effects of reducing the duration of untreated psychosis. Arch Gen Psychiatry 2008; 65:634–640.
5. Reynolds GP et al. Effect of 5-HT1A receptor gene polymorphism on negative and depressive symptom response to antipsychotic treatment of drug-naive psychotic patients. Am J Psychiatry 2006; 163:1826–1829.
6. Leucht S et al. Second-generation versus first-generation antipsychotic drugs for schizophrenia: a meta-analysis. Lancet 2009; 373:31–41.
7. Erhart SM et al. Treatment of schizophrenia negative symptoms: future prospects. Schizophr Bull 2006; 32:234–237.
8. Boyer P et al. Treatment of negative symptoms in schizophrenia with amisulpride. Br J Psychiatry 1995; 166:68–72.
9. Danion JM et al. Improvement of schizophrenic patients with primary negative symptoms treated with amisulpride. Amisulpride Study Group. Am J Psychiatry 1999; 156:610–616.
10. Speller JC et al. One-year, low-dose neuroleptic study of in-patients with chronic schizophrenia characterised by persistent negative symptoms. Amisulpride v. haloperidol. Br J Psychiatry 1997; 171:564–568.
11. Sirota P et al. Quetiapine versus olanzapine for the treatment of negative symptoms in patients with schizophrenia. Hum Psychopharmacol 2006; 21:227–234.

Schizophrenia

12. Olie JP et al. Ziprasidone and amisulpride effectively treat negative symptoms of schizophrenia: results of a 12-week, double-blind study. Int Clin Psychopharmacol 2006; 21:143–151.
13. Lecrubier Y et al. The treatment of negative symptoms and deficit states of chronic schizophrenia: olanzapine compared to amisulpride and placebo in a 6-month double-blind controlled clinical trial. Acta Psychiatr Scand 2006; 114:319–327.
14. Lindenmayer JP et al. A randomized controlled trial of olanzapine versus haloperidol in the treatment of primary negative symptoms and neurocognitive deficits in schizophrenia. J Clin Psychiatry 2007; 68:368–379.
15. Goff DC et al. Folate, homocysteine, and negative symptoms in schizophrenia. Am J Psychiatry 2004; 161:1705–1708.
16. Sumiyoshi T et al. Prediction of the ability of clozapine to treat negative symptoms from plasma glycine and serine levels in schizophrenia. Int J Neuropsychopharmacol 2005; 8:451–455.
17. Rummel C et al. Antidepressants for the negative symptoms of schizophrenia. Cochrane Database Syst Rev 2006; 3:CD005581.
18. Sepehry AA et al. Selective serotonin reuptake inhibitor (SSRI) add-on therapy for the negative symptoms of schizophrenia: a meta-analysis. J Clin sychiatry 2007; 68:604–610.
19. Lin A et al. Selegiline in the treatment of negative symptoms of schizophrenia. Prog Neurother Neuropsychopharmacol 2006; 1:121–131.
20. Amiri A et al. Efficacy of selegiline add on therapy to risperidone in the treatment of the negative symptoms of schizophrenia: a double-blind randomized placebo-controlled study. Hum Psychopharmacol 2008; 23:79–86.
21. Ko YH et al. Short-term testosterone augmentation in male schizophrenics: a randomized, double-blind, placebo-controlled trial. J Clin Psychopharmacol 2008; 28:375–383.
22. Zhang ZJ et al. Beneficial effects of ondansetron as an adjunct to haloperidol for chronic, treatment-resistant schizophrenia: a double-blind, randomized, placebo-controlled study. Schizophr Res 2006; 88:102–110.
23. Doruk A et al. A placebo-controlled study of extract of ginkgo biloba added to clozapine in patients with treatment-resistant schizophrenia. Int Clin Psychopharmacol 2008; 23:223–227.
24. Novak T et al. The double-blind sham-controlled study of high-frequency rTMS (20 Hz) for negative symptoms in schizophrenia: Negative results. Neuro Endocrinol Lett 2006; 27:209–213.
25. Mogg A et al. Repetitive transcranial magnetic stimulation for negative symptoms of schizophrenia: a randomized controlled pilot study. Schizophr Res 2007; 93:221–228.
26. Prikryl R et al. Treatment of negative symptoms of schizophrenia using repetitive transcranial magnetic stimulation in a double-blind, randomized controlled study. Schizophr Res 2007; 95:151–157.
27. Krivoy A et al. Addition of memantine to antipsychotic treatment in schizophrenia inpatients with residual symptoms: A preliminary study. Eur Neuropsychopharmacol 2008; 18:117–121.
28. Keefe RSE et al. Efficacy and safety of donepezil in patients with schizophrenia or schizoaffective disorder: significant placebo/practice effects in a 12-week, randomized, double-blind, placebo-controlled trial. Neuropsychopharmacology 2007; 33:1217–1228.
29. Mazeh D et al. Donepezil for negative signs in elderly patients with schizophrenia: an add-on, double-blind, crossover, placebo-controlled study. Int Psychogeriatr 2006; 18:429–436.
30. Pierre JM et al. A randomized, double-blind, placebo-controlled trial of modafinil for negative symptoms in schizophrenia. J Clin Psychiatry 2007; 68:705–710.
31. Potvin S et al. A meta-analysis of negative symptoms in dual diagnosis schizophrenia. Psychol Med 2006; 36:431–440.

Antipsychotic prophylaxis

First episode of psychosis

A placebo-controlled study showed that when no active prophylactic treatment is given, 57% of first-episode patients have relapsed at 1 year[1]. After 1–2 years of being well on antipsychotic medication, the risk of relapse remains high (figures of 10–15% per month have been quoted), but this area is less well researched[2,3]. Although the current consensus is that antipsychotics should be prescribed for 1–2 years after a first episode of schizophrenia[4,5], Gitlan et al.[6] found that withdrawing antipsychotic treatment in line with this consensus led to a relapse rate of almost 80% after one year medication-free and 98% after 2 years. Other studies in first-episode patients have found that discontinuing antipsychotics increases the risk of relapse 5-fold[7] and confirmed that only a small minority of patients who discontinue remain well 1–2 years later[8].

In practice, a firm diagnosis of schizophrenia is rarely made after a first episode and the majority of prescribers and/or patients will have at least attempted to stop antipsychotic treatment within one year[9]. It is vital that patients, carers and keyworkers are aware of the early signs of relapse and how to access help. Antipsychotics should not be considered the only intervention. Psychosocial and psychological interventions are clearly also important[10,11].

Multi-episode schizophrenia

The majority of those who have one episode of schizophrenia will go on to have further episodes. With each subsequent episode, the baseline level of functioning deteriorates[12] and the majority of this decline is seen in the first decade of illness. Suicide risk (10%) is also concentrated in the first decade of illness. Antipsychotic drugs, when taken regularly, protect against relapse in the short, medium and long term[13]. Those who receive targeted antipsychotics (i.e. only when symptoms re-emerge) have a worse outcome than those who receive prophylactic antipsychotics[14,15] and the risk of TD may also be higher. The figure below depicts the relapse rate in a large cohort of patients with psychotic illness, the majority of whom had already experienced multiple episodes[16]. All had originally received or were still receiving treatment with typical antipsychotics. Note that many of the studies included in this data set were old and unstandardised diagnostic criteria were used. Variable definitions of relapse and short follow-up periods were the norm and the use of other psychotropic drugs were not controlled for.

Figure   Effect of prophylactic antipsychotics

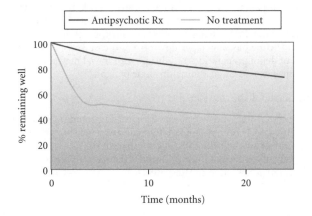

There are some data to support reduced relapse rates with depot antipsychotics compared with oral treatment although differences may not be apparent until the second year of treatment[10].

There is some evidence to support improved long-term outcomes with SGAs; a meta-analysis that contained data for 2032 patients concluded that the risk of relapse with SGAs is less than that associated with FGAs[17]. Note that lack of relapse is not the same as good functioning[10].

This apparent advantage for SGAs may not be a class effect and may not hold when appropriate doses of FGAs are used. For example, in a one-year maintenance RCT in first-episode patients, haloperidol (2–4 mg) and risperidone (2–4 mg) were found to be equally effective. Risperidone was not better tolerated overall[18].

Patients with schizophrenia may receive a number of sequential antipsychotic drugs during the maintenance phase[19]; such switching is at least partially due to a combination of suboptimal efficacy and poor tolerability. In both CATIE[20] and SOHO[21,22], the attrition rate from olanzapine was lower than the attrition rate from other antipsychotic drugs, suggesting that olanzapine may be more effective than other antipsychotic drugs (except clozapine). Note though that olanzapine is associated with a high propensity for metabolic side-effects.

Adherence to antipsychotic treatment
Amongst people with schizophrenia, non-adherence with antipsychotic treatment is high; only 10 days after discharge from hospital up to 25% are partially or non-adherent, rising to 50% at 1 year and 75% at 2 years[23]. Not only does non-adherence increase the risk of relapse, it may also increase the severity of relapse and the duration of hospitalisation[23]. The risk of suicide attempts also increases 4-fold[23].

Dose for prophylaxis
Many patients probably receive higher doses than necessary (particularly of the older drugs) when acutely psychotic[24,25]. In the longer term a balance needs to be made between effectiveness and side-effects. Lower doses of the older drugs (8 mg haloperidol/day or equivalent) are, when compared with higher doses, associated with less severe side-effects[26], better subjective state and better community adjustment[27]. Very low doses increase the risk of psychotic relapse[24,28]. There are no data to support the use of lower than standard doses of the newer drugs as prophylaxis. Doses that are acutely effective should generally be continued as prophylaxis[29].

How and when to stop[30]
The decision to stop antipsychotic drugs requires a thorough risk–benefit analysis for each patient. Withdrawal of antipsychotic drugs after long-term treatment should be gradual and closely monitored. The relapse rate in the first 6 months after abrupt withdrawal is double that seen after gradual withdrawal (defined as slow taper down over at least 3 weeks for oral antipsychotics or abrupt withdrawal of depot preparations)[31]. Abrupt withdrawal may also lead to discontinuation symptoms (e.g. headache, nausea, insomnia) in some patients[32].

The following factors should be considered[30]:

· Is the patient symptom-free, and if so, for how long? Long-standing, non-distressing symptoms which have not previously been responsive to medication may be excluded.
· What is the severity of side-effects (EPS, TD, obesity, etc.)?
· What was the previous pattern of illness? Consider the speed of onset, duration and severity of episodes and any danger posed to self and others.

- Has dosage reduction been attempted before, and, if so, what was the outcome?
- What are the patient's current social circumstances? Is it a period of relative stability, or are stressful life events anticipated?
- What is the social cost of relapse (e.g. is the patient the sole breadwinner for a family)?
- Is the patient/carer able to monitor symptoms, and, if so, will they seek help?

As with first-episode patients, patients, carers and keyworkers should be aware of the early signs of relapse and how to access help. Those with a history of aggressive behaviour or serious suicide attempts and those with residual psychotic symptoms should be considered for life-long treatment.

Key points that patients should know
- Antipsychotics do not 'cure' schizophrenia. They treat symptoms in the same way that insulin treats diabetes.
- Long-term treatment is required to prevent relapses.
- Family interventions[11] and CBT[10] increase the chance of staying well.
- Many antipsychotic drugs are available. Different drugs suit different patients. Perceived side-effects should always be discussed, so that the best tolerated drug can be found.
- Antipsychotics should not be stopped suddenly.

References

1. Crow TJ et al. The Northwick Park study of first episodes of schizophrenia 11. A randomised controlled trial of prophylactic neuroleptic treatment. Br J Psychiatry 1986; 148:120–127.
2. Nuechterlein KH et al. The early course of schizophrenia and long-term maintenance neuroleptic therapy. Arch Gen Psychiatry 1995; 52:203–205.
3. Davis JM et al. Depot antipsychotic drugs. Place in therapy. Drugs 1994; 47:741–773.
4. Sheitman BB et al. The evaluation and treatment of first-episode psychosis. Schizophr Bull 1997; 23:653–661.
5. American Psychiatric Association. Practice guideline for the treatment of patients with schizophrenia. Am J Psychiatry 1997;154 Suppl 4:1–63.
6. Gitlin M et al. Clinical outcome following neuroleptic discontinuation in patients with remitted recent-onset schizophrenia. Am J Psychiatry 2001; 158:1835–1842.
7. Robinson D et al. Predictors of relapse following response from a first episode of schizophrenia or schizoaffective disorder. Arch Gen Psychiatry 1999; 56:241–247.
8. Wunderink L et al. Guided discontinuation versus maintenance treatment in remitted first-episode psychosis: relapse rates and functional outcome. J Clin Psychiatry 2007; 68:654–661.
9. Professional attitudes in the UK towards neuroleptic maintenance therapy in schizophrenia. Psychiatr Bull 1997; 21:394–397.
10. Schooler NR. Relapse prevention and recovery in the treatment of schizophrenia. J Clin Psychiatry 2006;67 Suppl 5:19–23.
11. Motlova L et al. Relapse prevention in schizophrenia: does group family psychoeducation matter? One-year prospective follow-up field study. Int J Psychiatry Clin Pract 2006; 10:38–44.
12. Wyatt RJ. Neuroleptics and the natural course of schizophrenia. Schizophr Bull 1991; 17:325–351.
13. Almerie MQ et al. Cessation of medication for people with schizophrenia already stable on chlorpromazine. Schizophr Bull 2008; 34:13–14.
14. Jolley AG et al. Trial of brief intermittent neuroleptic prophylaxis for selected schizophrenic outpatients: clinical and social outcome at two years. Br Med J 1990; 301:837–842.
15. Herz MI et al. Intermittent vs maintenance medication in schizophrenia. Two-year results. Arch Gen Psychiatry 1991; 48:333–339.
16. Gilbert PL et al. Neuroleptic withdrawal in schizophrenic patients. A review of the literature. Arch Gen Psychiatry 1995; 52:173–188.
17. Leucht S et al. Relapse prevention in schizophrenia with new-generation antipsychotics: a systematic review and exploratory meta-analysis of randomized, controlled trials. Am J Psychiatry 2003; 160:1209–1222.
18. Gaebel W et al. Maintenance treatment with risperidone or low-dose haloperidol in first-episode schizophrenia: 1-year results of a randomized controlled trial within the German Research Network on Schizophrenia. J Clin Psychiatry 2007; 68:1763–1774.
19. Burns T et al. Maintenance antipsychotic medication patterns in outpatient schizophrenia patients: a naturalistic cohort study. Acta Psychiatr Scand 2006; 113:126–134.
20. Lieberman JA et al. Effectiveness of antipsychotic drugs in patients with chronic schizophrenia. N Engl J Med 2005; 353:1209–1223.
21. Haro JM et al. Three-year antipsychotic effectiveness in the outpatient care of schizophrenia: observational versus randomized studies results. Eur Neuropsychopharmacol 2007; 17:235–244.
22. Haro JM et al. Antipsychotic type and correlates of antipsychotic treatment discontinuation in the outpatient treatment of schizophrenia. Eur Psychiatry 2006; 21:41–47.
23. Leucht S et al. Epidemiology, clinical consequences, and psychosocial treatment of nonadherence in schizophrenia. J Clin Psychiatry 2006;67 Suppl 5:3–8.
24. Baldessarini RJ et al. Significance of neuroleptic dose and plasma level in the pharmacological treatment of psychoses. Arch Gen Psychiatry 1988; 45:79–90.
25. Harrington M et al. The results of a multi-centre audit of the prescribing of antipsychotic drugs for in-patients in the UK. Psychiatr Bull 2002; 26:414–418.
26. Geddes J et al. Atypical antipsychotics in the treatment of schizophrenia: systematic overview and meta-regression analysis. Br Med J 2000; 321: 1371–1376.
27. Hogarty GE et al. Dose of fluphenazine, familial expressed emotion, and outcome in schizophrenia. Results of a two-year controlled study. Arch Gen Psychiatry 1988; 45:797–805.

28. Marder SR et al. Low- and conventional-dose maintenance therapy with fluphenazine decanoate. Two-year outcome. Arch Gen Psychiatry 1987; 44: 518–521.
29. Rouillon F et al. Strategies of treatment with olanzapine in schizophrenic patients during stable phase: results of a pilot study. Eur Neuropsychopharmacol 2008; 18:646–652.
30. Wyatt RJ. Risks of withdrawing antipsychotic medications. Arch Gen Psychiatry 1995; 52:205–208.
31. Viguera AC et al. Clinical risk following abrupt and gradual withdrawal of maintenance neuroleptic treatment. Arch Gen Psychiatry 1997; 54:49–55.
32. Chouinard G et al. Withdrawal symptoms after long-term treatment with low-potency neuroleptics. J Clin Psychiatry 1984; 45:500–502.

Further reading

Bosveld-van Haandel LJM et al. Reasoning about the optimal duration of prophylactic antipsychotic medication in schizophrenia: evidence arguments. Acta Psychiatr Scand 2001; 103:335–346.
Csernansky JG et al. Relapse and rehospitalisation rates in patients with schizophrenia: effects of second generation antipsychotics. CNS Drugs 2002; 16: 473–484.
National Institute for Health and Clinical Excellence. Schizophrenia: core interventions in the treatment and management of schizophrenia in adults in primary and secondary care (update). 2009. http://www.nice.org.uk/.

Refractory schizophrenia

Clozapine – dosing regimen

Many of the adverse effects of clozapine are dose-dependent and associated with speed of titration. Adverse effects also tend to be more common at the beginning of therapy. To minimise these problems it is important to start treatment at a low dose and to increase dosage slowly.

Clozapine should normally be started at a dose of 12.5 mg once a day, at night. Blood pressure should be monitored hourly for 6 hours because of the hypotensive effect of clozapine. This monitoring is not usually necessary if the first dose is given at night. On day 2, the dose can be increased to 12.5 mg twice daily. If the patient is tolerating clozapine, the dose can be increased by 25–50 mg a day, until a dose of 300 mg a day is reached. This can usually be achieved in 2–3 weeks. Further dosage increases should be made slowly in increments of 50–100 mg each week. A plasma level of 350 µg/l should be aimed for to ensure an adequate trial, but response may occur at lower plasma levels. The average (there is substantial variation) dose at which this plasma level is reached varies according to gender and smoking status. The range is approximately 250 mg/day (female non-smoker) to 550 mg/day (male smoker)[1]. The total clozapine dose should be divided and, if sedation is a problem, the larger portion of the dose can be given at night.

The following table is a suggested starting regimen for clozapine. This is a cautious regimen – more rapid increases have been used in exceptional circumstances. Slower titration may be necessary where sedation is severe. If the patient is not tolerating a particular dose, decrease to one that was previously tolerated. If the adverse effect resolves, increase the dose again but at a slower rate. If for any reason a patient misses fewer than 2 days' clozapine, restart at the dose prescribed before the event. Do not administer extra tablets to catch up. If more than 2 days are missed, restart at 12.5 mg once daily and increase slowly (but at a faster rate than in drug-naïve patients).

Table	Suggested starting regimen for clozapine (in-patients)	
Day	*Morning dose (mg)*	*Evening dose (mg)*
1	–	12.5
2	12.5	12.5
3	25	25
4	25	25
5	25	50
6	25	50
7	50	50
8	50	75
9	75	75
10	75	100
11	100	100
12	100	125
13	125	125[a]
14	125	150
15	150	150
18	150	200[b]
21	200	200
28	200	250[c]

[a]Target dose for female non-smokers (250 mg/day)
[b]Target dose for male non-smokers (350 mg/day)
[c]Target dose for female smokers (450 mg/day)

Reference

1. Rostami-Hodjegan A et al. Influence of dose, cigarette smoking, age, sex, and metabolic activity on plasma clozapine concentrations: a predictive model and nomograms to aid clozapine dose adjustment and to assess compliance in individual patients. J Clin Psychopharmacol 2004; 24:70–78.

Optimising clozapine treatment

Using clozapine alone

Target dose (Note that dose is best adjusted according to patient tolerability)	• Average dose in UK is around 450 mg/day[1] • Response usually seen in the range 150–900 mg/day[2] • Lower doses required in the elderly, females and non-smokers, and in those prescribed certain enzyme inhibitors[3,4]
Plasma levels	• Most studies indicate that threshold for response is in the range 350–420 µg/l[5,6] Threshold may be as high as 500 µg/l[7] (see Chapter 1) • In male smokers who cannot achieve therapeutic plasma levels, metabolic inhibitors (fluvoxamine for example[8]) can be co-prescribed but extreme caution is required • Importance of norclozapine levels not established but clozapine/ norclozapine ratio may aid assessment of recent compliance

Clozapine augmentation

Clozapine 'augmentation' has become common practice because inadequate response to clozapine alone is a frequent clinical event. The evidence base supporting augmentation strategies is weak and not nearly sufficient to allow the development of any algorithm or schedule of treatment options. In practice, the result of clozapine augmentation is often disappointing and substantial changes in symptom severity are rarely observed. This clinical impression is supported by the equivocal results of many studies, which suggest a small effect size at best. Meta-analyses of antipsychotic augmentation suggest no effect[9], a small effect in long-term studies[10] or, in the largest meta-analysis, a very small effect overall[11].

It is recommended that all augmentation attempts are carefully monitored and, if no clear benefit is forthcoming, abandoned after 3–6 months. The addition of another drug to clozapine treatment might be expected to worsen overall adverse effect burden and so continued ineffective treatment is not appropriate. In some cases, the addition of an augmenting agent may reduce the severity of some adverse effects (e.g. weight gain, dyslipidaemia – see below) or allow a reduction in clozapine dose. The addition of aripiprazole to clozapine may be particularly effective in reversing metabolic effects[12].

The table below shows suggested treatment options (in alphabetical order) where 3–6 months of optimised clozapine alone has provided unsatisfactory benefit.

Table Suggested options for augmenting clozapine

Option	Comment
Add amisulpride[13–18] (400–800 mg/day)	• Some evidence and experience suggests amisulpride augmentation may be worthwhile. Only one small RCT. May allow clozapine dose reduction[19]
Add aripiprazole[12,20–24] (15–30 mg/day)	• Very limited evidence of therapeutic benefit. Improves metabolic parameters
Add haloperidol (2 mg/day)	• Modest evidence of benefit[25]
Add lamotrigine[26–28] (25–300 mg/day)	• May be useful in partial or non-responders. May reduce alcohol consumption[29]. Several negative reports[30,31] but meta-analysis suggests moderate effect size[32]
Add omega-3 triglycerides[33,34] (2–3 g EPA daily)	• Modest, and contested, evidence to support efficacy in non- or partial responders to antipsychotics, including clozapine
Add risperidone[35,36] (2–6 mg/day)	• Supported by a randomised, controlled trial but there are two negative RCTs each with minuscule response rates[37,38]. Small number of reports of increases in clozapine plasma levels
Add sulpiride[39] (400 mg/day)	• May be useful in partial or non-responders. Supported by a randomised trial

Notes:
- Always consider the use of mood-stabilisers and/or antidepressants especially where mood disturbance is thought to contribute to symptoms[40,41]
- Topiramate has also been suggested, either to augment clozapine and/or to induce weight loss. It may be effective as augmentation[42,43] but can worsen psychosis in some individuals[27,44]
- Other options include adding pimozide[45] and olanzapine[46]. Neither is recommended: pimozide has important cardiac toxicity and the addition of olanzapine is expensive and poorly supported. There is some evidence supporting ziprasidone augmentation of clozapine[47–49]. One small RCT supports the use of ginkgo biloba[50]

References

1. Taylor D et al. A prescription survey of the use of atypical antipsychotics for hospital patients in the UK. Int J Psychiatry Clin Pract 2000; 4:41–46.
2. Murphy B et al. Maintenance doses for clozapine. Psychiatr Bull 1998; 22:12–14.
3. Taylor D. Pharmacokinetic interactions involving clozapine. Br J Psychiatry 1997; 171:109–112.
4. Lane HY et al. Effects of gender and age on plasma levels of clozapine and its metabolites: analyzed by critical statistics. J Clin Psychiatry 1999; 60:36–40.
5. Taylor D et al. The use of clozapine plasma levels in optimising therapy. Psychiatr Bull 1995; 19:753–755.
6. Spina E et al. Relationship between plasma concentrations of clozapine and norclozapine and therapeutic response in patients with schizophrenia resistant to conventional neuroleptics. Psychopharmacology 2000; 148:83–89.
7. Perry PJ. Therapeutic drug monitoring of antipsychotics. Psychopharmacol Bull 2001; 35:19–29.
8. Papetti F et al. [Clozapine-resistant schizophrenia related to an increased metabolism and benefit of fluvoxamine: four case reports]. Encephale 2007; 33:811–818.
9. Barbui C et al. Does the addition of a second antipsychotic drug improve clozapine treatment? Schizophr Bull 2009; 35:458–468.
10. Paton C et al. Augmentation with a second antipsychotic in patients with schizophrenia who partially respond to clozapine: a meta-analysis. J Clin Psychopharmacol 2007; 27:198–204.
11. Taylor DM et al. Augmentation of clozapine with a second antipsychotic – a meta-analysis of randomized, placebo-controlled studies. Acta Psychiatr Scand 2009; 119:419–425.
12. Fleischhacker WW et al. Weight change on aripiprazole-clozapine combination in schizophrenic patients with weight gain and suboptimal response on clozapine: 16-week double-blind study. Eur Psychiatry 2008;23 Suppl 2:S114–S115.
13. Matthiasson P et al. Relationship between dopamine D2 receptor occupancy and clinical response in amisulpride augmentation of clozapine non-response. J Psychopharmacol 2001; 15:S41.
14. Munro J et al. Amisulpride augmentation of clozapine: an open non-randomized study in patients with schizophrenia partially responsive to clozapine. Acta Psychiatr Scand 2004; 110:292–298.
15. Zink M et al. Combination of clozapine and amisulpride in treatment-resistant schizophrenia – case reports and review of the literature. Pharmacopsychiatry 2004; 37:26–31.
16. Ziegenbein M et al. Augmentation of clozapine with amisulpride in patients with treatment-resistant schizophrenia. An open clinical study. German J Psychiatry 2006; 9:17–21.
17. Kampf P et al. Augmentation of clozapine with amisulpride: a promising therapeutic approach to refractory schizophrenic symptoms. Pharmacopsychiatry 2005; 38:39–40.
18. Assion HJ et al. Amisulpride augmentation in patients with schizophrenia partially responsive or unresponsive to clozapine. A randomized, double-blind, placebo-controlled trial. Pharmacopsychiatry 2008; 41:24–28.

19. Croissant B et al. Reduction of side-effects by combining clozapine with amisulpride: case report and short review of clozapine-induced hypersalivation – a case report. Pharmacopsychiatry 2005; 38:38–39.
20. Lim S et al. Possible increased efficacy of low-dose clozapine when combined with aripiprazole. J Clin Psychiatry 2004; 65:1284–1285.
21. Clarke LA et al. Clozapine augmentation with aripiprazole for negative symptoms. J Clin Psychiatry 2006; 67:675–676.
22. Ziegenbein M et al. Combination of clozapine and aripiprazole: a promising approach in treatment-resistant schizophrenia. Aust N Z J Psychiatry 2005; 39:840–841.
23. Henderson DC et al. An exploratory open-label trial of aripiprazole as an adjuvant to clozapine therapy in chronic schizophrenia. Acta Psychiatr Scand 2006; 113:142–147.
24. Chang JS et al. Aripiprazole augmentation in clozapine-treated patients with refractory schizophrenia: an 8-week, randomized, double-blind, placebo-controlled trial. J Clin Psychiatry 2008; 69:720–731.
25. Rajarethinam R et al. Augmentation of clozapine partial responders with conventional antipsychotics. Schizophr Res 2003; 60:97–98.
26. Dursun SM et al. Clozapine plus lamotrigine in treatment-resistant schizophrenia. Arch Gen Psychiatry 1999; 56:950.
27. Dursun SM et al. Augmenting antipsychotic treatment with lamotrigine or topiramate in patients with treatment-resistant schizophrenia: a naturalistic case-series outcome study. J Psychopharmacol 2001; 15:297–301.
28. Tiihonen J et al. Lamotrigine in treatment-resistant schizophrenia: a randomized placebo-controlled crossover trial. Biol Psychiatry 2003; 54: 1241–1248.
29. Kalyoncu A et al. Use of lamotrigine to augment clozapine in patients with resistant schizophrenia and comorbid alcohol dependence: a potent anti-craving effect? J Psychopharmacol 2005; 19:301–305.
30. Goff DC et al. Lamotrigine as add-on therapy in schizophrenia: results of 2 placebo-controlled trials. J Clin Psychopharmacol 2007; 27:582–589.
31. Heck AH et al. Addition of lamotrigine to clozapine in inpatients with chronic psychosis. J Clin Psychiatry 2005; 66:1333.
32. Tiihonen J et al. The efficacy of lamotrigine in clozapine-resistant schizophrenia: a systematic review and meta-analysis. Schizophr Res 2009; 109:10–14.
33. Peet M et al. Double-blind placebo controlled trial of N-3 polyunsaturated fatty acids as an adjunct to neuroleptics. Schizophr Res 1998; 29:160–161.
34. Puri BK et al. Sustained remission of positive and negative symptoms of schizophrenia following treatment with eicosapentaenoic acid. Arch Gen Psychiatry 1998; 55:188–189.
35. Josiassen RC et al. Clozapine augmented with risperidone in the treatment of schizophrenia: a randomized, double-blind, placebo-controlled trial. Am J Psychiatry 2005; 162:130–136.
36. Raskin S et al. Clozapine and risperidone: combination/augmentation treatment of refractory schizophrenia: a preliminary observation. Acta Psychiatr Scand 2000; 101:334–336.
37. Anil Yagcioglu AE et al. A double-blind controlled study of adjunctive treatment with risperidone in schizophrenic patients partially responsive to clozapine: efficacy and safety. J Clin Psychiatry 2005; 66:63–72.
38. Honer WG et al. Clozapine alone versus clozapine and risperidone with refractory schizophrenia. N Engl J Med 2006; 354:472–482.
39. Shiloh R et al. Sulpiride augmentation in people with schizophrenia partially responsive to clozapine. A double-blind, placebo-controlled study. Br J Psychiatry 1997; 171:569–573.
40. Citrome L. Schizophrenia and valproate. Psychopharmacol Bull 2003;37 Suppl 2:74–88.
41. Tranulis C et al. Somatic augmentation strategies in clozapine resistance – what facts? Clin Neuropharmacol 2006; 29:34–44.
42. Tiihonen J et al. Topiramate add-on in treatment-resistant schizophrenia: a randomized, double-blind, placebo-controlled, crossover trial. J Clin Psychiatry 2005; 66:1012–1015.
43. Afshar H et al. Topiramate add-on treatment in schizophrenia: a randomised double-blind, placebo-controlled clinical trial. J Psychopharmacol 2009; 23:157–162.
44. Millson RC et al. Topiramate for refractory schizophrenia. Am J Psychiatry 2002; 159:675.
45. Friedman J et al. Pimozide augmentation for the treatment of schizophrenic patients who are partial responders to clozapine. Biol Psychiatry 1997; 42:522–523.
46. Gupta S et al. Olanzapine augmentation of clozapine. Ann Clin Psychiatry 1998; 10:113–115.
47. Zink M et al. Combination of ziprasidone and clozapine in treatment-resistant schizophrenia. Hum Psychopharmacol 2004; 19:271–273.
48. Ziegenbein M et al. Clozapine and ziprasidone: a useful combination in patients with treatment-resistant schizophrenia. J Neuropsychiatry Clin Neurosci 2006; 18:246–247.
49. Ziegenbein M et al. Combination of clozapine and ziprasidone in treatment-resistant schizophrenia: an open clinical study. Clin Neuropharmacol 2005; 28:220–224.
50. Doruk A et al. A placebo-controlled study of extract of ginkgo biloba added to clozapine in patients with treatment-resistant schizophrenia. Int Clin Psychopharmacol 2008; 23:223–227.

Further reading

Correll CU et al. Antipsychotic combinations vs monotherapy in schizophrenia: a meta-analysis of randomized controlled trials. Schizophr Bull 2009; 35:443–457.

Kontaxakis VP et al. Randomized controlled augmentation trials in clozapine-resistant schizophrenic patients: a critical review. Eur Psychiatry 2005; 20:409–415.

Kontaxakis VP et al. Case studies of adjunctive agents in clozapine-resistant schizophrenic patients. Clin Neuropharmacol 2005; 28:50–53.

Mouaffak F et al. Augmentation strategies of clozapine with antipsychotics in the treatment of ultraresistant schizophrenia. Clin Neuropharmacol 2006; 29:28–33.

Remington G et al. Augmenting strategies in clozapine-resistant schizophrenia. CNS Drugs 2006; 20:171.

Refractory schizophrenia – alternatives to clozapine

Clozapine is the established treatment of choice in refractory schizophrenia. Where treatment resistence is established, clozapine treatment should not normally be delayed or withheld. The practice of using successive antipsychotics (or the latest) instead of clozapine is widespread but not supported by any cogent research. Where clozapine cannot be used (because of toxicity or patient refusal) other drugs or drug combinations may be tried (see below) but outcome is usually disappointing. Available data do not allow the drawing of any distinction between treatment regimens but it seems wise to use single drugs before trying multiple drug regimens. Many of the treatments listed below are somewhat experimental and some of the compounds difficult to obtain (e.g. glycine, D-serine). Before using any of the regimens outlined, readers should consult primary literature cited.

Table Alternatives to clozapine
(Treatments are listed in alphabetical order: no preference is implied by position in table)

Treatment	Comments
Allopurinol 300–600mg/day (+ **antipsychotic**)[1–4]	Increases adenosinergic transmission which may reduce effects of dopamine. Three positive RCTs[1,2,4]
Amisulpride[5] (up to 1200mg/day)	Single, small open study
Aripiprazole[6,7] (15–30mg/day)	Single randomized controlled study indicating moderate effect in patients resistant to risperidone or olanzapine (+ others). Higher doses (60mg/day) have been used[8]
CBT[9]	Non-drug therapies should always be considered
Celexcoxib + risperidone[10] (400mg + 6mg/day)	COX-2 inhibitors modulate immune response and may prevent glutamate-related cell death. One RCT showed useful activity in all main symptom domains
Donepezil 5–10mg/day (+ **antipsychotic**)[11–13]	Three RCTs, one negative[12], two positive[11,13], suggesting a small effect on cognitive and negative symptoms
D-alanine 100mg/kg/day (+ **antipsychotic**)[14]	Glycine (NMDA) agonist. One positive RCT
D-cycloserine 50mg/week (+ **antipsychotic**)[15]	One RCT suggests small improvement in negative symptoms
D-serine 30mg/kg/day (+ **olanzapine**)[16]	Glycine (NMDA) agonist. One positive RCT
ECT[17–20]	Open studies suggest moderate effect. Often reserved for last-line treatment in practice
Ginkgo biloba (+ **antipsychotic**)[21,22]	Possibly effective in combination with haloperidol. Unlikely to give rise to additional adverse effects but clinical experience limited
Mianserin + FGA 30mg/day[23]	$5HT_2$ antagonist. One, small positive RCT
Mirtazapine 30mg/day (+ **antipsychotic**)[24–26]	$5HT_2$ antagonist. Two RCTs, one negative[25], one positive[24]. Effect seems to be mainly on positive symptoms
N-acetylcysteine 2g/day (+ **antipsychotic**)[27]	One RCT suggests small benefits in negative symptoms and rates of akathisia

Table Alternatives to clozapine (Cont.)

Treatment	Comments
Olanzapine[28–33] 5–25mg/day	Supported by some well conducted trials but clinical experience disappointing. Some patients show moderate response
Olanzapine[34–40] 30–60mg/day	Contradictory findings in the literature but possibly effective. Expensive and unlicensed. High dose olanzapine is not atypical[41] and can be poorly tolerated[42] with gross metabolic changes[40]
Olanzapine + amisulpride[43] (up to 800mg/day)	Small open study suggests benefit
Olanzapine + aripiprazole[44]	Single case report suggests benefit
Olanzapine + glycine[45] (0.8g/kg/day)	Small, double-blind crossover trial suggests clinically relevant improvement in negative symptoms
Olanzapine + lamotrigine[46,47] (up to 400mg/day)	Reports contradictory and rather unconvincing. Reasonable theoretical basis for adding lamotrigine which is usually well tolerated
Olanzapine + risperidone[48] (various doses)	Small study suggests some patients may benefit from combined therapy after sequential failure of each drug alone
Olanzapine + sulpiride[49] (600mg/day)	Some evidence that this combination improves mood symptoms
Omega-3-triglycerides[50,51]	Suggested efficacy but data very limited
Ondansetron 8mg/day (+ antipsychotic)[52,53]	Two positive RCTs suggesting some effect on negative symptoms
Propentofylline + risperidone[54] (900mg + 6mg/day)	One RCT suggests some activity against postive symptoms
Quetiapine[55–58]	Very limited evidence and clinical experience not encouraging. High doses (>1200mg/day) have been used
Quetiapine + haloperidol[59]	Two case reports
Risperidone[60–62] 4–8mg/day	Doubtful efficacy in true treatment-refractory schziophrenia but some supporting evidence. May also be tried in combination with glycine[45] or lamotrigine[46] or indeed with other atypicals[63]
Ritanserin + risperidone (12mg + 6mg/day)[64]	$5HT_{2A/2C}$ antagonist. One RCT suggests small effect on negative symptoms
Sarcosine (2g/day)[65,66] (+ antipsychotic)	Enhances glycine action. Supported by two RCTs
Topiramate (300mg/day) (+ antipsychotic)[67]	Small effect shown in single RCT
Transcranial magnetic stimulation[68,69]	Probably not effective
Valproate[70]	Doubtful effect but may be useful where there is a clear affective component
Ziprasidone 80–160mg/day[71–73]	Two good RCTs. One[73] suggests superior efficacy to chlorpromazine in refractory schziophrenia, the other[71] suggests equivalence to clozapine in subjects with treatment intolerance/resistance

References

1. Akhondzadeh S et al. Beneficial antipsychotic effects of allopurinol as add-on therapy for schizophrenia: a double blind, randomized and placebo controlled trial. Prog Neuropsychopharmacol Biol Psychiatry 2005; 29:253–259.
2. Brunstein MG et al. A clinical trial of adjuvant allopurinol therapy for moderately refractory schizophrenia. J Clin Psychiatry 2005; 66:213–219.
3. Buie LW et al. Allopurinol as Adjuvant Therapy in Poorly Responsive or Treatment Refractory Schizophrenia (December). Ann Pharmacother 2006.
4. Dickerson FB et al. A double-blind trial of adjunctive allopurinol for schizophrenia. Schizophr Res 2009; 109:66–69.
5. Kontaxakis VP et al. Switching to amisulpride monotherapy for treatment-resistant schizophrenia. Eur Psychiatry 2006; 21: 214–217.
6. Kungel M et al. Efficacy and tolerability of aripiprazole compared to perphenazine in treatment-resistant schizophrenia. Pharmacopsychiatry 2003; 36:165.
7. Hsu WY et al. Aripiprazole in treatment-refractory schizophrenia. J Psychiatr Pract 2009; 15:221–226.
8. Crossman AM et al. Tolerability of high-dose aripiprazole in treatment-refractory schizophrenic patients. J Clin Psychiatry 2006; 67:1158–1159.
9. Valmaggia LR et al. Cognitive-behavioural therapy for refractory psychotic symptoms of schizophrenia resistant to atypical antipsychotic medication. Randomised controlled trial. Br J Psychiatry 2005; 186:324–330.
10. Akhondzadeh S et al. Celecoxib as adjunctive therapy in schizophrenia: a double-blind, randomized and placebo-controlled trial. Schizophr Res 2007; 90:179–185.
11. Lee BJ et al. A 12-week, double-blind, placebo-controlled trial of donepezil as an adjunct to haloperidol for treating cognitive impairments in patients with chronic schizophrenia. J Psychopharmacol 2007; 21:421–427.
12. Keefe RSE et al. Efficacy and safety of donepezil in patients with schizophrenia or schizoaffective disorder: significant placebo/practice effects in a 12-week, randomized, double-blind, placebo-controlled trial. Neuropsychopharmacology 2007; 33:1217–1228.
13. Akhondzadeh S et al. A 12-week, double-blind, placebo-controlled trial of donepezil adjunctive treatment to risperidone in chronic and stable schizophrenia. Prog Neuropsychopharmacol Biol Psychiatry 2008; 32:1810–1815.
14. Tsai GE et al. D-alanine added to antipsychotics for the treatment of schizophrenia. Biol Psychiatry 2006; 59:230–234.
15. Goff DC et al. Once-weekly D-cycloserine effects on negative symptoms and cognition in schizophrenia: an exploratory study. Schizophr Res 2008; 106:320–327.
16. Heresco-Levy U et al. D-serine efficacy as add-on pharmacotherapy to risperidone and olanzapine for treatment-refractory schizophrenia. Biol Psychiatry 2005; 57:577–585.
17. Chanpattana W et al. Combined ECT and neuroleptic therapy in treatment-refractory schizophrenia: prediction of outcome. Psychiatry Res 2001; 105:107–115.
18. Tang WK et al. Efficacy of electroconvulsive therapy in treatment-resistant schizophrenia: a prospective open trial. Prog Neuropsychopharmacol Biol Psychiatry 2003; 27:373–379.
19. Chanpattana W et al. Acute and maintenance ECT with flupenthixol in refractory schizophrenia: sustained improvements in psychopathology, quality of life, and social outcomes. Schizophr Res 2003; 63:189–193.
20. Chanpattana W et al. ECT for treatment-resistant schizophrenia: a response from the far East to the UK. NICE report. J ECT 2006; 22:4–12.
21. Zhou D et al. The effects of classic antipsychotic haloperidol plus the extract of ginkgo biloba on superoxide dismutase in patients with chronic refractory schizophrenia. Chin Med J 1999; 112:1093–1096.
22. Zhang XY et al. A double-blind, placebo-controlled trial of extract of Ginkgo biloba added to haloperidol in treatment-resistant patients with schizophrenia. J Clin Psychiatry 2001; 62:878–883.
23. Shiloh R et al. Mianserin or placebo as adjuncts to typical antipsychotics in resistant schizophrenia. Int Clin Psychopharmacol 2002; 17:59–64.
24. Joffe G et al. Add-on mirtazapine enhances antipsychotic effect of first generation antipsychotics in schizophrenia: A double-blind, randomized, placebo-controlled trial. Schizophr Res 2009; 108:245–251.
25. Berk M et al. Mirtazapine add-on therapy in the treatment of schizophrenia with atypical antipsychotics: a double-blind, randomised, placebo-controlled clinical trial. Hum Psychopharmacol 2009; 24:233–238.
26. Delle CR et al. Add-on mirtazapine enhances effects on cognition in schizophrenic patients under stabilized treatment with clozapine. Exp Clin Psychopharmacol 2007; 15:563–568.
27. Berk M et al. N-acetyl cysteine as a glutathione precursor for schizophrenia--a double-blind, randomized, placebo-controlled trial. Biol Psychiatry 2008; 64:361–368.
28. Breier A et al. Comparative efficacy of olanzapine and haloperidol for patients with treatment-resistant schizophrenia. Biol Psychiatry 1999; 45: 403–411.
29. Conley RR et al. Olanzapine compared with chlorpromazine in treatment-resistant schizophrenia. Am J Psychiatry 1998; 155:914–920.
30. Sanders RD et al. An open trial of olanzapine in patients with treatment-refractory psychoses. J Clin Psychopharmacol 1999; 19:62–66.
31. Taylor D et al. Olanzapine in practice: a prospective naturalistic study. Psychiatr Bull 1999; 23:178–180.
32. Bitter I et al. Olanzapine versus clozapine in treatment-resistant or treatment-intolerant schizophrenia. Prog Neuropsychopharmacol Biol Psychiatry 2004; 28:173–180.
33. Tollefson GD et al. Double-blind comparison of olanzapine versus clozapine in schizophrenic patients clinically eligible for treatment with clozapine. Biol Psychiatry 2001; 49:52–63.
34. Sheitman BB et al. High-dose olanzapine for treatment-refractory schizophrenia. Am J Psychiatry 1997; 154:1626.
35. Fanous A et al. Schizophrenia and schizoaffective disorder treated with high doses of olanzapine. J Clin Psychopharmacol 1999; 19:275–276.
36. Dursun SM et al. Olanzapine for patients with treatment-resistant schizophrenia: a naturalistic case-series outcome study. Can J Psychiatry 1999; 44: 701–704.
37. Conley RR et al. The efficacy of high-dose olanzapine versus clozapine in treatment-resistant schizophrenia: a double-blind crossover study. J Clin Psychopharmacol 2003; 23:668–671.
38. Kumra S et al. Clozapine and "high-dose" olanzapine in refractory early-onset schizophrenia: a 12-week randomized and double-blind comparison. Biol Psychiatry 2008; 63:524–529.
39. Kumra S et al. Clozapine versus "high-dose" olanzapine in refractory early-onset schizophrenia: an open-label extension study. J Child Adolesc Psychopharmacol 2008; 18:307–316.
40. Meltzer HY et al. A randomized, double-blind comparison of clozapine and high-dose olanzapine in treatment-resistant patients with schizophrenia. J Clin Psychiatry 2008; 69:274–285.
41. Bronson BD et al. Adverse effects of high-dose olanzapine in treatment-refractory schizophrenia. J Clin Psychopharmacol 2000; 20:382–384.
42. Kelly DL et al. Adverse effects and laboratory parameters of high-dose olanzapine vs. clozapine in treatment-resistant schizophrenia. Ann Clin Psychiatry 2003; 15:181–186.
43. Zink M et al. Combination of amisulpride and olanzapine in treatment-resistant schizophrenic psychoses. Eur Psychiatry 2004; 19:56–58.
44. Duggal HS. Aripirazole-olanzapine combination for treatment of schizophrenia. Can J Psychiatry 2004; 49:151.
45. Heresco-Levy U et al. High-dose glycine added to olanzapine and risperidone for the treatment of schizophrenia. Biol Psychiatry 2004; 55:165–171.
46. Kremer I et al. Placebo-controlled trial of lamotrigine added to conventional and atypical antipsychotics in schizophrenia. Biol Psychiatry 2004; 56: 441–446.
47. Dursun SM et al. Augmenting antipsychotic treatment with lamotrigine or topiramate in patients with treatment-resistant schizophrenia: a naturalistic case-series outcome study. J Psychopharmacol 2001; 15:297–301.

48. Suzuki T et al. Effectiveness of antipsychotic polypharmacy for patients with treatment refractory schizophrenia: an open-label trial of olanzapine plus risperidone for those who failed to respond to a sequential treatment with olanzapine, quetiapine and risperidone. Hum Psychopharmacol 2008; 23: 455–463.
49. Kotler M et al. Sulpiride augmentation of olanzapine in the management of treatment-resistant chronic schizophrenia: evidence for improvement of mood symptomatology. Int Clin Psychopharmacol 2004; 19:23–26.
50. Mellor JE et al. Omega-3 fatty acid supplementation in schizophrenic patients. Hum Psychopharmacol 1996; 11:39–46.
51. Puri BK et al. Sustained remission of positive and negative symptoms of schizophrenia following treatment with eicosapentaenoic acid. Arch Gen Psychiatry 1998; 55:188–189.
52. Zhang ZJ et al. Beneficial effects of ondansetron as an adjunct to haloperidol for chronic, treatment-resistant schizophrenia: a double-blind, randomized, placebo-controlled study. Schizophr Res 2006; 88:102–110.
53. Akhondzadeh S et al. Added ondansetron for stable schizophrenia: A double blind, placebo controlled trial. Schizophr Res 2009; 107:206–212.
54. Salimi S et al. A placebo controlled study of the propentofylline added to risperidone in chronic schizophrenia. Prog Neuropsychopharmacol Biol Psychiatry 2008; 32:726–732.
55. Reznik I et al. Long-term efficacy and safety of quetiapine in treatment-refractory schizophrenia: A case report. Int J Psychiatry Clin Pract 2000; 4:77–80.
56. De Nayer A et al. Efficacy and tolerability of quetiapine in patients with schizophrenia switched from other antipsychotics. Int J Psychiatry Clin Pract 2003; 7:66.
57. Larmo I et al. Efficacy and tolerability of quetiapine in patients with schizophrenia who switched from haloperidol, olanzapine or risperidone. Hum Psychopharmacol 2005; 20:573–581.
58. Boggs DL et al. Quetiapine at high doses for the treatment of refractory schizophrenia. Schizophr Res 2008; 101:347–348.
59. Aziz MA et al. Remission of positive and negative symptoms in refractory schizophrenia with a combination of haloperidol and quetiapine: Two case studies. J Psychiatr Pract 2006; 12:332–336.
60. Breier AF et al. Clozapine and risperidone in chronic schizophrenia: effects on symptoms, parkinsonian side effects, and neuroendocrine response. Am J Psychiatry 1999; 156:294–298.
61. Bondolfi G et al. Risperidone versus clozapine in treatment-resistant chronic schizophrenia: a randomized double-blind study. The Risperidone Study Group. Am J Psychiatry 1998; 155:499–504.
62. Conley RR et al. Risperidone, quetiapine, and fluphenazine in the treatment of patients with therapy-refractory schizophrenia. Clin Neuropharmacol 2005; 28:163–168.
63. Lerner V et al. Combination of "atypical" antipsychotic medication in the management of treatment-resistant schizophrenia and schizoaffective disorder. Prog Neuropsychopharmacol Biol Psychiatry 2004; 28:89–98.
64. Akhondzadeh S et al. Effect of ritanserin, a 5HT2A/2C antagonist, on negative symptoms of schizophrenia: a double-blind randomized placebo-controlled study. Prog Neuropsychopharmacol Biol Psychiatry 2008; 32:1879–1883.
65. Lane HY et al. Sarcosine or D-serine add-on treatment for acute exacerbation of schizophrenia: a randomized, double-blind, placebo-controlled study. Arch Gen Psychiatry 2005; 62:1196–1204.
66. Tsai G et al. Glycine transporter I inhibitor, N-methylglycine (sarcosine), added to antipsychotics for the treatment of schizophrenia. Biol Psychiatry 2004; 55:452–456.
67. Tiihonen J et al. Topiramate add-on in treatment-resistant schizophrenia: a randomized, double-blind, placebo-controlled, crossover trial. J Clin Psychiatry 2005; 66:1012–1015.
68. Franck N et al. Left temporoparietal transcranial magnetic stimulation in treatment-resistant schizophrenia with verbal hallucinations. Psychiatry Res 2003; 120:107–109.
69. Fitzgerald PB et al. A double-blind sham-controlled trial of repetitive transcranial magnetic stimulation in the treatment of refractory auditory hallucinations. J Clin Psychopharmacol 2005; 25:358–362.
70. Basan A et al. Valproate as an adjunct to antipsychotics for schizophrenia: a systematic review of randomized trials. Schizophr Res 2004; 70:33–37.
71. Sacchetti E et al. Ziprasidone vs clozapine in schizophrenia patients refractory to multiple antipsychotic treatments: the MOZART study. Schizophr Res 2009; 110:80–89.
72. Loebel AD et al. Ziprasidone in treatment-resistant schizophrenia: a 52-week, open-label continuation study. J Clin Psychiatry 2007; 68:1333–1338.
73. Kane JM et al. Efficacy and tolerability of ziprasidone in patients with treatment-resistant schizophrenia. Int Clin Psychopharmacol 2006; 21:21–28.

Schizophrenia

Further reading

Henderson DC et al. Switching from clozapine to olanzapine in treatment-refractory schizophrenia: safety, clinical efficacy, and predictors of response. J Clin Psychiatry 1998; 59: 585–588.
Lindenmayer JP et al. Olanzapine in refractory schizophrenia after failure of typical or atypical antipsychotic treatment: an open-label switch study. J Clin Psychiatry 2002; 63: 931–935.
Still DJ et al. Effects of switching inpatients with treatment-resistant schizophrenia from clozapine to risperidone. Psychiatr Serv 1996; 47: 1382–1384.

Clozapine – management of common adverse effects

Clozapine has a wide range of adverse effects many of which are serious or potentially life-threatening. The table below describes some more common adverse effects; tables on the following pages deal with rare and serious events.

Table

Adverse effect	Time course	Action
Sedation	First few months. May persist, but usually wears off	Give smaller dose in the morning. Reduce dose if necessary – check plasma level
Hypersalivation	First few months. May persist, but sometimes wears off. Often very troublesome at night	Give hyoscine 300 µg (Kwells) sucked and swallowed at night. Pirenzepine[1] (not licensed in the UK) up to 100 mg/day can be tried (see section on hypersalivation)
Constipation	Usually persists	Recommend high-fibre diet. Bulk-forming laxatives and stimulants should be used. Effective treatment or prevention of constipation is essential as death may result[2–5]
Hypotension	First 4 weeks	Advise patient to take time when standing up. Reduce dose or slow down rate of increase. If severe, consider moclobemide and Bovril[6], or fludrocortisone
Hypertension	First 4 weeks, sometimes longer	Monitor closely and increase dose as slowly as is necessary. Hypotensive therapy (e.g. atenolol 25 mg/day) is sometimes necessary[7]
Tachycardia	First 4 weeks, but sometimes persists	Very common in early stages of treatment but usually benign. Tachycardia, if persistent at rest and associated with fever, hypotension or chest pain, may indicate myocarditis[8,9] (see section on serious adverse effects of clozapine). Referral to a cardiologist is advised. Clozapine should be stopped if tachycardia occurs in the context of chest pain or heart failure. Benign sinus tachycardia can be treated with atenolol
Weight gain	Usually during the first year of treatment	Dietary counselling is essential. Advice may be more effective if given before weight gain occurs. Weight gain is common and often profound (>10 lb)
Fever	First 3 weeks	Clozapine induces inflammatory response (increased C-reactive protein and interleukin-6)[10,11]. Give antipyretic but check FBC. Reduce rate of dose titration[12]. This fever is not usually related to blood dyscrasias[13,14] but beware myocarditis (see following section)
Seizures	May occur at any time[15]	Dose-/dose increase-related. Consider prophylactic valproate* if on high dose or with high plasma level (500 µg/l +). After a seizure: withhold clozapine for one day; restart at reduced dose; give sodium valproate. EEG abnormalities are common in those on clozapine[16]
Nausea	First 6 weeks	May give anti-emetic. Avoid prochlorperazine and metoclopramide if previous EPSEs

Table   (Cont.)

Adverse effect	Time course	Action
Nocturnal enuresis	May occur at any time	Try manipulating dose schedule. Avoid fluids before bedtime. May resolve spontaneously[17], but may persist for months or years[18]. In severe cases, desmopressin is usually effective[19] but is not without risk: hyponatraemia may result[20]. Anticholinergic agents may be effective[21] but support for this approach is weak
Neutropenia/ agranulocytosis	First 18 weeks (but may occur at any time)	Stop clozapine; admit to hospital if agranulocytosis confirmed

*Usual dose is 1000–2000 mg/day. Plasma levels may be useful as a rough guide to dosing – aim for 50–100 mg/l. Use of modified-release preparation (Epilim Chrono) may aid compliance: can be given once-daily and may be better tolerated

References

1. Fritze J et al. Pirenzepine for clozapine-induced hypersalivation. Lancet 1995; 346:1034.
2. Townsend G et al. Case report: rapidly fatal bowel ischaemia on clozapine treatment. BMC Psychiatry 2006; 6:43.
3. Rege S et al. Life-threatening constipation associated with clozapine. Australas Psychiatry 2008; 16:216–219.
4. Leung JS et al. Rapidly fatal clozapine-induced intestinal obstruction without prior warning signs. Aust N Z J Psychiatry 2008; 42:1073–1074.
5. Palmer SE et al. Life-threatening clozapine-induced gastrointestinal hypomotility: an analysis of 102 cases. J Clin Psychiatry 2008; 69:759–768.
6. Taylor D et al. Clozapine-induced hypotension treated with moclobemide and Bovril. Br J Psychiatry 1995; 167:409–410.
7. Henderson DC et al. Clozapine and hypertension: a chart review of 82 patients. J Clin Psychiatry 2004; 65:686–689.
8. Committee on Safety of Medicines. Clozapine and cardiac safety: updated advice for prescribers. Curr Prob Pharmacovigilance 2002; 28:8.
9. Hagg S et al. Myocarditis related to clozapine treatment. J Clin Psychopharmacol 2001; 21:382–388.
10. Kohen I et al. Increases in C-reactive protein may predict recurrence of clozapine-induced fever. Ann Pharmacother 2009; 43:143–146.
11. Kluge M et al. Effects of clozapine and olanzapine on cytokine systems are closely linked to weight gain and drug-induced fever. Psychoneuroendocrinology 2009; 34:118–128.
12. Pui-yin CJ et al. The incidence and characteristics of clozapine- induced fever in a local psychiatric unit in Hong Kong. Can J Psychiatry 2008; 53:857–862.
13. Tham JC et al. Clozapine-induced fevers and 1-year clozapine discontinuation rate. J Clin Psychiatry 2002; 63:880–884.
14. Tremeau F et al. Spiking fevers with clozapine treatment. Clin Neuropharmacol 1997; 20:168–170.
15. Pacia SV et al. Clozapine-related seizures: experience with 5,629 patients. Neurology 1994; 44:2247–2249.
16. Centorrino F et al. EEG abnormalities during treatment with typical and atypical antipsychotics. Am J Psychiatry 2002; 159:109–115.
17. Warner JP et al. Clozapine and urinary incontinence. Int Clin Psychopharmacol 1994; 9:207–209.
18. Jeong SH et al. A 2-year prospective follow-up study of lower urinary tract symptoms in patients treated with clozapine. J Clin Psychopharmacol 2008; 28:618–624.
19. Steingard S. Use of desmopressin to treat clozapine-induced nocturnal enuresis. J Clin Psychiatry 1994; 55:315–316.
20. Sarma S et al. Severe hyponatraemia associated with desmopressin nasal spray to treat clozapine-induced nocturnal enuresis. Aust N Z J Psychiatry 2005; 39:949.
21. Praharaj SK et al. Amitriptyline for clozapine-induced nocturnal enuresis and sialorrhoea. Br J Clin Pharmacol 2007; 63:128–129.

Further reading

Iqbal MM et al. Clozapine: a clinical review of adverse effects and management. Ann Clin Psychiatry 2003; 15:33–48.
Lieberman JA. Maximizing clozapine therapy: managing side-effects. J Clin Psychiatry 1998;59 (Suppl. 3):38–43.

Clozapine – uncommon or unusual adverse effects

Pharmacoepidemiological monitoring of clozapine is more extensive than with any other drug. Awareness of adverse effects related to clozapine treatment is therefore enhanced. The table below gives brief details of unusual or uncommon adverse effects of clozapine reported since its relaunch in 1990.

Table	
Adverse effect	*Comment*
Agranulocytosis/ neutropenia (delayed)[1-3]	Occasional reports of apparent clozapine-related blood dyscrasia even after 1 year of treatment
Colitis[4,5]	A few reports in the literature, but clear causative link to clozapine in one case. Any severe or chronic diarrhoea should prompt specialist referral
Delirium[6,7]	Reported to be fairly common, but rarely seen in practice if dose is titrated slowly and plasma level determinations are used
Eosinophilia[8,9]	Reasonably common but significance unclear. Some suggestion that eosinophilia predicts neutropenia but this is disputed. May be associated with colitis and related symptoms[5]
Heat stroke[10]	Occasional case reported. May be mistaken for NMS
Hepatic failure/enzyme abnormalities[11,12]	Benign changes in LFTs are common (up to 50% of patients) but worth monitoring because of the very small risk of fulminant hepatic failure. Rash may be associated with clozapine-related hepatitis[13]
Ocular pigmentation[14]	Single case report
Pancreatitis[15]	Rare reports of asymptomatic and symptomatic pancreatitis sometimes associated with eosinophilia. Some authors recommend monitoring serum amylase in all patients treated with clozapine
Pericardial effusion[16,17]	Several reports in the literature. Symptoms include fatigue, dyspnoea and tachycardia. Use echocardiogram to confirm/rule out effusion
Pneumonia[18,19]	Very rarely results from saliva aspiration. Some cases of fatal pneumonia reported. Infections in general may be more common in those on clozapine[20]. Note that respiratory infections may give rise to elevated clozapine levels[21,22]. (Possibly an artefact: smoking usually ceases during an infection)
Thrombocytopenia[23]	Few data but apparently fairly common. Probably transient and clinically unimportant
Vasculitis[24]	One report in the literature in which patient developed confluent erythematous rash on lower limbs

References

1. Thompson A et al. Late onset neutropenia with clozapine. Can J Psychiatry 2004; 49:647–648.
2. Bhanji NH et al. Late-onset agranulocytosis in a patient with schizophrenia after 17 months of clozapine treatment. J Clin Psychopharmacol 2003; 23:522–523.
3. Sedky K et al. Clozapine-induced agranulocytosis after 11 years of treatment (Letter). Am J Psychiatry 2005; 162:814.
4. Hawe R et al. Response to clozapine-induced microscopic colitis: a case report and review of the literature. J Clin Psychopharmacol 2008; 28:454–455.
5. Karmacharya R et al. Clozapine-Induced Eosinophilic Colitis (Letter). Am J Psychiatry 2005; 162:1386–1388.
6. Centorrino F et al. Delirium during clozapine treatment: incidence and associated risk factors. Pharmacopsychiatry 2003; 36:156–160.
7. Shankar BR. Clozapine-induced delirium. J Neuropsychiatry Clin Neurosci 2008; 20:239–240.
8. Hummer M et al. Does eosinophilia predict clozapine induced neutropenia? Psychopharmacology 1996; 124:201–204.
9. Ames D et al. Predictive value of eosinophilia for neutropenia during clozapine treatment. J Clin Psychiatry 1996; 57:579–581.
10. Kerwin RW et al. Heat stroke in schizophrenia during clozapine treatment: rapid recognition and management. J Psychopharmacol 2004; 18:121–123.
11. Erdogan A et al. Management of marked liver enzyme increase during clozapine treatment: a case report and review of the literature. Int J Psychiatry Med 2004; 34:83–89.
12. Macfarlane B et al. Fatal acute fulminant liver failure due to clozapine: a case report and review of clozapine-induced hepatotoxicity. Gastroenterology 1997; 112:1707–1709.
13. Fong SY et al. Clozapine-induced toxic hepatitis with skin rash. J Psychopharmacol 2005; 19:107.
14. Borovik AM et al. Ocular pigmentation associated with clozapine. Med J Aust 2009; 190:210–211.
15. Bergemann N et al. Asymptomatic pancreatitis associated with clozapine. Pharmacopsychiatry 1999; 32:78–80.
16. Raju P et al. Pericardial effusion in patients with schizophrenia: are they on clozapine? Emerg Med J 2008; 25:383–384.
17. Dauner DG et al. Clozapine-induced pericardial effusion. J Clin Psychopharmacol 2008; 28:455–456.
18. Hinkes R et al. Aspiration pneumonia possibly secondary to clozapine-induced sialorrhea. J Clin Psychopharmacol 1996; 16:462–463.
19. Taylor DM et al. Reasons for discontinuing clozapine: matched, case-control comparison with risperidone long-acting injection. Br J Psychiatry 2009; 194:165–167.
20. Landry P et al. Increased use of antibiotics in clozapine-treated patients. Int Clin Psychopharmacol 2003; 18:297–298.
21. Raaska K et al. Bacterial pneumonia can increase serum concentration of clozapine. Eur J Clin Pharmacol 2002; 58:321–322.
22. de Leon J et al. Serious respiratory infections can increase clozapine levels and contribute to side-effects: a case report. Prog Neuropsychopharmacol Biol Psychiatry 2003; 27:1059–1063.
23. Jagadheesan K et al. Clozapine-induced thrombocytopenia: a pilot study. Hong Kong J Psychiatry 2003; 13:12–15.
24. Penaskovic KM et al. Clozapine-induced allergic vasculitis (Letter). Am J Psychiatry 2005; 162:1543–1542.

Schizophrenia

65

Clozapine – serious haematological and cardiovascular adverse effects

Agranulocytosis, thromboembolism, cardiomyopathy and myocarditis

Clozapine is a somewhat toxic drug, but it may reduce overall mortality in schizophrenia, largely because of a reduction in the rate of suicide[1–3]. Clozapine can cause serious, life-threatening adverse effects, of which agranulocytosis is the best known. In the UK, the risk of death from agranulocytosis is probably less than 1 in 10 000 patients exposed (Novartis report 4 deaths from 47 000 exposed)[4]. Risk is well managed by the approved clozapine-monitoring systems.

A possible association between clozapine and thromboembolism has been suggested[5]. Initially, Walker et al[1] uncovered a risk of fatal pulmonary embolism of 1 in 4500 – about 20 times the risk in the population as a whole. Following a case report of non-fatal pulmonary embolism possibly related to clozapine[6], data from the Swedish authorities were published[7]. Twelve cases of venous thromboembolism were described, of which five were fatal. The risk of thromboembolism was estimated to be 1 in 2000 to 1 in 6000 patients treated. Thromboembolism may be related to clozapine's observed effects on antiphospholipid antibodies[8] and platelet aggregation[9]. It seems most likely to occur in the first 3 months of treatment but can occur at any time. Other antipsychotics are also strongly linked to thromboembolism[10–16].

With all drugs, the causes of thromboembolism are probably multifactorial[11]. Encouraging exercise and ensuring good hydration are essential precautionary measures[17].

It has also been suggested that clozapine is associated with myocarditis and cardiomyopathy. Australian data initially identified 23 cases (15 myocarditis, 8 cardiomyopathy), of which 6 were fatal[18]. Risk of death from either cause was estimated from these data to be 1 in 1300. Similar findings were reported in New Zealand[19]. Myocarditis seems to occur within 6–8 weeks of starting clozapine (median 3 weeks[20]); cardiomyopathy may occur later in treatment (median 9 months[20]) but both may occur at any time. It is notable that other data sources give rather different risk estimates: in Canada the risk of fatal myocarditis was estimated to be 1 in 12 500; in the USA, 1 in 67 000[21]. Conversely, another Australian study identified nine cases of possible (non-fatal) myocarditis in 94 patients treated[22]. The most recent Australian study estimated the risk of myocarditis to be around 1% of those treated (in whom 1 in 10 died)[23].

Despite this uncertainty over incidence, patients should be closely monitored for signs of myocarditis especially in the first few months of treatment[24]. Symptoms include tachycardia, fever, flu-like symptoms, fatigue, dyspnoea and chest pain[25]. Signs include ECG changes (ST depression), enlarged heart on radiography/echo and eosinophilia. Many of these symptoms occur in patients on clozapine not developing myocarditis[26]. Nonetheless, signs of heart failure should provoke immediate cessation of clozapine. Rechallenge has been successfully completed[22] (the use of beta-blockers and ACE inhibitors may help[27,28]) but recurrence is possible[29,30]. Cardiomyopathy should be suspected in any patient showing signs of heart failure, which should provoke immediate cessation of clozapine and referral. Presentation of cardiomyopathy varies somewhat[31,32] so any reported symptoms of palpitations, sweating and breathing difficulties should be closely investigated.

Note also that, despite an overall reduction in mortality, younger patients may have an increased risk of sudden death[33], perhaps because of clozapine-induced ECG changes[34]. The overall picture remains very unclear but caution is required. There may, of course, be similar problems with other antipsychotics[35–37].

Summary

- Overall mortality may be lower for those on clozapine than in schizophrenia as a whole
- Risk of fatal agranulocytosis is less than 1 in 5000 patients treated in the UK
- Risk of fatal pulmonary embolism is estimated to be around 1 in 4500 patients treated
- Risk of fatal myocarditis or cardiomyopathy may be as high as 1 in 1000 patients
- Careful monitoring is essential during clozapine treatment, particularly during the first 3 months

References

1. Walker AM et al. Mortality in current and former users of clozapine. Epidemiology 1997; 8:671–677.
2. Munro J et al. Active monitoring of 12760 clozapine recipients in the UK and Ireland. Br J Psychiatry 1999; 175:576–580.
3. Tiihonen J et al. 11-year follow-up of mortality in patients with schizophrenia: a population-based cohort study (FIN11 study). Lancet 2009; Epub ahead of print-DOI:10.1016/SO140–6736(09)60742-X.
4. Thuillier S. Clozapine and agranulocytosis. 2006. (Personal Communication.)
5. Paciullo CA. Evaluating the association between clozapine and venous thromboembolism. Am J Health Syst Pharm 2008; 65:1825–1829.
6. Lacika S et al. Pulmonary embolus possibly associated with clozapine treatment (Letter). Can J Psychiatry 1999; 44:396–397.
7. Hagg S et al. Association of venous thromboembolism and clozapine. Lancet 2000; 355:1155–1156.
8. Davis S et al. Antiphospholipid antibodies associated with clozapine treatment. Am J Hematol 1994; 46:166–167.
9. Axelsson S et al. In vitro effects of antipsychotics on human platelet adhesion and aggregation and plasma coagulation. Clin Exp Pharmacol Physiol 2007; 34:775–780.
10. Liperoti R et al. Venous thromboembolism among elderly patients treated with atypical and conventional antipsychotic agents. Arch Intern Med 2005; 165:2677–2682.
11. Lacut K. Association between antipsychotic drugs, antidepressant drugs, and venous thromboembolism. Clin Adv Hematol Oncol 2008; 6:887–890.
12. Borras L et al. Pulmonary thromboembolism associated with olanzapine and risperidone. J Emerg Med 2008; 35:159–161.
13. Maly R et al. Four cases of venous thromboembolism associated with olanzapine. Psychiatry Clin Neurosci 2009; 63:116–118.
14. Hagg S et al. Associations between venous thromboembolism and antipsychotics. A study of the WHO database of adverse drug reactions. Drug Saf 2008; 31:685–694.
15. Lacut K et al. Association between antipsychotic drugs, antidepressant drugs and venous thromboembolism: results from the EDITH case-control study. Fundam Clin Pharmacol 2007; 21:643–650.
16. Zink M et al. A case of pulmonary thromboembolism and rhabdomyolysis during therapy with mirtazapine and risperidone. J Clin Psychiatry 2006; 67:835.
17. Maly R et al. Assessment of risk of venous thromboembolism and its possible prevention in psychiatric patients. Psychiatry Clin Neurosci 2008; 62:3–8.
18. Killian JG et al. Myocarditis and cardiomyopathy associated with clozapine. Lancet 1999; 354:1841–1845.
19. Hill GR et al. Clozapine and myocarditis: a case series from the New Zealand Intensive Medicines Monitoring Programme. N Z Med J 2008; 121:68–75.
20. La Grenade L et al. Myocarditis and cardiomyopathy associated with clozapine use in the United States (Letter). N Engl J Med 2001; 345:224–225.
21. Warner B et al. Clozapine and sudden death. Lancet 2000; 355:842.
22. Reinders J et al. Clozapine-related myocarditis and cardiomyopathy in an Australian metropolitan psychiatric service. Aust N Z J Psychiatry 2004; 38:915–922.
23. Haas SJ et al. Clozapine-associated myocarditis: a review of 116 cases of suspected myocarditis associated with the use of clozapine in Australia during 1993–2003. Drug Saf 2007; 30:47–57.
24. Marder SR et al. Physical health monitoring of patients with schizophrenia. Am J Psychiatry 2004; 161:1334–1349.
25. Annamraju S et al. Early recognition of clozapine-induced myocarditis. J Clin Psychopharmacol 2007; 27:479–483.
26. Wehmeier PM et al. Chart review for potential features of myocarditis, pericarditis, and cardiomyopathy in children and adolescents treated with clozapine. J Child Adolesc Psychopharmacol 2004; 14:267–271.
27. Rostagno C et al. Beta-blocker and angiotensin-converting enzyme inhibitor may limit certain cardiac adverse effects of clozapine. Gen Hosp Psychiatry 2008; 30:280–283.
28. Floreani J et al. Successful re-challenge with clozapine following development of clozapine-induced cardiomyopathy. Aust N Z J Psychiatry 2008; 42:747–748.
29. Roh S et al. Cardiomyopathy associated with clozapine. Exp Clin Psychopharmacol 2006; 14:94–98.
30. Masopust J et al. Repeated occurrence of clozapine-induced myocarditis in a patient with schizoaffective disorder and comorbid Parkinson's disease. Neuro Endocrinol Lett 2009; 30:19–21.
31. Pastor CA et al. Masked clozapine-induced cardiomyopathy. J Am Board Fam Med 2008; 21:70–74.
32. Sagar R et al. Clozapine-induced cardiomyopathy presenting as panic attacks. J Psychiatr Pract 2008; 14:182–185.
33. Modai I et al. Sudden death in patients receiving clozapine treatment: a preliminary investigation. J Clin Psychopharmacol 2000; 20:325–327.
34. Kang UG et al. Electrocardiographic abnormalities in patients treated with clozapine. J Clin Psychiatry 2000; 61:441–446.
35. Thomassen R et al. Antipsychotic drugs and venous thromboembolism (Letter). Lancet 2000; 356:252.
36. Hagg S et al. Antipsychotic-induced venous thromboembolism: a review of the evidence. CNS Drugs 2002; 16:765–776.
37. Coulter DM et al. Antipsychotic drugs and heart muscle disorder in international pharmacovigilance: data mining study. BMJ 2001; 322:1207–1209.

Further reading

Razminia M et al. Clozapine induced myopericarditis: early recognition improves clinical outcome. Am J Ther 2006; 13:274–276.
Wehmeier PM et al. Myocarditis, pericarditis and cardiomyopathy in patients treated with clozapine. J Clin Pharm Ther 2005; 30:91–96.

Clozapine, neutropenia and lithium

Risk of clozapine-induced neutropenia

Around 2.7% of patients treated with clozapine develop neutropenia. Of these, half do so within the first 18 weeks of treatment and three-quarters by the end of the first year[1]. Risk factors[1] include being Afro-Caribbean (77% increase in risk) and young (17% decrease in risk per decade increase in age), and having a low baseline white cell count (WCC) (31% increase in risk for each 1×10^9/l drop). Risk is not dose-related. Approximately, 0.8% will developed agranulocytosis. The mechanism of clozapine-induced neutropenia/agranulocytosis is unclear and it is possible that immune-mediated and direct cytotoxic effects may both be important. The mechanism may differ between individuals and also between mild and severe forms of marrow suppression[2]. One third of patients who stop clozapine because they have developed neutropenia or agranulocytosis will develop a blood dyscrasia on rechallenge. In almost all cases, the second reaction will occur more rapidly, be more severe and last longer than the first[3].

Benign ethnic neutropenia (BEN)

After being released from the bone marrow, neutrophils can either circulate freely in the bloodstream or be deposited next to vessel walls (margination)[4]. All of these neutrophils are available to fight infection. The proportion of marginated neutrophils is greater in people of Afro-Caribbean or African origin than in Caucasians, leading to lower apparent white cell counts (WCC) in the former. This is benign ethnic neutropenia.

Many patients develop neutropenia on clozapine but not all are clozapine-related or even pathological. Benign ethnic neutropenia very probably accounts for a proportion of observed or apparent clozapine-associated neutropenias (hence higher rates among Afro-Caribbeans). Distinguishing between true clozapine toxicity and neutropenia unrelated to clozapine is not possible with certainty but some factors are important. True clozapine-induced neutropenia generally occurs early in treatment. White cell counts are normal to begin with but then fall precipitantly (over 1–2 weeks or less) and recover slowly once clozapine is withdrawn. In benign ethnic neutropenia, WCCs are generally low and may frequently fall below the lower limit of normal. This pattern may be observed before, during and after the use of clozapine. Of course, true clozapine-induced neutropenia can occur in the context of benign ethnic neutropenia. Partly because of this, any iatrogenic manipulation of WCCs in benign ethnic neutropenia carries significant risk.

Effect of lithium on the WCC

Lithium increases the neutrophil count and total WCC both acutely[5] and chronically[6]. The magnitude of this effect is poorly quantified, but a mean neutrophil count of 11.9 x 10^9/l has been reported in lithium-treated patients[5] and a mean rise in neutrophil count of 2 x 10^9/l was seen in clozapine-treated patients after the addition of lithium[7]. This effect does not seem to be clearly dose-related[5,6] although a minimum lithium serum level of 0.4 mmol/l may be required[8]. The mechanism is not completely understood: both stimulation of granulocyte-macrophage colony-stimulating factor (GM-CSF)[9] and demargination[7] have been suggested. Lithium has been successfully used to raise the WCC during cancer chemotherapy[10–12]. White cells are fully formed and function normally – there is no 'left shift'.

Case reports

Lithium has been used to increase the WCC in patients who have developed neutropenia with clozapine, thus allowing clozapine treatment to continue. Several case reports in adults[8,13–17] and in children[18] have been published. All patients had serum lithium levels of >0.6 mmol/l. Lithium has also been reported to speed up the recovery of the WCC when prescribed after the development of clozapine-induced agranulocytosis[8]. In a case series (n = 25) of patients who had stopped clozapine because of a blood dyscrasia and were rechallenged in the presence of lithium, only one developed a subsequent dyscrasia; a far lower proportion than would be expected[19] (see above).

Other potential benefits of lithium–clozapine combinations

Combinations of clozapine and lithium may improve symptoms in schizoaffective patients[7] and refractory bipolar illness[20,21]. There are no data pertaining to schizophrenia.

Potential risks

At least 0.8% of clozapine-treated patients develop agranulocytosis, which is potentially fatal. Over 80% of cases develop within the first 18 weeks of treatment[1]. Risk factors include increasing age and Asian race[1]. Some patients may be genetically predisposed[22]. Although the timescale and individual risk factors for the development of agranulocytosis are different from those associated with neutropenia, it is impossible to be certain in any given patient that neutropenia is not a precursor to agranulocytosis. Lithium does not seem to protect against true clozapine-induced agranulocytosis: One case of fatal agranulocytosis has occurred with this combination[23] and a second case of agranulocytosis has been reported where the bone marrow was resistant to treatment with GM-CSF[24]. Note also that up to 20% of patients who receive clozapine–lithium combinations develop neurological symptoms typical of lithium toxicity despite lithium levels being maintained well within the therapeutic range[7,25].

The use of lithium to elevate WCC in patients with clear prior clozapine-induced neutropenia is not recommended. Lithium should only be used to elevate WCC where it is strongly felt that prior neutropenic episodes were unrelated to clozapine.

The patient's individual clinical circumstances should be considered. In particular, patients in whom the first dyscrasia:

- Was inconsistent with previous WCCs (i.e. not part of a pattern of repeated low WCCs)
- Occurred within the first 18 weeks of treatment
- Was severe (neutrophils < 0.5 x 10^9/1), and
- Was prolonged

should be considered to be very high risk if rechallenged with clozapine. Generally re-exposure to clozapine should not be attempted.

Management of patients with:

- Low initial WCC (< 4 × 109/l) or neutrophils (< 2.5 × 109/l)

or

- Clozapine-associated leucopenia (WCC < 3 × 10^9/l) or neutropenia (neutrophils < 1.5 0^9/l) thought to be linked to benign ethnic neutropenia. Such patients will be of African or Middle Eastern descent, have no history of susceptibility to infection and have morphologically normal white blood cells

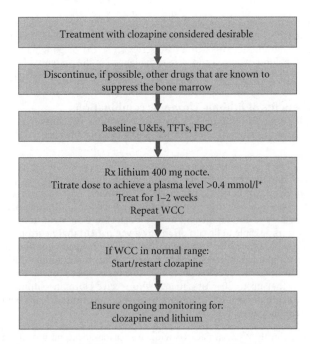

Treatment with clozapine considered desirable

↓

Discontinue, if possible, other drugs that are known to suppress the bone marrow

↓

Baseline U&Es, TFTs, FBC

↓

Rx lithium 400 mg nocte.
Titrate dose to achieve a plasma level >0.4 mmol/l*
Treat for 1–2 weeks
Repeat WCC

↓

If WCC in normal range:
Start/restart clozapine

↓

Ensure ongoing monitoring for:
clozapine and lithium

NB: Lithium does not protect against agranulocytosis: if the WCC continues to fall despite lithium treatment, consideration should be given to discontinuing clozapine. Particular vigilance is required in high-risk patients during the first 18 weeks of treatment.
*Higher plasma levels may be appropriate for patients who have an affective component to their illness.

References

1. Munro J et al. Active monitoring of 12760 clozapine recipients in the UK and Ireland. Br J Psychiatry 1999; 175:576–580.
2. Whiskey E et al. Restarting clozapine after neutropenia: evaluating the possibilities and practicalities. CNS Drugs 2007; 21:25–35.
3. Dunk LR et al. Rechallenge with clozapine following leucopenia or neutropenia during previous therapy. Br J Psychiatry 2006; 188:255–263.
4. Abramson N et al. Leukocytosis: basics of clinical assessment. Am Fam Physician 2000; 62:2053–2060.
5. Lapierre G et al. Lithium carbonate and leukocytosis. Am J Hosp Pharm 1980; 37:1525–1528.
6. Carmen J et al. The effects of lithium therapy on leukocytes: a 1-year follow-up study. J Natl Med Assoc 1993; 85:301–303.
7. Small JG et al. Tolerability and efficacy of clozapine combined with lithium in schizophrenia and schizoaffective disorder. J Clin Psychopharmacol 2003; 23:223–228.
8. Blier P et al. Lithium and clozapine-induced neutropenia/agranulocytosis. Int Clin Psychopharmacol 1998; 13:137–140.
9. Ozdemir MA et al. Lithium-induced hematologic changes in patients with bipolar affective disorder. Biol Psychiatry 1994; 35:210–213.
10. Johnke RM et al. Accelerated marrow recovery following total-body irradiation after treatment with vincristine, lithium or combined vincristine-lithium. Int J Cell Cloning 1991; 9:78–88.
11. Greco FA et al. Effect of lithium carbonate on the neutropenia caused by chemotherapy: a preliminary clinical trial. Oncology 1977; 34:153–155.
12. Ridgway D et al. Enhanced lymphocyte response to PHA among leukopenia patients taking oral lithium carbonate. Cancer Invest 1986; 4:513–517.
13. Adityanjee A. Modification of clozapine-induced leukopenia and neutropenia with lithium carbonate. Am J Psychiatry 1995; 152:648–649.
14. Silverstone PH. Prevention of clozapine-induced neutropenia by pretreatment with lithium. J Clin Psychopharmacol 1998; 18:86–88.
15. Boshes RA et al. Initiation of clozapine therapy in a patient with preexisting leukopenia: a discussion of the rationale of current treatment options. Ann Clin Psychiatry 2001; 13:233–237.
16. Papetti F et al. Treatment of clozapine-induced granulocytopenia with lithium (two observations). Encephale 2004; 30:578–582.
17. Kutscher EC et al. Clozapine-induced leukopenia successfully treated with lithium. Am J Health Syst Pharm 2007; 64:2027–2031.
18. Sporn A et al. Clozapine-induced neutropenia in children: management with lithium carbonate. J Child Adolesc Psychopharmacol 2003; 13:401–404.
19. Kanaan RA et al. Lithium and clozapine rechallenge: a restrospective case analysis. J Clin Psychiatry 2006; 67:756–760.
20. Suppes T et al. Clozapine treatment of nonpsychotic rapid cycling bipolar disorder: a report of three cases. Biol Psychiatry 1994; 36:338–340.
21. Puri BK et al. Low-dose maintenance clozapine treatment in the prophylaxis of bipolar affective disorder. Br J Clin Pract 1995; 49:333–334.
22. Dettling M et al. Further evidence of human leukocyte antigen-encoded susceptibility to clozapine-induced agranulocytosis independent of ancestry. Pharmacogenetics 2001; 11:135–141.
23. Gerson SL et al. Polypharmacy in fatal clozapine-asscoaited agranulocytosis. Lancet 1991; 338:262–263.
24. Valevski A et al. Clozapine-lithium combined treatment and agranulocytosis. Int Clin Psychopharmacol 1993; 8:63–65.
25. Blake LM et al. Reversible neurologic symptoms with clozapine and lithium. J Clin Psychopharmacol 1992; 12:297–299.

Further reading

Paton C et al. Managing clozapine-induced neutropenia with lithium. Psychiatr Bull 2005; 29:186–188.

Clozapine-related hypersalivation

Clozapine is well known to be causally associated with apparent hypersalivation (drooling, particularly at night). This seems to be chiefly problematic in the early stages of treatment and is probably dose-related. Clinical observation suggests that hypersalivation reduces in severity over time (usually several months) but may persist. Clozapine-induced hypersalivation is socially embarrassing and potentially life-threatening[1], so treatment is a matter of some urgency.

The pharmacological basis of clozapine-related hypersalivation remains unclear[2]. Suggested mechanisms include muscarinic M_4 agonism, adrenergic α_2 antagonism and inhibition of the swallowing reflex[3,4]. The last of these is supported by trials which suggest that saliva production is not increased in clozapine-treated patients[5,6].

Whatever the mechanism, drugs which reduce saliva production are likely to diminish the severity of this adverse effect. The table below describes drug treatments so far examined.

Table Clozapine-related hypersalivation – Summary

Treatment	Comments
Amisulpride 400 mg/day[7]	Supported by one, small positive RCT
Amitriptyline 75–100 mg/day[8,9]	Limited literature support. Adverse effects may be troublesome
Atropine eye drops (1%) given sublingually[10] or as solution (1 mg/10 ml) used as a mouthwash	Limited literature support. Rarely used
Benzhexol (trihexyphenidyl) 5–15 mg/day[11]	Small, open study suggests useful activity. Used in some centres but may impair cognitive function.
Benzatropine 2 mg/day + terazosin 2 mg/day[12]	Combination shown to be better than either drug alone Not widely used
Botulinum toxin[13] (Botox)	Effective in treating sialorrhoea associated with neurological disorders. Single case report of success in clozapine-treated patient
Clonidine 0.1 mg patch weekly or 0.1 mg orally at night[14,15]	α_2 partial agonist. Limited literature support. May exacerbate psychosis and depression
Glycopyrrolate 0.5 mg to 4 mg BD[16,17]	Case reports only. Worsens constipation
Hyoscine 0.3 mg sucked and swallowed up to 3 times daily	Peripheral and central anticholinergic. Very widely used but no published data available on oral treatment. May cause cognitive impairment, drowsiness and constipation. Patches also used[18,19]
Ipratropium Nasal spray (0.03% or 0.06%) – given sublingually[20,21] or intranasally[21]	Limited literature support. Rarely used
Lofexidine 0.2 mg twice daily[22]	α_2 agonist. Very few data. May exacerbate psychosis and depression
Pirenzepine 25–100 mg/day[23–25]	Selective M_1, M_4 antagonist. Does not affect clozapine metabolism Extensive clinical experience suggests efficacy in some but randomised trial suggested no effect. Still widely used. Does not have a UK licence for any indication
Propantheline 7.5 mg at night[26]	Peripheral anticholinergic. No central effects. Two Chinese RCTs (one positive)
Quetiapine[27]	May reduce hypersalivation by allowing lower doses of clozapine to be used
Sulpiride 150–300 mg/day[28]	Supported by one, small positive RCT

References

1. Hinkes R et al. Aspiration pneumonia possibly secondary to clozapine-induced sialorrhea. J Clin Psychopharmacol 1996; 16:462–463.
2. Praharaj SK et al. Clozapine-induced sialorrhea: pathophysiology and management strategies. Psychopharmacology 2006; 185:265–273.
3. Davydov L et al. Clozapine-induced hypersalivation. Ann Pharmacother 2000; 34:662–665.
4. Rogers DP et al. Therapeutic options in the treatment of clozapine-induced sialorrhea. Pharmacotherapy 2000; 20:1092–1095.
5. Rabinowitz T et al. The effect of clozapine on saliva flow rate: a pilot study. Biol Psychiatry 1996; 40:1132–1134.
6. Ben Aryeh H et al. Salivary flow-rate and composition in schizophrenic patients on clozapine: subjective reports and laboratory data. Biol Psychiatry 1996; 39:946–949.
7. Kreinin A et al. Amisulpride treatment of clozapine-induced hypersalivation in schizophrenia patients: a randomized, double-blind, placebo-controlled cross-over study. Int Clin Psychopharmacol 2006; 21:99–103.
8. Copp P et al. Amitriptyline in clozapine-induced sialorrhoea. Br J Psychiatry 1991; 159:166.
9. Praharaj SK et al. Amitriptyline for clozapine-induced nocturnal enuresis and sialorrhoea. Br J Clin Pharmacol 2007; 63:128–129.
10. Antonello C et al. Clozapine and sialorrhea: a new intervention for this bothersome and potentially dangerous side-effect. J Psychiatry Neurosci 1999; 24:250.
11. Spivak B et al. Trihexyphenidyl treatment of clozapine-induced hypersalivation. Int Clin Psychopharmacol 1997; 12:213–215.
12. Reinstein M et al. Comparative efficacy and tolerability of benzatropine and terazosin in the treatment of hypersalivation secondary to clozapine. Clin Drug Invest 1999; 17:97–102.
13. Kahl KG et al. Botulinum toxin as an effective treatment of clozapine-induced hypersalivation. Psychopharmacology 2004; 173:229–230.
14. Grabowski J. Clonidine treatment of clozapine-induced hypersalivation. J Clin Psychopharmacol 1992; 12:69–70.
15. Praharaj SK et al. Is clonidine useful for treatment of clozapine-induced sialorrhea? J Psychopharmacol 2005; 19:426–428.
16. Duggal HS. Glycopyrrolate for clozapine-induced sialorrhea. Prog Neuropsychopharmacol Biol Psychiatry 2007; 31:1546–1547.
17. Robb AS et al. Glycopyrrolate for treatment of clozapine-induced sialorrhea in three adolescents. J Child Adolesc Psychopharmacol 2008; 18:99–107.
18. McKane JP et al. Hyoscine patches in clozapine-induced hypersalivation. Psychiatr Bull 2001; 25:277–278.
19. Gaftanyuk O et al. Scolpolamine patch for clozapine-induced sialorrhea. Psychiatr Serv 2004; 55:318.
20. Calderon J et al. Potential use of ipatropium bromide for the treatment of clozapine-induced hypersalivation: a preliminary report. Int Clin Psychopharmacol 2000; 15:49–52.
21. Freudenreich O et al. Clozapine-induced sialorrhea treated with sublingual ipratropium spray: a case series. J Clin Psychopharmacol 2004; 24:98–100.
22. Corrigan FM et al. Clozapine-induced hypersalivation and the alpha 2 adrenoceptor. Br J Psychiatry 1995; 167:412.
23. Fritze J et al. Pirenzepine for clozapine-induced hypersalivation. Lancet 1995; 346:1034.
24. Bai YM et al. Therapeutic effect of pirenzepine for clozapine-induced hypersalivation: a randomized, double-blind, placebo-controlled, cross-over study. J Clin Psychopharmacol 2001; 21:608–611.
25. Schneider B et al. Reduction of clozapine-induced hypersalivation by pirenzepine is safe. Pharmacopsychiatry 2004; 37:43–45.
26. Syed Sheriff RJ et al. Pharmacological interventions for clozapine-induced hypersalivation. Schizophr Bull 2008; 34:611–612.
27. Reinstein MJ et al. Use of quetiapine to manage patients who experienced adverse effects with clozapine. Clin Drug Invest 2003; 23:63–67.
28. Kreinin A et al. Sulpiride addition for the treatment of clozapine-induced hypersalivation: preliminary study. Isr J Psychiatry Relat Sci 2005; 42:61–63.

Further reading

Sockalingam S et al. Clozapine-induced hypersalivation: a review of treatment strategies. Can J Psychiatry 2007; 52:377–384.

Schizophrenia

Clozapine and chemotherapy

The use of clozapine with agents which cause neutropenia is formally contra-indicated. Most chemotherapy treatments cause significant bone marrow suppression. When the white blood cell count drops below $3.0 \times 10^9/l$ clozapine is usually discontinued; this is an important safety precaution outlined in the SPC. In many patients it can be predicted that chemotherapy will reduce the white blood cell count below this level, irrespective of the use of clozapine.

If possible clozapine should be discontinued before chemotherapy. However, this will place most patients at high risk of relapse or deterioration which may impact upon the patient's capacity to consent to chemotherapy. This poses a therapeutic dilemma in patients prescribed clozapine and requiring chemotherapy.

There are a number of case reports supporting continuing clozapine during chemotherapy[1-11]. Before initiating chemotherapy in a patient who takes clozapine it is essential to put in place a treatment plan that is agreed with all relevant staff involved in the patient's care, and of course, the patient themself; this will include the oncologist/physician, psychiatrist, pharmacist and the clozapine monitoring service. Plans should be made in advance for the action that should be taken when the white blood count drops below the normally accepted minimum. This plan should cover the frequency of haematological monitoring, increased vigilance regarding the clinical consequences of neutropenia/agranulocytosis, if and when clozapine should be stopped, and the place of 'antidote' medication such as lithium and granulocyte-colony stimulating factor (G-CSF).

The clozapine monitoring service will ask the psychiatrist to sign an 'unlicensed use' form and will request additional blood monitoring. Complications appear to be rare but there is one case report of neutropenia persisting for 6 months after doxorubicin, radiotherapy and clozapine[7]. G-CSF has been used to treat agranulocytosis associated with chemotherapy and clozapine in combination[8]. Risks of life-threatening blood dyscrasia are probably lowest in those who have received clozapine for longer than a year in whom clozapine-induced neutropenia would be highly unusual.

Summary

- If possible clozapine should be discontinued before starting chemotherapy
- The risk of relapse or deterioration must be considered before discontinuing clozapine
- If the patient's mental state deteriorates they may retract their consent for chemotherapy
- When clozapine is continued during chemotherapy a collaborative approach between the oncologist, psychiatrist, pharmacy, patient and clozapine monitoring service is strongly recommended

References

1. Wesson ML et al. Continuing clozapine despite neutropenia. Br J Psychiatry 1996; 168:217–220.
2. Bareggi C et al. Clozapine and full-dose concomitant chemoradiation therapy in a schizophrenic patient with nasopharyngeal cancer. Tumori 2002; 88:59–60.
3. Avnon M et al. Clozapine, cancer, and schizophrenia. Am J Psychiatry 1993; 150:1562–1563.
4. Hundertmark J et al. Reintroduction of clozapine after diagnosis of lymphoma. Br J Psychiatry 2001; 178:576.
5. McKenna RC et al. Clozapine and chemotherapy. Hosp Community Psychiatry 1994; 45:831.
6. Haut FA. Clozapine and chemotherapy. J Drug Dev Clin Pract 1995; 7:237–239.
7. Rosenstock J. Clozapine therapy during cancer treatment. Am J Psychiatry 2004; 161:175.
8. Lee SY et al. Combined antitumor chemotherapy in a refractory schizophrenic receiving clozapine (Korean). J Korean Neuropsychiatr Assoc 2000; 39:234–239.
9. Rosenberg I et al. Restarting clozapine treatment during ablation chemotherapy and stem cell transplant for Hodgkin's lymphoma. Am J Psychiatry 2007; 164:1438–1439.
10. Goulet K et al. Case report: clozapine given in the context of chemotherapy for lung cancer. Psychooncology 2008; 17:512–516.
11. Frieri T et al. Maintaining clozapine treatment during chemotherapy for non-Hodgkin's lymphoma. Prog Neuropsychopharmacol Biol Psychiatry 2008; 32:1611–1612.

Guidelines for the initiation of clozapine for patients based in the community

Some points to check before starting:

- Is the patient likely to be adherent with oral medication?
- Has the patient understood the need for regular blood tests?
- Is it possible for the patient to be seen every day during the early titration phase?
- Is the patient able to attend the team base or pharmacy to collect medication every week?
- Does the patient need medication delivered to their home?
- Is the patient's GP aware that they are starting clozapine?

Mandatory blood monitoring and registration

- Register with the relevant monitoring service.
- Perform baseline blood tests (WCC and differential count) before starting clozapine.
- Further blood testing continues weekly for the first 18 weeks and then every 2 weeks for the remainder of the year. After that, the blood monitoring is usually done monthly.

Dosing

Starting clozapine in the community requires a slow and flexible titration schedule. Prior antipsychotics should be slowly discontinued.

There are two basic methods for starting clozapine in the community. One is to give the first dose in the morning in clinic and then monitor as usual for 6 hours. The patient is then allowed home and the process repeated the next day. On the second day the patient takes home a night-time dose. The second method involves giving the first dose before retiring, so avoiding the need for close physical monitoring immediately after administration. This dosing schedule is described in the table below. (This is a very cautious schedule: most patients will tolerate faster titration.) All initiations should take place on a Monday and Tuesday so that adequate staffing and monitoring are assured.

Table	Suggested titration regimen – clozapine in the community			
Day	*Day of the week*	*Morning dose (mg)*	*Evening dose (mg)*	*Percentage dose of previous antipsychotic*
1	Monday	–	6.25	100
2	Tuesday	6.25	6.25	
3	Wednesday	6.25	6.25	
4	Thursday	6.25	12.5	
5	Friday	12.5	12.5	
6	Saturday	12.5	12.5	
7	Sunday	12.5	12.5	
8	Monday	12.5	25	
9	Tuesday	12.5	25	
10	Wednesday	25	25	
11	Thursday	25	37.5	
12	Friday	25	37.5	
13	Saturday	25	37.5	
14	Sunday	25	37.5	
15	Monday	37.5	37.5	75
16	Tuesday	37.5	37.5	
17	Wednesday	37.5	50	
18	Thursday	37.5	50	
19	Friday	50	50	
20	Saturday	50	50	
21	Sunday	50	50	
22	Monday	50	75	
23	Tuesday	50	75	
24	Wednesday	75	75	
25	Thursday	75	75	
26	Friday	75	100	50
27	Saturday	75	100	
28	Sunday	75	100	

Futher increments should be 25 mg/day until target dose is reached (use plasma levels).

Switching from other antipsychotics
- The switching regimen will be largely dependent on the patient's mental state.
- Consider additive side-effects of the antipsychotics (e.g. hypotension, sedation effect on QTc interval).
- Consider drug interactions (e.g. some SSRIs may increase clozapine levels).
- All depots, sertindole, pimozide and ziprasidone should be stopped before clozapine is started.
- Other antipsychotics and clozapine may be cross-tapered with varying degrees of caution. ECG monitoring is prudent when clozapine is co-prescribed with other drugs known to affect QT interval.

Acute monitoring requirements

- After the first dose, monitor BP, temperature and pulse hourly for at least 3 (preferably 6) hours afterwards. (This may not be necessary if the first dose is given at bedtime.) Thereafter, the patient should be seen at least once a day and all three parameters should be monitored before and after the morning dose.
- Continue daily monitoring for at least 2 weeks or until there are no unacceptable adverse effects. Alternate day monitoring may then be undertaken until a stable dose is reached. Thereafter monitor at time of blood testing.
- The formal carer (usually the Community Psychiatric Nurse) should inform the prescriber if:
  - temperature rises above 38°C (this is very common and is not a good reason, on its own, for stopping clozapine)
  - pulse is >100 bpm (also common but may rarely be linked to myocarditis)
  - postural drop of >30 mmHg
  - patient is clearly over-sedated
  - any other adverse effect is intolerable.

A doctor should see the patient at least once a week for the first month to assess mental and physical state.

Additional monitoring requirements

Baseline	1 month	3 months	4–6 months	12 months
Weight, lipids	Weight	Weight, lipids	Weight, lipids	Weight, lipids
Plasma glucose	Plasma glucose		Plasma glucose	Plasma glucose
LFTs			LFTs	
BMI, waist	BMI, waist	BMI, waist	BMI, waist	BMI, waist

Where available, consider also use of ECG (benefit not established but see above). Oral glucose tolerance test is preferred to plasma glucose. If fasting sampling not possible, draw random sample and test for glucose and HbA_{1C}.

Adverse effects

- Sedation and hypotension are common at the start of treatment. These effects can usually be managed by reducing the dose or slowing the rate of titration (see section on common adverse effects).
- Many other adverse effects associated with clozapine can also be managed by dose reduction.

Serious cardiac adverse effects

Patients who have persistent tachycardia at rest, especially during the first 2 months of treatment, should be closely observed for other signs or symptoms of myocarditis. These include palpitations, fever, arrhythmia, symptoms mimicking myocardial infarction, chest pain and other unexplained symptoms of heart failure (see section on serious adverse effects).

In patients with suspected clozapine-induced myocarditis or cardiomyopathy, the drug must be stopped and the patient referred to a cardiologist. If clozapine-induced myocarditis or cardiomyopathy is confirmed, the patient must not normally be re-exposed to clozapine.

Further reading

Lovett L. Initiation of clozapine treatment at home. Prog Neurol Psychiatry 2004; 8:19–21.
O'Brien A. Starting clozapine in the community: a UK perspective. CNS Drugs 2004; 18:845–852.

Omega-3 fatty acid (fish oils) in schizophrenia

Fish oils contain the omega-3 fatty acids, eicosapentanoic acid (EPA) and docosahexanoic acid (DHA). These compounds are thought to be involved in maintaining neuronal membrane structure, in the modulation of membrane proteins and in the production of prostaglandins and leukot-rienes[1]. They have been suggested as treatments for a variety of psychiatric illnesses[2,3] but most research relates to their use in schizophrenia, where case reports[4–6], case series[7] and prospective trials suggest useful efficacy (see the following table).

On balance, evidence suggests that EPA (2–3 g daily) is a worthwhile option in schizophrenia when added to standard treatment, particularly clozapine[8,9]. However, doubt still remains over the true extent of the beneficial effect derived from fish oils, and research in this area has dwindled in the last few years[9,10]. Set against doubts over efficacy are the observations that fish oils are relatively cheap, well tolerated (mild GI symptoms may occur) and benefit physical health[1,11–14].

Fish oils are therefore very tentatively recommended for the treatment of residual symptoms of schizophrenia but particularly in patients responding poorly to clozapine. Careful assessment of response is important and fish oils may be withdrawn if no effect is observed after 3 months' treatment, unless required for their beneficial metabolic effects.

Table A summary of the evidence – fish oils in schizophrenia

References	n	Design	Outcome
Mellor et al. 1995[15]	20	Open label evaluation of fish oil (EPA+DHA) added to usual medication	Significant improvement in symptoms
Peet et al. 2001[16]	45	Double-blind, randomised comparison of EPA (2 g daily), DHA and placebo (12 weeks)	EPA significantly more effective than DHA or placebo
Peet et al. 2001[16]	26	Double-blind, randomised comparison of EPA (2 g daily) or placebo as sole drug treatment (12 weeks)	All 12 patients given placebo required conventional antipsychotic treatment; 8 of 14 given EPA required antipsychotics. EPA more effective
Fenton et al. 2001[17]	87	Double-blind, randomised comparison of EPA (3 g daily) and placebo added to standard drug treatment (16 weeks)	No differences between EPA and placebo
Peet & Horrobin 2002[18]	115	Double-blind randomised comparison of ethyl-EPA (1, 2 or 4 g/day) and placebo added to antipsychotic treatment conventional, atypical or clozapine) (12 weeks)	Ethyl-EPA significantly improved response in patients receiving clozapine. 2 g/day most effective dose
Emsley et al. 2002[19]	40	Double-blind, randomised comparison of EPA (3 g daily) and placebo added to standard drug treatment (12 weeks)	EPA associated with significantly greater reduction in symptoms and tardive dyskinesia (9 patients in each group received clozapine)

The recommended dose is

Omacor (460 mg EPA) 5 capsules daily
or
Maxepa (170 mg EPA) 10 capsules daily

References

1. Fenton WS et al. Essential fatty acids, lipid membrane abnormalities, and the diagnosis and treatment of schizophrenia. Biol Psychiatry 2000; 47:8–21.
2. Freeman MP. Omega-3 fatty acids in psychiatry: a review. Ann Clin Psychiatry 2000; 12:159–165.
3. Ross BM et al. Omega-3 fatty acids as treatments for mental illness: which disorder and which fatty acid? Lipids Health Dis 2007; 6:21.
4. Richardson AJ et al. Red cell and plasma fatty acid changes accompanying symptom remission in a patient with schizophrenia treated with eicosapentaenoic acid. Eur Neuropsychopharmacol 2000; 10:189–193.
5. Puri BK et al. Eicosapentaenoic acid treatment in schizophrenia associated with symptom remission, normalisation of blood fatty acids, reduced neuronal membrane phospholipid turnover and structural brain changes. Int J Clin Pract 2000; 54:57–63.
6. Su KP et al. Omega-3 fatty acids as a psychotherapeutic agent for a pregnant schizophrenic patient. Eur Neuropsychopharmacol 2001; 11:295–299.
7. Sivrioglu EY et al. The impact of omega-3 fatty acids, vitamins E and C supplementation on treatment outcome and side-effects in schizophrenia patients treated with haloperidol: an open-label pilot study. Prog Neuropsychopharmacol Biol Psychiatry 2007; 31:1493–1499.
8. Emsley R et al. Clinical potential of omega-3 fatty acids in the treatment of schizophrenia. CNS Drugs 2003; 17:1081–1091.
9. Joy CB et al. Polyunsaturated fatty acid supplementation for schizophrenia. Cochrane Database Syst Rev 2006; 3:CD001257.
10. Peet M. Omega-3 polyunsaturated fatty acids in the treatment of schizophrenia. Isr J Psychiatry Relat Sci 2008; 45:19–25.
11. Scorza FA et al. Omega-3 fatty acids and sudden cardiac death in schizophrenia: if not a friend, at least a great colleague. Schizophr Res 2007; 94: 375–376.
12. Caniato RN et al. Effect of omega-3 fatty acids on the lipid profile of patients taking clozapine. Aust N Z J Psychiatry 2006; 40:691–697.
13. Emsley R et al. Safety of the omega-3 fatty acid, eicosapentaenoic acid (EPA) in psychiatric patients: results from a randomized, placebo-controlled trial. Psychiatry Res 2008; 161:284–291.
14. Das UN. Essential fatty acids and their metabolites could function as endogenous HMG-CoA reductase and ACE enzyme inhibitors, anti-arrhythmic, anti-hypertensive, anti-atherosclerotic, anti-inflammatory, cytoprotective, and cardioprotective molecules. Lipids Health Dis 2008; 7:37.
15. Mellor JE et al. Schizophrenic symptoms and dietary intake of n-3 fatty acids. Schizophr Res 1995; 18:85–86.
16. Peet M et al. Two double-blind placebo-controlled pilot studies of eicosapentaenoic acid in the treatment of schizophrenia. Schizophr Res 2001; 49: 243–251.
17. Fenton WS et al. A placebo-controlled trial of omega-3 fatty acid (ethyl eicosapentaenoic acid) supplementation for residual symptoms and cognitive impairment in schizophrenia. Am J Psychiatry 2001; 158:2071–2074.
18. Peet M et al. A dose-ranging exploratory study of the effects of ethyl-eicosapentaenoate in patients with persistent schizophrenic symptoms. J Psychiatr Res 2002; 36:7–18.
19. Emsley R et al. Randomized, placebo-controlled study of ethyl-eicosapentaenoic acid as supplemental treatment in schizophrenia. Am J Psychiatry 2002; 159:1596–1598.

Extrapyramidal side-effects

Table Most common extrapyramidal side-effects

	Dystonia (uncontrolled muscular spasm)	Pseudo-parkinsonism (tremor, etc.)	Akathisia (restlessness)[1]	Tardive dyskinesia (abnormal movements)
Signs and symptoms[2]	Muscle spasm in any part of the body, e.g. • Eyes rolling upwards (oculogyric crisis) • Head and neck twisted to the side (torticollis) The patient may be unable to swallow or speak clearly. In extreme cases, the back may arch or the jaw dislocate Acute dystonia can be both painful and very frightening	• Tremor and/or rigidity • Bradykinesia (decreased facial expression, flat monotone voice, slow body movements, inability to initiate movement) • Bradyphrenia (slowed thinking) • Salivation Pseudoparkinsonism can be mistaken for depression or the negative symptoms of schizophrenia	A subjectively unpleasant state of inner restlessness where there is a strong desire or compulsion to move • Foot stamping when seated • Constantly crossing/ uncrossing legs • Rocking from foot to foot • Constantly pacing up and down Akathisia can be mistaken for psychotic agitation and has been (weakly) linked with suicide and aggression towards others[3]	A wide variety of movements can occur such as: • Lip smacking or chewing • Tongue protrusion (fly catching) • Choreiform hand movements (pill rolling or piano playing) • Pelvic thrusting Severe orofacial movements can lead to difficulty speaking, eating or breathing. Movements are worse when under stress
Rating scales	No specific scale. Small component of general EPS scales	Simpson–Angus EPS Rating Scale[4]	Barnes Akathisia Scale[5]	Abnormal Involuntary Movement Scale[6] (AIMS)
Prevalence (with older drugs)	Approximately 10%[7], but more common[8]: • In young males • In the neuroleptic-naive • With high potency drugs (e.g. haloperidol) Dystonic reactions are rare in the elderly	Approximately 20%[9], but more common in: • Elderly females • Those with pre-existing neurological damage (head injury, stroke, etc.)	Approximately 25%[10], less with atypicals In decreasing order: aripiprazole, risperidone, olanzapine, quetiapine and clozapine[11]	5% of patients per year of antipsychotic exposure[12]. More common in: • Elderly women • Those with affective illness • Those who have had acute EPS early on in treatment

Time taken to develop	Acute dystonia can occur within hours of starting antipsychotics (minutes if the IM or IV route is used) Tardive dystonia occurs after months to years of antipsychotic treatment	Days to weeks after antipsychotic drugs are started or the dose is increased	Acute akathisia occurs within hours to weeks of starting antipsychotics or increasing the dose. Tardive akathisia takes longer to develop and can persist after antipsychotics have been withdrawn	Months to years Approximately 50% of cases are reversible[12]
Treatment	Anticholinergic drugs given orally, IM or IV depending on the severity of symptoms[8] • Remember the patient may be unable to swallow • Response to IV administration will be seen within 5 minutes • Response to IM administration takes around 20 minutes • Tardive dystonia may respond to ECT[13] • Where symptoms do not respond to simpler measures including switching to an antipsychotic with a low propensity for EPS, botulinuim toxin may be effective[14]	Several options are available depending on the clinical circumstances: • Reduce the antipsychotic dose • Change to an atypical drug (as antipsychotic monotherapy) • Prescribe an anticholinergic. The majority of patients do not require long-term anticholinergics. Use should be reviewed at least every 3 months. Do not prescribe at night (symptoms usually absent during sleep)	• Reduce the antipsychotic dose • Change to an atypical drug • A reduction in symptoms may be seen with: propranolol 30–80mg/day, clonazepam (low dose) $5HT_2$ antagonists such as: cyproheptadine[13], mirtazapine[15], trazodone[16], mianserin[17], and cyproheptadine[13] may help, as may diphenhydramine[18] All are unlicenced for this indication Anticholinergics are generally unhelpful[19]	• Stop anticholinergic if prescribed • Reduce dose of antipsychotic • Change to an atypical drug[20–23] • Clozapine is the antipsychotic most likely to be associated with resolution of symptoms[24] • For other treatment options see section on tardive dyskinesia

ANTICHOLINERGIC (A'TGY: BENZOTROPIN, BIPERIDEN, PROCYCLIDIN, ORFENADRIN

EXTP?

EPS are:

- dose-related
- more likely with high-potency typicals
- uncommon with atypicals.

Patients who experience one type of EPS may be more vulnerable to developing others[25].

References

1. Barnes TRE. The Barnes akathisia scale – revisited. J Psychopharmacol 2003; 17:365–370.
2. Gervin M et al. Assessment of drug-related movement disorders in schizophrenia. Adv Psychiatr Treat 2000; 6:332–341.
3. Leong GB et al. Neuroleptic-induced akathisia and violence: a review. J Forensic Sci 2003; 48:187–189.
4. Simpson GM et al. A rating scale for extrapyramidal side-effects. Acta Psychiatr Scand 1970; 212:11–19.
5. Barnes TRE. A rating scale for drug-induced akathisia. Br J Psychiatry 1989; 154:672–676.
6. Guy W. ECDEU Assessment Manual for Psychopharmacology. Washington, DC: US Department of Health, Education, and Welfare 1976;534–537.
7. American Psychiatric Association. Practice guideline for the treatment of patients with schizophrenia. Am J Psychiatry 1997;154 Suppl 4:1–63.
8. van Harten PN et al. Acute dystonia induced by drug treatment. Br Med J 1999; 319:623–626.
9. Bollini P et al. Antipsychotic drugs: is more worse? A meta-analysis of the published randomized control trials. Psychol Med 1994; 24:307–316.
10. Halstead SM et al. Akathisia: prevalence and associated dysphoria in an in-patient population with chronic schizophrenia. Br J Psychiatry 1994; 164: 177–183.
11. Hirose S. The causes of underdiagnosing akathisia. Schizophr Bull 2003; 29:547–558.
12. American Psychiatric Association. Tardive Dyskinesia: A task force report of the American Psychiatric Association. Hosp Community Psychiatry 1993; 44:190.
13. Miller CH et al. Managing antipsychotic-induced acute and chronic akathisia. Drug Saf 2000; 22:73–81.
14. Hennings JM et al. Successful treatment of tardive lingual dystonia with botulinum toxin: case report and review of the literature. Prog Neuropsychopharmacol Biol Psychiatry 2008; 32:1167–1171.
15. Poyurovsky M et al. Efficacy of low-dose mirtazapine in neuroleptic-induced akathisia: a double-blind randomized placebo-controlled pilot study. J Clin Psychopharmacol 2003; 23:305–308.
16. Stryjer R et al. Treatment of neuroleptic-induced akathisia with the 5-HT2A antagonist trazodone. Clin Neuropharmacol 2003; 26:137–141.
17. Stryjer R et al. Mianserin for the rapid improvement of chronic akathisia in a schizophrenia patient. Eur Psychiatry 2004; 19:237–238.
18. Vinson DR. Diphenhydramine in the treatment of akathisia induced by prochlorperazine. J Emerg Med 2004; 26:265–270.
19. Lima AR et al. Anticholinergics for neuroleptic-induced acute akathisia. Cochrane Database Syst Rev 2004; CD003727.
20. Glazer WM. Expected incidence of tardive dyskinesia associated with atypical antipsychotics. J Clin Psychiatry 2000;61 Suppl 4:21–26.
21. Kinon BJ et al. Olanzapine treatment for tardive dyskinesia in schizophrenia patients: a prospective clinical trial with patients randomized to blinded dose reduction periods. Prog Neuropsychopharmacol Biol Psychiatry 2004; 28:985–996.
22. Bai YM et al. Risperidone for severe tardive dyskinesia: a 12-week randomized, double-blind, placebo-controlled study. J Clin Psychiatry 2003; 64: 1342–1348.
23. Tenback DE et al. Effects of antipsychotic treatment on tardive dyskinesia: a 6-month evaluation of patients from the European Schizophrenia Outpatient Health Outcomes (SOHO) Study. J Clin Psychiatry 2005; 66:1130–1133.
24. Simpson GM. The treatment of tardive dyskinesia and tardive dystonia. J Clin Psychiatry 2000;61 Suppl 4:39–44.
25. Kim JH et al. Prevalence and characteristics of subjective akathisia, objective akathisia, and mixed akathisia in chronic schizophrenic subjects. Clin Neuropharmacol 2003; 26:312–316.

Further reading

Dayalu P et al. Antipsychotic-induced extrapyramidal symptoms and their management. Expert Opin Pharmacother 2008; 9:1451–1462.

El Sayeh HG et al. Non-neuroleptic catecholaminergic drugs for neuroleptic-induced tardive dyskinesia. Cochrane Database Syst Rev 2006; CD000458.

Margolese HC et al. Tardive dyskinesia in the era of typical and atypical antipsychotics. Part 2: Incidence and management strategies in patients with schizophrenia. Can J Psychiatry 2005; 50:703–714.

McGrath JJ et al. Neuroleptic reduction and/or cessation and neuroleptics as specific treatments for tardive dyskinesia. Cochrane Database Syst Rev 2000; CD000459.

Hyperprolactinaemia

Dopamine inhibits prolactin release and so dopamine antagonists can be expected to increase prolactin plasma levels. All antipsychotics cause measurable changes in prolactin but some do not normally increase prolactin above the normal range at standard doses. These drugs are clozapine, olanzapine, quetiapine, aripiprazole and ziprasidone[1-5]. Even with these drugs (particularly olanzapine and ziprasidone), raised prolactin and prolactin-related symptoms are occasionally reported[6-9]. With all drugs, the degree of prolactin elevation is probably dose-related[10].

Hyperprolactinaemia is often superficially asymptomatic (that is, the patient does not spontaneously report problems) and there is evidence that hyperprolactinaemia does not affect subjective quality of life[11]. Nonetheless, persistent elevation of plasma prolactin is associated with a number of adverse consequences. These include sexual dysfunction[12-15] (but note that other pharmacological activities also give rise to sexual dysfunction), reductions in bone mineral density[16-20], menstrual disturbances[2,21], breast growth and galactorrhoea[21], suppression of the hypothalamic-pituitary-gonadal axis[22] and a possible increase in the risk of breast cancer[2,23-25].

Prolactin concentration interpretation[26]
- Take blood sample at least one hour after waking or eating.
- Minimise stress during venepuncture (stress elevates plasma prolactin).
- Treatment of hyperprolactinaemia depends more on symptoms and long-term risk than on measured plasma level.

Normal	Women	0–25 ng/ml	(~ 0–530 mIU/l)
	Men	0–20 ng/ml	(~ 0–424 mIU/l)
Need for re-test, if prolactin concentration		25–100 ng/ml	(~ 530–2120 mIU/l)
Need referral for tests to rule out prolactinoma if prolactin concentration		>150 ng/ml	(>3180 mIU/l)

Treatment
For most patients with symptomatic hyperprolactinaemia, a switch to a non prolactin-elevating drug is the first choice[2,15,27,28]. An alternative is to add aripiprazole to existing treatment[29-32] – hyperprolactinaemia and related symptoms are reported to improve fairly promptly following the addition of aripiprazole. When switching, symptoms tend to resolve slowly and symptom severity does not always reflect prolactin changes[27]. Genetic differences may play a part[33].

For patients who need to remain on a prolactin-elevating antipsychotic, dopamine agonists may be effective[3,27,34]. Amantadine, carbergoline and bromocriptine have all been used, but each has the potential to worsen psychosis (although this has not been reported in trials). A herbal remedy – Peony Glycyrrhiza Decoction – has also been shown to be effective[35].

Table	Established antipsychotics not usually associated with hyperprolactinaemia
	Aripiprazole
	Clozapine
	Olanzapine
	Quetiapine
	Ziprasidone

References

1. David SR et al. The effects of olanzapine, risperidone, and haloperidol on plasma prolactin levels in patients with schizophrenia. Clin Ther 2000; 22:1085–1096.
2. Haddad PM et al. Antipsychotic-induced hyperprolactinaemia: mechanisms, clinical features and management. Drugs 2004; 64:2291–2314.
3. Hamner MB et al. Hyperprolactinaemia in antipsychotic-treated patients: guidelines for avoidance and management. CNS Drugs 1998; 10:209–222.
4. Bushe C et al. Comparison of metabolic and prolactin variables from a six-month randomised trial of olanzapine and quetiapine in schizophrenia. J Psychopharmacol 2009; In Press.
5. Byerly MJ et al. Effects of aripiprazole on prolactin levels in subjects with schizophrenia during cross-titration with risperidone or olanzapine: Analysis of a randomized, open-label study. Schizophr Res 2009; 107:218–222.
6. Melkersson K. Differences in prolactin elevation and related symptoms of atypical antipsychotics in schizophrenic patients. J Clin Psychiatry 2005; 66:761–767.
7. Kopecek M et al. Ziprasidone-induced galactorrhea: a case report. Neuro Endocrinol Lett 2005; 26:69–70.
8. Buhagiar K et al. Quetiapine-induced hyperprolactinemic galactorrhea in an adolescent male. German J Psychiatry 2006; 9:118–120.
9. Johnsen E et al. Antipsychotic-induced hyperprolactinemia: a cross-sectional survey. J Clin Psychopharmacol 2008; 28:686–690.
10. Staller J. The effect of long-term antipsychotic treatment on prolactin. J Child Adolesc Psychopharmacol 2006; 16:317–326.
11. Kaneda Y. The impact of prolactin elevation with antipsychotic medications on subjective quality of life in patients with schizophrenia. Clin Neuropharmacol 2003; 26:182–184.
12. Bobes J et al. Frequency of sexual dysfunction and other reproductive side-effects in patients with schizophrenia treated with risperidone, olanzapine, quetiapine, or haloperidol: the results of the EIRE study. J Sex Marital Ther 2003; 29:125–147.
13. Smith S. Effects of antipsychotics on sexual and endocrine function in women: implications for clinical practice. J Clin Psychopharmacol 2003; 23: S27–S32.
14. Spollen JJ, III et al. Prolactin levels and erectile function in patients treated with risperidone. J Clin Psychopharmacol 2004; 24:161–166.
15. Knegtering R et al. A randomized open-label study of the impact of quetiapine versus risperidone on sexual functioning. J Clin Psychopharmacol 2004; 24:56–61.
16. Halbreich U et al. Accelerated osteoporosis in psychiatric patients: possible pathophysiological processes. Schizophr Bull 1996; 22:447–454.
17. Becker D et al. Risperidone, but not olanzapine, decreases bone mineral density in female premenopausal schizophrenia patients. J Clin Psychiatry 2003; 64:761–766.
18. Meaney AM et al. Reduced bone mineral density in patients with schizophrenia receiving prolactin raising anti-psychotic medication. J Psychopharmacol 2003; 17:455–458.
19. Meaney AM et al. Effects of long-term prolactin-raising antipsychotic medication on bone mineral density in patients with schizophrenia. Br J Psychiatry 2004; 184:503–508.
20. Kishimoto T et al. Antipsychotic-induced hyperprolactinemia inhibits the hypothalamo-pituitary-gonadal axis and reduces bone mineral density in male patients with schizophrenia. J Clin Psychiatry 2008; 69:385–391.
21. Wieck A et al. Antipsychotic-induced hyperprolactinaemia in women: pathophysiology, severity and consequences. Selective literature review. Br J Psychiatry 2003; 182:199–204.
22. Smith S et al. The effects of antipsychotic-induced hyperprolactinaemia on the hypothalamic-pituitary-gonadal axis. J Clin Psychopharmacol 2002; 22:109–114.
23. Halbreich U et al. Are chronic psychiatric patients at increased risk for developing breast cancer? Am J Psychiatry 1996; 153:559–560.
24. Wang PS et al. Dopamine antagonists and the development of breast cancer. Arch Gen Psychiatry 2002; 59:1147–1154.
25. Harvey PW et al. Adverse effects of prolactin in rodents and humans: breast and prostate cancer. J Psychopharmacol 2008; 22:20–27.
26. Holt RI. Medical causes and consequences of hyperprolactinaemia. A context for psychiatrists. J Psychopharmacol 2008; 22:28–37.
27. Duncan D et al. Treatment of psychotropic-induced hyperprolactinaemia. Psychiatr Bull 1995; 19:755–757.
28. Anghelescu I et al. Successful switch to aripiprazole after induction of hyperprolactinemia by ziprasidone: a case report. J Clin Psychiatry 2004; 65: 1286–1287.
29. Shim JC et al. Adjunctive treatment with a dopamine partial agonist, aripiprazole, for antipsychotic-induced hyperprolactinemia: a placebo-controlled trial. Am J Psychiatry 2007; 164:1404–1410.
30. Lorenz RA et al. Resolution of haloperidol-induced hyperprolactinemia with aripiprazole. J Clin Psychopharmacol 2007; 27:524–525.
31. Lu ML et al. Time course of the changes in antipsychotic-induced hyperprolactinemia following the switch to aripiprazole. Prog Neuropsychopharmacol Biol Psychiatry 2008; 32:1978–1981.
32. Mir A et al. Change in sexual dysfunction with aripiprazole: a switching or add-on study. J Psychopharmacol 2008; 22:244–253.
33. Young RM et al. Prolactin levels in antipsychotic treatment of patients with schizophrenia carrying the DRD2*A1 allele. Br J Psychiatry 2004; 185: 147–151.
34. Cavallaro R et al. Cabergoline treatment of risperidone-induced hyperprolactinemia: a pilot study. J Clin Psychiatry 2004; 65:187–190.
35. Yuan HN et al. A randomized, crossover comparison of herbal medicine and bromocriptine against risperidone-induced hyperprolactinemia in patients with schizophrenia. J Clin Psychopharmacol 2008; 28:264–370.

Algorithm for the treatment of antipsychotic-induced akathisia

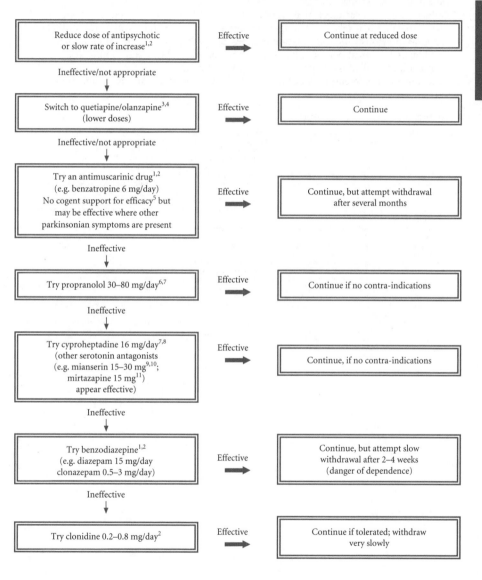

Reduce dose of antipsychotic or slow rate of increase[1,2]	**Effective** →	Continue at reduced dose

Ineffective/not appropriate ↓

Switch to quetiapine/olanzapine[3,4] (lower doses)	**Effective** →	Continue

Ineffective/not appropriate ↓

Try an antimuscarinic drug[1,2] (e.g. benzatropine 6 mg/day) No cogent support for efficacy[5] but may be effective where other parkinsonian symptoms are present	**Effective** →	Continue, but attempt withdrawal after several months

Ineffective ↓

Try propranolol 30–80 mg/day[6,7]	**Effective** →	Continue if no contra-indications

Ineffective ↓

Try cyproheptadine 16 mg/day[7,8] (other serotonin antagonists (e.g. mianserin 15–30 mg[9,10]; mirtazapine 15 mg[11]) appear effective)	**Effective** →	Continue, if no contra-indications

Ineffective ↓

Try benzodiazepine[1,2] (e.g. diazepam 15 mg/day clonazepam 0.5–3 mg/day)	**Effective** →	Continue, but attempt slow withdrawal after 2–4 weeks (danger of dependence)

Ineffective ↓

Try clonidine 0.2–0.8 mg/day[2]	**Effective** →	Continue if tolerated; withdraw very slowly

Notes:

- Akathisia is sometimes difficult to diagnose with certainty. A careful history of symptoms, medication and illicit substance use is essential. Note that severe akathisia may be linked to violent or suicidal behaviour[12–14].
- Evaluate efficacy of each treatment option over at least 1 month. Some effect may be seen after a few days but it may take much longer to become apparent in those with chronic akathisia.
- Withdraw previously ineffective treatments before starting the next option in the algorithm.
- Combinations of treatment may be used in refractory cases if carefully monitored.
- Consider tardive akathisia in patients on long-term therapy.
- Other possible treatments include vitamin B6[10,15], diphenhydramine[16] and zolmitriptan[17,18].

References

1. Fleischhacker WW et al. The pharmacologic treatment of neuroleptic-induced akathisia. J Clin Psychopharmacol 1990; 10:12–21.
2. Sachdev P. The identification and management of drug-induced akathisia. CNS Drugs 1995; 4:28–46.
3. Kumar R et al. Akathisia and second-generation antipsychotic drugs. Curr Opin Psychiatry 2009; 22:293–299.
4. Miller DD et al. Extrapyramidal side-effects of antipsychotics in a randomised trial. Br J Psychiatry 2008; 193:279–288.
5. Rathbone J et al. Anticholinergics for neuroleptic-induced acute akathisia. Cochrane Database Syst Rev 2006; CD003727.
6. Adler L et al. A controlled assessment of propranolol in the treatment of neuroleptic-induced akathisia. Br J Psychiatry 1986; 149:42–45.
7. Fischel T et al. Cyproheptadine versus propranolol for the treatment of acute neuroleptic-induced akathisia: a comparative double-blind study. J Clin Psychopharmacol 2001; 21:612–615.
8. Weiss D et al. Cyproheptadine treatment in neuroleptic-induced akathisia. Br J Psychiatry 1995; 167:483–486.
9. Poyurovsky M et al. Treatment of neuroleptic-induced akathisia with the 5-HT2 antagonist mianserin. Double-blind, placebo-controlled study. Br J Psychiatry 1999; 174:238–242.
10. Miodownik C et al. Vitamin B6 versus mianserin and placebo in acute neuroleptic-induced akathisia: a randomized, double-blind, controlled study. Clin Neuropharmacol 2006; 29:68–72.
11. Poyurovsky M et al. Low-dose mirtazapine: a new option in the treatment of antipsychotic-induced akathisia. A randomized, double-blind, placebo- and propranolol-controlled trial. Biol Psychiatry 2006; 59:1071–1077.
12. Drake RE et al. Suicide attempts associated with akathisia. Am J Psychiatry 1985; 142:499–501.
13. Azhar MZ et al. Akathisia-induced suicidal behaviour. Eur Psychiatry 1992; 7:239–241.
14. Hansen L. A critical review of akathisia, and its possible association with suicidal behaviour. Hum Psychopharmacol 2001; 16:495–505.
15. Lerner V et al. Vitamin B6 treatment in acute neuroleptic-induced akathisia: a randomized, double-blind, placebo-controlled study. J Clin Psychiatry 2004; 65:1550–1554.
16. Friedman BW et al. A randomized trial of diphenhydramine as prophylaxis against metoclopramide-induced akathisia in nauseated emergency department patients. Ann Emerg Med 2009; 53:379–385.
17. Gross-Isseroff R et al. The 5-HT1D receptor agonist zolmitriptan for neuroleptic-induced akathisia: an open label preliminary study. Int Clin Psychopharmacol 2005; 20:23–25.
18. Avital A et al. Zolmitriptan compared to propranolol in the treatment of acute neuroleptic-induced akathisia: a comparative double-blind study. Eur Neuropsychopharmacol 2009; 19:476–482.

Treatment of tardive dyskinesia (TD)

Tardive dyskinesia is now a somewhat less commonly encountered problem than in previous decades, probably because of the introduction and widespread use of SGAs[1–4]. Treatment of established TD is often unsuccessful, so prevention and early detection are essential. TD is associated with more severe psychopathology[5] and higher mortality[6].

There is fairly good evidence that some newer 'atypical' antipsychotics are less likely to cause TD[7–11] although TD certainly does occur with these drugs[12–17]. The observation that SGAs produce less TD than typical drugs is consistent with the long-held belief that early acute movement disorders and akathisia predict later TD[18–20]. Note, also, that TD can occur after minuscule doses of conventional drugs (and in the absence of portentous acute movement disorder[21]) and following the use of other dopamine antagonists such as metoclopramide[22].

Treatment – first steps

Most authorities recommend the withdrawal of any anticholinergic drugs and a reduction in the dose of antipsychotic as initial steps in those with early signs of TD[23,24] (dose reduction may initially worsen TD). Cochrane, however found little support for this approach[25]. It has now become common practice to withdraw the antipsychotic prescribed when TD was first observed and to substitute another drug. The use of clozapine[23] is probably best supported in this regard, but quetiapine, another weak striatal dopamine antagonist, is also effective[26–32]. Olanzapine is also an option,[33,34] while there are a few supporting data for risperidone[35] and aripiprazole[36,37].

Treatment – additional agents

Switching or withdrawing antipsychotics is not always effective and so additional agents are often used. The table below describes the most frequently prescribed add-on drugs for TD.

Drug	Comments
Tetrabenazine[38]	Only licensed treatment for TD in UK. Has antipsychotic properties but reported to be depressogenic. Drowsiness and akathisia also occur[39]. Dose is 25–200 mg/day
Benzodiazepines[23,24]	Widely used and considered effective but Cochrane review suggests benzodiazepines are 'experimental'[40]. Intermittant use may be necessary to avoid tolerance to effects. Most used are clonazepam 1–4 mg/day and diazepam 6–25 mg/day
Vitamin E[41,42]	Numerous studies but efficacy remains to be conclusively established. Dose is in the range 400–1600 IU/day. (IU to mg equivalence varies – see individual product information)

Schizophrenia

Treatment – other possible options

The large number of proposed treatments for TD undoubtedly reflects the somewhat limited effectiveness of standard remedies. The following table lists some of these putative treatments in alphabetical order. Supporting evidence is at best modest in each case.

Drug	Comments
Amino acids[43]	Use is supported by a small randomised, placebo-controlled trial. Low risk of toxicity
Botulinum toxin[44–46]	Case reports of success for localised dyskinesia
Calcium antagonists[47]	A few published studies but not widely used. Cochrane is dismissive
Donepezil[48–50]	Supported by a single open study and case series. One negative RCT (n = 12). Dose is 10 mg/day
Fish oils[51,52]	Very limited support for use of EPA at dose of 2 g/day
Gabapentin[53]	Data derived almost entirely from a single research group. Adds weight to theory that GABAergic mechansims improve TD. Dose is 900–1200 mg/day
Levetiracetam[54–56]	Two published reports. One RCT. Dose up to 3000 mg/day
Melatonin[57]	Use is supported by a well conducted trial. Usually well tolerated. Dose is 10 mg/day
Naltrexone[58]	May be effective when added to benzodiazepines. Well tolerated. Dose is 200 mg/day
Ondansetron[59,60]	Limited evidence but low toxicity. Dose – up to 12 mg/day
Pyridoxine[61]	Supported by a well conducted trial. Dose – up to 400 mg/day
Quercetin[62]	Plant compound which is thought to be an antioxidant. No human studies in TD but widely used in other conditions
Sodium oxybate[63]	One case report. Dose was 8 g/day
Transcranial magnetic stimulation[64] (rTMS)	Single case report

References

1. Halliday J et al. Nithsdale Schizophrenia Surveys 23: movement disorders. 20-year review. Br J Psychiatry 2002; 181:422–427.
2. Kane JM. Tardive dyskinesia circa 2006. Am J Psychiatry 2006; 163:1316–1318.
3. de Leon J. The effect of atypical versus typical antipsychotics on tardive dyskinesia: a naturalistic study. Eur Arch Psychiatry Clin Neurosci 2007; 257:169–172.
4. Eberhard J et al. Tardive dyskinesia and antipsychotics: a 5-year longitudinal study of frequency, correlates and course. Int Clin Psychopharmacol 2006; 21:35–42.
5. Ascher-Svanum H et al. Tardive dyskinesia and the 3-year course of schizophrenia: results from a large, prospective, naturalistic study. J Clin Psychiatry 2008; 69:1580–1588.
6. Chong SA et al. Mortality rates among patients with schizophrenia and tardive dyskinesia. J Clin Psychopharmacol 2009; 29:5–8.
7. Beasley C et al. Randomised double-blind comparison of the incidence of tardive dyskinesia in patients with schizophrenia during long-term treatment with olanzapine or haloperidol. Br J Psychiatry 1999; 174:23–30.
8. Glazer WM. Expected incidence of tardive dyskinesia associated with atypical antipsychotics. J Clin Psychiatry 2000;61 Suppl 4:21–26.
9. Correll CU et al. Lower risk for tardive dyskinesia associated with second-generation antipsychotics: a systematic review of 1-year studies. Am J Psychiatry 2004; 161:414–425.
10. Dolder CR et al. Incidence of tardive dyskinesia with typical versus atypical antipsychotics in very high risk patients. Biol Psychiatry 2003; 53:1142–1145.
11. Correll CU et al. Tardive dyskinesia and new antipsychotics. Curr Opin Psychiatry 2008; 21:151–156.
12. Karama S et al. Tardive dyskinesia following brief exposure to risperidone – a case study (Letter). Eur Psychiatry 2004; 19:391–392.
13. Gafoor R et al. Three case reports of emergent dyskinesia with clozapine. Eur Psychiatry 2003; 18:260–261.
14. Bhanji NH et al. Tardive dyskinesia associated with olanzapine in a neuroleptic-naive patient with schizophrenia (Letter). Can J Psychiatry 2004; 49:343.
15. Keck ME et al. Ziprasidone-related tardive dyskinesia. Am J Psychiatry 2004; 161:175–176.
16. Maytal G et al. Aripiprazole-related tardive dyskinesia. CNS Spectr 2006; 11:435–439.
17. Fountoulakis KN et al. Amisulpride-induced tardive dyskinesia. Schizophr Res 2006; 88:232–234.
18. Sachdev P. Early extrapyramidal side-effects as risk factors for later tardive dyskinesia: a prospective study. Aust N Z J Psychiatry 2004; 38:445–449.

19. Miller DD et al. Clinical correlates of tardive dyskinesia in schizophrenia: baseline data from the CATIE schizophrenia trial. Schizophr Res 2005; 80:33–43.
20. Tenback DE et al. Evidence that early extrapyramidal symptoms predict later tardive dyskinesia: a prospective analysis of 10,000 patients in the European Schizophrenia Outpatient Health Outcomes (SOHO) Study. Am J Psychiatry 2006; 163:1438–1440.
21. Oosthuizen PP et al. Incidence of tardive dyskinesia in first-episode psychosis patients treated with low-dose haloperidol. J Clin Psychiatry 2003; 64:1075–1080.
22. Kenney C et al. Metoclopramide, an increasingly recognized cause of tardive dyskinesia. J Clin Pharmacol 2008; 48:379–384.
23. Duncan D et al. Tardive dyskinesia: how is it prevented and treated? Psychiatr Bull 1997; 21:422–425.
24. Simpson GM. The treatment of tardive dyskinesia and tardive dystonia. J Clin Psychiatry 2000;61 Suppl 4:39–44.
25. Soares-Weiser K et al. Neuroleptic reduction and/or cessation and neuroleptics as specific treatments for tardive dyskinesia. Cochrane Database Syst Rev 2006; CD000459.
26. Vesely C et al. Remission of severe tardive dyskinesia in a schizophrenic patient treated with the atypical antipsychotic substance quetiapine. Int Clin Psychopharmacol 2000; 15:57–60.
27. Alptekin K et al. Quetiapine-induced improvement of tardive dyskinesia in three patients with schizophrenia. Int Clin Psychopharmacol 2002; 17: 263–264.
28. Nelson MW et al. Adjunctive quetiapine decreases symptoms of tardive dyskinesia in a patient taking risperidone. Clin Neuropharmacol 2003; 26: 297–298.
29. Emsley R et al. A single-blind, randomized trial comparing quetiapine and haloperidol in the treatment of tardive dyskinesia. J Clin Psychiatry 2004; 65:696–701.
30. Bressan RA et al. Atypical antipsychotic drugs and tardive dyskinesia: relevance of D2 receptor affinity. J Psychopharmacol 2004; 18:124–127.
31. Sacchetti E et al. Quetiapine, clozapine, and olanzapine in the treatment of tardive dyskinesia induced by first-generation antipsychotics: a 124-week case report. Int Clin Psychopharmacol 2003; 18:357–359.
32. Gourzis P et al. Quetiapine in the treatment of focal tardive dystonia induced by other atypical antipsychotics: a report of 2 cases. Clin Neuropharmacol 2005; 28:195–196.
33. Soutullo CA et al. Olanzapine in the treatment of tardive dyskinesia: a report of two cases. J Clin Psychopharmacol 1999; 19:100–101.
34. Kinon BJ et al. Olanzapine treatment for tardive dyskinesia in schizophrenia patients: a prospective clinical trial with patients randomized to blinded dose reduction periods. Prog Neuropsychopharmacol Biol Psychiatry 2004; 28:985–996.
35. Bai YM et al. Risperidone for severe tardive dyskinesia: a 12-week randomized, double-blind, placebo-controlled study. J Clin Psychiatry 2003; 64: 1342–1348.
36. Duggal HS. Aripiprazole-induced improvement in tardive dyskinesia. Can J Psychiatry 2003; 48:771–772.
37. Grant MJ et al. Possible improvement of neuroleptic-associated tardive dyskinesia during treatment with aripiprazole. Ann Pharmacother 2005; 39:1953.
38. Jankovic J et al. Long-term effects of tetrabenazine in hyperkinetic movement disorders. Neurology 1997; 48:358–362.
39. Kenney C et al. Long-term tolerability of tetrabenazine in the treatment of hyperkinetic movement disorders. Mov Disord 2007; 22:193–197.
40. Bhoopathi PS et al. Benzodiazepines for neuroleptic-induced tardive dyskinesia. Cochrane Database Syst Rev 2006; 3:CD000205.
41. Adler LA et al. Vitamin E treatment for tardive dyskinesia: adrenoceptor. Br J Psychiatry 1995; 167:412.
42. Zhang XY et al. The effect of vitamin E treatment on tardive dyskinesia and blood superoxide dismutase: a double-blind placebo-controlled trial. J Clin Psychopharmacol 2004; 24:83–86.
43. Richardson MA et al. Efficacy of the branched-chain amino acids in the treatment of tardive dyskinesia in men. Am J Psychiatry 2003; 160:1117–1124.
44. Tarsy D et al. An open-label study of botulinum toxin A for treatment of tardive dystonia. Clin Neuropharmacol 1997; 20:90–93.
45. Brashear A et al. Comparison of treatment of tardive dystonia and idiopathic cervical dystonia with botulinum toxin type A. Mov Disord 1998; 13: 158–161.
46. Hennings JM et al. Successful treatment of tardive lingual dystonia with botulinum toxin: case report and review of the literature. Prog Neuropsychopharmacol Biol Psychiatry 2008; 32:1167–1171.
47. Soares-Weiser K et al. Calcium channel blockers for neuroleptic-induced tardive dyskinesia. Cochrane Database Syst Rev 2004; CD000206.
48. Caroff SN et al. Treatment of tardive dyskinesia with donepezil. J Clin Psychiatry 2001; 62:128–129.
49. Bergman J et al. Beneficial effect of donepezil in the treatment of elderly patients with tardive movement disorders. J Clin Psychiatry 2005; 66:107–110.
50. Ogunmefun A et al. Effect of donepezil on tardive dyskinesia. J Clin Psychopharmacol 2009; 29:102–104.
51. Emsley R et al. The effects of eicosapentaenoic acid in the treatment of tardive dyskinesia: a randomized, placebo-controlled trial. Schizophr Res 2006; 84:112–120.
52. Vaddadi K et al. Tardive dyskinesia and essential fatty acids. Int Rev Psychiatry 2006; 18:133–143.
53. Hardoy MC et al. Gabapentin in antipsychotic-induced tardive dyskinesia: results of 1-year follow-up. J Affect Disord 2003; 75:125–130.
54. McGavin CL et al. Levetiracetam as a treatment for tardive dyskinesia: a case report. Neurology 2003; 61:419.
55. Meco G et al. Levetiracetam in tardive dyskinesia. Clin Neuropharmacol 2006; 29:265–268.
56. Woods SW et al. Effects of levetiracetam on tardive dyskinesia: a randomized, double-blind, placebo-controlled study. J Clin Psychiatry 2008; 69: 546–554.
57. Shamir E et al. Melatonin treatment for tardive dyskinesia: a double-blind, placebo-controlled, crossover study. Arch Gen Psychiatry 2001; 58: 1049–1052.
58. Wonodi I et al. Naltrexone treatment of tardive dyskinesia in patients with schizophrenia. J Clin Psychopharmacol 2004; 24:441–445.
59. Sirota P et al. Use of the selective serotonin 3 receptor antagonist ondansetron in the treatment of neuroleptic-induced tardive dyskinesia. Am J Psychiatry 2000; 157:287–289.
60. Naidu PS et al. Reversal of neuroleptic-induced orofacial dyskinesia by 5-HT3 receptor antagonists. Eur J Pharmacol 2001; 420:113–117.
61. Lerner V et al. Vitamin B(6) in the treatment of tardive dyskinesia: a double-blind, placebo-controlled, crossover study. Am J Psychiatry 2001; 158: 1511–1514.
62. Naidu PS et al. Reversal of haloperidol-induced orofacial dyskinesia by quercetin, a bioflavonoid. Psychopharmacology 2003; 167:418–423.
63. Berner JE. A case of sodium oxybate treatment of tardive dyskinesia and bipolar disorder. J Clin Psychiatry 2008; 69:862.
64. Brambilla P et al. Transient improvement of tardive dyskinesia induced with rTMS. Neurology 2003; 61:1155.

Further reading

Paleacu D et al. Tetrabenazine treatment in movement disorders. Clin Neuropharmacol 2004; 27:230–233.

Schizophrenia

Neuroleptic malignant syndrome (NMS)

NMS is a rare but potentially serious or even fatal adverse effect of all antipsychotics. NMS is a syndrome largely of sympathetic hyperactivity occurring as a result of dopaminergic antagonism in the context of psychological stressors and genetic predisposition[1]. Although widely seen as an acute, severe syndrome, NMS may, in many cases, have few signs and symptoms; 'full-blown' NMS may thus represent the extreme of a range of non-malignant related symptoms[2]. Certainly, asymptomatic rises in plasma creatine kinase (CK) are fairly common[3].

The incidence and mortality rate of NMS are difficult to establish and probably vary as drug use changes and recognition increases. It has been estimated that fewer than 1% of all patients treated with conventional antipsychotics will experience NMS[4]. Incidence figures for SGA drugs are not available, but all have been reported to be associated with the syndrome[5–12], even newer drugs like ziprasidone[13,14], aripiprazole[15–18], paliperidone[19] and risperidone injection[20]. Mortality may be lower with SGAs[21]. NMS is also very rarely seen with other drugs such as antidepressants[22–25] and lithium[26]. Combinations of antipsychotics and SSRIs[27] and cholinesterase inhibitors[28,29] may increase the risk of NMS.

Table	Neuroleptic malignant syndrome
Signs and symptoms[1,4,30,31] (presentation varies considerably)[32]	Fever, diaphoresis, rigidity, confusion, fluctuating consciousness
	Fluctuating blood pressure, tachycardia
	Elevated creatine kinase, leukocytosis, altered liver function tests
Risk factors[30,31,33–35]	High-potency typical drugs, recent or rapid dose increase, rapid dose reduction, abrupt withdrawal of anticholinergics
	Psychosis, organic brain disease, alcoholism, Parkinson's disease, hyperthyroidism, psychomotor agitation, mental retardation
	Agitation, dehydration
Treatments[4,30,36–39]	**In the psychiatric unit:**
	Withdraw antipsychotics, monitor temperature, pulse, BP. Consider benzodiazepines if not already prescribed – IM lorazepam has been used[40]
	In the medical/A&E unit:
	Rehydration, bromocriptine + dantrolene, sedation with benzodiazepines, artificial ventilation if required
	L-dopa, apomorphine, and carbamazepine have also been used, among many other drugs. Consider ECT for treatment of psychosis
Restarting antipsychotics[30,36,41]	Antipsychotic treatment will be required in most instances and rechallenge is associated with acceptable risk
	Stop antipsychotics for at least 5 days, preferably longer. Allow time for symptoms and signs to resolve completely
	Begin with very small dose and increase very slowly with close monitoring of temperature, pulse and blood pressure. CK monitoring may be used, but is controversial[31,42]. Close monitoring of physical and biochemical parameters is effective in reducing progression to full-blown NMS[43,44].
	Consider using an antipsychotic structurally unrelated to that associated with NMS or a drug with low dopamine affinity (quetiapine or clozapine). Aripiprazole may also be considered[45]
	Avoid depots and high potency conventional antipsychotics

References

1. Gurrera RJ. Sympathoadrenal hyperactivity and the etiology of neuroleptic malignant syndrome. Am J Psychiatry 1999; 156:169–180.
2. Bristow MF et al. How "malignant" is the neuroleptic malignant syndrome? BMJ 1993; 307:1223–1224.
3. Meltzer HY et al. Marked elevations of serum creatine kinase activity associated with antipsychotic drug treatment. Neuropsychopharmacology 1996; 15:395–405.
4. Guze BH et al. Current concepts. Neuroleptic malignant syndrome. N Engl J Med 1985; 313:163–166.
5. Sing KJ et al. Neuroleptic malignant syndrome and quetiapine (Letter). Am J Psychiatry 2002; 159:149–150.
6. Suh H et al. Neuroleptic malignant syndrome and low-dose olanzapine (Letter). Am J Psychiatry 2003; 160:796.
7. Gallarda T et al. Neuroleptic malignant syndrome in an 72-year-old-man with Alzheimer's disease: A case report and review of the literature. Eur Neuropsychopharmacol 2000;10 (Suppl 3):357.
8. Stanley AK et al. Possible neuroleptic malignant syndrome with quetiapine. Br J Psychiatry 2000; 176:497.
9. Sierra-Biddle D et al. Neuroleptic malignant syndrome and olanzapine. J Clin Psychopharmacol 2000; 20:704–705.
10. Hasan S et al. Novel antipsychotics and the neuroleptic malignant syndrome: a review and critique. Am J Psychiatry 1998; 155:1113–1116.
11. Tsai JH et al. Zotepine-induced catatonia as a precursor in the progression to neuroleptic malignant syndrome. Pharmacotherapy 2005; 25:1156–1159.
12. Gortney JS et al. Neuroleptic malignant syndrome secondary to quetiapine. Ann Pharmacother 2009; 43:785–791.
13. Leibold J et al. Neuroleptic malignant syndrome associated with ziprasidone in an adolescent. Clin Ther 2004; 26:1105–1108.
14. Borovicka MC et al. Ziprasidone- and lithium-induced neuroleptic malignant syndrome. Ann Pharmacother 2006; 40:139–142.
15. Spalding S et al. Aripiprazole and atypical neuroleptic malignant syndrome. J Am Acad Child Adolesc Psychiatry 2004; 43:1457–1458.
16. Chakraborty N et al. Aripiprazole and neuroleptic malignant syndrome. Int Clin Psychopharmacol 2004; 19:351–353.
17. Rodriguez OP et al. A case report of neuroleptic malignant syndrome without fever in a patient given aripiprazole. J Okla State Med Assoc 2006; 99:435–438.
18. Srephichit S et al. Neuroleptic malignant syndrome and aripiprazole in an antipsychotic-naive patient. J Clin Psychopharmacol 2006; 26:94–95.
19. Duggal HS. Possible neuroleptic malignant syndrome associated with paliperidone. J Neuropsychiatry Clin Neurosci 2007; 19:477–478.
20. Mall GD et al. Catatonia and mild neuroleptic malignant syndrome after initiation of long-acting injectable risperidone: case report. J Clin Psychopharmacol 2008; 28:572–573.
21. Ananth J et al. Neuroleptic malignant syndrome and atypical antipsychotic drugs. J Clin Psychiatry 2004; 65:464–470.
22. Kontaxakis VP et al. Neuroleptic malignant syndrome after addition of paroxetine to olanzapine. J Clin Psychopharmacol 2003; 23:671–672.
23. Young C. A case of neuroleptic malignant syndrome and serotonin disturbance. J Clin Psychopharmacol 1997; 17:65–66.
24. June R et al. Neuroleptic malignant syndrome associated with nortriptyline. Am J Emerg Med 1999; 17:736–737.
25. Lu TC et al. Neuroleptic malignant syndrome after the use of venlafaxine in a patient with generalized anxiety disorder. J Formos Med Assoc 2006; 105:90–93.
26. Gill J et al. Acute lithium intoxication and neuroleptic malignant syndrome. Pharmacotherapy 2003; 23:811–815.
27. Stevens DL. Association between selective serotonin-reuptake inhibitors, second-generation antipsychotics, and neuroleptic malignant syndrome. Ann Pharmacother 2008; 42:1290–1297.
28. Stevens DL et al. Olanzapine-associated neuroleptic malignant syndrome in a patient receiving concomitant rivastigmine therapy. Pharmacotherapy 2008; 28:403–405.
29. Warwick TC et al. Neuroleptic malignant syndrome variant in a patient receiving donepezil and olanzapine. Nat Clin Pract Neurol 2008; 4:170–174.
30. Levenson JL. Neuroleptic malignant syndrome. Am J Psychiatry 1985; 142:1137–1145.
31. Hermesh H et al. High serum creatinine kinase level: possible risk factor for neuroleptic malignant syndrome. J Clin Psychopharmacol 2002; 22:252–256.
32. Picard LS et al. Atypical neuroleptic malignant syndrome: diagnostic controversies and considerations. Pharmacotherapy 2008; 28:530–535.
33. Viejo LF et al. Risk factors in neuroleptic malignant syndrome. A case-control study. Acta Psychiatr Scand 2003; 107:45–49.
34. Spivak B et al. Neuroleptic malignant syndrome during abrupt reduction of neuroleptic treatment. Acta Psychiatr Scand 1990; 81:168–169.
35. Spivak B et al. Neuroleptic malignant syndrome associated with abrupt withdrawal of anticholinergic agents. Int Clin Psychopharmacol 1996; 11:207–209.
36. Olmsted TR. Neuroleptic malignant syndrome: guidelines for treatment and reinstitution of neuroleptics. South Med J 1988; 81:888–891.
37. Shoop SA et al. Carbidopa/levodopa in the treatment of neuroleptic malignant syndrome (Letter). Ann Pharmacother 1997; 31:119.
38. Terao T. Carbamazepine in the treatment of neuroleptic malignant syndrome (Letter). Biol Psychiatry 1999; 45:381–382.
39. Lattanzi L et al. Subcutaneous apomorphine for neuroleptic malignant syndrome. Am J Psychiatry 2006; 163:1450–1451.
40. Francis A et al. Is lorazepam a treatment for neuroleptic malignant syndrome? CNS Spectr 2000; 5:54–57.
41. Wells AJ et al. Neuroleptic rechallenge after neuroleptic malignant syndrome: case report and literature review. Drug Intel Clin Pharm 1988; 22:475–480.
42. Klein JP et al. Massive creatine kinase elevations with quetiapine: report of two cases. Pharmacopsychiatry 2006; 39:39–40.
43. Shiloh R et al. Precautionary measures reduce risk of definite neuroleptic malignant syndrome in newly typical neuroleptic-treated schizophrenia inpatients. Int Clin Psychopharmacol 2003; 18:147–149.
44. Hatch CD et al. Failed challenge with quetiapine after neuroleptic malignant syndrome with conventional antipsychotics. Pharmacotherapy 2001; 21:1003–1006.
45. Trutia A et al. Neuroleptic rechallenge with aripiprazole in a patient with previously documented neuroleptic malignant syndrome. J Psychiatr Pract 2008; 14:398–402.

Catatonia

Catatonia is a disorder characterised by movement abnormalities usually associated with schizophrenia, mood disorders and, less frequently, general medical conditions. A number of neurological disorders, endocrine and metabolic disorders, infections, drug withdrawal and toxic drug states can precipitate catatonic symptoms[1-3]. The clinical picture is characterised by marked psychomotor disturbance that may involve motoric immobility or excessive motor activity, extreme negativism, mutism, peculiarities of voluntary movement, echolalia or echopraxia.

The term lethal catatonia has now been replaced by malignant catatonia, which is used when motor symptoms of catatonia are accompanied by autonomic instability or hyperthermia. This potentially fatal condition cannot be distinguished either clinically or by laboratory testing from neuroleptic malignant syndrome (NMS), leading to the conclusion that NMS is a variant form of malignant catatonia[4]. In addition, both catatonia and antipsychotic treatment are recognised as a risk factor for the development of NMS[5].

Prompt treatment of catatonia is crucial and may prevent complications, which include, dehydration, venous thrombosis, pulmonary embolism and pneumonia[6]. Numerous studies and case reports indicate that benzodiazepines are rapidly effective, safe and easily administered and are therefore regarded as first-line treatment[7]. They may act by increasing GABAergic transmission or reducing levels of brain-derived neurotropic factor[8]. There is most experience with lorazepam. Many patients will respond to standard doses (up to 4 mg daily), but repeated and higher doses (between 8 and 24 mg per day of lorazepam) may be needed[9]. Approximately 80% of catatonic patients will respond to benzodiazepine treatment and response is usually seen within 3–7 days.

Patients with schizophrenia are somewhat less likely to respond to benzodiazepines, with response in the range of 40–50%[7]. A double-blind, placebo-controlled, cross-over trial with lorazepam up to 6 mg/day demonstrated no effect on catatonic symptoms in patients with chronic schizophrenia[10]. If catatonic symptoms do not resolve rapidly with lorazepam, ECT treatment is indicated[11]. The response of catatonic symptoms to ECT is about 85%. The effect of ECT is probably greater than that seen with benzodiazepines[12]. As with benzodiazepines, response to ECT may be lower in patients with schizophrenia than in patients with mood disorders.

The use of antipsychotics in patients with catatonic symptoms is controversial. Some authors recommend that antipsychotics should be avoided altogether in catatonic patients, although there are case reports of successful treatment with aripiprazole, risperidone, olanzapine, ziprasidone and clozapine[13-18]. During the acute phase of catatonia, the use of an antipsychotic should be avoided, more so in cases of malignant catatonia where their use may be harmful. In patients with chronic persistent catatonic symptoms, treatment of the underlying cause is necessary. SGAs, because of their reduced potential for inducing movement disorders, may be used in those patients with schizophrenia who have a predisposition to catatonia, although clinicians should be vigilant to the signs of NMS and be ready for prompt discontinuation of any antipsychotic. Quetiapine is cautiously recommended in these patients on the basis that it is a weak D_2 antagonist with a short half-life.

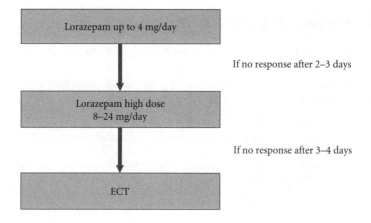

Lorazepam up to 4 mg/day

If no response after 2–3 days

Lorazepam high dose
8–24 mg/day

If no response after 3–4 days

ECT

References

1. Lee J et al. Catatonia and psychosis associated with sibutramine: a case report and pathophysiologic correlation. J Psychosom Res 2008; 64:107–109.
2. Bastiampillai T et al. Clozapine-withdrawal catatonia. Aust N Z J Psychiatry 2009; 43:283–284.
3. Gunduz A et al. Postictal catatonia in a schizophrenic patient and electroconvulsive treatment. J ECT 2008; 24:166–167.
4. Taylor MA et al. Catatonia in psychiatric classification: a home of its own. Am J Psychiatry 2003; 160:1233–1241.
5. White DA et al. Catatonia: harbinger of the neuroleptic malignant syndrome. Br J Psychiatry 1991; 158:419–421.
6. Petrides G et al. Synergism of lorazepam and electroconvulsive therapy in the treatment of catatonia. Biol Psychiatry 1997; 42:375–381.
7. Rosebush PI et al. Catatonia: re-awakening to a forgotten disorder. Mov Disord 1999; 14:395–397.
8. Huang TL et al. Lorazepam reduces the serum brain-derived neurotrophic factor level in schizophrenia patients with catatonia. Prog Neuropsychopharmacol Biol Psychiatry 2009; 33:158–159.
9. Fink M et al. Neuroleptic malignant syndrome is malignant catatonia, warranting treatments efficacious for catatonia. Prog Neuropsychopharmacol Biol Psychiatry 2006; 30:1182–1183.
10. Ungvari GS et al. Lorazepam for chronic catatonia: a randomized, double-blind, placebo-controlled cross-over study. Psychopharmacology 1999; 142:393–398.
11. Bush G et al. Catatonia. II. Treatment with lorazepam and electroconvulsive therapy. Acta Psychiatr Scand 1996; 93:137–143.
12. Hawkins JM et al. Somatic treatment of catatonia. Int J Psychiatry Med 1995; 25:345–369.
13. Van Den EF et al. The use of atypical antipsychotics in the treatment of catatonia. Eur Psychiatry 2005; 20:422–429.
14. Caroff SN et al. Movement disorders associated with atypical antipsychotic drugs. J Clin Psychiatry 2002;63 Suppl 4:12–19.
15. Guzman CS et al. Treatment of periodic catatonia with atypical antipsychotic, olanzapine. Psychiatry Clin Neurosci 2008; 62:482.
16. Babington PW et al. Treatment of catatonia with olanzapine and amantadine. Psychosomatics 2007; 48:534–536.
17. Bastiampillai T et al. Catatonia resolution and aripiprazole. Aust N Z J Psychiatry 2008; 42:907.
18. Strawn JR et al. Successful treatment of catatonia with aripiprazole in an adolescent with psychosis. J Child Adolesc Psychopharmacol 2007; 17: 733–735.

Antipsychotics and hypertension

There are two ways in which antipsychotic drugs may be associated with the development or worsening of hypertension:

- Slow steady rise in blood pressure over time. This may be associated with weight gain. Being overweight increases the risk of developing hypertension. The magnitude of the effect has been modelled using the Framingham data; for every 30 people who gain 4 kg, one will develop hypertension over the next 10 years[1]. Note that this is a very modest weight gain, the majority of patients treated with some antipsychotics gain more than this, increasing further the risk of developing hypertension.
- Unpredictable rapid sharp increase in blood pressure on starting a new drug or increasing the dose. Increases in blood pressure occur shortly after starting, ranging from within hours of the first dose to a month. The information below relates to the pharmacological mechanism behind this and the antipsychotic drugs that are most implicated.

Postural hypotension is commonly associated with antipsychotic drugs that are antagonists at postsynaptic adrenergic α_1 receptors. Examples include clozapine, chlorpromazine, quetiapine and risperidone. Some antipsychotics are also antagonists at pre-synaptic α_2 adrenergic receptors; this can lead to increased release of norepinephrine, increased vagal activity and vaso-constriction. As all antipsychotics that are antagonists at α_2 receptors are also antagonists at α_1 receptors, the end result for any given patient can be difficult to predict, but for a very small number it can be hypertension. Some antipsychotics are more commonly implicated than others, but individual patient factors are undoubtedly also important.

Receptor binding studies have demonstrated that clozapine, olanzapine and risperidone have the highest affinity for α_2 adrenergic receptors[2] so it could be predicted that these drugs would be most likely to cause hypertension. Most case reports implicate clozapine[3-9] with some clearly describing normal blood pressure before clozapine was introduced, a sharp rise during treatment and return to normal when clozapine was discontinued. Blood pressure has also been reported to rise again on rechallenge and increased plasma catecholamines have been noted in some cases. Single case reports also implicate aripiprazole[10], sulpiride[11], risperidone[8], quetiapine[8] and ziprasidone[12].

Data available through the CSM yellow card system indicate that clozapine is the antipsychotic drug most associated with hypertension. There are a small number of reports with aripiprazole, olanzapine, quetiapine and risperidone[13].

No antipsychotic is contra-indicated in essential hypertension but extreme care is needed when clozapine is prescribed. Concomitant treatment with SSRIs may increase risk of hypertension, possibly via inhibition of the metabolism of the antipsychotic[8]. It is also (theoretically) possible that α_2 antagonism may be at least partially responsible for clozapine-induced tachycardia and nausea[14].

References

1. Fontaine KR et al. Estimating the consequences of anti-psychotic induced weight gain on health and mortality rate. Psychiatry Res 2001; 101:277–288.
2. Abi-Dargham A et al. Mechanisms of action of second generation antipsychotic drugs in schizophrenia: insights from brain imaging studies. Eur Psychiatry 2005; 20:15–27.
3. Gupta S et al. Paradoxical hypertension associated with clozapine. Am J Psychiatry 1994; 151:148.
4. Krentz AJ et al. Drug Points: Pseudophaeochromocytoma syndrome associated with clozapine. BMJ 2001; 322:1213.
5. George TP et al. Hypertension after initiation of clozapine. Am J Psychiatry 1996; 153:1368–1369.
6. Prasad SE et al. Pseudophaeochromocytoma associated with clozapine treatment. Ir J Psychol Med 2003; 20:132–134.
7. Shiwach RS. Treatment of clozapine induced hypertension and possible mechanisms. Clin Neuropharmacol 1998; 21:139–140.
8. Coulter D. Atypical antipsychotics may cause hypertension. 2003. http://www.medsafe.govt.nz/
9. Li JK et al. Clozapine: a mimicry of phaeochromocytoma. Aust N Z J Psychiatry 1997; 31:889–891.
10. Borras L et al. Hypertension and aripiprazole. Am J Psychiatry 2005; 162:2392.
11. Mayer RD et al. Acute hypertensive episode induced by sulpiride – a case report. Hum Psychopharmacol 1989; 4:149–150.
12. Villanueva N et al. Probable association between ziprasidone and worsening hypertension. Pharmacotherapy 2006; 26:1352–1357.
13. Medicines and Healthcare Products Regulatory Agency. Reporting suspected adverse drug reactions. http://www.mhra.gov.uk/home
14. Pandharipande P et al. Alpha-2 agonists: can they modify the outcomes in the Postanesthesia Care Unit? Curr Drug Targets 2005; 6:749–754.

Schizophrenia

Antipsychotic-induced weight gain

Antipsychotics have long been recognised as weight-inducing agents. Suggested mechanisms include $5HT_{2C}$ antagonism, H_1 antagonism, hyperprolactinaemia and increased serum leptin (leading to leptin desensitisation)[1–4]. There is no evidence that drugs exert any direct metabolic effect: weight gain seems to result from increased food intake and, in some cases, reduced energy expenditure[5,6]. Risk of weight gain appears to be related to clinical response[7] and may also have a genetic basis[8,9].

All available antipsychotics have been associated with weight gain, although mean weight gained varies substantially between drugs. With all drugs, some patients gain no weight. Assessment of relative risk is made difficult by the poor quality of available data and the relative scarcity of long-term data. The following table suggests approximate relative risk of weight gain and mean weight gain[10–12].

See following section for advice on treating drug-induced weight gain.

Table Antipsychotic-induced weight gain

Drug	Risk/extent of weight gain
Clozapine Olanzapine	High
Chlorpromazine Iloperidone Quetiapine Risperidone Zotepine	Moderate
Amisulpride Asenapine Aripiprazole Bifeprunox Haloperidol Sulpiride Trifluoperazine Ziprasidone	Low

References

1. Monteleone P, Fabrazzo M, Tortorella A et al. Pronounced early increase in circulating leptin predicts a lower weight gain during clozapine treatment. J Clin Psychopharmacol 2002; 22:424–426.
2. Herran A, Garcia-Unzueta MT, Amado JA et al. Effects of long-term treatment with antipsychotics on serum leptin levels. Br J Psychiatry 2001; 179:59–62.
3. McIntyre RS, Mancini DA, Basile VS. Mechanisms of antipsychotic-induced weight gain. J Clin Psychiatry 2001;62 Suppl 23:23–29.
4. Kroeze WK, Hufeisen SJ, Popadak BA et al. H1-histamine receptor affinity predicts short-term weight gain for typical and atypical antipsychotic drugs. Neuropsychopharmacology 2003; 28:519–526.
5. Virkkunen M, Wahlbeck K, Rissanen A et al. Decrease of energy expenditure causes weight increase in olanzapine treatment – a case study. Pharmacopsychiatry 2002; 35:124–126.
6. Sharpe JK, Stedman TJ, Byrne NM et al. Energy expenditure and physical activity in clozapine use: implications for weight management. Aust N Z J Psychiatry 2006; 40:810–814.
7. Czobor P, Volavka J, Sheitman B et al. Antipsychotic-induced weight gain and therapeutic response: a differential association. J Clin Psychopharmacol 2002; 22:244–251.
8. Basile VS, Masellis M, McIntyre RS et al. Genetic dissection of atypical antipsychotic-induced weight gain: novel preliminary data on the pharmacogenetic puzzle. J Clin Psychiatry 2001;62 Suppl 23:45–66.
9. Reynolds GP, Zhang Z, Zhang X. Polymorphism of the promoter region of the serotonin 5-HT(2C) receptor gene and clozapine-induced weight gain. Am J Psychiatry 2003; 160:677–679.
10. Allison D, Mentore J, Heo M et al. Antipsychotic-induced weight gain: A comprehensive research synthesis. Am J Psychiatry 1999; 156:1686–1696.
11. Bishara D et al. Upcoming agents for the treatment of schizophrenia. Mechanism of action, efficacy and tolerability. Drugs 2008; 68:2269–2296.
12. Taylor DM, McAskill R. Atypical antipsychotics and weight gain – a systematic review. Acta Psychiatr Scand 2000; 101:416–432

Further reading

Consensus Development Conference on Antipsychotic Drugs and Obesity and Diabetes. Diabetes Care 2004; 27:596–601.

Treatment of drug-induced weight gain

Weight gain is an important adverse effect of nearly all antipsychotics with obvious consequences for self-image, morbidity and mortality. Prevention and treatment are therefore matters of clinical urgency.

Patients starting antipsychotic treatment or changing drugs should, as an absolute minimum, be weighed and their weight clearly recorded. Estimates of body mass index and waist circumference should, ideally, also be made at baseline and later at least every 6 months[1]. Weekly monitoring of weight is recommended early in treatment – for the first 3 months at least. There is evidence that very few UK patients have anywhere near adequate monitoring of weight[2]. Clearly, monitoring of weight parameters is essential to assess the value of preventative and remedial measures.

Most of the relevant literature in this area relates to attempts at reversing antipsychotic-related weight gain[3]. There are relatively few data suggesting that early interventions can prevent weight gain[4–6] although this seems a more sensible approach.

When weight gain occurs, initial options involve switching drugs or instituting behavioural programmes (or both). Switching always presents a risk of relapse but there is fairly strong support for switching to aripiprazole[7–11] or ziprasidone[12,13] as a method for reversing weight gain. It is possible that switching to other drugs with a low propensity for weight gain is also beneficial[14,15]. Another option is to add aripiprazole to existing treatment – weight loss has been observed when aripiprazole was added to clozapine[16–18].

A variety of behavioural methods have been proposed and evaluated with fairly good results[19]. Methods include calorie restriction[20], low-glycaemic-index diet[21], Weight Watchers[22] and diet/exercise programmes[3,5,6,23–26]. Pharmacological methods should be considered only where behavioural methods or switching have failed or where obesity presents clear, immediate physical risk to the patient. Some options are described in the table.

Table   Drug treatment of antipsychotic-induced weight gain

Drug	Comments
Amantadine[27–30] (100–300 mg/day)	May attenuate olanzapine-related weight gain. Seems to be well tolerated. May (theoretically, at least) exacerbate psychosis
Bupropion[31,32] (amfebutamone)	Seems to be effective in obesity when combined with calorie-restricted diets. Few data of its effects on drug-induced weight gain. Note that pharmacology is essentially that of a dual-acting antidepressant. Caution in patients with bipolar illness
Fluoxetine[33,34] (and other SSRIs)	Probably not effective
H$_2$ antagonists[35–38] (e.g. nizatidine 300 mg BD or famotidine 40 mg/day)	Some positive studies but most negative. Effect, if any, is small. Few data supporting a reversal of weight gain
Metformin[39–45] (500 mg tds)	Now a substantial database supporting the use of metformin in both reducing and reversing weight gain caused by antipsychotics (mainly olanzapine). Beneficial effects on other metabolic parameters. Some negative studies. Ideal for those with weight gain and diabetes
Methylcellulose (1500 mg ac)	Old-fashioned and rather unpalatable preparation. No data in drug-induced weight gain but formerly fairly widely used. Also acts as a laxative so may be suitable for clozapine-related weight gain
Orlistat[46–50] (120 mg tds ac/pc)	Reliable effect in obesity, especially when combined with calorie restriction. Few published data in drug-induced weight gain but widely used with some success. Failure to adhere to a low-fat diet will result in fatty diarrhoea and possible malabsorbtion of orally administered medication
Phenylpropanolamine[51]	Probably not effective
Reboxetine[52] (4 mg daily)	Attenuates olanzapine-induced weight gain. No data on weight reduction
Rimonabant[53,54]	Undoubted effect on weight and metabolic parameters in 'medical' populations. Few data in psychiatric population except to suggest that rimonabant is not antipsychotic[54]. Animal data suggest useful effect on antidepressant-induced weight gain[53]. Licence now suspended due to association with depression and suicide[55]
Sibutramine[48,56] (10–15 mg daily)	Effective, with one positive RCT[57]. Tachycardia, insomnia and hypertension may be problematic. Note that the SPC lists 'psychiatric illness' as a contra-indication. Panic and psychosis have been reported
Topiramate[58–67] (Up to 300 mg daily)	Reliably reduces weight even when drug-induced, but data are mainly observational. Problems may arise because of topiramate's propensity for causing sedation, confusion and cognitive impairment. May be antipsychotic[68]
Zonisamide[69] (400–600 mg/day)	Newer antiepileptic drug with weight reducing properties. No data on drug-induced weight gain

References

1. Marder SR et al. Physical health monitoring of patients with schizophrenia. Am J Psychiatry 2004; 161:1334–1349.
2. Paton C et al. Obesity, dyslipidaemias and smoking in an inpatient population treated with antipsychotic drugs. Acta Psychiatr Scand 2004; 110: 299–305.
3. Kwon JS et al. Weight management program for treatment-emergent weight gain in olanzapine-treated patients with schizophrenia or schizoaffective disorder: A 12-week randomized controlled clinical trial. J Clin Psychiatry 2006; 67:547–553.

4. Littrell KH et al. The effects of an educational intervention on antipsychotic-induced weight gain. J Nurs Scholarsh 2003; 35:237–241.

5. Mauri M et al. Effects of an educational intervention on weight gain in patients treated with antipsychotics. J Clin Psychopharmacol 2006; 26:462–466.

6. Alvarez-Jimenez M et al. Attenuation of antipsychotic-induced weight gain with early behavioral intervention in drug-naive first-episode psychosis patients: A randomized controlled trial. J Clin Psychiatry 2006; 67:1253–1260.

7. Casey DE et al. Switching patients to aripiprazole from other antipsychotic agents: a multicenter randomized study. Psychopharmacology 2003; 166: 391–399.

8. De Hert M et al. A case series: evaluation of the metabolic safety of aripiprazole. Schizophr Bull 2007; 33:823–830.

9. Lin SK et al. Reversal of antipsychotic-induced hyperprolactinemia, weight gain, and dyslipidemia by aripiprazole: A case report. J Clin Psychiatry 2006; 67:1307.

10. Newcomer JW et al. A multicenter, randomized, double-blind study of the effects of aripiprazole in overweight subjects with schizophrenia or schizoaffective disorder switched from olanzapine. J Clin Psychiatry 2008; 69:1046–1056.

11. Kim SH et al. Metabolic impact of switching antipsychotic therapy to aripiprazole after weight gain: a pilot study. J Clin Psychopharmacol 2007; 27:365–368.

12. Weiden PJ et al. Improvement in indices of health status in outpatients with schizophrenia switched to ziprasidone. J Clin Psychopharmacol 2003; 23:595–600.

13. Montes JM et al. Improvement in antipsychotic-related metabolic disturbances in patients with schizophrenia switched to ziprasidone. Prog Neuropsychopharmacol Biol Psychiatry 2007; 31:383–388.

14. Gupta S et al. Weight decline in patients switching from olanzapine to quetiapine. Schizophr Res 2004; 70:57–62.

15. Ried LD et al. Weight change after an atypical antipsychotic switch. Ann Pharmacother 2003; 37:1381–1386.

16. Englisch S et al. Combined antipsychotic treatment involving clozapine and aripiprazole. Prog Neuropsychopharmacol Biol Psychiatry 2008; 32: 1386–1392.

17. Schorr SG et al. A 12-month follow-up study of treating overweight schizophrenic patients with aripiprazole. Acta Psychiatr Scand 2008; 118:246–250.

18. Fleischhacker WW et al. Weight change on aripiprazole-clozapine combination in schizophrenic patients with weight gain and suboptimal response on clozapine: 16-week double-blind study. Eur Psychiatry 2008;23 Suppl 2:S114–S115.

19. Werneke U et al. Behavioural management of antipsychotic-induced weight gain: a review. Acta Psychiatr Scand 2003; 108:252–259.

20. Cohen S et al. Weight gain with risperidone among patients with mental retardation: effect of calorie restriction. J Clin Psychiatry 2001; 62:114–116.

21. Smith H et al. Low glycaemic index diet in patients prescribed clozapine: pilot study. Psychiatr Bull 2004; 28:292–294.

22. Ball MP et al. A program for treating olanzapine-related weight gain. Psychiatr Serv 2001; 52:967–969.

23. Pendlebury J et al. Evaluation of a behavioural weight management programme for patients with severe mental illness: 3 year results. Hum Psychopharmacol 2005; 20:447–448.

24. Vreeland B et al. A program for managing weight gain associated with atypical antipsychotics. Psychiatr Serv 2003; 54:1155–1157.

25. Ohlsen RI et al. A dedicated nurse-led service for antipsychotic-induced weight gain: An evaluation. Psychiatr Bull 2004; 28:164–166.

26. Chen CK et al. Effects of a 10-week weight control program on obese patients with schizophrenia or schizoaffective disorder: a 12-month follow up. Psychiatry Clin Neurosci 2009; 63:17–22.

27. Floris M et al. Effect of amantadine on weight gain during olanzapine treatment. Eur Neuropsychopharmacol 2001; 11:181–182.

28. Gracious BL et al. Amantadine treatment of psychotropic-induced weight gain in children and adolescents: case series. J Child Adolesc Psychopharmacol 2002; 12:249–257.

29. Bahk WM et al. Open label study of the effect of amantadine on weight gain induced by olanzapine. Psychiatry Clin Neurosci 2004; 58:163–167.

30. Deberdt W et al. Amantadine for weight gain associated with olanzapine treatment. Eur Neuropsychopharmacol 2005; 15:13–21.

31. Gadde KM et al. Bupropion for weight loss: an investigation of efficacy and tolerability in overweight and obese women. Obes Res 2001; 9:544–551.

32. Jain AK et al. Bupropion SR vs. placebo for weight loss in obese patients with depressive symptoms. Obes Res 2002; 10:1049–1056.

33. Poyurovsky M et al. Olanzapine-induced weight gain in patients with first-episode schizophrenia: a double-blind, placebo-controlled study of fluoxetine addition. Am J Psychiatry 2002; 159:1058–1060.

34. Bustillo JR et al. Treatment of weight gain with fluoxetine in olanzapine-treated schizophrenic outpatients. Neuropsychopharmacology 2003; 28: 527–529.

35. Cavazzoni P et al. Nizatidine for prevention of weight gain with olanzapine: a double-blind placebo-controlled trial. Eur Neuropsychopharmacol 2003; 13:81–85.

36. Pae CU et al. Effect of nizatidine on olanzapine-associated weight gain in schizophrenic patients in Korea: a pilot study. Hum Psychopharmacol 2003; 18:453–456.

37. Poyurovsky M et al. The effect of famotidine addition on olanzapine-induced weight gain in first-episode schizophrenia patients: a double-blind placebo-controlled pilot study. Eur Neuropsychopharmacol 2004; 14:332–336.

38. Atmaca M et al. Nizatidine for the treatment of patients with quetiapine-induced weight gain. Hum Psychopharmacol 2004; 19:37–40.

39. Morrison JA et al. Metformin for weight loss in pediatric patients taking psychotropic drugs. Am J Psychiatry 2002; 159:655–657.

40. Mogul HR et al. Long-term (2–4 year) weight reduction with metformin plus carbohydrate-modified diet in euglycemic, hyperinsulinemic, midlife women (Syndrome W). Heart Dis 2003; 5:384–392.

41. Baptista T et al. Metformin for prevention of weight gain and insulin resistance with olanzapine: a double-blind placebo-controlled trial. Can J Psychiatry 2006; 51:192–196.

42. Klein DJ et al. A randomized, double-blind, placebo-controlled trial of metformin treatment of weight gain associated with initiation of atypical antipsychotic therapy in children and adolescents. Am J Psychiatry 2006; 163:2072–2079.

43. Wu RR et al. Lifestyle intervention and metformin for treatment of antipsychotic-induced weight gain: a randomized controlled trial. JAMA 2008; 299:185–193.

44. Wu RR et al. Metformin addition attenuates olanzapine-induced weight gain in drug-naive first-episode schizophrenia patients: a double-blind, placebo-controlled study. Am J Psychiatry 2008; 165:352–358.

45. Baptista T et al. Metformin plus sibutramine for olanzapine-associated weight gain and metabolic dysfunction in schizophrenia: a 12-week double-blind, placebo-controlled pilot study. Psychiatry Res 2008; 159:250–253.

46. Sjostrom L et al. Randomised placebo-controlled trial of orlistat for weight loss and prevention of weight regain in obese patients. European Multicentre Orlistat Study Group. Lancet 1998; 352:167–172.

47. Hilger E et al. The effect of orlistat on plasma levels of psychotropic drugs in patients with long-term psychopharmacotherapy. J Clin Psychopharmacol 2002; 22:68–70.

48. Werneke U et al. Options for pharmacological management of obesity in patients treated with atypical antipsychotics. Int Clin Psychopharmacol 2002; 17:145–160.

49. Pavlovic ZM. Orlistat in the treatment of clozapine-induced hyperglycemia and weight gain. Eur Psychiatry 2005; 20:520.

50. Carpenter LL et al. A case series describing orlistat use in patients on psychotropic medications. Med Health R I 2004; 87:375–377.

51. Borovicka MC et al. Phenylpropanolamine appears not to promote weight loss in patients with schizophrenia who have gained weight during clozapine treatment. J Clin Psychiatry 2002; 63:345–348.

52. Poyurovsky M et al. Attenuation of olanzapine-induced weight gain with reboxetine in patients with schizophrenia: a double-blind, placebo-controlled study. Am J Psychiatry 2003; 160:297–302.

53. Gobshtis N et al. Antidepressant-induced undesirable weight gain: Prevention with rimonabant without interference with behavioral effectiveness. Eur J Pharmacol 2007; 554:155–163.

54. Meltzer HY et al. Placebo-controlled evaluation of four novel compounds for the treatment of schizophrenia and schizoaffective disorder. Am J Psychiatry 2004; 161:975–984.
55. Taylor D. Withdrawal of Rimonabant--walking the tightrope of 21st century pharmaceutical regulation? Curr Drug Saf 2009; 4:2–4.
56. Arterburn DE et al. The efficacy and safety of sibutramine for weight loss: a systematic review. Arch Intern Med 2004; 164:994–1003.
57. Henderson DC et al. A double-blind, placebo-controlled trial of sibutramine for olanzapine-associated weight gain. Am J Psychiatry 2005; 162: 954–962.
58. Binkley K et al. Sibutramine and panic attacks. Am J Psychiatry 2002; 159:1793–1794.
59. Taflinski T et al. Sibutramine-associated psychotic episode. Am J Psychiatry 2000; 157:2057–2058.
60. Dursun SM et al. Clozapine weight gain, plus topiramate weight loss. Can J Psychiatry 2000; 45:198.
61. Levy E et al. Topiramate produced weight loss following olanzapine-induced weight gain in schizophrenia. J Clin Psychiatry 2002; 63:1045.
62. Van Ameringen M et al. Topiramate treatment for SSRI-induced weight gain in anxiety disorders. J Clin Psychiatry 2002; 63:981–984.
63. Appolinario JC et al. Topiramate use in obese patients with binge eating disorder: an open study. Can J Psychiatry 2002; 47:271–273.
64. Chengappa KN et al. Changes in body weight and body mass index among psychiatric patients receiving lithium, valproate, or topiramate: an open-label, nonrandomized chart review. Clin Ther 2002; 24:1576–1584.
65. Pavuluri MN et al. Topiramate plus risperidone for controlling weight gain and symptoms in preschool mania. J Child Adolesc Psychopharmacol 2002; 12:271–273.
66. Cates ME et al. Efficacy of add-on topiramate therapy in psychiatric patients with weight gain. Ann Pharmacother 2008; 42:505–510.
67. Egger C et al. Influence of topiramate on olanzapine-related weight gain in women: an 18-month follow-up observation. J Clin Psychopharmacol 2007; 27:475–478.
68. Afshar H et al. Topiramate add-on treatment in schizophrenia: a randomised, double-blind, placebo-controlled clinical trial. J Psychopharmacol 2009; 23:157–162.
69. Gadde KM et al. Zonisamide for weight loss in obese adults: a randomized controlled trial. JAMA 2003; 289:1820–1825.

Further reading

Baptista T et al. Pharmacological management of atypical antipsychotic-induced weight gain. CNS Drugs 2008; 22:477–495.

Psychotropic-related QT prolongation

Introduction

Many psychotropic drugs are associated with ECG changes and it is probable that certain drugs are causally linked to serious ventricular arrhythmia and sudden cardiac death. Specifically, some antipsychotics block cardiac potassium channels and are linked to prolongation of the cardiac QT interval, a risk factor for the ventricular arrhythmia torsade de pointes, which is occasionally fatal. Case-control studies have suggested that the use of most antipsychotics is associated with an increase in the rate of sudden cardiac death[1-6]. This risk is probably a result of the arrhythmogenic potential of antipsychotics[7,8]. Overall risk is clearly dose-related and, although low, it is substantially higher than the risk of fatal agranulocytosis with clozapine[7]. Tricyclic antidepressants are sodium channel antagonists which prolong QRS interval and QT interval, effects which are usually evident only following overdose[9,10].

ECG monitoring of drug-induced changes in mental health settings is complicated by a number of factors. Psychiatrists may have limited expertise in ECG interpretation, for example. (Self-reading, computerised ECG devices are available and to some extent compensate for some lack of expertise.) In addition, ECG machines may not be as readily available in all clinical areas as they are in general medicine. Also, time for ECG determination may not be available in many areas (e.g. out-patients). Lastly, ECG determination may be difficult to perform in acutely disturbed, physically uncooperative patients.

ECG monitoring is essential for all patients prescribed antipsychotics. An estimate of QTc interval should be made on admission to in-patient units (note that this is recommended in the NICE schizophrenia guideline[11]) on discharge, and yearly thereafter.

QT prolongation

- The cardiac QT interval (usually cited as QTc – QT corrected for heart rate) is a useful, but imprecise indicator of risk of torsade de pointes and of increased cardiac mortality[12]. Different correction factors and methods may give markedly different values[13].
- There is some controversy over the exact association between QTc and risk of arrhythmia. Very limited evidence suggests that risk is exponentially related to the extent of prolongation beyond normal limits (440 ms for men; 470 ms for women), although there are well-known exceptions which appear to disprove this theory[14]. Rather stronger evidence links QTc values over 500 ms to a clearly increased risk of arrhythmia[15]. Despite these uncertainties, QTc determination remains an important measure in estimating risk of arrhythmia and sudden death.
- QTc measurements and evaluation are complicated by:
  - difficulty in determining the end of the T wave, particularly where U waves are present (this applies both to manual and self-reading ECG machines)[15]
  - normal physiological variation in QTc interval: QT varies with gender, time of day, food intake, alcohol intake, menstrual cycle, ECG lead, etc.[13,14]
  - variation in the extent of drug-induced prolongation of QTc because of changes in plasma levels. QTc prolongation is most prominent at peak drug plasma levels and least obvious at trough levels[13,14].

Other ECG changes

Tricyclics and other antidepressants may prolong the QRS interval, particularly in overdose. Other reported antipsychotic-induced changes include atrial fibrillation, giant P waves, T-wave changes and heart block[14].

Quantifying risk

Drugs are categorised here according to data available on their effects on the cardiac QTc interval (as calculated by Bazett's correction formula). 'No-effect' drugs are those with which QTc prolongation has not been reported either at therapeutic doses or in overdose. 'Low-effect' drugs are those for which severe QTc prolongation has been reported only following overdose or where only small average increases (<10 ms) have been observed at clinical doses. 'Moderate-effect' drugs are those which have been observed to prolong QTc by >10 ms on average when given at normal

(Continued)

Table Psychotropics – effect on QTc[13,14,17–36]	
No effect	**Moderate effect**
Aripiprazole	Chlorpromazine
Paliperidone (but note warning in SPC)	Iloperidone
	Melperone
SSRIs (except citalopram)	Quetiapine
Reboxetine	Ziprasidone
Nefazodone	Zotepine
Mirtazapine	
MAOIs	TCAs
Carbamazepine	**High effect**
Gabapentin	Any intravenous antipsychotic
Lamotrigine	Haloperidol
Valproate	Methadone
	Pimozide
Benzodiazepines	Sertindole
Low effect	Any drug or combination of drugs used in
Amisulpride	doses exceeding recommended maximum
Clozapine	
Flupentixol	**Unknown effect**
Fluphenazine	Loxapine
Perphenazine	Pipothiazine
Prochlorperazine	Trifluoperazine
Olanzapine*	Zuclopenthixol
Risperidone	
Sulpiride	Anticholinergic drugs (procyclidine, benzhexol, etc.)
Bupropion	
Citalopram	
Moclobemide	
Venlafaxine	
Trazodone	
Lithium	

*Isolated cases of QTc prolongation[21,37] demonstrated effect on I_{Kr}[38], other data suggest no effect on QT_C[14,19,20,39].

clinical doses or where ECG monitoring is officially recommended in some circumstances. 'High-effect' drugs are those for which extensive average QTc prolongation (usually >20 ms at normal clinical doses) has been noted or where ECG monitoring is mandated by the manufacturer's data sheet.

Note that effect on QTc may not necessarily equate directly to risk of torsade de pointes or sudden death[16], although this is often assumed. Note also that categorisation is inevitably approximate given the problems associated with QTc measurements.

Other risk factors

A number of physiological/pathological factors are associated with an increased risk of QT changes and of arrhythmia (Table 1) and many non-psychotropic drugs are linked to QT prolongation (Table 2)[15].

Table 1 Physiological risk factors for QTc prolongation and arrhythmia
Cardiac
Long QT syndrome
Bradycardia
Ischaemic heart disease
Myocarditis
Myocardial infarction
Left ventricular hypertrophy
Metabolic
Hypokalaemia
Hypomagnesaemia
Hypocalcaemia
Others
Extreme physical exertion
Stress or shock
Anorexia nervosa
Extremes of age – children and elderly may be more susceptible to QT changes
Female gender
Note: Hypokalaemia-related QTc prolongation is more commonly observed in acute psychotic admissions[40]. Also, be aware that there are a number of physical and genetic factors which may not be discovered on routine examination but which probably predispose patients to arrhythmia[41,42].

Table 2 Non-psychotropics associated with QT prolongation	
Antibiotics	**Antiarrhythmics**
Erythromycin	Quinidine
Clarithromycin	Disopyramide
Ampicillin	Procainamide
Co-trimoxazole	Sotalol
Pentamidine	Amiodarone
(Some 4 quinolones affect QTc – see	Bretylium
manufacturers' literature)	
Antimalarials	**Others**
Chloroquine	Amantadine
Mefloquine	Cyclosporin
Quinine	Diphenhydramine
	Hydroxyzine
	Nicardipine
	Tamoxifen

Note: β_2 agonists and sympathomimetics may provoke torsade de pointes in patients with prolonged QTc.

ECG monitoring
Measure QTc in all patients prescribed antipsychotics:

* on admission
* before discharge and at yearly check-up.

Actions to be taken

* **QTc <440 ms (men) or <470 ms (women)**
  No action required unless abnormal T-wave morphology – consider referral to cardiologist if in doubt.
* **QTc >440 ms (men) or >470 ms (women) but <500 ms**
  Consider reducing dose or switching to drug of lower effect; repeat ECG and consider referral to cardiologist.
* **QTc >500 ms**
  Stop suspected causative drug(s) and switch to drug of lower effect; refer to cardiologist immediately.
* **Abnormal T- wave morphology**
  Review treatment. Consider reducing dose or switching to drug of lower effect. Refer to cardiologist immediately.

Metabolic inhibition
The effect of drugs on the QTc interval is usually plasma level-dependent. Drug interactions are therefore important, especially when metabolic inhibition results in increased plasma levels of the drug affecting QTc. Commonly used metabolic inhibitors include fluvoxamine, fluoxetine, paroxetine and valproate.

Other cardiovascular risk factors

The risk of drug-induced arrhythmia and sudden cardiac death with psychotropics is an important consideration. With respect to cardiovascular disease, note that other risk factors such as smoking, obesity and impaired glucose tolerance, present a much greater risk to patient morbidity and mortality than the uncertain outcome of QT changes. See relevant sections for discussion of these problems.

Summary

* In the absence of conclusive data, assume all antipsychotics are linked to sudden cardiac death
* Prescribe the lowest dose possible and avoid polypharmacy/metabolic interactions
* Perform ECG on admission, before discharge and at yearly check-up

Schizophrenia

References

1. Reilly JG et al. Thioridazine and sudden unexplained death in psychiatric in-patients. Br J Psychiatry 2002; 180:515–522.
2. Ray WA et al. Antipsychotics and the risk of sudden cardiac death. Arch Gen Psychiatry 2001; 58:1161–1167.
3. Hennessy S et al. Cardiac arrest and ventricular arrhythmia in patients taking antipsychotic drugs: cohort study using administrative data. BMJ 2002; 325:1070.
4. Straus SM et al. Antipsychotics and the risk of sudden cardiac death. Arch Intern Med 2004; 164:1293–1297.
5. Liperoti R et al. Conventional and atypical antipsychotics and the risk of hospitalization for ventricular arrhythmias or cardiac arrest. Arch Intern Med 2005; 165:696–701.
6. Ray WA et al. Atypical antipsychotic drugs and the risk of sudden cardiac death. N Engl J Med 2009; 360:225–235.
7. Schneeweiss S et al. Antipsychotic agents and sudden cardiac death – how should we manage the risk? N Engl J Med 2009; 360:294–296.
8. Nakagawa S et al. Antipsychotics and risk of first-time hospitalization for myocardial infarction: a population-based case-control study. J Intern Med 2006; 260:451–458.
9. Cohen H et al. Antidepressant poisoning and treatment: a review and case illustration. J Pharm Pract 1997; 10:249–270.
10. Whyte IM et al. Relative toxicity of venlafaxine and selective serotonin reuptake inhibitors in overdose compared to tricyclic antidepressants. QJM 2003; 96:369–374.
11. National Institute for Health and Clinical Excellence. Schizophrenia: core interventions in the treatment and management of schizophrenia in adults in primary and secondary care (update). 2009. http://www.nice.org.uk/
12. Malik M et al. Evaluation of drug-induced QT interval prolongation: implications for drug approval and labelling. Drug Saf 2001; 24:323–351.
13. Haddad PM et al. Antipsychotic-related QTc prolongation, torsade de pointes and sudden death. Drugs 2002; 62:1649–1671.
14. Taylor DM. Antipsychotics and QT prolongation. Acta Psychiatr Scand 2003; 107:85–95.
15. Botstein P. Is QT interval prolongation harmful? A regulatory perspective. Am J Cardiol 1993; 72:50B–52B.
16. Witchel HJ et al. Psychotropic drugs, cardiac arrhythmia, and sudden death. J Clin Psychopharmacol 2003; 23:58–77.
17. Glassman AH et al. Antipsychotic drugs: prolonged QTc interval, torsade de pointes, and sudden death. Am J Psychiatry 2001; 158:1774–1782.
18. Warner B et al. Investigation of the potential of clozapine to cause torsade de pointes. Adverse Drug React Toxicol Rev 2002; 21:189–203.
19. Harrigan EP et al. A randomized evaluation of the effects of six antipsychotic agents on QTc, in the absence and presence of metabolic inhibition. J Clin Psychopharmacol 2004; 24:62–69.
20. Lindborg SR et al. Effects of intramuscular olanzapine vs. haloperidol and placebo on QTc intervals in acutely agitated patients. Psychiatry Res 2003; 119:113–123.
21. Dineen S et al. QTc prolongation and high-dose olanzapine (Letter). Psychosomatics 2003; 44:174–175.
22. Gupta S et al. Quetiapine and QTc issues: a case report (Letter). J Clin Psychiatry 2003; 64:612–613.
23. Su KP et al. A pilot cross-over design study on QTc interval prolongation associated with sulpiride and haloperidol. Schizophr Res 2003; 59:93–94.
24. Lin CH et al. Predictive factors for QTc prolongation in schizophrenic patients taking antipsychotics. J Formos Med Assoc 2004; 103:437–441.
25. Chong SA et al. Prolonged QTc intervals in medicated patients with schizophrenia. Hum Psychopharmacol 2003; 18:647–649.
26. Krantz MJ et al. Dose-related effects of methadone on QT prolongation in a series of patients with torsade de pointes. Pharmacotherapy 2003; 23:802–805.
27. Gil M et al. QT prolongation and torsades de pointes in patients infected with human immunodeficiency virus and treated with methadone. Am J Cardiol 2003; 92:995–997.
28. Piguet V et al. QT interval prolongation in patients on methadone with concomitant drugs (Letter). J Clin Psychopharmacol 2004; 24:446–448.
29. Stollberger C et al. Antipsychotic drugs and QT prolongation. Int Clin Psychopharmacol 2005; 20:243–251.
30. Isbister GK et al. Amisulpride deliberate self-poisoning causing severe cardiac toxicity including QT prolongation and torsades de pointes. Med J Aust 2006; 184:354–356.
31. Ward DI. Two cases of amisulpride overdose: A cause for prolonged QT syndrome. Emerg Med Australas 2005; 17:274–276.
32. Vieweg WV et al. Torsade de pointes in a patient with complex medical and psychiatric conditions receiving low-dose quetiapine. Acta Psychiatr Scand 2005; 112:318–322.
33. Huang BH et al. Sulpiride induced torsade de pointes. Int J Cardiol 2007; 118:e100–e102.
34. Kane JM et al. Long-term efficacy and safety of iloperidone: results from 3 clinical trials for the treatment of schizophrenia. J Clin Psychopharmacol 2008; 28:S29–S35.
35. Kim MD et al. Blockade of HERG human K+ channel and IKr of guinea pig cardiomyocytes by prochlorperazine. Eur J Pharmacol 2006; 544:82–90.
36. Meltzer H et al. Efficacy and tolerability of oral paliperidone extended-release tablets in the treatment of acute schizophrenia: pooled data from three 6-week placebo-controlled studies. J Clin Psychiatry 2006; 69:817–829.

37. Su KP et al. Olanzapine-induced QTc prolongation in a patient with Wolff-Parkinson-White syndrome. Schizophr Res 2004; 66:191–192.
38. Morissette P et al. Olanzapine prolongs cardiac repolarization by blocking the rapid component of the delayed rectifier potassium current. J Psychopharmacol 2007; 21:735–741.
39. Bar KJ et al. Influence of olanzapine on QT variability and complexity measures of heart rate in patients with schizophrenia. J Clin Psychopharmacol 2008; 28:694–698.
40. Hatta K et al. Prolonged QT interval in acute psychotic patients. Psychiatry Res 2000; 94:279–285.
41. Priori SG et al. Low penetrance in the long-QT syndrome: clinical impact. Circulation 1999; 99:529–533.
42. Frassati D et al. Hidden cardiac lesions and psychotropic drugs as a possible cause of sudden death in psychiatric patients: a report of 14 cases and review of the literature. Can J Psychiatry 2004; 49:100–105.

Further reading

Abdelmawla N et al. Sudden cardiac death and antipsychotics. Part 1: Risk factors and mechanisms. Adv Psychiatr Treat 2006; 12:35–44.
Sicouri S et al. Sudden cardiac death secondary to antidepressant and antipsychotic drugs. Expert Opin Drug Saf 2008; 7:181–194.
Titier K et al. Atypical antipsychotics – from potassium channels to torsade de pointes and sudden death. Drug Safety 2005; 28:35–51.

Schizophrenia

Antipsychotics, diabetes and impaired glucose tolerance

Schizophrenia
Schizophrenia seems to be associated with relatively high rates of insulin resistance and diabetes[1,2] – an observation that predates the discovery of effective antipsychotics[3–5].

Antipsychotics
Data relating to diabetes and antipsychotic use are numerous but less than perfect[6–9]. The main problem is that incidence and prevalence studies assume full or uniform screening for diabetes. Neither assumption is likely to be correct[6]. Many studies do not account for other factors affecting risk of diabetes[9]. Small differences between drugs are therefore difficult to substantiate but may in any case be ultimately unimportant: risk is probably increased for all those with schizophrenia receiving any antipsychotic.

The mechanisms involved in the development of antipsychotic-related diabetes are unclear, but may include $5HT_{2A}/5HT_{2C}$ antagonism, increased lipids, weight gain and leptin resistance[10].

First-generation antipsychotics
Phenothiazine derivatives have long been associated with impaired glucose tolerance and diabetes[11]. Diabetes prevalence rates were reported to have substantially increased following the introduction and widespread use of conventional drugs[12]. Prevalence of impaired glucose tolerance seems to be higher with aliphatic phenothiazines than with fluphenazine or haloperidol[13]. Hyperglycaemia has also been reported with other conventional drugs, such as loxapine[14], and other data confirm an association with haloperidol[15]. Some data suggest that FGAs are no different from SGAs in their propensity to cause diabetes[16,17], whereas others suggest a modest but statistically significant excess incidence of diabetes with SGAs[18].

Second-generation antipsychotics
Clozapine
Clozapine has been strongly linked to hyperglycaemia, impaired glucose tolerance and diabetic ketoacidosis[19]. The risk of diabetes appears to be higher with clozapine than with other SGAs and conventional drugs, especially in younger patients[20–23], although this is not a consistent finding[24,25].

As many as a third of patients may develop diabetes after 5 years of treatment[26]. Many cases of diabetes are noted in the first 6 months of treatment and some occur within 1 month[27], some after many years[25]. Death from ketoacidosis has also been reported[27]. Diabetes associated with clozapine is not necessarily linked to obesity or to family history of diabetes[19,28].

Clozapine appears to increase plasma levels of insulin in a clozapine-level-dependent fashion[29,30]. It has been shown to be more likely than typical drugs to increase plasma glucose and insulin following oral glucose challenge[31]. Much clozapine-related diabetes may go unnoticed[32]. Testing for diabetes is essential given the high prevalence of diabetes in people receiving clozapine[33].

Olanzapine
Like clozapine, olanzapine has been strongly linked to impaired glucose tolerance, diabetes and diabetic ketoacidosis[34]. Olanzapine and clozapine appear to directly induce insulin resistance[35,36]. Risk of diabetes has also been reported to be higher than with FGA drugs[37], again with a particular risk in younger patients[21]. The time course of development of diabetes has not been established but impaired glucose tolerance seems to occur even in the absence of obesity and family history of diabetes[19,28]. Olanzapine is probably more diabetogenic than risperidone[38–42].

Olanzapine is associated with plasma levels of glucose and insulin higher than those seen with conventional drugs (after oral glucose load)[31,43].

Risperidone

Risperidone has been linked mainly in case reports to impaired glucose tolerance[44], diabetes[45] and ketoacidosis[46]. The number of reports of such adverse effects is substantially smaller than with either clozapine or olanzapine[47]. At least one study has suggested that changes in fasting glucose are significantly less common with risperidone than with olanzapine[38] but other studies have detected no difference[48].

Risperidone seems no more likely than FGA drugs to be associated with diabetes[21,37,39], although there may be an increased risk in patients under 40 years of age[21]. Risperidone has, however, been observed adversely to affect fasting glucose and plasma glucose (following glucose challenge) compared with levels seen in healthy volunteers (but not compared with patients taking conventional drugs)[31].

Quetiapine

Like risperidone, quetiapine has been linked to cases of new-onset diabetes and ketoacidosis[49,50]. Again, the number of reports is much fewer than with olanzapine or clozapine. Quetiapine appears to be more likely than conventional drugs to be associated with diabetes[21,51]. Two studies showed quetiapine to be equal to olanzapine in incidence of diabetes[48,52]. Inexplicably, quetiapine may ameliorate clozapine-related diabetes when given in conjunction with clozapine[53].

Other SGAs

Amisulpride appears not to elevate plasma glucose[54] and seems not to be associated with diabetes[55]. Data for aripiprazole[56–59] and ziprasidone[60,61] suggest that neither drug alters glucose homeostasis. Aripiprazole may even reverse diabetes caused by other drugs[62] (although ketoacidosis has been reported with aripiprazole[63–65]). These three drugs are cautiously recommended for those with a history of or predisposition to diabetes mellitus or as an alternative to other antipsychotics known to be diabetogenic.

Predicting antipsychotic-related diabetes

Risk of diabetes is increased to a much greater extent in younger adults than in the elderly[66] (in whom antipsychotics may show no increased risk[67]). First-episode patients seem particularly prone to the development of diabetes when given a variety of antipsychotics[68–70]. During treatment, rapid weight gain and a rise in plasma triglycerides seem to predict the development of diabetes[71].

Monitoring

Diabetes is a growing problem in western society and has a strong association with obesity, (older) age, (lower) educational achievement and certain racial groups[72,73]. Diabetes markedly increases cardiovascular mortality, largely as a consequence of atherosclerosis[74]. Likewise, the use of antipsychotics also increases cardiovascular mortality[75–77]. Intervention to reduce plasma glucose levels and minimise other risk factors (obesity, hypercholesterolaemia) is therefore essential[78].

There is no clear consensus on diabetes-monitoring practice for those receiving antipsychotics[79]. Given the known parlous state of testing for diabetes in the UK[6,80,81] and elsewhere[82,83], arguments over precisely which tests are done and when seem redundant. There is an overwhelming need to improve monitoring by any means and so any tests for diabetes are supported – urine glucose and random plasma glucose included.

Ideally, though, all patients should have oral glucose tolerance tests (OGTT) performed as this is the most sensitive method of detection[84]. Fasting plasma glucose (FPG) tests are less sensitive but recommended[85]. Fasting tests are often difficult to obtain in acutely ill, disorganised patients, so measurement of random plasma glucose in conjunction with glycosylated haemoglobin (HbA$_{1C}$) may also be used (fasting not required). Frequency of monitoring should then be determined by physical factors (e.g. weight gain) and known risk factors (e.g. family history of diabetes, lipid abnormalities). The absolute minimum is yearly testing for diabetes for all patients.

Schizophrenia

Recommended monitoring		
	Ideally	*Minimum*
Baseline	OGTT or FPG	Urine glucose (UG) Random plasma glucose (RPG)
Continuation	All drugs: OGTT or FPG Every 12 months	UG or RPG every 12 months
	For clozapine and olanzapine or if other risk factors present: OGTT or FPC after one month, then every 4–6 months	

References

1. Schimmelbusch WH et al. The positive correlation between insulin resistance and duration of hospitalization in untreated schizophrenia. Br J Psychiatry 1971; 118:429–436.
2. Waitzkin L. A survey for unknown diabetics in a mental hospital. I. Men under age fifty. Diabetes 1966; 15:97–104.
3. Kasanin J. The blood sugar curve in mental disease. II. The schizophrenia (dementia praecox) groups. Arch Neurol Psychiatry 1926; 16:414–419.
4. Braceland FJ et al. Delayed action of insulin in schizophrenia. Am J Psychiatry 1945; 102:108–110.
5. Kohen D. Diabetes mellitus and schizophrenia: historical perspective. Br J Psychiatry Suppl 2004; 47:S64–S66.
6. Taylor D et al. Testing for diabetes in hospitalised patients prescribed antipsychotic drugs. Br J Psychiatry 2004; 185:152–156.
7. Haddad PM. Antipsychotics and diabetes: review of non-prospective data. Br J Psychiatry Suppl 2004; 47:S80–S86.
8. Bushe C et al. Association between atypical antipsychotic agents and type 2 diabetes: review of prospective clinical data. Br J Psychiatry 2004; 184: S87–S93.
9. Gianfrancesco F et al. The influence of study design on the results of pharmacoepidemiologic studies of diabetes risk with antipsychotic therapy. Ann Clin Psychiatry 2006; 18:9–17.
10. Buchholz S et al. Atypical antipsychotic-induced diabetes mellitus: an update on epidemiology and postulated mechanisms. Intern Med J 2008; 38: 602–606.
11. Arneson GA. Phenothiazine derivatives and glucose metabolism. J Neuropsychiatr 1964; 5:181.
12. Lindenmayer JP et al. Hyperglycemia associated with the use of atypical antipsychotics. J Clin Psychiatry 2001;62 Suppl 23:30–38.
13. Keskiner A et al. Psychotropic drugs, diabetes and chronic mental patients. Psychosomatics 1973; 14:176–181.
14. Tollefson G et al. Nonketotic hyperglycemia associated with loxapine and amoxapine: case report. J Clin Psychiatry 1983; 44: 347–348.
15. Lindenmayer JP et al. Changes in glucose and cholesterol levels in patients with schizophrenia treated with typical or atypical antipsychotics. Am J Psychiatry 2003; 160:290–296.
16. Carlson C et al. Diabetes mellitus and antipsychotic treatment in the United Kingdom. Eur Neuropsychopharmacol 2006; 16:366–375.
17. Ostbye T et al. Atypical antipsychotic drugs and diabetes mellitus in a large outpatient population: a retrospective cohort study. Pharmacoepidemiol Drug Saf 2005; 14:407–415.
18. Smith M et al. First- v. second-generation antipsychotics and risk for diabetes in schizophrenia: systematic review and meta-analysis. Br J Psychiatry 2008; 192:406–411.
19. Mir S et al. Atypical antipsychotics and hyperglycaemia. Int Clin Psychopharmacol 2001; 16:63–74.
20. Lund BC et al. Clozapine use in patients with schizophrenia and the risk of diabetes, hyperlipidemia, and hypertension: a claims-based approach. Arch Gen Psychiatry 2001; 58:1172–1176.
21. Sernyak MJ et al. Association of diabetes mellitus with use of atypical neuroleptics in the treatment of schizophrenia. Am J Psychiatry 2002; 159: 561–566.
22. Gianfrancesco FD et al. Differential effects of risperidone, olanzapine, clozapine, and conventional antipsychotics on type 2 diabetes: findings from a large health plan database. J Clin Psychiatry 2002; 63:920–930.
23. Guo JJ et al. Risk of diabetes mellitus associated with atypical antipsychotic use among patients with bipolar disorder: A retrospective, population-based, case-control study. J Clin Psychiatry 2006; 67:1055–1061.
24. Wang PS et al. Clozapine use and risk of diabetes mellitus. J Clin Psychopharmacol 2002; 22:236–243.
25. Sumiyoshi T et al. A comparison of incidence of diabetes mellitus between atypical antipsychotic drugs: a survey for clozapine, risperidone, olanzapine, and quetiapine (Letter). J Clin Psychopharmacol 2004; 24:345–348.
26. Henderson DC et al. Clozapine, diabetes mellitus, weight gain, and lipid abnormalities: A five-year naturalistic study. Am J Psychiatry 2000; 157: 975–981.
27. Koller E et al. Clozapine-associated diabetes. Am J Med 2001; 111:716–723.
28. Sumiyoshi T et al. The effect of hypertension and obesity on the development of diabetes mellitus in patients treated with atypical antipsychotic drugs (Letter). J Clin Psychopharmacol 2004; 24:452–454.
29. Melkersson KI et al. Different influences of classical antipsychotics and clozapine on glucose-insulin homeostasis in patients with schizophrenia or related psychoses. J Clin Psychiatry 1999; 60:783–791.
30. Melkersson K. Clozapine and olanzapine, but not conventional antipsychotics, increase insulin release in vitro. Eur Neuropsychopharmacol 2004; 14:115–119.
31. Newcomer JW et al. Abnormalities in glucose regulation during antipsychotic treatment of schizophrenia. Arch Gen Psychiatry 2002; 59:337–345.
32. Sernyak MJ et al. Undiagnosed hyperglycemia in clozapine-treated patients with schizophrenia. J Clin Psychiatry 2003; 64:605–608.

33. Lamberti JS et al. Diabetes mellitus among outpatients receiving clozapine: prevalence and clinical-demographic correlates. J Clin Psychiatry 2005; 66:900–906.
34. Wirshing DA et al. Novel antipsychotics and new onset diabetes. Biol Psychiatry 1998; 44:778–783.
35. Engl J et al. Olanzapine impairs glycogen synthesis and insulin signaling in L6 skeletal muscle cells. Mol Psychiatry 2005; 10:1089–1096.
36. Vestri HS et al. Atypical antipsychotic drugs directly impair insulin action in adipocytes: effects on glucose transport, lipogenesis, and antilipolysis. Neuropsychopharmacology 2007; 32:765–772.
37. Koro CE et al. Assessment of independent effect of olanzapine and risperidone on risk of diabetes among patients with schizophrenia: population based nested case-control study. BMJ 2002; 325:243.
38. Meyer JM. A retrospective comparison of weight, lipid, and glucose changes between risperidone- and olanzapine-treated inpatients: metabolic outcomes after 1 year. J Clin Psychiatry 2002; 63:425–433.
39. Gianfrancesco F et al. Antipsychotic-induced type 2 diabetes: evidence from a large health plan database. J Clin Psychopharmacol 2003; 23:328–335.
40. Leslie DL et al. Incidence of newly diagnosed diabetes attributable to atypical antipsychotic medications. Am J Psychiatry 2004; 161:1709–1711.
41. Duncan E et al. Relative risk of glucose elevation during antipsychotic exposure in a Veterans Administration population. Int Clin Psychopharmacol 2007; 22:1–11.
42. Meyer JM et al. Change in metabolic syndrome parameters with antipsychotic treatment in the CATIE Schizophrenia Trial: prospective data from phase 1. Schizophr Res 2008; 101:273–286.
43. Ebenbichler CF et al. Olanzapine induces insulin resistance: results from a prospective study. J Clin Psychiatry 2003; 64:1436–1439.
44. Mallya A et al. Resolution of hyperglycemia on risperidone discontinuation: a case report. J Clin Psychiatry 2002; 63:453–454.
45. Wirshing DA et al. Risperidone-associated new-onset diabetes. Biol Psychiatry 2001; 50:148–149.
46. Croarkin PE et al. Diabetic ketoacidosis associated with risperidone treatment? Psychosomatics 2000; 41:369–370.
47. Koller EA et al. Risperidone-associated diabetes mellitus: a pharmacovigilance study. Pharmacotherapy 2003; 23:735–744.
48. Lambert BL et al. Diabetes risk associated with use of olanzapine, quetiapine, and risperidone in veterans health administration patients with schizophrenia. Am J Epidemiol 2006; 164:672–681.
49. Henderson DC. Atypical antipsychotic-induced diabetes mellitus: how strong is the evidence? CNS Drugs 2002; 16:77–89.
50. Koller EA et al. A survey of reports of quetiapine-associated hyperglycemia and diabetes mellitus. J Clin Psychiatry 2004; 65:857–863.
51. Citrome L et al. Relationship between antipsychotic medication treatment and new cases of diabetes among psychiatric inpatients. Psychiatr Serv 2004; 55:1006–1013.
52. Bushe C et al. Comparison of metabolic and prolactin variables from a six-month randomised trial of olanzapine and quetiapine in schizophrenia. J Psychopharmacol 2009; In Press.
53. Reinstein MJ et al. Effect of clozapine-quetiapine combination therapy on weight and glycaemic control. Clin Drug Invest 1999; 18:99–104.
54. Vanelle JM et al. A double-blind randomised comparative trial of amisulpride versus olanzapine for 2 months in the treatment of subjects with schizophrenia and comorbid depression. Eur Psychiatry 2006; 21:523–530.
55. De Hert MA et al. Prevalence of the metabolic syndrome in patients with schizophrenia treated with antipsychotic medication. Schizophr Res 2006; 83:87–93.
56. Keck PE Jr et al. Aripiprazole: a partial dopamine D2 receptor agonist antipsychotic. Expert Opin Investig Drugs 2003; 12:655–662.
57. Pigott TA et al. Aripiprazole for the prevention of relapse in stabilized patients with chronic schizophrenia: a placebo-controlled 26-week study. J Clin Psychiatry 2003; 64:1048–1056.
58. van Winkel et al. Major changes in glucose metabolism, including new-onset diabetes, within 3 months after initiation of or switch to atypical antipsychotic medication in patients with schizophrenia and schizoaffective disorder. J Clin Psychiatry 2008; 69:472–479.
59. Baker RA et al. Atypical antipsychotic drugs and diabetes mellitus in the US Food and Drug Administration Adverse Event Database: A Systematic Bayesian Signal Detection Analysis. Psychopharmacol Bull 2009; 42:11–31.
60. Simpson GM et al. Randomized, controlled, double-blind multicenter comparison of the efficacy and tolerability of ziprasidone and olanzapine in acutely ill inpatients with schizophrenia or schizoaffective disorder. Am J Psychiatry 2004; 161:1837–1847.
61. Sacher J et al. Effects of olanzapine and ziprasidone on glucose tolerance in healthy volunteers. Neuropsychopharmacology 2008; 33:1633–1641.
62. De Hert M et al. A case series: evaluation of the metabolic safety of aripiprazole. Schizophr Bull 2007; 33:823–830.
63. Church CO et al. Diabetic ketoacidosis associated with aripiprazole. Diabet Med 2005; 22:1440–1443.
64. Reddymasu S et al. Elevated lipase and diabetic ketoacidosis associated with aripiprazole. JOP 2006; 7:303–305.
65. Campanella LM et al. Severe hyperglycemic hyperosmolar nonketotic coma in a nondiabetic patient receiving aripiprazole. Ann Emerg Med 2009; 53:264–266.
66. Hammerman A et al. Antipsychotics and diabetes: an age-related association. Ann Pharmacother 2008; 42:1316–1322.
67. Albert SG et al. Atypical antipsychotics and the risk of diabetes in an elderly population in long-term care: a retrospective nursing home chart review study. J Am Med Dir Assoc 2009; 10:115–119.
68. De HM et al. Typical and atypical antipsychotics differentially affect long-term incidence rates of the metabolic syndrome in first-episode patients with schizophrenia: a retrospective chart review. Schizophr Res 2008; 101:295–303.
69. Saddichha S et al. Metabolic syndrome in first episode schizophrenia – a randomized double-blind controlled, short-term prospective study. Schizophr Res 2008; 101:266–272.
70. Saddichha S et al. Diabetes and schizophrenia – effect of disease or drug? Results from a randomized, double-blind, controlled prospective study in first-episode schizophrenia. Acta Psychiatr Scand 2008; 117:342–347.
71. Reaven GM et al. In search of moderators and mediators of hyperglycemia with atypical antipsychotic treatment. J Psychiatr Res 2009; 43:997–1002.
72. Mokdad AH et al. The continuing increase of diabetes in the US. Diabetes Care 2001; 24:412.
73. Mokdad AH et al. Diabetes trends in the U.S.: 1990–1998. Diabetes Care 2000; 23:1278–1283.
74. Beckman JA et al. Diabetes and atherosclerosis: epidemiology, pathophysiology, and management. JAMA 2002; 287:2570–2581.
75. Henderson DC et al. Clozapine, diabetes mellitus, hyperlipidemia, and cardiovascular risks and mortality: results of a 10-year naturalistic study. J Clin Psychiatry 2005; 66:1116–1121.
76. Lamberti JS et al. Prevalence of the metabolic syndrome among patients receiving clozapine. Am J Psychiatry 2006; 163:1273–1276.
77. Goff DC et al. A comparison of ten-year cardiac risk estimates in schizophrenia patients from the CATIE study and matched controls. Schizophr Res 2005; 80:45–53.
78. Haupt DW et al. Hyperglycemia and antipsychotic medications. J Clin Psychiatry 2001;62 Suppl 27:15–26.
79. Cohn TA et al. Metabolic monitoring for patients treated with antipsychotic medications. Can J Psychiatry 2006; 51:492–501.
80. Barnes TR et al. A UK audit of screening for the metabolic side-effects of antipsychotics in community patients. Schizophr Bull 2007; 33:1397–1403.
81. Barnes TR et al. Screening for the metabolic syndrome in community psychiatric patients prescribed antipsychotics: a quality improvement programme. Acta Psychiatr Scand 2008; 118:26–33.
82. Morrato EH et al. Metabolic screening after the ADA's Consensus Statement on Antipsychotic Drugs and Diabetes. Diabetes Care 2009; 32:1037–1042.
83. Haupt DW et al. Prevalence and predictors of lipid and glucose monitoring in commercially insured patients treated with second-generation antipsychotic agents. Am J Psychiatry 2009; 166:345–353.
84. De Hert M et al. Oral glucose tolerance tests in treated patients with schizophrenia. Data to support an adaptation of the proposed guidelines for monitoring of patients on second generation antipsychotics? Eur Psychiatry 2006; 21:224–226.
85. Marder SR et al. Physical health monitoring of patients with schizophrenia. Am J Psychiatry 2004; 161:1334–1349.

Antipsychotics and dyslipidaemia

Morbidity and mortality from cardiovascular disease are higher in people with schizophrenia than in the general population[1]. Dyslipidaemia is an established risk factor for cardiovascular disease along with obesity, hypertension, smoking, diabetes and sedentary lifestyle. The majority of patients with schizophrenia have several of these risk factors and can be considered at 'high risk' of developing cardiovascular disease. Dyslipidaemia is treatable and intervention is known to reduce morbidity and mortality[2]. Aggressive treatment is particularly important in people with diabetes, the prevalence of which is increased 2- to 3-fold over population norms in people with schizophrenia (see section on diabetes).

Effect of antipsychotic drugs on lipids

First-generation antipsychotics

Phenothiazines are known to be associated with increases in triglycerides and low-density lipoprotein (LDL) cholesterol and decreases in high-density lipoprotein (HDL)[3] cholesterol, but the magnitude of these effects is poorly quantified[4]. Haloperidol seems to have minimal effect on lipid profiles[3].

Second-generation antipsychotics

Although there are relatively more data pertaining to some atypicals, they are derived from a variety of sources and are reported in different ways, making it difficult to compare drugs directly. While cholesterol levels can rise, the most profound effect of these drugs seems to be on triglycerides. Raised triglycerides are in general, associated with obesity and diabetes. From the available data, olanzapine would seem to have the greatest propensity to increase lipids; quetiapine, moderate propensity; and risperidone, moderate or minimal propensity. There are few data for other atypicals. Aripiprazole and ziprasidone have minimal adverse effect on blood lipids[5–8] and may even reverse dyslipidaemias associated with previous antipsychotics[9].

Olanzapine has been shown to increase triglyceride levels by 40% over the short (12 weeks) and medium (16 months) term[10,11]. Levels may continue to rise for up to a year[12]. Up to two-thirds of olanzapine-treated patients have raised triglycerides[13] and just under 10% may develop severe hypertriglyceridaemia[14]. While weight gain with olanzapine is generally associated with both increases in cholesterol[11,15] and triglycerides[14], severe hypertriglyceridaemia can occur independently of weight gain[14]. In one study, patients treated with olanzapine and risperidone gained a similar amount of weight, but in olanzapine patients serum triglyceride levels increased by four times as much (80 mg/dl) as in risperidone patients (20 mg/dl)[14]. Quetiapine[16] seems to have more modest effects than olanzapine, although data are conflicting[17].

A case-control study conducted in the UK found that patients with schizophrenia who were treated with olanzapine were five times more likely to develop hyperlipidaemia than controls and three times more likely to develop hyperlipidaemia than patients receiving typical antipsychotics[18]. Risperidone-treated patients could not be distinguished from controls.

Clozapine

Mean triglyceride levels have been shown to double and cholesterol levels to increase by at least 10% after 5 years' treatment with clozapine[19]. Patients treated with clozapine have triglyceride levels that are almost double those of patients who are treated with typical antipsychotics[20,21]. Cholesterol levels do not seem to be significantly different.

Particular care should be taken before prescribing clozapine, olanzapine, quetiapine and possibly phenothiazines for patients who are obese, diabetic or known to have pre-existing hyperlipidaemia[22].

Screening

All patients should have their lipids measured at baseline. Those prescribed clozapine, olanzapine, quetiapine or phenothiazines should ideally have their serum lipids measured every 3 months for the first year of treatment[12]. Those prescribed other antipsychotics should have their lipids measured after 3 months then annually. Clinically significant changes in cholesterol are unlikely over the short term but triglycerides can increase dramatically[23]. In practice, dyslipidaemia is widespread in patients taking long-term antipsychotics irrespective of drug prescribed or diagnosis[24]. Severe hypertriglyceridemia (fasting level of >5 mmol/l) is a risk factor for pancreatitis. Note that antipsychotic-induced dyslipidaemia can occur independent of weight gain[25].

Treatment of dyslipidaemia

If moderate to severe hyperlipidaemia develops during antipsychotic treatment, a switch to another antipsychotic less likely to cause this problem should be considered in the first instance. Although not recommended as a strategy in patients with treatment-resistant illness, clozapine-induced hypertriglyceridaemia has been shown to reverse after a switch to risperidone[26]. This may hold true with other switching regimens but data are scarce[27]. Aripiprazole seems at present to be the treatment of choice in those with prior antipsychotic-induced dyslipidaemia[28].

Patients with raised cholesterol may benefit from dietary advice, lifestyle changes and/or treatment with statins[29]. Risk tables and treatment guidelines can be found in the *British National Formulary* (*BNF*). Evidence supports the treatment of cholesterol concentrations as low as 4 mmol/l in high-risk patients[30] and this is the highest level recommended by NICE for secondary prevention of cardiovascular events[31]. NICE makes no recommendations on target levels for primary prevention. Coronary heart disease and stroke risk can be reduced by a third by reducing cholesterol to as low as 3.5 mmol/l[2]. When triglycerides alone are raised, diets low in saturated fats, and the taking of fish oil and fibrates are effective treatments[12,32]. Such patients should be screened for IGT and diabetes. Note the suggested effective use of fish oils in some psychiatric conditions.

Summary

Monitoring	
Drug	*Suggested monitoring*
Clozapine Olanzapine Quetiapine Phenothiazines	Fasting lipids at baseline then every 3 months for a year, then annually
Other antipsychotics	Fasting lipids at baseline and at 3 months, and then annually

References

1.   Brown S et al. Causes of the excess mortality of schizophrenia. Br J Psychiatry 2000; 177:212–217.
2.   Durrington P. Dyslipidaemia. Lancet 2003; 362:717–731.
3.   Sasaki J et al. Lipids and apolipoproteins in patients treated with major tranquilizers. Clin Pharmacol Ther 1985; 37:684–687.
4.   Henkin Y et al. Secondary dyslipidemia. Inadvertent effects of drugs in clinical practice. JAMA 1992; 267:961–968.
5.   Olfson M et al. Hyperlipidemia following treatment with antipsychotic medications. Am J Psychiatry 2006; 163:1821–1825.
6.   L'Italien GJ et al. Comparison of metabolic syndrome incidence among schizophrenia patients treated with aripiprazole versus olanzapine or placebo. J Clin Psychiatry 2007; 68:1510–1516.
7.   Fenton WS et al. Medication-induced weight gain and dyslipidemia in patients with schizophrenia. Am J Psychiatry 2006; 163:1697–1704.

8. Meyer JM et al. Change in metabolic syndrome parameters with antipsychotic treatment in the CATIE Schizophrenia Trial: prospective data from phase 1. Schizophr Res 2008; 101:273–286.
9. De Hert M et al. A case series: evaluation of the metabolic safety of aripiprazole. Schizophr Bull 2007; 33:823–830.
10. Sheitman BB et al. Olanzapine-induced elevation of plasma triglyceride levels. Am J Psychiatry 1999; 156:1471–1472.
11. Osser DN et al. Olanzapine increases weight and serum triglyceride levels. J Clin Psychiatry 1999; 60:767–770.
12. Meyer JM. Effects of atypical antipsychotics on weight and serum lipid levels. J Clin Psychiatry 2001;62 Suppl 27:27–34.
13. Melkersson KI et al. Elevated levels of insulin, leptin, and blood lipids in olanzapine-treated patients with schizophrenia or related psychoses. J Clin Psychiatry 2000; 61:742–749.
14. Meyer JM. Novel antipsychotics and severe hyperlipidemia. J Clin Psychopharmacol 2001; 21:369–374.
15. Kinon BJ et al. Long-term olanzapine treatment: weight change and weight-related health factors in schizophrenia. J Clin Psychiatry 2001; 62:92–100.
16. Atmaca M et al. Serum leptin and triglyceride levels in patients on treatment with atypical antipsychotics. J Clin Psychiatry 2003; 64:598–604.
17. de LJ et al. A clinical study of the association of antipsychotics with hyperlipidemia. Schizophr Res 2007; 92:95–102.
18. Koro CE et al. An assessment of the independent effects of olanzapine and risperidone exposure on the risk of hyperlipidemia in schizophrenic patients. Arch Gen Psychiatry 2002; 59:1021–1026.
19. Henderson DC et al. Clozapine, diabetes mellitus, weight gain, and lipid abnormalities: A five-year naturalistic study. Am J Psychiatry 2000; 157: 975–981.
20. Ghaeli P et al. Serum triglyceride levels in patients treated with clozapine. Am J Health Syst Pharm 1996; 53:2079–2081.
21. Spivak B et al. Diminished suicidal and aggressive behavior, high plasma norepinephrine levels, and serum triglyceride levels in chronic neuroleptic-resistant schizophrenic patients maintained on clozapine. Clin Neuropharmacol 1998; 21:245–250.
22. Baptista T et al. Novel antipsychotics and severe hyperlipidemia: comments on the Meyer paper. J Clin Psychopharmacol 2002; 22:536–537.
23. Meyer JM et al. The effects of antipsychotic therapy on serum lipids: a comprehensive review. Schizophr Res 2004; 70:1–17.
24. Paton C et al. Obesity, dyslipidaemias and smoking in an inpatient population treated with antipsychotic drugs. Acta Psychiatr Scand 2004; 110: 299–305.
25. Birkenaes AB et al. Dyslipidemia independent of body mass in antipsychotic-treated patients under real-life conditions. J Clin Psychopharmacol 2008; 28:132–137.
26. Ghaeli P et al. Elevated serum triglycerides in clozapine resolve with risperidone. Pharmacotherapy 1995; 15:382–385.
27. Weiden PJ. Switching antipsychotics as a treatment strategy for antipsychotic-induced weight gain and dyslipidemia. J Clin Psychiatry 2007;68 Suppl 4:34–39.
28. Newcomer JW et al. A multicenter, randomized, double-blind study of the effects of aripiprazole in overweight subjects with schizophrenia or schizoaffective disorder switched from olanzapine. J Clin Psychiatry 2008; 69:1046–1056.
29. Ojala K et al. Statins are effective in treating dyslipidemia among psychiatric patients using second-generation antipsychotic agents. J Psychopharmacol 2008; 22:33–38.
30. Heart Protection Study Collaborative Group. MRC/BHF Heart Protection Study of cholesterol lowering with simvastatin in 20,536 high-risk individuals: a randomised placebo-controlled trial. Lancet 2002; 360:7–22.
31. National Institute for Health and Clinical Excellence. Lipid modification: cardiovascular risk assessment and the modification of blood lipids for the primary and secondary prevention of cardiovascular disease. Clinical Guidance 67. 2008. http://www.nice.org.uk/
32. Caniato RN et al. Effect of omega-3 fatty acids on the lipid profile of patients taking clozapine. Aust N Z J Psychiatry 2006; 40:691–697.

Further reading

American Diabetes Association, American Psychiatric Association, American Association of Clinical Endocrinologists et al. Consensus development conference on antipsychotic drugs and obesity and diabetes. J Clin Psychiatry 2004; 65:267–272.
Bushe C et al. The potential impact of antipsychotics on lipids in schizophrenia: is there enough evidence to confirm a link? J Psychopharmacol 2005; 19:76–83.
Young IS. Lipids for psychiatrists – an overview. J Psychopharmacol 2005; 19:66–75.

Antipsychotics and sexual dysfunction

Primary sexual disorders are common, although reliable normative data are lacking[1]. Reported prevalence rates vary depending on the method of data collection (low numbers with spontaneous reports, increasing with confidential questionnaires and further still with direct questioning[2]). Physical illness, psychiatric illness, substance misuse and prescribed drug treatment can all cause sexual dysfunction[2].

Baseline sexual functioning should be determined if possible (questionnaires may be useful) because sexual function can affect quality of life[3] and affect compliance with medication (sexual dysfunction is one of the major causes of treatment dropout)[4]. Complaints of sexual dysfunction may also indicate progression or inadequate treatment of underlying medical or psychiatric conditions[5,6]. It may also be due to drug treatment where intervention may greatly improve quality of life[7].

The human sexual response

There are four phases of the human sexual response, as detailed in the table below[2,8–10].

Table	The human sexual response
Desire	• Related to testosterone levels in men • Possibly increased by dopamine and decreased by prolactin • Psychosocial context and conditioning significantly affect desire
Arousal	• Influenced by testosterone in men and oestrogen in women • Other potential mechanisms include: central dopamine stimulation, modulation of the cholinergic/adrenergic balance, peripheral α_1 agonism and nitric oxide pathways • Physical pathology such as hypertension or diabetes can have a significant effect
Orgasm	• May be related to oxytocin • Inhibition of orgasm may be caused by an increase in serotonin activity, as well as α_1 blockade
Resolution	• Occurs passively after orgasm
Note: Many other hormones and neurotransmitters may interact in a complex way at each phase.	

Effects of psychosis

Sexual dysfunction is a problem in first-episode schizophrenia[11] and up to 82% of men and 96% of women with established illness report problems with associated reductions in quality of life[3]. Men[12] complain of reduced desire, inability to achieve an erection and premature ejaculation whereas women complain more generally about reduced enjoyment[12,13]. Women with psychosis are known to have reduced fertility[14]. People with psychosis are less able to develop good psycho-sexual relationships and, for some, treatment with an antipsychotic can improve sexual functioning[15]. Assessment of sexual functioning can clearly be difficult in someone who is psychotic. The Arizona Sexual Experience Scale (ASEX) may be useful in this respect[16].

Effects of antipsychotic drugs

Sexual dysfunction has been reported as a side-effect of all antipsychotics[7], and up to 45% of people taking conventional antipsychotics experience sexual dysfunction[17]. Individual suscepti-bility varies and all effects are reversible. Antipsychotics decrease dopaminergic transmission, which in itself can decrease libido but may also increase prolactin levels via negative feedback. This can cause amenorrhoea in women and a lack of libido, breast enlargement and galactorrhoea in both men and women[18]. The overall propensity of an antipsychotic to cause sexual dysfunction is similar to its propensity to raise prolactin, i.e. risperidone > haloperidol > olanzapine > quetiapine

> aripiprazole[5,19]. Aripiprazole is relatively free of sexual side-effects when used as monotherapy[20] and possibly also in combination with another antipsychotic[21,22].

Anticholinergic effects can cause disorders of arousal[23] and drugs that block peripheral α_1 receptors cause particular problems with erection and ejaculation in men[7]. Drugs that are antagonists at both peripheral α_1 receptors and cholinergic receptors can cause priapism[24]. Antipsychotic-induced sedation and weight gain may reduce sexual desire[24]. These principles can be used to predict the sexual side-effects of different antipsychotic drugs (see table below).

Table Sexual adverse effects of antipsychotics

Drug	Type of problem
Phenothiazines	• Hyperprolactinaemia and anticholinergic effects. Reports of delayed orgasm at lower doses followed by normal orgasm but without ejaculation at higher doses[13] • Most problems occur with thioridazine (which can also reduce testosterone levels)[25] • Priapism has been reported with thioridazine, risperidone and chlorpromazine (probably due to α_1 blockade)[26–28]
Thioxanthenes	• Arousal problems and anorgasmia[15]
Haloperidol	• Similar problems to the phenothiazines[29] but anticholinergic effects reduced[26]
Olanzapine	• Possibly less sexual dysfunction due to relative lack of prolactin-related effects[29] • Priapism reported rarely[30,31]
Risperidone	• Potent elevator of serum prolactin • Less anticholinergic • Specific peripheral α_1 adrenergic blockade leads to a moderately high reported incidence of ejaculatory problems such as retrograde ejaculation[32,33] • Priapism reported rarely[24]
Sulpiride/ amisulpride	• Potent elevators of serum prolactin[17]
Quetiapine	• No effect on serum prolactin[34] • Possibly associated with low risk of sexual dysfunction[35–38], but studies are conflicting[39,40]
Clozapine	• Significant α_1 adrenergic blockade and anticholinergic effects[41]. No effect on prolactin[42] • Probably fewer problems than with typical antipsychotics[43]
Aripiprazole	• No effect on prolactin or α_1 receptors. No reported adverse effects on sexual function. Improves sexual function in those switched from other antipsychotics[20,22,44]

Treatment

Before attempting to treat sexual dysfunction, a thorough assessment is essential to determine the most likely cause. Assuming that physical pathology has been excluded, the following principles apply.

Spontaneous remission may occasionally occur[24]. The most obvious first step is to decrease the dose or discontinue the offending drug where appropriate. The next step is to switch to a different drug that is less likely to cause the specific sexual problem experienced (see table above). If this fails or is not practicable, 'antidote' drugs can be tried: for example, cyproheptadine (a 5HT$_2$ antagonist at doses of 4–16 mg/day) has been used to treat SSRI-induced sexual dysfunction but sedation is a common side-effect. Amantadine, bupropion, buspirone, bethanechol and yohimbine have all been used with varying degrees of success but have a number of unwanted side-effects and interactions with other drugs (see opposite). Given that hyperprolactinaemia may contribute to sexual dysfunction, selegiline (enhances dopamine activity) has been tested in an RCT. This was negative[45]. Testosterone patches have been shown to increase libido in women, although note though that breast cancer risk may be significantly increased[46,47].

(*Continued*)

115

Table Remedial treatments for psychotropic-induced sexual dysfunction

Drug	Pharmacology	Potential treatment for	Side-effects
Alprostadil[1,9]	Prostaglandin	Erectile dysfunction	Pain, fibrosis, hypotension, priapism
Amantadine[1,48]	Dopamine agonist	Prolactin-induced reduction in desire and arousal (dopamine increases libido and facilitates ejaculation)	Return of psychotic symptoms, GI effects, nervousness, insomnia, rash
Bethanechol[49]	Cholinergic or cholinergic potentiation of adrenergic neurotransmission	Anticholinergic induced arousal problems and anorgasmia (from TCAs, antipsychotics, etc.)	Nausea and vomiting, colic, bradycardia, blurred vision, sweating
Bromocriptine[7]	Dopamine agonist	Prolactin-induced reduction in desire and arousal	Return of psychotic symptoms, GI effects
Bupropion[50]	Noradrenaline and dopamine reuptake inhibitor	SSRI-induced sexual dysfunction (evidence poor)	Concentration problems, reduced sleep, tremor
Buspirone[51]	$5HT_{1a}$ partial agonist	SSRI-induced sexual dysfunction, particularly decreased libido and anorgasmia	Nausea, dizziness, headache
Cyproheptadine[1,51,52]	$5HT_2$ antagonist	Sexual dysfunction caused by increased serotonin transmission (e.g. SSRIs), particularly anorgasmia	Sedation and fatigue. Reversal of the therapeutic effect of antidepressants
Sildenafil[9,53–56]	Phosphodiesterase inhibitor	Erectile dysfunction of any aetiology. Anorgasmia in women. Effective when prolactin raised	Mild headaches, dizziness, nasal congestion
Yohimbine[1,9,57–59]	Central and peripheral α_2 adrenoceptor antagonist	SSRI-induced sexual dysfunction, particularly erectile dysfunction, decreased libido and anorgasmia (evidence poor)	Anxiety, nausea, fine tremor, increased BP, sweating, fatigue

Note: The use of the drugs listed above should ideally be under the care or supervision of a specialist in sexual dysfunction.

(Cont.)

The evidence base supporting the use of 'antidotes' is poor[24].

Drugs such as sildenafil (Viagra) or alprostadil (Caverject) are effective only in the treatment of erectile dysfunction. In the UK they are available for prescription by GPs for a limited number of medical indications, not including psychosis or antipsychotic-induced impotence[60]. Psychological approaches used by sexual dysfunction clinics may be difficult for clients with mental health problems to engage in[7].

References

1. Baldwin DS et al. Effects of antidepressant drugs on sexual function. Int J Psychiatry Clin Pract 1997; 1:47–58.
2. Pollack MH et al. Genitourinary and sexual adverse effects of psychotropic medication. Int J Psychiatry Med 1992; 22:305–327.
3. Olfson M et al. Male sexual dysfunction and quality of life in schizophrenia. J Clin Psychiatry 2005; 66:331–338.
4. Montejo AL et al. Incidence of sexual dysfunction associated with antidepressant agents: a prospective multicenter study of 1022 outpatients. Spanish Working Group for the Study of Psychotropic-Related Sexual Dysfunction. J Clin Psychiatry 2001;62 Suppl 3:10–21.
5. Baggaley M. Sexual dysfunction in schizophrenia: focus on recent evidence. Hum Psychopharmacol 2008; 23:201–209.
6. Ucok A et al. Sexual dysfunction in patients with schizophrenia on antipsychotic medication. Eur Psychiatry 2007; 22:328–333.
7. Segraves RT. Effects of psychotropic drugs on human erection and ejaculation. Arch Gen Psychiatry 1989; 46:275–284.
8. Stahl SM. The psychopharmacology of sex, Part 1: Neurotransmitters and the 3 phases of the human sexual response. J Clin Psychiatry 2001; 62:80–81.
9. Garcia-Reboll L et al. Drugs for the treatment of impotence. Drugs Aging 1997; 11:140–151.
10. deGroat WC et al. Physiology of male sexual function. Ann Intern Med 1980; 92:329–331.
11. Bitter I et al. Antipsychotic treatment and sexual functioning in first-time neuroleptic-treated schizophrenic patients. Int Clin Psychopharmacol 2005; 20:19–21.
12. Macdonald S et al. Nithsdale Schizophrenia Surveys 24: sexual dysfunction. Case-control study. Br J Psychiatry 2003; 182:50–56.
13. Smith S. Effects of antipsychotics on sexual and endocrine function in women: implications for clinical practice. J Clin Psychopharmacol 2003; 23: S27–S32.
14. Howard LM et al. The general fertility rate in women with psychotic disorders. Am J Psychiatry 2002; 159:991–997.
15. Aizenberg D et al. Sexual dysfunction in male schizophrenic patients. J Clin Psychiatry 1995; 56:137–141.
16. Byerly MJ et al. An empirical evaluation of the Arizona sexual experience scale and a simple one-item screening test for assessing antipsychotic-related sexual dysfunction in outpatients with schizophrenia and schizoaffective disorder. Schizophr Res 2006; 81:311–316.
17. Smith SM et al. Sexual dysfunction in patients taking conventional antipsychotic medication. Br J Psychiatry 2002; 181:49–55.
18. Anon. Adverse effects of the atypical antipsychotics. Collaborative Working Group on Clinical Trial Evaluations. J Clin Psychiatry 1998;59 Suppl 12:17–22.
19. Knegtering H et al. Are sexual side-effects of prolactin-raising antipsychotics reducible to serum prolactin? Psychoneuroendocrinology 2008; 33: 711–717.
20. Hanssens L et al. The effect of antipsychotic medication on sexual function and serum prolactin levels in community-treated schizophrenic patients: results from the Schizophrenia Trial of Aripiprazole (STAR) study (NCT00237913). BMC Psychiatry 2008; 8:95.
21. Mir A et al. Change in sexual dysfunction with aripiprazole: a switching or add-on study. J Psychopharmacol 2008; 22:244–253.
22. Byerly MJ et al. Effects of aripiprazole on prolactin levels in subjects with schizophrenia during cross-titration with risperidone or olanzapine: Analysis of a randomized, open-label study. Schizophr Res 2009; 107:218–222.
23. Aldridge SA. Drug-induced sexual dysfunction. Clin Pharm 1982; 1:141–147.
24. Baldwin D et al. Sexual side-effects of antidepressant and antipsychotic drugs. Adv Psychiatr Treat 2003; 9:202–210.
25. Kotin J et al. Thioridazine and sexual dysfunction. Am J Psychiatry 1976; 133:82–85.
26. Mitchell JE et al. Antipsychotic drug therapy and sexual dysfunction in men. Am J Psychiatry 1982; 139:633–637.
27. Loh C et al. Risperidone-induced retrograde ejaculation: case report and review of the literature. Int Clin Psychopharmacol 2004; 19:111–112.
28. Thompson JW, Jr. et al. Psychotropic medication and priapism: a comprehensive review. J Clin Psychiatry 1990; 51:430–433.
29. Crawford AM et al. The acute and long-term effect of olanzapine compared with placebo and haloperidol on serum prolactin concentrations. Schizophr Res 1997; 26:41–54.
30. Eli Lilly and Company Limited. Summary of Product Characteristics Zyprexa 2.5mg, 5mg, 7.5mg, 10mg, 15mg, and 20mg coated tablets. Zyprexa Velotab 5mg, 10mg, 15mg, and 20mg orodispersible tablets. 2009. http://emc.medicines.org.uk/
31. Dossenbach M et al. Effects of atypical and typical antipsychotic treatments on sexual function in patients with schizophrenia: 12-month results from the Intercontinental Schizophrenia Outpatient Health Outcomes (IC-SOHO) study. Eur Psychiatry 2006; 21:251–258.
32. Tran PV et al. Double-blind comparison of olanzapine versus risperidone in the treatment of schizophrenia and other psychotic disorders. J Clin Psychopharmacol 1997; 17:407–418.
33. Raja M. Risperidone-induced absence of ejaculation. Int Clin Psychopharmacol 1999; 14:317–319.
34. Peuskens J et al. A comparison of quetiapine and chlorpromazine in the treatment of schizophrenia. Acta Psychiatr Scand 1997; 96:265–273.
35. Bobes J et al. Frequency of sexual dysfunction and other reproductive side-effects in patients with schizophrenia treated with risperidone, olanzapine, quetiapine, or haloperidol: the results of the EIRE study. J Sex Marital Ther 2003; 29:125–147.
36. Byerly MJ et al. An open-label trial of quetiapine for antipsychotic-induced sexual dysfunction. J Sex Marital Ther 2004; 30:325–332.
37. Knegtering R et al. A randomized open-label study of the impact of quetiapine versus risperidone on sexual functioning. J Clin Psychopharmacol 2004; 24:56–61.
38. Montejo Gonzalez AL et al. A 6-month prospective observational study on the effects of quetiapine on sexual functioning. J Clin Psychopharmacol 2005; 25:533–538.
39. Atmaca M et al. A new atypical antipsychotic: quetiapine-induced sexual dysfunctions. Int J Impot Res 2005; 17:201–203.
40. Kelly DL et al. A randomized double-blind 12-week study of quetiapine, risperidone or fluphenazine on sexual functioning in people with schizophrenia. Psychoneuroendocrinology 2006; 31:340–346.
41. Coward DM. General pharmacology of clozapine. Br J Psychiatry 1992; 160:5–11.
42. Meltzer HY et al. Effect of clozapine on human serum prolactin levels. Am J Psychiatry 1979; 136:1550–1555.
43. Aizenberg D et al. Comparison of sexual dysfunction in male schizophrenic patients maintained on treatment with classical antipsychotics versus clozapine. J Clin Psychiatry 2001; 62:541–544.
44. Rykmans V et al. A comparision of switching strategies from risperidone to aripiprazole in patients with schizophrenia with insufficient efficacy/ tolerability on risperidone (cn138–169). Eur Psychiatry 2008; 23:S111.

Schizophrenia

45. Kodesh A et al. Selegiline in the treatment of sexual dysfunction in schizophrenic patients maintained on neuroleptics: a pilot study. Clin Neuropharmacol 2003; 26:193–195.
46. Davis SR et al. Testosterone for low libido in postmenopausal women not taking estrogen. New Engl J Med 2008; 359:2005–2017.
47. Schover LR. Androgen therapy for loss of desire in women: is the benefit worth the breast cancer risk? Fertil Steril 2008; 90:129–140.
48. Valevski A et al. Effect of amantadine on sexual dysfunction in neuroleptic-treated male schizophrenic patients. Clin Neuropharmacol 1998; 21:355–357.
49. Gross MD. Reversal by bethanechol of sexual dysfunction caused by anticholinergic antidepressants. Am J Psychiatry 1982; 139:1193–1194.
50. Masand PS et al. Sustained-release bupropion for selective serotonin reuptake inhibitor-induced sexual dysfunction: a randomized, double-blind, placebo-controlled, parallel-group study. Am J Psychiatry 2001; 158:805–807.
51. Rothschild AJ. Sexual side-effects of antidepressants. J Clin Psychiatry 2000;61 Suppl 11:28–36.
52. Lauerma H. Successful treatment of citalopram-induced anorgasmia by cyproheptadine. Acta Psychiatr Scand 1996; 93:69–70.
53. Nurnberg HG et al. Sildenafil for women patients with antidepressant-induced sexual dysfunction. Psychiatr Serv 1999; 50:1076–1078.
54. Salerian AJ et al. Sildenafil for psychotropic-induced sexual dysfunction in 31 women and 61 men. J Sex Marital Ther 2000; 26:133–140.
55. Nurnberg HG et al. Treatment of antidepressant-associated sexual dysfunction with sildenafil: a randomized controlled trial. JAMA 2003; 289:56–64.
56. Gopalakrishnan R et al. Sildenafil in the treatment of antipsychotic-induced erectile dysfunction: a randomized, double-blind, placebo-controlled, flexible-dose, two-way crossover trial. Am J Psychiatry 2006; 163:494–499.
57. Jacobsen FM. Fluoxetine-induced sexual dysfunction and an open trial of yohimbine. J Clin Psychiatry 1992; 53:119–122.
58. Michelson D et al. Mirtazapine, yohimbine or olanzapine augmentation therapy for serotonin reuptake-associated female sexual dysfunction: a randomized, placebo controlled trial. J Psychiatr Res 2002; 36:147–152.
59. Woodrum ST et al. Management of SSRI-induced sexual dysfunction. Ann Pharmacother 1998; 32:1209–1215.
60. Department of Health. HSC 1999/117: The new NHS guidance on out of area treatments. 1999. http://www.dh.gov.uk/

Further reading

Meco G et al. Sexual dysfunction in Parkinson's disease. Parkinsonism Relat Disord 2008; 14:451–456.
Tenback DE et al. Tardive dyskinesia in schizophrenia is associated with prolactin-related sexual disturbances. Neuropsychopharmacology 2006; 31:1832–1837.

Schizophrenia

Antipsychotic-induced hyponatraemia

Hyponatraemia can occur in the context of:

- **Water intoxication** where water consumption exceeds the maximal renal clearance capacity. Serum and urine osmolality are low. Cross-sectional studies of chronically ill, hospitalised, psychiatric patients have found the prevalence of water intoxication to be approximately 5%[1,2]. A longitudinal study found that 10% of severely ill patients with a diagnosis of schizophrenia had episodic hyponatraemia secondary to fluid overload[3].The primary aetiology is poorly understood. It has been postulated that it may be driven, at least in part, by an extreme compensatory response to the anticholinergic side-effects of antipsychotic drugs[4].
- **Drug-induced syndrome of inappropriate antidiuretic hormone** (SIADH) where the kidney retains an excessive quantity of solute-free water. Serum osmolality is low and urine osmolality relatively high. The prevalence of SIADH is estimated to be as high as 11% in acutely ill psychiatric patients[5]. Risk factors for antidepressant-induced SIADH (increasing age, female gender, medical co-morbidity and polypharmacy) seem to be less relevant in the population of patients treated with antipsychotic drugs[6]. SIADH usually develops in the first few weeks of treatment with the offending drug. Phenothiazines, haloperidol, pimozide, risperidone, quetiapine, olanzapine, aripiprazole and clozapine have all been implicated[6,7]. Note, however, that the literature consists entirely of case reports and case series. Desmopressin use (for clozapine-induced enuresis) can also result in hyponatraemia[8].
- **Severe hyperlipidaemia and/or hyperglycaemia** lead to secondary increases in plasma volume and 'pseudohyponatraemia'[4]. Both are more common in people treated with antipsychotic drugs than in the general population and should be excluded as causes.

Mild to moderate hyponatraemia presents as confusion, nausea, headache and lethargy. As the plasma sodium falls, these symptoms become increasingly severe and seizures and coma can develop.

Monitoring of plasma sodium is probably not strictly necessary for all those receiving antipsychotics, but is desirable. Signs of confusion of lethargy should provoke thorough diagnostic analysis, including plasma sodium determination.

Table Treatment[4,5]

Cause of hyponatraemia	Antipsychotic drugs implicated	Treatment
Water intoxication (serum and urine osmolality low)	Only very speculative evidence to support drugs as a cause Core part of illness in a minority of patients (e.g. psychotic polydipsia)	• Fluid restriction with careful monitoring of serum sodium, particularly diurnal variation (Na drops as the day progresses). Refer to specialist medical care if Na < 125 mmol/l. Note that the use of IV saline to correct hyponatraemia has been reported to precipitate rhabdomyolysis[9] • Consider treatment with clozapine: shown to increase plasma osmolality into the normal range and increase urine osmolality (not usually reaching the normal range)[10]. These effects are consistent with reduced fluid intake. This effect is not clearly related to improvements in mental state[11] • There are both[6] positive and negative reports for olanzapine[12] and risperidone[13] and one positive case report for quetiapine[14]. Compared with clozapine, the evidence base is weak • There is no evidence that either reducing or increasing the dose of an antipsychotic results in improvements in serum sodium in water-intoxicated patients[15] • Demeclocycline should not be used (exerts its effect by interfering with ADH and increasing water excretion, already at capacity in these patients)
SIADH (serum osmolality low; urine osmolality relatively high)	All antipsychotic drugs	• If mild, fluid restriction with careful monitoring of serum sodium. Refer to specialist medical care if Na < 125 mmol/l • Switching to a different antipsychotic drug. There are insufficient data available to guide choice. Be aware that cross-sensitivity may occur (the individual may be predisposed and the choice of drug relatively less important) • Consider demeclocycline (see *BNF* for details) • Lithium may be effective[6] but is a potentially toxic drug. Remember that hyponatraemia predisposes to lithium toxicity

A new class of drugs in development called vaptans (non-peptide arginine-vasopression antagonists) shows promise in the treatment of hyponatraemia of varying aetiology, including that caused by SIADH. They are also known as aquaretics because they induce a highly hypotonic diuresis[16].

References

1. de Leon J et al. Polydipsia and water intoxication in psychiatric patients: a review of the epidemiological literature. Biol Psychiatry 1994; 35:408–419.
2. Patel JK. Polydipsia, hyponatremia, and water intoxication among psychiatric patients. Hosp Community Psychiatry 1994; 45:1073–1074.
3. de Leon J. Polydipsia – a study in a long-term psychiatric unit. Eur Arch Psychiatry Clin Neurosci 2003; 253:37–39.
4. Siegel AJ et al. Primary and drug-induced disorders of water homeostasis in psychiatric patients: principles of diagnosis and management. Harv Rev Psychiatry 1998; 6:190–200.
5. Siegler EL et al. Risk factors for the development of hyponatremia in psychiatric inpatients. Arch Intern Med 1995; 155:953–957.
6. Madhusoodanan S et al. Hyponatraemia associated with psychotropic medications. A review of the literature and spontaneous reports. Adverse Drug React Toxicol Rev 2002; 21:17–29.
7. Bachu K et al. Aripiprazole-induced syndrome of inappropriate antidiuretic hormone secretion (SIADH). Am J Ther 2006; 13:370–372.
8. Sarma S et al. Severe hyponatraemia associated with desmopressin nasal spray to treat clozapine-induced nocturnal enuresis. Aust N Z J Psychiatry 2005; 39:949.
9. Zaidi AN. Rhabdomyolysis after correction of hyponatremia in psychogenic polydipsia possibly complicated by ziprasidone. Ann Pharmacother 2005; 39:1726–1731.
10. Canuso CM et al. Clozapine restores water balance in schizophrenic patients with polydipsia-hyponatremia syndrome. J Neuropsychiatry Clin Neurosci 1999; 11:86–90.
11. Spears NM et al. Clozapine treatment in polydipsia and intermittent hyponatremia. J Clin Psychiatry 1996; 57:123–128.
12. Littrell KH et al. Effects of olanzapine on polydipsia and intermittent hyponatremia. J Clin Psychiatry 1997; 58:549.
13. Kawai N et al. Risperidone failed to improve polydipsia-hyponatremia of the schizophrenic patients. Psychiatry Clin Neurosci 2002; 56:107–110.
14. Montgomery JH et al. Adjunctive quetiapine treatment of the polydipsia, intermittent hyponatremia, and psychosis syndrome: a case report. J Clin Psychiatry 2003; 64:339–341.
15. Canuso CM et al. Does minimizing neuroleptic dosage influence hyponatremia? Psychiatry Res 1996; 63:227–229.
16. Decaux G et al. Non-peptide arginine-vasopressin antagonists: the vaptans. Lancet 2008; 371:1624–1632.

Schizophrenia

Antipsychotics: relative adverse effects – a rough guide

Drug	Sedation	Weight gain	Extra-pyramidal	Anti-cholinergic	Hypotension	Prolactin elevation
Amisulpride	–	+	+	–	–	+++
Aripiprazole	–	+/–	+/–	–	–	–
Asenapine	–	+/–	+/–	–	–	+/–
Benperidol	+	+	+++	+	+	+++
Bifeprunox	–	+/–	+/–	–	–	–
Chlorpromazine	+++	++	++	++	+++	+++
Clozapine	+++	+++	–	+++	+++	–
Flupentixol	+	++	++	++	+	+++
Fluphenazine	+	+	+++	++	+	+++
Haloperidol	+	+	+++	+	+	+++
Iloperidone	–	++	+	–	+	–
Loxapine	++	+	+++	+	++	+++
Olanzapine	++	+++	+/–	+	+	+
Paliperidone	+	++	+	+	++	+++
Perphenazine	+	+	+++	+	+	+++
Pimozide	+	+	+	+	+	+++
Pipotiazine	++	++	++	++	++	+++
Promazine	+++	++	+	++	++	++
Quetiapine	++	++	–	+	++	–
Risperidone	+	++	+	+	++	+++
Sertindole	–	+	–	–	+++	+/–
Sulpiride	–	+	+	–	–	+++
Trifluoperazine	+	+	+++	+/–	+	+++
Ziprasidone	+	+/–	+/–	–	+	+/–
Zotepine	+++	++	+	+	++	++ +
Zuclopenthixol	++	++	++	++	+	+++

Key: +++ High incidence/severity
    ++ Moderate
    + Low
    – Very low

Note: the table above is made up of approximate estimates of relative incidence and/or severity, based on clinical experience, manufacturers' literature and published research. This is a rough guide – see individual sections for more precise information.

Other sides-effects not mentioned in this table do occur. Please see dedicated sections on other side-effects included in this book for more information.

Schizophrenia

chapter 3

Bipolar disorder

Valproate

Mechanism of action[1]

Valproate is a simple branched-chain fatty acid. Its mechanism of action is complex and not fully understood. Valproate inhibits the catabolism of GABA, reduces the turnover of arachidonic acid, activates the extracellular signal-regulated kinase (ERK) pathway thus altering synaptic plasticity, interferes with intracellular signalling, promotes BDNF expression and reduces levels of protein kinase C. Recent research has focused on the ability of valproate to alter the expression of multiple genes that are involved in transcription regulation, cytoskeletal modifications and ion homeostasis. Other mechanisms that have been proposed include depletion of inositol and indirect effects on non-GABA pathways through inhibition of voltage-gated sodium channels.

There is a growing literature relating to the potential use of valproate as an adjunctive treatment in several types of cancer; the relevant mechanism of action being inhibition of histone deacetylase[2,3].

Formulations

Valproate is available in the UK in three forms: sodium valproate and valproic acid (licensed for the treatment of epilepsy), and semi-sodium valproate, licensed for the treatment of acute mania. Both semi-sodium and sodium valproate are metabolised to valproic acid, which is responsible for the pharmacological activity of all three preparations[4]. Clinical studies of the treatment of affective disorders variably use sodium valproate, semi-sodium valproate, 'valproate' or valproic acid. The great majority have used semi-sodium valproate.

In the US, valproic acid is widely used in the treatment of bipolar illness[5], and in the UK sodium valproate is widely used. It is important to remember that doses of sodium valproate and semi-sodium valproate are not equivalent; a slightly higher (approximately 10%) dose is required if sodium valproate is used to allow for the extra sodium content.

It is unclear if there is any difference in efficacy between valproic acid, valproate semi-sodium and sodium valproate. One large US quasi-experimental study found that inpatients who initially received the semi-sodium preparation had a hospital stay that was a third longer than patients who initially received valproic acid[6]. Note that sodium valproate controlled-release (Epilim Chrono) can be administered as a once-daily dose whereas other sodium and semi-sodium valproate preparations require at least twice-daily administration.

Indications

Randomised controlled trials (RCTs) have shown valproate to be effective in the treatment of **mania**[7,8], with a response rate of 50% and a NNT of 2–4[9]. One RCT found lithium to be more effective overall than valproate[8] but a large (n = 300) randomised open trial of 12 weeks' duration found lithium and valproate to be equally effective in the treatment of acute mania[10]. Valproate may be effective in patients who have failed to respond to lithium; in a small placebo-controlled RCT (n = 36) in patients who had failed to respond to or could not tolerate lithium, the median decrease in Young Mania Rating Scale scores was 54% in the valproate group and 5% in the placebo group[11]. It may be less effective than olanzapine as an adjunctive treatment to lithium in acute mania[12].

Open studies and two small randomised placebo-controlled studies[13,14] suggest that valproate may have some efficacy in **bipolar depression** although further data are required[9]. The attrition rate in all of these studies was high (a feature of all bipolar studies).

Although open label studies suggest that valproate is effective in the **prophylaxis** of bipolar affective disorder[15], RCT data are limited[16,17]. Bowden et al[18] found no difference between lithium, valproate and placebo in the primary outcome measure, time to any mood episode, although valproate was superior to lithium and placebo on some secondary outcome measures. This study can be criticised for including patients who were 'not ill enough' and for not lasting 'long enough' (1 year). In another RCT[16], which lasted for 47 weeks, there was no difference in relapse rates between valproate and olanzapine. The study had no placebo arm and the attrition rate was high, so is difficult to interpret. A post-hoc analysis of data from this study found that patients with rapid-cycling illness had a better very early response to valproate than to olanzapine but that this advantage was not maintained[17]. Outcomes with respect to manic symptoms for those who did not have a rapid-cycling illness were better at 1 year with olanzapine than valproate. In a further 20-month RCT of lithium versus valproate in patients with rapid-cycling illness, both the relapse and attrition rates were high, and no difference in efficacy between valproate and lithium was apparent[19].

NICE recommends valproate as a first-line option for the treatment of acute episodes of mania, in combination with an antidepressant for the treatment of acute episodes of depression, and for prophylaxis[20].

Valproate is sometimes used to treat aggressive behaviours of variable aetiology[21]. One small RCT (n = 16) failed to detect any advantage for risperidone augmented with valproate over risperidone alone in reducing hostility in patients with schizophrenia[22]. A mirror-image study found that, in patients with schizophrenia or bipolar disorder in a secure setting, valproate decreased agitation[23].

There is a small positive placebo-controlled RCT of valproate in generalized anxiety disorder[24].

Plasma levels

The pharmacokinetics of valproate are complex, following a three-compartmental model and showing protein-binding saturation. Plasma level monitoring is supposedly of more limited use than with lithium or carbamazepine. There may be a linear association between valproate serum levels and response in acute mania, with serum levels <55 mg/L being no more effective than placebo and levels >94 mg/L being associated with the most robust response[25]. Note that this is the top of the reference range (for epilepsy) that is quoted on laboratory forms. Optimal serum levels during the maintenance phase are unknown, but are likely to be at least 50 mg/L[26]. Achieving therapeutic plasma levels rapidly using a loading dose regimen is generally well tolerated. Plasma levels can also be used to detect non-compliance or toxicity.

Adverse effects
Valproate can cause both gastric irritation and hyperammonaemia[27], both of which can lead to nausea. Lethargy and confusion can occasionally occur with starting doses above 750 mg/day. Weight gain can be significant[28], particularly when valproate is used in combination with clozapine. Valproate causes dose-related tremor in up to a quarter of patients[29]. In the majority of these patients it is intention/postural tremor that is problematic, but a very small proportion develop Parkinsonism associated with cognitive decline; these symptoms are reversible when valproate is discontinued[30].

Hair loss with curly regrowth and peripheral oedema can occur, as can thrombocytopenia, leuco-penia, red cell hypoplasia and pancreatitis[31]. Valproate can cause hyperandrogenism in women[32] and has been linked with the development of polycystic ovaries; the evidence supporting this association is conflicting. Valproate is a major human teratogen (see Pregnancy section, Chapter 7). Valproate may very rarely cause fulminant hepatic failure. Young children receiving multiple anticonvulsants are most at risk. Any patient with raised LFTs (common in early treatment[33]) should be evaluated clinically and other markers of hepatic function such as albumin and clotting time should be checked.

Many side effects of valproate are dose-related (peak plasma-level related) and increase in frequency and severity when the plasma level is >100 mg/L. The once-daily Chrono form of sodium valproate does not produce as high peak plasma levels as the conventional formulation, and so may be better tolerated.

Note that valproate is eliminated mainly through the kidneys, partly in the form of ketone bodies, and may give a false-positive urine test for ketones.

Pre-treatment tests
Baseline FBC, LFTs and weight or BMI are recommended by NICE.

On-treatment monitoring
NICE recommend that a FBC and LFTs should be repeated after 6 months, and that BMI should be monitored. Valproate SPCs recommend more frequent LFTs during the first 6 months with albumin and clotting measured if enzyme levels are abnormal.

Discontinuation
It is unknown if abrupt discontinuation of valproate worsens the natural course of bipolar illness in the same way as lithium does. One small naturalistic retrospective study suggests that it might[34]. Until further data are available, if valproate is to be discontinued, it should be done slowly.

Use in women of childbearing age
Valproate is an established human teratogen. NICE recommend that alternative anticonvulsants are to be preferred in women with epilepsy[35] and that valproate should not be routinely used to treat bipolar illness in women of childbearing age[20].

The SPCs for sodium valproate and semi-sodium valproate[36,37] state that:

- These drugs should not be initiated in women of childbearing potential without specialist advice (from a neurologist or psychiatrist)
- Women who are trying to conceive and require valproate, should be prescribed prophylactic folate.

Women who have mania are likely to be sexually disinhibited. The risk of unplanned pregnancy is likely to be above population norms (where 50% of pregnancies are unplanned). If valproate cannot be avoided, adequate contraception should be ensured and prophylactic folate prescribed.

The teratogenic potential of valproate is not widely appreciated and many women of childbearing age are not advised of the need for contraception or prophylactic folate[38,39]. Valproate may also cause impaired cognitive function in children exposed to valproate in utero[40].

Interactions with other drugs

Valproate is highly protein bound and can be displaced by other protein-bound drugs, such as aspirin, leading to toxicity. Aspirin also inhibits the metabolism of valproate; a dose of at least 300 mg aspirin is required[41]. Other, less strongly protein-bound drugs such as warfarin can be displaced by valproate, leading to higher free levels and toxicity.

Valproate is hepatically metabolised; drugs that inhibit CYP enzymes can increase valproate levels (e.g. erythromycin, fluoxetine and cimetidine). Valproate can increase the plasma levels of some drugs, possibly by inhibition/competitive inhibition of their metabolism. Examples include TCAs (particularly clomipramine[42]), lamotrigine[43], quetiapine[44], warfarin[45] and phenobarbital. Valproate may also significantly lower plasma olanzapine concentrations; the mechanism is unknown[46].

Pharmacodynamic interactions also occur. The anticonvulsant effect of valproate is antagonised by drugs that lower the seizure threshold (e.g. antipsychotics). Weight gain can be exacerbated by other drugs such as clozapine and olanzapine.

Table	Valproate: prescribing and monitoring
Indications	Mania, hypomania, bipolar depression (with an antidepressant) and prophylaxis of bipolar affective disorder. May reduce aggression in a range of psychiatric disorders (data weak)
	Note that sodium valproate is licensed only for epilepsy and semi-sodium valproate only for acute mania
Pre-valproate work up	FBC and LFTs. Baseline measure of weight desirable
Prescribing	Titrate dose upwards against response and side effects. Loading doses can be used and are generally well tolerated. Note that CR sodium valproate (Epilim Chrono) can be given once daily. All other formulations must be administered at least twice daily
	Plasma levels can be used to assure adequate dosing and treatment compliance. Blood should be taken immediately before the next dose
Monitoring	As a minimum, FBC and LFTs after 6 months
	Weight (or BMI) should also be monitored
Stopping	Reduce slowly over at least 1 month

References

1. Rosenberg G. The mechanisms of action of valproate in neuropsychiatric disorders: can we see the forest for the trees? Cell Mol Life Sci 2007; 64: 2090–103.
2. Kuendgen A et al. Valproic acid for the treatment of myeloid malignancies. Cancer 2007; 110:943–54.
3. Atmaca A et al. Valproic acid (VPA) in patients with refractory advanced cancer: a dose escalating phase I clinical trial. Br J Cancer 2007; 97:177–82.
4. Fisher C et al. Sodium valproate or valproate semisodium: is there a difference in the treatment of bipolar disorder? Psychiatr Bull 2003; 27:446–8.
5. Iqbal SU et al. Divalproex sodium vs. valproic acid: drug utilization patterns, persistence rates and predictors of hospitalization among VA patients diagnosed with bipolar disorder. J Clin Pharm Ther 2007; 32:625–32.
6. Wassef AA et al. Lower effectiveness of divalproex versus valproic acid in a prospective, quasi-experimental clinical trial involving 9,260 psychiatric admissions. Am J Psychiatry 2005; 162:330–9.
7. Bowden CL et al. Efficacy of divalproex vs lithium and placebo in the treatment of mania. The Depakote Mania Study Group. JAMA 1994; 271:918–24.
8. Freeman TW et al. A double-blind comparison of valproate and lithium in the treatment of acute-mania. Am J Psychiatry 1992; 149:108–11.
9. Nasrallah HA et al. Carbamazepine and valproate for the treatment of bipolar disorder: a review of the literature. J Affect Disord 2006; 95:69–78.
10. Bowden C et al. A 12-week, open, randomized trial comparing sodium valproate to lithium in patients with bipolar I disorder suffering from a manic episode. Int Clin Psychopharmacol 2008; 23:254–62.
11. Pope HG Jr et al. Valproate in the treatment of acute mania. A placebo-controlled study. Arch Gen Psychiatry 1991; 48:62–8.
12. Maina G et al. Valproate or olanzapine add-on to lithium: an 8-week, randomized, open-label study in Italian patients with a manic relapse. J Affect Disord 2007; 99:247–51.
13. Davis LL et al. Divalproex in the treatment of bipolar depression: a placebo-controlled study. J Affect Disord 2005; 85:259–66.
14. Ghaemi SN et al. Divalproex in the treatment of acute bipolar depression: a preliminary double-blind, randomized, placebo-controlled pilot study. J Clin Psychiatry 2007; 68:1840–4.
15. Calabrese JR et al. Spectrum of efficacy of valproate in 55 patients with rapid-cycling bipolar disorder. Am J Psychiatry 1990; 147:431–4.
16. Tohen M et al. Olanzapine versus divalproex sodium for the treatment of acute mania and maintenance of remission: a 47-week study. Am J Psychiatry 2003; 160:1263–71.
17. Suppes T et al. Rapid versus non-rapid cycling as a predictor of response to olanzapine and divalproex sodium for bipolar mania and maintenance of remission: post hoc analyses of 47-week data. J Affect Disord 2005; 89:69–77.
18. Bowden CL et al. A randomized, placebo-controlled 12-month trial of divalproex and lithium in treatment of outpatients with bipolar I disorder. Divalproex Maintenance Study Group. Arch Gen Psychiatry 2000; 57:481–9.
19. Calabrese JR et al. A 20-month, double-blind, maintenance trial of lithium versus divalproex in rapid-cycling bipolar disorder. Am J Psychiatry 2005; 162:2152–61.
20. National Institute for Health and Clinical Excellence. Bipolar disorder. The management of bipolar disorder in adults, children and adolescents, in primary and secondary care. Clinical Guidance 38. http://www.nice.org.uk. 2006.
21. Lindenmayer JP et al. Use of sodium valproate in violent and aggressive behaviors: a critical review. J Clin Psychiatry 2000; 61:123–8.
22. Citrome L et al. Risperidone alone versus risperidone plus valproate in the treatment of patients with schizophrenia and hostility. Int Clin Psychopharmacol 2007; 22:356–62.
23. Gobbi G et al. Efficacy of topiramate, valproate, and their combination on aggression/agitation behavior in patients with psychosis. J Clin Psychopharmacol 2006; 26:467–73.
24. Aliyev NA et al. Valproate (depakine-chrono) in the acute treatment of outpatients with generalized anxiety disorder without psychiatric comorbidity: randomized, double-blind placebo-controlled study. Eur Psychiatry 2008; 23:109–14.
25. Allen MH et al. Linear relationship of valproate serum concentration to response and optimal serum levels for acute mania. Am J Psychiatry 2006; 163:272–5.
26. Taylor D et al. Doses of carbamazepine and valproate in bipolar affective disorder. Psychiatr Bull 1997; 21:221–3.
27. Segura-Bruna N et al. Valproate-induced hyperammonemic encephalopathy. Acta Neurol Scand 2006; 114:1–7.
28. El-Khatib F et al. Valproate, weight gain and carbohydrate craving: a gender study. Seizure 2007; 16:226–32.
29. Zadikoff C et al. Movement disorders in patients taking anticonvulsants. J Neurol Neurosurg Psychiatry 2007; 78:147–51.
30. Ristic AJ et al. The frequency of reversible parkinsonism and cognitive decline associated with valproate treatment: a study of 364 patients with different types of epilepsy. Epilepsia 2006; 47:2183–5.
31. Gerstner T et al. Valproic acid-induced pancreatitis: 16 new cases and a review of the literature. J Gastroenterol 2007; 42:39–48.
32. Joffe H et al. Valproate is associated with new-onset oligoamenorrhea with hyperandrogenism in women with bipolar disorder. Biol Psychiatry 2006; 59:1078–86.
33. Bjornsson E. Hepatotoxicity associated with antiepileptic drugs. Acta Neurol Scand 2008; 118:281–90.
34. Franks MA et al. Bouncing back: is the bipolar rebound phenomenon peculiar to lithium? A retrospective naturalistic study. J Psychopharmacol 2008; 22:452–6.
35. National Institute for Clinical Excellence. The clinical effectiveness and cost effectiveness of newer drugs for epilepsy in adults. Technology Appraisal 76. 2004. http://www.nice.org.uk
36. Sanofi-Aventis. Summary of Product Characteristics. Epilim. 2009. http://emc.medicines.org.uk/
37. Sanofi-Aventis. Summary of Product Characteristics. Depakote tablets. 2009. http://emc.medicines.org.uk/
38. James L et al. Informing patients of the teratogenic potential of mood stabilising drugs; a case notes review of the practice of psychiatrists. J Psychopharmacol 2007; 21:815–19.
39. James L et al. Mood stabilizers and teratogenicity – prescribing practice and awareness amongst practising psychiatrists. J Ment Health 2009; 18:137–43.
40. Meador KJ et al. Cognitive function at 3 years of age after fetal exposure to antiepileptic drugs. N Engl J Med 2009; 360:1597–605.
41. Sandson NB et al. An interaction between aspirin and valproate: the relevance of plasma protein displacement drug–drug interactions. Am J Psychiatry 2006; 163:1891–6.
42. Fehr C et al. Increase in serum clomipramine concentrations caused by valproate. J Clin Psychopharmacol 2000; 20:493–4.
43. Morris RG et al. Clinical study of lamotrigine and valproic acid in patients with epilepsy: using a drug interaction to advantage? Ther Drug Monit 2000; 22:656–60.
44. Aichhorn W et al. Influence of age, gender, body weight and valproate comedication on quetiapine plasma concentrations. Int Clin Psychopharmacol 2006; 21:81–5.
45. Gunes A et al. Inhibitory effect of valproic acid on cytochrome P450 2C9 activity in epilepsy patients. Basic Clin Pharmacol Toxicol 2007; 100:383–6.
46. Bergemann N et al. Valproate lowers plasma concentration of olanzapine. J Clin Psychopharmacol 2006; 26:432–4.

Lithium

Mechanism of action

Lithium is an element that is very similar to sodium. The ubiquitous nature of sodium in the human body, its involvement in a wide range of biological processes, and the potential for lithium to alter these processes has made it extremely difficult to ascertain the key mechanism(s) of action of lithium in regulating mood. For example, there is some evidence that people with bipolar illness have higher intracellular concentrations of sodium and calcium than controls and that lithium can reduce these. Reduced activity of sodium-dependent intracellular second-messenger systems has been demonstrated, as have modulation of dopamine and serotonin neurotransmitter pathways, reduced activity of protein kinase C and reduced turnover of arachidonic acid. Lithium may also have neuroprotective effects, possibly mediated through its effects on NMDA pathways. For a recent review see Marmol (2008)[1]. It is notable that literature pertaining to the possible neuroprotective effect of lithium reports largely on either in vitro or animal studies. The clinical literature is dominated by reports of neurotoxicity[2].

Indications

Lithium is effective in the treatment of *moderate to severe mania* with a NNT of 6[3]. Its use for this indication is limited by the fact that it usually takes at least a week to achieve a response[4] and that the co-administration of antipsychotics may increase the risk of neurological side effects. It can also be difficult to achieve therapeutic plasma levels rapidly and monitoring can be problematic if the patient is uncooperative.

The main indication for lithium is in the *prophylaxis of bipolar affective disorder* where it reduces both the number and the severity of relapses[5]. Lithium is more effective at preventing manic than depressive relapse[6]; the NNT to prevent relapse into mania or depression has been calculated to be 10 and 14 respectively[6]. Lithium also offers some protection against antidepressant-induced hypomania. It is recommended by NICE that a mood-stabiliser should be prescribed prophylactically (1) after a single manic episode that was associated with significant risk and adverse consequences, (2) in the case of bipolar I illness, two or more acute episodes or (3) in the case of bipolar II illness, significant functional impairment, frequent episodes or significant risk of suicide[7]. NICE supports the use of lithium as a first-line mood-stabiliser.

Lithium *augmentation of an antidepressant* in patients with unipolar depression is recommended by NICE as a next-step treatment in patients who have not responded to standard antidepressant drugs[8]. A recent meta-analysis found lithium to be three times as effective as placebo for this indication with a NNT of 5[9], although the response rate in STAR-D was more modest (see section on refractory depression).

The effectiveness of lithium in treating mood disorders does not go unchallenged. For a review, see Moncrieff[10].

Lithium is also used to treat aggressive[11] and self-mutilating behaviour, to both prevent and treat steroid-induced psychosis[12] and to raise the white blood cell count in patients receiving clozapine.

Lithium and suicide

It is estimated that 15% of people with bipolar disorder take their own life[13]. A meta-analysis of clinical trials concluded that lithium reduced by 80% the risk of both attempted and completed suicide in patients with bipolar illness[14], and two large database studies have shown that lithium-treated patients were less likely to complete suicide than patients treated with divalproex[15] or with other mood-stabilising drugs (valproate, gabapentin, carbamazepine)[16].

In patients with unipolar depression, lithium also seems to protect against suicide; the effect size being similar to that found in bipolar illness[17]. The mechanism of this protective effect is unknown.

Plasma levels

A recent systematic review of the relationship between plasma levels and response in patients with bipolar illness concluded that the minimum effective plasma level for prophylaxis is 0.4 mmol/L, with the optimal range being 0.6–0.75 mmol/L. Levels above 0.75 mmol/L offer additional protection only against manic symptoms[7,18]. Changes in plasma levels seem to worsen the risk of relapse[19]. The optimal plasma level range for patients who have unipolar depression is less clear[9].

Children and adolescents may require higher plasma levels than adults to ensure that an adequate concentration of lithium is present in the CNS[20].

Lithium is rapidly absorbed from the gastrointestinal tract but has a long distribution phase. Blood samples for plasma lithium level estimations should be taken 10–14 hours (ideally 12) post dose in patients who are prescribed a single daily dose of a prolonged release preparation at bedtime[21].

Formulations

There is no clinically significant difference in the pharmacokinetics of the two most widely prescribed brands of lithium in the UK: Priadel and Camcolit. Other preparations should not be assumed to be bioequivalent and should be prescribed by brand.

- Lithium carbonate 400 mg tablets each contain 10.8 mmol/lithium
- Lithium citrate liquid is available in two strengths and should be administered twice daily:
  - 5.4 mmol/5 ml is equivalent to 200 mg lithium carbonate
  - 10.8 mmol/5 ml is equivalent to 400 mg lithium carbonate.

Lack of clarity over which liquid preparation is intended when prescribing can lead to the patient receiving a sub-therapeutic or toxic dose.

Adverse effects

Most side effects are dose (plasma level) related. These include mild gastrointestinal upset, fine tremor, polyuria and polydipsia. Polyuria may occur more frequently with twice-daily dosing[22]. Propranolol can be useful in lithium-induced tremor. Some skin conditions such as psoriasis and acne can be aggravated by lithium therapy. Lithium can also cause a metallic taste in the mouth, ankle oedema and weight gain.

Lithium can cause a reduction in urinary concentrating capacity – nephrogenic diabetes insipidus – hence the occurrence of thirst and polyuria. This effect is usually reversible in the short to medium term but may be irreversible after long-term treatment (>15 years)[21,22]. Lithium treatment can also lead to a reduction in the glomerular filtration rate[23] and although in the majority of patients this effect is considered to be benign[24], a recent large cross-sectional study found that a third of young people prescribed lithium had an e-GFR of <60 ml/min (chronic kidney disease stage 3)[23]. A very small number of patients may develop interstitial nephritis. Lithium levels of >0.8 mmol/L are associated with a higher risk of renal toxicity[18].

In the longer term, lithium increases the risk of hypothyroidism; in middle-aged women, the risk may be up to 20%[25]. A case has been made for testing thyroid autoantibodies in this group before starting lithium (to better estimate risk) and for measuring TFTs more frequently in the first year of treatment[26]. Hypothyroidism is easily treated with thyroxine. TFTs usually return to normal when lithium is discontinued. Lithium also increases the risk of hyperparathyroidism, and some recommend that calcium levels should be monitored in patients on long-term treatment[26]. Clinical consequences of chronically increased serum calcium include renal stones, osteoporosis, dyspepsia, hypertension and renal impairment[26].

Lithium toxicity

Toxic effects reliably occur at levels >1.5 mmol/L and usually consist of gastrointestinal effects (increasing anorexia, nausea and diarrhoea) and CNS effects (muscle weakness, drowsiness, ataxia, course tremor and muscle twitching). Above 2 mmol/L, increased disorientation and seizures usually occur, which can progress to coma, and ultimately death. In the presence of more severe symptoms, osmotic or forced alkaline diuresis should be used (note, NEVER thiazide or loop diuretics). Above 3 mmol/L peritoneal or haemodialysis is often used. These plasma levels are only a guide and individuals vary in their susceptibility to symptoms of toxicity.

Most **risk factors for toxicity** involve changes in sodium levels or the way the body handles sodium. For example, low-salt diets, dehydration, drug interactions (see summary table) and some uncommon physical illnesses such as Addison's disease.

Information relating to the symptoms of toxicity and the common risk factors should always be given to patients when treatment with lithium is initiated. This information should be repeated at appropriate intervals to make sure that it is clearly understood.

Pre-treatment tests

Before prescribing lithium, renal, thyroid and cardiac function should be checked. As a minimum, e-GFR[27] and TFTs should be checked. An ECG is also recommended in patients who have risk factors for, or existing cardiovascular disease. A baseline measure of weight is also desirable.

Lithium is a human teratogen. Women of childbearing age should be advised to use a reliable form of contraception. See section on psychotropics and pregnancy (Chapter 7).

On-treatment monitoring[7]

As a minimum, plasma lithium should be checked every 3 months. e-GFR and TFTs should be checked every 6 months. More frequent tests may be required in those who are prescribed interacting drugs. Weight (or BMI) should also be monitored.

Discontinuation

Intermittent treatment with lithium may worsen the natural course of bipolar illness. A much greater than expected incidence of manic relapse is seen in the first few months after discontinuing lithium[28], even in patients who have been symptom-free for as long as 5 years[29]. This has led to recommendations that lithium treatment should not be started unless there is a clear intention to continue it for at least 3 years[30]. This advice has obvious implications for initiating lithium treatment against a patient's will (or in a patient known to be non-compliant with medication) during a period of acute illness.

The risk of relapse **may** be reduced by decreasing the dose gradually over a period of at least a month[31], and avoiding incremental serum level reductions of >0.2 mmol/L[18]. In contrast with these recommendations, a recent naturalistic study found that, in patients who had been in remission for at least 2 years and had discontinued lithium very slowly, the recurrence rate was at least three times greater than in patients who continued lithium; significant survival differences persisted for many years. Patients maintained on high lithium levels prior to discontinuation were particularly prone to relapse[32].

One large US study based on prescription records found that half of those prescribed lithium took almost all of their prescribed doses, a quarter took between 50 and 80%, and the remaining quarter took less than 50%; in addition one-third of patients took lithium for less than 6 months in total[33]. It is clear that sub-optimal adherence limits the effectiveness of lithium in clinical practice. One database study suggested the extent to which lithium was taken was directly related to the risk of suicide (more prescriptions = lower suicide rate)[34].

Less convincing data support the emergence of depressive symptoms in bipolar patients after lithium discontinuation[28]. There are few data relating to patients with unipolar depression.

Table Lithium: prescribing and monitoring	
Indications	Mania, hypomania, prophylaxis of bipolar affective disorder and recurrent depression reduces aggression and suicidality
Pre-lithium work up	e-GFR and TFTs. ECG recommended in patients who have risk factors for, or existing cardiovascular disease
	Baseline measure of weight desirable
Prescribing	Start at 400 mg at night (200 mg in the elderly). Plasma level after 7 days, then 7 days after every dose change until the desired level is reached (0.4 mmol/L may be effective in unipolar depression, 0.6–1.0 mmol/L in bipolar illness, slightly higher levels in difficult to treat mania)
	Blood should be taken 12 hours after the last dose. Take care when prescribing liquid preparations to clearly specify the strength required
Monitoring	Plasma lithium every 3 months. e-GFR and TFTs every 6 months. More frequent tests may be required in those who are prescribed interacting drugs. Weight (or BMI) should also be monitored
Stopping	Reduce slowly over at least 1 month
	Avoid incremental reductions in plasma levels of >0.2 mmol/L

Interactions with other drugs[35,36]
Because of lithium's relatively narrow therapeutic index, pharmacokinetic interactions with other drugs can precipitate lithium toxicity. Most clinically significant interactions are with drugs that alter renal sodium handling.

ACE inhibitors: ACE inhibitors can (1) reduce thirst which can lead to mild dehydration, and (2) increase renal sodium Na loss leading to increased Na re-absorption by the kidney, leading to an increase in lithium plasma levels. The magnitude of this effect is variable; from no increase to a four-fold increase. The full effect can take several weeks to develop. The risk seems to be increased in patients with heart failure, dehydration and renal impairment (presumably because of changes in fluid balance/handling). In the elderly, ACE inhibitors increase seven-fold the risk of hospitalisation due to lithium toxicity. ACE inhibitors can also precipitate renal failure so, if co-prescribed with lithium, more frequent monitoring of e-GFR and plasma lithium is required.

The following drugs are ACE inhibitors: captopril, cilazapril enalapril, fosinopril, imidapril, lisinopril, moexipril, perindopril, quinapril, ramipril and trandolapril.

Care is also required with **angiotensin 11 receptor antagonists;** candesartan, eprosartan, irbesartan, losartan, olmesartan, telmisartan and valsartan.

Diuretics: Diuretics can reduce the renal clearance of lithium, the magnitude of this effect being greater with thiazide than loop diuretics. Lithium levels usually rise within 10 days of a *thiazide diuretic* being prescribed; the magnitude of the rise is unpredictable and can vary from 25% to 400%. The following drugs are thiazide (or related) diuretics: bendroflumethiazide, chlortalidone, cyclopenthiazide, indapamide, metolazone and xipamide.

Although there are case reports of lithium toxicity induced by *loop diuretics*, many patients receive this combination of drugs without apparent problems. The risk of an interaction seems to be greatest in the first month after the loop diuretic has been prescribed and extra lithium plasma level monitoring during this time is recommended if these drugs are co-prescribed. Loop diuretics can increase Na loss and subsequent re-absorption by the kidney. Patients taking loop diuretics may also have been advised to restrict their salt intake; this may contribute to the risk of lithium toxicity in these individuals. The following drugs are loop diuretics: bumetanide, furosemide and torasemide.

Anti-inflammatory drugs (NSAIDs)
NSAIDs inhibit the synthesis of renal prostaglandins, thereby reducing renal blood flow and possibly increasing renal re-absorption of sodium and therefore lithium. The magnitude of the rise is unpredictable for any given patient; case reports vary from around 10% to over 400%. The onset of effect also seems to be variable; from a few days to several months. Risk appears to be increased in those patients who have impaired renal function, renal artery stenosis or heart failure and who are dehydrated or on a low-salt diet. There are a growing number of case reports of an interaction between lithium and COX-2 inhibitors.

NSAIDs (or COX-2 inhibitors) can be combined with lithium but; (1) they should be prescribed regularly NOT PRN, and; (2) more frequent plasma lithium monitoring is essential.

Some NSAIDs can be purchased without a prescription, so it is particularly important that patients are aware of the potential for interaction.

The following drugs are NSAIDs or COX-2 inhibitors: aceclofenac, acemetacin, celecoxib, dexibu-profen, dexketoprofen, diclofenac, diflunisal, etodolac, etoricoxib, fenbufen, fenoprofen, flurbiprofen, ibuprofen, indometacin, ketoprofen, lumiracoxib, mefenamic acid, meloxicam, nabumetone, naproxen, piroxicam, sulindac, tenoxicam and tiaprofenic acid.

Carbamazepine: There are rare reports of neurotoxicity when carbamazepine is combined with lithium. Most are old and in the context of treatment involving high plasma lithium levels. It is of note though that carbamazepine can cause hyponatraemia, which may in turn lead to lithium retention and toxicity. Similarly, rare reports of CNS toxicity implicate *SSRIs*, another group of drugs that can cause hyponatraemia.

Table Lithium: clinically relevant drug interactions

Drug group	Magnitude of effect	Timescale of effect	Additional information
ACE inhibitors	• Unpredictable • Up to 4-fold increases in [Li]	Develops over several weeks	• 7-fold increased risk of hospitalisation for lithium toxicity in the elderly • **Angiotension II receptor antagonists** may be associated with similar risk
Thiazide diuretics	• Unpredictable • Up to 4-fold increases in [Li]	Usually apparent in first 10 days	• Loop diuretics are safer • Any effect will be apparent in the first month
NSAIDs	• Unpredictable • From 10% to >4-fold increases in [Li]	Variable; few days to several months	• NSAIDs are widely used on a PRN basis • Can be bought without a prescription • COX-2 inhibitors likely to carry the same risk

Bipolar disorder

References

1. Marmol F. Lithium: Bipolar disorder and neurodegenerative diseases Possible cellular mechanisms of the therapeutic effects of lithium. Prog Neuropsychopharmacol Biol Psychiatry 2008; 32:1761–71.
2. Fountoulakis KN et al. A systematic review of existing data on long-term lithium therapy: neuroprotective or neurotoxic? Int J Neuropsychopharmacol 2008; 11:269–87.
3. Storosum JG et al. Magnitude of effect of lithium in short-term efficacy studies of moderate to severe manic episode. Bipolar Disord 2007; 9:793–8.
4. Ferrier IN et al. Lithium therapy. Adv Psychiatr Treat 1995; 1:102–10.
5. Tondo L et al. Long-term clinical effectiveness of lithium maintenance treatment in types I and II bipolar disorders. Br J Psychiatry Suppl 2001; 41:s184–90.
6. Geddes JR et al. Long-term lithium therapy for bipolar disorder: systematic review and meta-analysis of randomized controlled trials. Am J Psychiatry 2004; 161:217–22.
7. National Institute for Health and Clinical Excellence. Bipolar disorder. The management of bipolar disorder in adults, children and adolescents, in primary and secondary care. Clinical Guidance 38. http://www.nice.org.uk. 2006
8. National Institute for Clinical Excellence. Depression: the treatment and management of depression in adults (update). 2009. http://www.nice.org.uk/.
9. Crossley NA et al. Acceleration and augmentation of antidepressants with lithium for depressive disorders: two meta-analyses of randomized, placebo-controlled trials. J Clin Psychiatry 2007; 68:935–40.
10. Moncrieff J. Lithium: evidence reconsidered. Br J Psychiatry 1997; 171:113–19.
11. Tyrer SP. Lithium and treatment of aggressive behaviour. Eur Neuropsychopharmacol 1994; 4:234–6.
12. Falk WE et al. Lithium prophylaxis of corticotropin-induced psychosis. JAMA 1979; 241:1011–12.
13. Harris EC et al. Excess mortality of mental disorder. Br J Psychiatry 1998; 173:11–53.
14. Baldessarini RJ et al. Decreased risk of suicides and attempts during long-term lithium treatment: a meta-analytic review. Bipolar Disord 2006; 8:625–39.
15. Goodwin FK et al. Suicide risk in bipolar disorder during treatment with lithium and divalproex. JAMA 2003; 290:1467–73.
16. Collins JC et al. Divalproex, lithium and suicide among Medicaid patients with bipolar disorder. J Affect Disord 2008; 107:23–8.
17. Guzzetta F et al. Lithium treatment reduces suicide risk in recurrent major depressive disorder. J Clin Psychiatry 2007; 68:380–3.
18. Severus WE et al. What is the optimal serum lithium level in the long-term treatment of bipolar disorder – a review? Bipolar Disord 2008; 10:231–7.
19. Perlis RH et al. Effect of abrupt change from standard to low serum levels of lithium: a reanalysis of double-blind lithium maintenance data. Am J Psychiatry 2002; 159:1155–9.
20. Moore CM et al. Brain-to-serum lithium ratio and age: an in vivo magnetic resonance spectroscopy study. Am J Psychiatry 2002; 159:1240–2.
21. Anon. Using lithium safely. Drug Ther Bull 1999; 37:22–4.
22. Bowen RC et al. Less frequent lithium administration and lower urine volume. Am J Psychiatry 1991; 148:189–92.
23. Bassilios N et al. Monitoring of glomerular filtration rate in lithium-treated outpatients – an ambulatory laboratory database surveillance. Nephrol Dial Transplant 2008; 23:562–5.
24. Gitlin M. Lithium and the kidney: an updated review. Drug Saf 1999; 20:231–43.
25. Johnston AM et al. Lithium-associated clinical hypothyroidism. Prevalence and risk factors. Br J Psychiatry 1999; 175:336–9.
26. Livingstone C et al. Lithium: a review of its metabolic adverse effects. J Psychopharmacol 2006; 20:347–55.
27. Morriss R et al. Lithium and eGFR: a new routinely available tool for the prevention of chronic kidney disease. Br J Psychiatry 2008; 193:93–5.
28. Cavanagh J et al. Relapse into mania or depression following lithium discontinuation: a 7-year follow-up. Acta Psychiatr Scand 2004; 109:91–5.
29. Yazici O et al. Controlled lithium discontinuation in bipolar patients with good response to long-term lithium prophylaxis. J Affect Disord 2004; 80:269–71.
30. Goodwin GM. Recurrence of mania after lithium withdrawal. Implications for the use of lithium in the treatment of bipolar affective disorder. Br J Psychiatry 1994; 164:149–52.
31. Baldessarini RJ et al. Effects of the rate of discontinuing lithium maintenance treatment in bipolar disorders. J Clin Psychiatry 1996; 57:441–8.
32. Biel MG et al. Continuation versus discontinuation of lithium in recurrent bipolar illness: a naturalistic study. Bipolar Disord 2007; 9:435–42.
33. Sajatovic M et al. Treatment adherence with lithium and anticonvulsant medications among patients with bipolar disorder. Psychiatr Serv 2007; 58:855–63.
34. Kessing LV et al. Suicide risk in patients treated with lithium. Arch Gen Psychiatry 2005; 62:860–6.
35. Stockley's Drug Interactions. [Online]. 2009. http://www.medicinescomplete.com
36. Juurlink DN et al. Drug-induced lithium toxicity in the elderly: a population-based study. J Am Geriatr Soc 2004; 52:794–8.

Carbamazepine

Mechanism of action[1]

Carbamazepine blocks voltage-dependent sodium channels thus inhibiting repetitive neuronal firing. It reduces glutamate release and decreases the turnover of dopamine and norepinephrine. Carbamazepine has a similar molecular structure to TCAs.

As well as blocking voltage-dependent sodium channels, oxcarbazepine also increases potassium conductance and modulates high-voltage-activated calcium channels.

Formulations

Carbamazepine is available as a liquid and chewable, immediate-release and controlled-release tablets. Conventional formulations generally have to be administered two to three times daily. The controlled-release preparation can be given once or twice daily, and the reduced fluctuation in serum levels usually leads to improved tolerability. This preparation has a lower bioavailability and an increase in dose of 10–15% may be required.

Indications

Carbamazepine is primarily used as an anticonvulsant in the treatment of grand mal and focal seizures. It is also used in the treatment of trigeminal neuralgia and, in the UK, is licensed for the treatment of bipolar illness in patients who do not respond to lithium.

With respect to the treatment of *mania*, two placebo-controlled randomised studies have found the extended-release formulation of carbamazepine to be effective; in both studies, the response rate in the carbamazepine arm was twice that in the placebo arm[2,3]. Carbamazepine was not particularly well tolerated; the incidence of dizziness, somnolence and nausea was high. Another study found carbamazepine alone to be as effective as carbamazepine plus olanzapine[4]. NICE does not recommend carbamazepine as a first-line treatment for mania[5].

Open studies suggest that carbamazepine monotherapy has some efficacy in *bipolar depression*[6]; note that the evidence base supporting other strategies is stronger (see section on bipolar depression). Carbamazepine may also be useful in *unipolar depression* either alone[7] or as an augmentation strategy[8].

Carbamazepine is generally considered to be less effective than lithium in the *prophylaxis* of bipolar illness[9]; several published studies report a low response rate and high drop-out rate. A blinded, randomised trial of carbamazepine versus lithium found lithium to be the superior prophylactic agent[10]; most of the lithium treatment failures occurred in the first 3 months of treatment, whereas relapses on carbamazepine occurred steadily at the rate of 40% per year. Lithium is considered to be superior to carbamazepine in reducing suicidal behaviour[11], although data are not consistent[12]. NICE considers carbamazepine to be a third-line prophylactic agent[5]. Two small studies suggest oxcarbazepine may have some prophylactic efficacy when used in combination with other mood-stabilising drugs[13,14].

There are data supporting the use of carbamazepine in the management of alcohol-withdrawal symptoms[15], although the high doses required initially are often poorly tolerated. Carbamazepine has also been used to manage aggressive behaviour in patients with schizophrenia[16]; the quality of data is weak and the mode of action unknown. There are a number of case reports and open case series that report on the use of carbamazepine in various psychiatric illnesses such as panic disorder, borderline personality disorder and episodic dyscontrol syndrome.

Plasma levels

When carbamazepine is used as an anticonvulsant, the therapeutic range is generally considered to be 4–12 mg/L, although the supporting evidence is not strong. In patients with affective illness, a dose of at least 600 mg/day and a plasma level of at least 7 mg/L may be required[17], although this is not a consistent finding[4,7,18]. Levels above 12 mg/L are associated with a higher side effect burden.

Carbamazepine serum levels vary markedly within a dosage interval. It is therefore important to sample at a point in time where levels are likely to be reproducible for any given individual. The most appropriate way of monitoring is to take a trough level before the first dose of the day.

Carbamazepine is a hepatic enzyme inducer that induces its own metabolism as well as that of other drugs. An initial plasma half-life of around 30 hours is reduced to around 12 hours on chronic dosing. For this reason, plasma levels should be checked 2–4 weeks after an increase in dose to ensure that the desired level is still being obtained.

Most published clinical trials that demonstrate the efficacy of carbamazepine as a mood-stabiliser use doses that are significantly higher (800–1200 mg/day) than those commonly prescribed in UK clinical practice[19].

Adverse effects[1]

The main side effects associated with carbamazepine therapy are dizziness, diplopia, drowsiness, ataxia, nausea and headaches. They can sometimes be avoided by starting with a low dose and increasing slowly. Avoiding high peak blood levels by splitting the dose throughout the day or using a controlled-release formulation may also help. Dry mouth, oedema and hyponatraemia are also common. Sexual dysfunction can occur, probably mediated through reduced testosterone levels[20]. Around 3% of patients treated with carbamazepine develop a generalised erythematous rash. Serious exfoliative dermatological reactions can rarely occur; vulnerability is genetically determined[21], and genetic testing of people of Han Chinese or Thai origin is recommended before carbamazepine is prescribed. Carbamazepine is a known human teratogen (see Chapter 7).

Carbamazepine commonly causes a chronic low white blood cell (WBC) count. One patient in 20,000 develops agranulocytosis and/or aplastic anaemia[22]. Raised ALP and GGT are common (a GGT of 2–3 times normal is rarely a cause for concern[23]). A delayed multi-organ hypersensitivity reaction rarely occurs, mainly manifesting itself as various skin reactions, a low WBC count, and abnormal LFTs. Fatalities have been reported[23,24]. There is no clear timescale for these events.

Pre-treatment tests

Baseline U&Es, FBC and LFTs are recommended by NICE. A baseline measure of weight is also desirable.

On-treatment monitoring

NICE recommends that U&Es, FBC and LFTs should be repeated after 6 months, and that weight (or BMI) should also be monitored.

Discontinuation

It is not known if abrupt discontinuation of carbamazepine worsens the natural course of bipolar illness in the same way as abrupt cessation of lithium does. In one small case series (n = 6), one patient developed depression within a month of discontinuation[25], while in another small case series (n = 4), three patients had a recurrence of their mood disorder within 3 months[26]. Until further data are available, if carbamazepine is to be discontinued, it should be done slowly.

Use in women of childbearing age

Carbamazepine is an established human teratogen (see Chapter 7).

Women who have mania are likely to be sexually disinhibited. The risk of unplanned pregnancy is likely to be above population norms (where 50% of pregnancies are unplanned). If carbamazepine cannot be avoided, adequate contraception should be ensured (note the interaction between carbamazepine and oral contraceptives outlined below) and prophylactic folate prescribed.

Interactions with other drugs[27–30]

Carbamazepine is a potent inducer of hepatic cytochrome P450 enzymes and is metabolised by CYP3A4. Plasma levels of most **antidepressants**, most **antipsychotics, benzodiazepines**, some **cholinesterase inhibitors, methadone, thyroxine, theophylline, oestrogens** and other steroids may be reduced by carbamazepine, resulting in treatment failure. Patients requiring contraception should either receive a preparation containing not less than 50 µg oestrogen or use a non-hormonal method. Drugs that inhibit CYP3A4 will increase carbamazepine plasma levels and may precipitate toxicity. Examples include **cimetidine, diltiazem, verapamil, erythromycin** and some **SSRIs**.

Pharmacodynamic interactions also occur. The anticonvulsant activity of carbamazepine is reduced by drugs that lower the seizure threshold (e.g. antipsychotics and antidepressants), the potential for carbamazepine to cause neutropenia may be increased by other drugs that have the potential to depress the bone marrow (e.g. clozapine), and the risk of hyponatraemia may be increased by other drugs that have the potential to deplete sodium (e.g. diuretics). Neurotoxicity has been reported when carbamazepine is used in combination with lithium. This is rare.

As carbamazepine is structurally similar to TCAs, in theory it should not be given within 14 days of discontinuing a MAOI.

Table	Carbamazepine: prescribing and monitoring
Indications	Mania (not first line), bipolar depression (evidence weak), unipolar depression (evidence weak), and prophylaxis of bipolar disorder (third line after antipsychotics and valproate). Alcohol withdrawal (may be poorly tolerated)
	Carbamazepine is licensed for the treatment of bipolar illness in patients who do not respond to lithium
Pre-carbamazepine work up	U&Es, FBC and LFTs. Baseline measure of weight desirable
Prescribing	Titrate dose upwards against response and side effects; start with 100–200 mg bd and aim for 400 mg bd (some patients will require higher doses)
	Note that the modified-release formulation (Tegretol Retard) can be given once to twice daily, is associated with less severe fluctuations in serum levels and is generally better tolerated
	Plasma levels can be used to assure adequate dosing and treatment compliance. Blood should be taken immediately before the next dose. Carbamazepine induces its own metabolism; serum levels (if used) should be re-checked a month after an increase in dose
Monitoring	As a minimum, U&Es, FBC and LFTs after 6 months
	Weight (or BMI) should also be monitored
Stopping	Reduce slowly over at least 1 month

References

1. Novartis Pharmaceuticals UK Ltd. Summary of Product Characteristics. Tegretol Retard Tablets 200 mg, 400 mg. 2009. http://emc.medicines.org.uk/
2. Weisler RH et al. A multicenter, randomized, double-blind, placebo-controlled trial of extended-release carbamazepine capsules as monotherapy for bipolar disorder patients with manic or mixed episodes. J Clin Psychiatry 2004; 65:478–84.
3. Weisler RH et al. Extended-release carbamazepine capsules as monotherapy for acute mania in bipolar disorder: a multicenter, randomized, double-blind, placebo-controlled trial. J Clin Psychiatry 2005; 66:323–30.
4. Tohen M et al. Olanzapine plus carbamazepine v. carbamazepine alone in treating manic episodes. Br J Psychiatry 2008; 192:135–43.
5. National Institute for Health and Clinical Excellence. Bipolar disorder. The management of bipolar disorder in adults, children and adolescents, in primary and secondary care. Clinical Guidance 38. http://www.nice.org.uk. 2006.
6. Dilsaver SC et al. Treatment of bipolar depression with carbamazepine: results of an open study. Biol Psychiatry 1996; 40:935–7.
7. Zhang ZJ et al. The effectiveness of carbamazepine in unipolar depression: a double-blind, randomized, placebo-controlled study. J Affect Disord 2008; 109:91–7.
8. Kramlinger KG et al. The addition of lithium to carbamazepine. Antidepressant efficacy in treatment-resistant depression. Arch Gen Psychiatry 1989; 46:794–800.
9. Nasrallah HA et al. Carbamazepine and valproate for the treatment of bipolar disorder: a review of the literature. J Affect Disord 2006; 95:69–78.
10. Hartong EG et al. Prophylactic efficacy of lithium versus carbamazepine in treatment-naive bipolar patients. J Clin Psychiatry 2003; 64:144–51.
11. Kleindienst N et al. Differential efficacy of lithium and carbamazepine in the prophylaxis of bipolar disorder: results of the MAP study. Neuropsychobiology 2000; 42 Suppl 1:2–10.
12. Yerevanian BI et al. Bipolar pharmacotherapy and suicidal behavior. Part I: Lithium, divalproex and carbamazepine. J Affect Disord 2007; 103:5–11.
13. Vieta E et al. A double-blind, randomized, placebo-controlled prophylaxis trial of oxcarbazepine as adjunctive treatment to lithium in the long-term treatment of bipolar I and II disorder. Int J Neuropsychopharmacol 2008; 11:445–52.
14. Conway CR et al. An open-label trial of adjunctive oxcarbazepine for bipolar disorder. J Clin Psychopharmacol 2006; 26:95–7.
15. Malcolm R et al. The effects of carbamazepine and lorazepam on single versus multiple previous alcohol withdrawals in an outpatient randomized trial. J Gen Intern Med 2002; 17:349–55.
16. Brieden T et al. Psychopharmacological treatment of aggression in schizophrenic patients. Pharmacopsychiatry 2002; 35:83–9.
17. Taylor D et al. Doses of carbamazepine and valproate in bipolar affective disorder. Psychiatr Bull 1997; 21:221–3.
18. Simhandl C et al. The comparative efficacy of carbamazepine low and high serum level and lithium carbonate in the prophylaxis of affective disorders. J Affect Disord 1993; 28:221–31.
19. Taylor DM et al. Prescribing and monitoring of carbamazepine and valproate – a case note review. Psychiatr Bull 2000; 24:174–7.
20. Lossius MI et al. Reversible effects of antiepileptic drugs on reproductive endocrine function in men and women with epilepsy – a prospective randomized double-blind withdrawal study. Epilepsia 2007; 48:1875–82.
21. Hung SI et al. Genetic susceptibility to carbamazepine-induced cutaneous adverse drug reactions. Pharmacogenet Genomics 2006; 16:297–306.
22. Kaufman DW et al. Drugs in the aetiology of agranulocytosis and aplastic anaemia. Eur J Haematol Suppl 1996; 60:23–30.
23. Bjornsson E. Hepatotoxicity associated with antiepileptic drugs. Acta Neurol Scand 2008; 118:281–90.
24. Ganeva M et al. Carbamazepine-induced drug reaction with eosinophilia and systemic symptoms (DRESS) syndrome: report of four cases and brief review. Int J Dermatol 2008; 47:853–60.
25. Macritchie KA et al. Does 'rebound mania' occur after stopping carbamazepine? A pilot study. J Psychopharmacol 2000; 14:266–8.
26. Franks MA et al. Bouncing back: is the bipolar rebound phenomenon peculiar to lithium? A retrospective naturalistic study. J Psychopharmacol 2008; 22:452–6.
27. Spina E et al. Clinical significance of pharmacokinetic interactions between antiepileptic and psychotropic drugs. Epilepsia 2002; 43 Suppl 2:37–44.
28. Patsalos PN et al. The importance of drug interactions in epilepsy therapy. Epilepsia 2002; 43:365–85.
29. Crawford P. Interactions between antiepileptic drugs and hormonal contraception. CNS Drugs 2002; 16:263–72.
30. Citrome L et al. Pharmacokinetics of aripiprazole and concomitant carbamazepine. J Clin Psychopharmacol 2007; 27:279–83.

Table Physical monitoring for people with bipolar disorder (based on NICE guidelines[1])

Test or measurement	Monitoring for all patients		Additional monitoring for specific drugs			
	Initial health check	Annual check up	Antipsychotics	Lithium	Valproate	Carbamazepine
Thyroid function	Yes	Yes		At start and every 6 months; more often if evidence of deterioration		
Liver function	Yes	Yes			At start and at 6 months	At start and at 6 months
Renal function	Yes	Yes		At start and at every 6 months; more often if evidence of deterioration or patient begins interacting drug		Urea and electrolytes every 6 months
Full blood count	Yes	Yes		Only if clinically indicated	At start and 6 months	At start and at 6 months
Blood (plasma) glucose	Yes	Yes	At start and then every 4–6 months (and at 1 month if taking olanzapine);			

Lipid profile	Yes	Over 40s only	At start and at 3 months; more often initially if evidence of elevated levels			
Blood pressure	Yes	Yes				
Prolactin	Children and adolescents only		At start and if symptoms of raised prolactin develop.			
ECG	If indicated by history or clinical picture		At start if there are risk factors for or existing cardiovascular disease (or haloperidol is prescribed)	At start if risk factors for or existing cardiovascular disease		
Weight and height	Yes		At start then frequently for 3 months then three monthly for first year	At start and when needed if the patient gains weight rapidly	At start and at 3 and 6 months	At start and at 6 months
Plasma levels of drug			One week after initiation and one week after every dose change until levels stable, then every 3 months	Titrate by effect and tolerability. Use plasma levels to assure adequate dosing and/or compliance	Two weeks after initiation and two weeks after dose change. Then every 6 months	

For patients on **lamotrigine**, do an annual health check, but no special monitoring tests are needed.

Reference

1. National Institute for Health and Clinical Excellence. Bipolar disorder. The management of bipolar disorder in adults, children and adolescents, in primary and secondary care. Clinical Guidance 38. http://www.nice.org.uk. 2006.

Treatment of acute mania or hypomania

Drug treatment is the mainstay of therapy for mania and hypomania. Both antipsychotics and so-called mood-stabilisers are effective. Sedative and anxiolytic drugs (e.g. benzodiazepines) may add to the effects of these drugs. Drug choice is made difficult by the dearth of useful comparative data[1] – no one drug can be recommended over another on efficacy grounds. The value of antipsychotic–mood-stabiliser combinations is established for those relapsing while on mood-stabilisers but unclear for those presenting on no treatment[2-6].

The diagram below outlines a treatment strategy for mania and hypomania. These recommendations are based on UK NICE guidelines[7], BAP guidelines[3], APA guidelines[4], UK NICE guidance on olanzapine and valproate[5], and individual references cited. Where an antipsychotic is recommended choose from those licensed for mania/bipolar disorder, i.e. most conventional drugs (see individual SPCs), aripiprazole, olanzapine, risperidone and quetiapine.

Treatment of acute mania or hypomania[2-17]

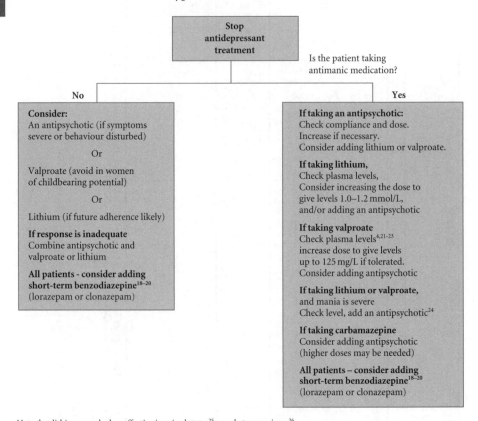

Note that lithium may be less effective in mixed states[25] or substance misuse[26].

Table   Mania: suggested doses

Drug	Dose
Lithium	400 mg/day, increasing every 5–7 days according to plasma levels
Valproate	As **semi sodium** – 250 mg three times daily increasing according to tolerability and plasma levels
	As **sodium valproate** slow release – 500 mg/day increasing as above
	Higher, so-called loading doses, have been used, both oral[27–29] and intravenous[30]. Dose is 20–30 mg/kg/day
Aripiprazole	15 mg/day increasing up to 30 mg/day as required[31,32]
Olanzapine	10 mg/day increasing to 15 mg or 20 mg as required
Risperidone	2 or 3 mg/day increased to 6 mg/day as required
Quetiapine	**IR** – 100 mg/day increasing to 800 mg/day as required (see SPC). Higher starting doses have been used[33]
	XL – 300 mg/day increasing to 600 mg/day on day two
Haloperidol	5–10 mg/day increasing to 15 mg/day if required
Lorazepam[19,20]	Up to 4 mg/day (some centres use higher doses)
Clonazepam[18,20]	Up to 8 mg/day

Table   Mania: other possible treatments

Treatment	Comments
Allopurinol[34] (600 mg/day)	Clear therapeutic effect when added to lithium in an RCT (n = 120)
Clozapine[35,36]	Established treatment option for refractory mania/bipolar disorder
Donepezil[37] (5–10 mg)	Probably not effective
Gabapentin[38–40] (up to 2400 mg/day)	Probably only effective by virtue of an anxiolytic effect. Rarely used. May be useful as prophylaxis[41]
Lamotrigine[42,43] (up to 200 mg/day)	Possibly effective but better efficacy in bipolar depression
Levetiracetam[44,45] (up to 4000 mg/day)	Possibly effective but controlled studies required
Oxcarbazepine[46–52] (around 300–3000 mg/day)	Probably effective acutely and as prophylaxis. One controlled study conducted (in youths) was negative[53]
Phenytoin[54] (300–400 mg/day)	Rarely used. Limited data
Ritanserin[55] (10 mg/day)	Supported by a single randomised, controlled trial. Well tolerated. May protect against EPS
Tamoxifen[56,57] (10–140 mg/day)	Probably effective. Two small RCTs. Dose–response relationship unclear
Topiramate[58–61] (up to 300 mg/day)	Possibly effective, even in refractory mania. Causes weight loss
Tryptophan depletion[62]	Supported by a small RCT
Ziprasidone[63]	Supported by a randomised, placebo-controlled study

Alphabetical order – no preference implied by order in the table.
Consult specialist and primary literature before using any treatment listed.

References

1. Smith LA et al. Pharmacological interventions for acute bipolar mania: a systematic review of randomized placebo-controlled trials. Bipolar Disord 2007; 9:551–60.
2. Smith LA et al. Acute bipolar mania: a systematic review and meta-analysis of co-therapy vs. monotherapy. Acta Psychiatr Scand 2007; 115:12–20.
3. Goodwin G. Evidence-based guidelines for treating bipolar disorder: revised second edition – recommendations from the British Association for Psychopharmacology. J Psychopharmacol 2009; 23:346–88.
4. American Psychiatric Association. Practice guideline for the treatment of patients with bipolar disorder. Am J Psychiatry 2002; 159 Suppl 4:1–50.
5. National Institute for Health and Clinical Excellence. The clinical effectiveness and cost effectiveness of new drugs for bi-polar disorder. Technical Appraisal 66. http://www.nice.org.uk. 2003.
6. Sachs GS. Decision tree for the treatment of bipolar disorder. J Clin Psychiatry 2003; 64 Suppl 8:35–40.
7. National Institute for Health and Clinical Excellence. Bipolar disorder. The management of bipolar disorder in adults, children and adolescents, in primary and secondary care. Clinical Guidance 38. http://www.nice.org.uk. 2006.
8. Tohen M et al. A 12-week, double-blind comparison of olanzapine vs haloperidol in the treatment of acute mania. Arch Gen Psychiatry 2003; 60:1218–26.
9. Baldessarini RJ et al. Olanzapine versus placebo in acute mania treatment responses in subgroups. J Clin Psychopharmacol 2003; 23:370–6.
10. Applebaum J et al. Intravenous fosphenytoin in acute mania. J Clin Psychiatry 2003; 64:408–9.
11. Sachs G et al. Quetiapine with lithium or divalproex for the treatment of bipolar mania: a randomized, double-blind, placebo-controlled study. Bipolar Disord 2004; 6:213–23.
12. Yatham LN et al. Quetiapine versus placebo in combination with lithium or divalproex for the treatment of bipolar mania. J Clin Psychopharmacol 2004; 24:599–606.
13. Yatham LN et al. Risperidone plus lithium versus risperidone plus valproate in acute and continuation treatment of mania. Int Clin Psychopharmacol 2004; 19:103–9.
14. Bowden CL et al. Risperidone in combination with mood stabilizers: a 10-week continuation phase study in bipolar I disorder. J Clin Psychiatry 2004; 65:707–14.
15. Hirschfeld RM et al. Rapid antimanic effect of risperidone monotherapy: a 3-week multicenter, double-blind, placebo-controlled trial. Am J Psychiatry 2004; 161:1057–65.
16. Bowden CL et al. A randomized, double-blind, placebo-controlled efficacy and safety study of quetiapine or lithium as monotherapy for mania in bipolar disorder. J Clin Psychiatry 2005; 66:111–21.
17. Khanna S et al. Risperidone in the treatment of acute mania: double-blind, placebo-controlled study. Br J Psychiatry 2005; 187:229–34.
18. Sachs GS et al. Adjunctive clonazepam for maintenance treatment of bipolar affective disorder. J Clin Psychopharmacol 1990; 10:42–7.
19. Modell JG et al. Inpatient clinical trial of lorazepam for the management of manic agitation. J Clin Psychopharmacol 1985; 5:109–13.
20. Curtin F et al. Clonazepam and lorazepam in acute mania: a Bayesian meta-analysis. J Affect Disord 2004; 78:201–8.
21. Goodwin GM et al. The British Association for Psychopharmacology guidelines for treatment of bipolar disorder: a summary. J Psychopharmacol 2003; 17:3–6.
22. Taylor D et al. Doses of carbamazepine and valproate in bipolar affective disorder. Psychiatr Bull 1997; 21:221–3.
23. Allen MH et al. Linear relationship of valproate serum concentration to response and optimal serum levels for acute mania. Am J Psychiatry 2006; 163:272–5.
24. Smith LA et al. Acute bipolar mania: a systematic review and meta-analysis of co-therapy vs. monotherapy. Acta Psychiatr Scand 2007; 115:12–20.
25. Swann AC et al. Lithium treatment of mania: clinical characteristics, specificity of symptom change, and outcome. Psychiatry Res 1986; 18:127–41.
26. Goldberg JF et al. A history of substance abuse complicates remission from acute mania in bipolar disorder. J Clin Psychiatry 1999; 60:733–40.
27. McElroy SL et al. A randomized comparison of divalproex oral loading versus haloperidol in the initial treatment of acute psychotic mania. J Clin Psychiatry 1996; 57:142–6.
28. Hirschfeld RM et al. Safety and tolerability of oral loading divalproex sodium in acutely manic bipolar patients. J Clin Psychiatry 1999; 60:815–18.
29. Hirschfeld RM et al. The safety and early efficacy of oral-loaded divalproex versus standard-titration divalproex, lithium, olanzapine, and placebo in the treatment of acute mania associated with bipolar disorder. J Clin Psychiatry 2003; 64:841–6.
30. Jagadheesan K et al. Acute antimanic efficacy and safety of intravenous valproate loading therapy: an open-label study. Neuropsychobiology 2003; 47:90–3.
31. Young AH et al. Aripiprazole monotherapy in acute mania: 12-week randomised placebo- and haloperidol-controlled study. Br J Psychiatry 2009; 194:40–8.
32. Keck PE et al. Aripiprazole monotherapy in the treatment of acute bipolar I mania: a randomized, double-blind, placebo- and lithium-controlled study. J Affect Disord 2009; 112:36–49.
33. Pajonk FG et al. Rapid dose titration of quetiapine for the treatment of acute schizophrenia and acute mania: a case series. J Psychopharmacol 2006; 20:119–24.
34. Machado-Vieira R et al. A double-blind, randomized, placebo-controlled 4-week study on the efficacy and safety of the purinergic agents allopurinol and dipyridamole adjunctive to lithium in acute bipolar mania. J Clin Psychiatry 2008; 69:1237–45.
35. Mahmood T et al. Clozapine in the management of bipolar and schizoaffective manic episodes resistant to standard treatment. Aust N Z J Psychiatry 1997; 31:424–6.
36. Green AI et al. Clozapine in the treatment of refractory psychotic mania. Am J Psychiatry 2000; 157:982–6.
37. Eden EA et al. A double-blind, placebo-controlled trial of adjunctive donepezil in treatment-resistant mania. Bipolar Disord 2006; 8:75–80.
38. Macdonald KJ et al. Newer antiepileptic drugs in bipolar disorder: rationale for use and role in therapy. CNS Drugs 2002; 16:549–62.
39. Cabras PL et al. Clinical experience with gabapentin in patients with bipolar or schizoaffective disorder: results of an open-label study. J Clin Psychiatry 1999; 60:245–8.
40. Pande AC et al. Gabapentin in bipolar disorder: a placebo-controlled trial of adjunctive therapy. Gabapentin Bipolar Disorder Study Group. Bipolar Disord 2000; 2 (3 Pt 2):249–55.
41. Vieta E et al. A double-blind, randomized, placebo-controlled, prophylaxis study of adjunctive gabapentin for bipolar disorder. J Clin Psychiatry 2006; 67:473–7.
42. Calabrese JR et al. Spectrum of activity of lamotrigine in treatment-refractory bipolar disorder. Am J Psychiatry 1999; 156:1019–23.
43. Bowden CL et al. A placebo-controlled 18-month trial of lamotrigine and lithium maintenance treatment in recently manic or hypomanic patients with bipolar I disorder. Arch Gen Psychiatry 2003; 60:392–400.
44. Grunze H et al. Levetiracetam in the treatment of acute mania: an open add-on study with an on-off-on design. J Clin Psychiatry 2003; 64:781–4.
45. Goldberg JF et al. Levetiracetam for acute mania (Letter). Am J Psychiatry 2002; 159:148.
46. Benedetti A et al. Oxcarbazepine as add-on treatment in patients with bipolar manic, mixed or depressive episode. J Affect Disord 2004; 79:273–7.
47. Lande RG. Oxcarbazepine: Efficacy, safety, and tolerability in the treatment of mania. Int J Psychiatry Clin Pract 2004; 8:37–40.
48. Ghaemi SN et al. Oxcarbazepine treatment of bipolar disorder. J Clin Psychiatry 2003; 64:943–5.
49. Pratoomsri W et al. Oxcarbazepine in the treatment of bipolar disorder: a review. Can J Psychiatry 2006; 51:540–5.
50. Juruena MF et al. Bipolar I and II disorder residual symptoms: oxcarbazepine and carbamazepine as add-on treatment to lithium in a double-blind, randomized trial. Prog Neuropsychopharmacol Biol Psychiatry 2009; 33:94–9.
51. Suppes T et al. Comparison of two anticonvulsants in a randomized, single-blind treatment of hypomanic symptoms in patients with bipolar disorder. Aust N Z J Psychiatry 2007; 41:397–402.

52. Vieta E et al. A double-blind, randomized, placebo-controlled prophylaxis trial of oxcarbazepine as adjunctive treatment to lithium in the long-term treatment of bipolar I and II disorder. Int J Neuropsychopharmacol 2008; 11:445–52.
53. Wagner KD et al. A double-blind, randomized, placebo-controlled trial of oxcarbazepine in the treatment of bipolar disorder in children and adolescents. Am J Psychiatry 2006; 163:1179–86.
54. Mishory A et al. Phenytoin as an antimanic anticonvulsant: a controlled study. Am J Psychiatry 2000; 157:463–5.
55. Akhondzadeh S et al. Ritanserin as an adjunct to lithium and haloperidol for the treatment of medication-naive patients with acute mania: a double blind and placebo controlled trial. BMC Psychiatry 2003; 3:7.
56. Zarate CA Jr et al. Efficacy of a protein kinase C inhibitor (tamoxifen) in the treatment of acute mania: a pilot study. Bipolar Disord 2007; 9:561–70.
57. Yildiz A et al. Protein kinase C inhibition in the treatment of mania: a double-blind, placebo-controlled trial of tamoxifen. Arch Gen Psychiatry 2008; 65:255–63.
58. Grunze HC et al. Antimanic efficacy of topiramate in 11 patients in an open trial with an on-off-on design. J Clin Psychiatry 2001; 62:464–8.
59. Yatham LN et al. Third generation anticonvulsants in bipolar disorder: a review of efficacy and summary of clinical recommendations. J Clin Psychiatry 2002; 63:275–83.
60. Vieta E et al. 1-year follow-up of patients treated with risperidone and topiramate for a manic episode. J Clin Psychiatry 2003; 64:834–9.
61. Vieta E et al. Use of topiramate in treatment-resistant bipolar spectrum disorders. J Clin Psychopharmacol 2002; 22:431–5.
62. Applebaum J et al. Rapid tryptophan depletion as a treatment for acute mania: a double-blind, pilot-controlled study. Bipolar Disord 2007; 9:884–7.
63. Keck PE Jr et al. Ziprasidone in the treatment of acute bipolar mania: a three-week, placebo-controlled, double-blind, randomized trial. Am J Psychiatry 2003; 160:741–8.

Table Drugs for acute mania: relative costs (May 2009)

Drug	Costs for 30 days' treatment	Comments
Lithium (Priadel) 800 mg/day	£2.01	Add cost of plasma level monitoring
Carbamazepine (Tegretol Retard) 800 mg/day	£11.18	Self-induction complicates acute treatment
Sodium valproate (Epilim Chrono) 1500 mg/day	£26.19	Not licensed for mania, but may be given once daily
Valproate semisodium (Depakote) 1500 mg/day	£24.29	Licensed for mania, but given two or three times daily
Aripiprazole (Abilify) 15 mg/day	£104.65	Non-sedative, but effective
Haloperidol (generic) 10 mg/day	£4.31	Most widely used typical antipsychotic
Olanzapine (Zyprexa) 15 mg/day	£127.69	Most widely used atypical
Quetiapine IR or XL (Seroquel) 600 mg/day	£170.00	Efficacy aspects across all phases of bipolar disorder
Risperidone (generic) 4 mg/day	£30.80	Non-sedative but effective

Antipsychotics in bipolar disorder

It is unhelpful to think of antipsychotic drugs as having only antipsychotic actions. Individual antipsychotics variously possess sedative, anxiolytic, antimanic and antidepressant properties. Some antipsychotics (quetiapine and olanzapine) show all of these activities. Antipsychotics are used in bipolar disorder to treat all aspects of the condition.

First-generation antipsychotics have long been used in mania and several studies support their use in a variety of hypomanic and manic presentations[1-3]. Their effectiveness seems to be enhanced by the addition of a mood-stabiliser[4,5]. In the longer-term treatment of bipolar disorder, typicals are widely used (presumably as prophylaxis)[6] but robust supporting data are absent[7]. The observation that typical antipsychotics can induce depression and tardive dyskinesia in bipolar patients militates against their long-term use[7-9].

Among atypical antipsychotics, olanzapine, risperidone, quetiapine and aripiprazole have been most robustly evaluated and are licensed in the UK for the treatment of mania. Olanzapine is probably most widely used. It is more effective than placebo in mania[10,11], and at least as effective as valproate semi-sodium[12,13] and lithium[14,15]. As with typical drugs, olanzapine may be most effective when used in combination with a mood-stabiliser[16,17] (although olanzapine + carbamazepine was no better than carbamazepine alone[18]). Data suggest olanzapine may offer benefits in longer-term treatment[19,20]; it may be more effective than lithium[21], and it is formally licensed as prophylaxis.

Clozapine seems to be effective in refractory bipolar conditions, including refractory mania[22-25]. Risperidone has shown efficacy in mania[26], particularly in combination with a mood-stabiliser[2,27]. Data relating to quetiapine[28-33] are compelling but those relating to amisulpride[34] and zotepine[35] are scarce. Aripiprazole is effective in mania[36-38], perhaps to a greater extent than haloperidol[39,40]. It has also been shown to be effective as an add-on agent[41] and in long-term prophylaxis[42].

References

1. Prien RF et al. Comparison of lithium carbonate and chlorpromazine in the treatment of mania. Report of the Veterans Administration and National Institute of Mental Health Collaborative Study Group. Arch Gen Psychiatry 1972; 26:146–53.
2. Sachs GS et al. Combination of a mood stabilizer with risperidone or haloperidol for treatment of acute mania: a double-blind, placebo-controlled comparison of efficacy and safety. Am J Psychiatry 2002; 159:1146–54.
3. McElroy SL et al. A randomized comparison of divalproex oral loading versus haloperidol in the initial treatment of acute psychotic mania. J Clin Psychiatry 1996; 57:142–6.
4. Chou JC et al. Acute mania: haloperidol dose and augmentation with lithium or lorazepam. J Clin Psychopharmacol 1999; 19:500–5.
5. Small JG et al. A placebo-controlled study of lithium combined with neuroleptics in chronic schizophrenic patients. Am J Psychiatry 1975; 132:1315–17.
6. Soares JC et al. Adjunctive antipsychotic use in bipolar patients: an open 6-month prospective study following an acute episode. J Affect Disord 1999; 56:1–8.
7. Keck PE Jr et al. Anticonvulsants and antipsychotics in the treatment of bipolar disorder. J Clin Psychiatry 1998; 59 Suppl 6:74–81.
8. Tohen M et al. Antipsychotic agents and bipolar disorder. J Clin Psychiatry 1998; 59 Suppl 1:38–48.
9. Zarate CA Jr et al. Double-blind comparison of the continued use of antipsychotic treatment versus its discontinuation in remitted manic patients. Am J Psychiatry 2004; 161:169–71.
10. Tohen M et al. Olanzapine versus placebo in the treatment of acute mania. Olanzapine HGEH Study Group. Am J Psychiatry 1999; 156:702–9.
11. Tohen M et al. Efficacy of olanzapine in acute bipolar mania: a double-blind, placebo-controlled study. The Olanzipine HGGW Study Group. Arch Gen Psychiatry 2000; 57:841–9.
12. Tohen M et al. Olanzapine versus divalproex in the treatment of acute mania. Am J Psychiatry 2002; 159:1011–17.
13. Tohen M et al. Olanzapine versus divalproex versus placebo in the treatment of mild to moderate mania: a randomized, 12-week, double-blind study. J Clin Psychiatry 2008; 69:1776–89.
14. Berk M et al. Olanzapine compared to lithium in mania: a double-blind randomized controlled trial. Int Clin Psychopharmacol 1999; 14:339–43.
15. Niufan G et al. Olanzapine versus lithium in the acute treatment of bipolar mania: a double-blind, randomized, controlled trial. J Affect Disord 2008; 105:101–8.
16. Tohen M et al. Efficacy of olanzapine in combination with valproate or lithium in the treatment of mania in patients partially nonresponsive to valproate or lithium monotherapy. Arch Gen Psychiatry 2002; 59:62–9.
17. Tohen M et al. Relapse prevention in bipolar I disorder: 18-month comparison of olanzapine plus mood stabiliser v. mood stabiliser alone. Br J Psychiatry 2004; 184:337–45.
18. Tohen M et al. Olanzapine plus carbamazepine v. carbamazepine alone in treating manic episodes. Br J Psychiatry 2008; 192:135–43.
19. Sanger TM et al. Long-term olanzapine therapy in the treatment of bipolar I disorder: an open-label continuation phase study. J Clin Psychiatry 2001; 62:273–81.
20. Vieta E et al. Olanzapine as long-term adjunctive therapy in treatment-resistant bipolar disorder. J Clin Psychopharmacol 2001; 21:469–73.

21. Tohen M et al. Olanzapine versus lithium in the maintenance treatment of bipolar disorder: a 12-month, randomized, double-blind, controlled clinical trial. Am J Psychiatry 2005; 162:1281–90.
22. Calabrese JR et al. Clozapine for treatment-refractory mania. Am J Psychiatry 1996; 153:759–64.
23. Green AI et al. Clozapine in the treatment of refractory psychotic mania. Am J Psychiatry 2000; 157:982–6.
24. Kimmel SE et al. Clozapine in treatment-refractory mood disorders. J Clin Psychiatry 1994; 55 Suppl B:91–3.
25. Chang JS et al. The effects of long-term clozapine add-on therapy on the rehospitalization rate and the mood polarity patterns in bipolar disorders. J Clin Psychiatry 2006; 67:461–7.
26. Segal J et al. Risperidone compared with both lithium and haloperidol in mania: a double-blind randomized controlled trial. Clin Neuropharmacol 1998; 21:176–80.
27. Vieta E et al. Risperidone in the treatment of mania: efficacy and safety results from a large, multicentre, open study in Spain. J Affect Disord 2002; 72:15–19.
28. Ghaemi SN et al. The use of quetiapine for treatment-resistant bipolar disorder: a case series. Ann Clin Psychiatry 1999; 11:137–40.
29. Sachs G et al. Quetiapine with lithium or divalproex for the treatment of bipolar mania: a randomized, double-blind, placebo-controlled study. Bipolar Disord 2004; 6:213–23.
30. Altamura AC et al. Efficacy and tolerability of quetiapine in the treatment of bipolar disorder: preliminary evidence from a 12-month open label study. J Affect Disord 2003; 76:267–71.
31. Yatham LN et al. Quetiapine versus placebo in combination with lithium or divalproex for the treatment of bipolar mania. J Clin Psychopharmacol 2004; 24:599–606.
32. Bowden CL et al. A randomized, double-blind, placebo-controlled efficacy and safety study of quetiapine or lithium as monotherapy for mania in bipolar disorder. J Clin Psychiatry 2005; 66:111–121.
33. McIntyre RS et al. Quetiapine or haloperidol as monotherapy for bipolar mania--a 12-week, double-blind, randomised, parallel-group, placebo-controlled trial. Eur Neuropsychopharmacol 2005; 15:573–585.
34. Vieta E et al. An open-label study of amisulpride in the treatment of mania. J Clin Psychiatry 2005; 66:575–8.
35. Amann B et al. Zotepine loading in acute and severely manic patients: a pilot study. Bipolar Disord 2005; 7:471–6.
36. Sachs G et al. Aripiprazole in the treatment of acute manic or mixed episodes in patients with bipolar I disorder: a 3-week placebo-controlled study. J Psychopharmacol 2006; 20:536–46.
37. Keck PE Monotherapy in the treatment of acute bipolar I mania: a randomized, double-blind, placebo- and lithium-controlled study. J Affect Disord 2009; 112:36–49.
38. Young AH et al. Aripiprazole monotherapy in acute mania: 12-week randomised placebo- and haloperidol-controlled study. The British Journal of Psychiatry 2009; 194:40–8.
39. Vieta E et al. Effectiveness of aripiprazole v. haloperidol in acute bipolar mania: double-blind, randomised, comparative 12-week trial. Br J Psychiatry 2005; 187:235–42.
40. Cipriani A et al. Haloperidol alone or in combination for acute mania. Cochrane Database Syst Rev 2006; 3:CD004362.
41. Vieta E et al. Efficacy of adjunctive aripiprazole to either valproate or lithium in bipolar mania patients partially nonresponsive to valproate/lithium monotherapy: a placebo-controlled study. Am J Psychiatry 2008; 165:1316–25.
42. Keck PE Jr et al. Aripiprazole monotherapy for maintenance therapy in bipolar I disorder: a 100-week, double-blind study versus placebo. J Clin Psychiatry 2007; 68:1480–91.

146

Bipolar depression

Bipolar depression is a common and debilitating disorder which differs from unipolar disorder in severity, timecourse, recurrence and response to drug treatment. Episodes of bipolar depression are, compared with unipolar depression, more rapid in onset, more frequent, more severe, shorter and more likely to involve reverse neurovegetative symptoms such as hyperphagia and hypersomnia[1,2]. Around 15% of people with bipolar disorder commit suicide[3], a statistic which aptly reflects the severity and frequency of depressive episodes. Bipolar depression entails greater socio-economic burden than both mania and unipolar depression[4].

The drug treatment of bipolar depression is somewhat controversial for two reasons. First, until recently there were few well-conducted, randomised, controlled trials reported in the literature and second, the condition entails consideration of lifelong outcome rather than discrete episode response[5]. We have some knowledge of the therapeutic effects of drugs in bipolar depressive episodes but more limited awareness of the therapeutic or deleterious effects of drugs in the longer term. In the UK, NICE recommends the initial use of an SSRI (in addition to an antimanic drug) or quetiapine (assuming an antipsychotic is not already prescribed)[6]. Second-line treatment is to switch to mirtazapine or venlafaxine or to add quetiapine, olanzapine or lithium to the antidepressant. The tables below give some broad guidance on treatment options in bipolar depression.

Table Bipolar depression – established treatments

Drug/regimen	Comments
Lithium[1,7–10]	Lithium is probably effective in treating bipolar depression but supporting data are confounded by cross-over designs incorporating abrupt switching to placebo. There is some evidence that lithium prevents depressive relapse but its effects on manic relapse are considered more robust. Fairly strong support for lithium in reducing suicidality in bipolar disorder[11,12]
Lithium and antidepressant[13–20]	Antidepressants are widely used in bipolar depression, particularly for breakthrough episodes occurring in those on mood-stabilisers. They appear to be effective, although there is a risk of cycle acceleration and/or switching. Recent studies suggest mood-stabilisers alone are just as effective as mood-stabilisers/antidepressant combination[21,22]. Tricyclics and MAOIs are usually avoided. SSRIs are generally recommended. Venlafaxine and bupropion (amfebutamone) have also been used. Venlafaxine may be more likely to induce a switch to mania[23,24]. There is limited evidence that antidepressants are effective only when lithium plasma levels are below 0.8 mmol/L
	Continuing antidepressant treatment after resolution of symptoms may protect against depressive relapse[25,26], although this is controversial
Lamotrigine[1,8,27–33]	Lamotrigine appears to be effective both as a treatment for bipolar depression and as prophylaxis against further episodes. It does not induce switching or rapid cycling. It is as effective as citalopram and causes less weight gain than lithium. Overall, the effect of lamotrigine is modest, with numerous failed trials[34,35]. It may be useful as an adjunct to lithium[36] or as an alternative to it in pregnancy[37]
	Treatment is complicated by the risk of rash, which is associated with speed of dose titration. The necessity for titration may limit clinical utility
	A further complication is the question of dose: 50 mg/day has efficacy, but 200 mg/day is probably better. In the USA doses of up to 1200 mg/day have been used (mean around 250 mg/day)
Olanzapine and fluoxetine[8,14,38–41]	This combination ('Symbyax®') is more effective than both placebo and olanzapine alone in treating bipolar depression. The dose is 6 and 25 mg or 12 and 50 mg/day (so presumably 5/20 mg and 10/40 mg are effective). May be more effective than lamotrigine. Reasonable evidence of prophylactic effect
Quetiapine[14,42–46]	Two large published RCTs have demonstrated clear efficacy for doses of 300 mg and 600 mg daily (as monotherapy) in bipolar I and bipolar II depression. An anxiolytic effect has also been shown
	As expected, quetiapine appears not to be associated with switching to mania. Longer-term data are very encouraging – quetiapine prevents relapse into depression and mania[47–51]. Quetiapine is probably the drug of choice in bipolar depression[52]

Table Bipolar depression – alternative treatments: refer to primary literature before using

Drug/regimen	Comments
Pramipexole[53,54]	Pramipexole is a dopamine agonist which is widely used in Parkinson's disease. Two small placebo-controlled trials suggest useful efficacy in bipolar depression. Effective dose averages around 1.7 mg/day. Both studies used pramipexole as an adjunct to existing mood-stabiliser treatment. Neither study detected an increased risk of switching to mania/hypomania (a theoretical consideration) but data are insufficient to exclude this possibility. Probably best reserved for specialist centres
Valproate[1,8,55,56–58]	Limited evidence of efficacy as monotherapy but recommended in some guidelines. Probably protects against depressive relapse but database is small
Carbamazepine[1,8,56,59]	Occasionally recommended but database is poor and effect modest. May have useful activity when added to other mood-stabilisers
Antidepressants[60–68]	'Unopposed' antidepressants (i.e. without mood-stabiliser protection) are generally avoided in bipolar depression because of the risk of switching. There is also evidence that they are relatively less effective in bipolar depression than in unipolar depression. Nonetheless short-term use of fluoxetine, venlafaxine and moclobemide seems reasonably effective and safe even as monotherapy. Overall, however, unopposed antidepressant treatment should be avoided, especially in bipolar I disorder. Even in combination with mood-stabilisers risks may outweigh benefits[21]

Table Bipolar depression – other possible treatments: seek specialist advice before using

Drug/regimen	Comments
Aripiprazole[69,70]	Limited support from open studies as add-on treatment
Gabapentin[1,71,72]	Open studies suggest modest effect when added to mood-stabilisers or antipsychotics. Doses average around 1750 mg/day. Anxiolytic effect may account for apparent effect in bipolar depression
Inositol[73]	Small, randomised, pilot study suggests that 12 g/day inositol is effective in bipolar depression
Modafinil[74]	One positive RCT as adjunct to mood-stabiliser. Dose is 100–200 mg/day
Riluzole[75]	Riluzole shares some pharmacological characteristics with lamotrigine. Database is limited to a single case report supporting use in bipolar depression
Thyroxine[76]	Limited evidence of efficacy as augmentation. Doses average around 300 µg/day
Mifepristone[77]	Some evidence of mood-elevating properties in bipolar depression. May also improve cognitive function. Dose is 600 mg/day
Zonisamide[78,79]	Supported by two small RCTs. Dose is 100–300 mg a day

References

1. Malhi GS et al. Bipolar depression: management options. CNS Drugs 2003; 17:9–25.
2. Perlis RH et al. Clinical features of bipolar depression versus major depressive disorder in large multicenter trials. Am J Psychiatry 2006; 163:225–31.
3. Haddad P et al. Pharmacological management of bipolar depression. Acta Psychiatr Scand 2002; 105:401–3.
4. Hirschfeld RM. Bipolar depression: the real challenge. Eur Neuropsychopharmacol 2004; 14 Suppl 2:S83–8.
5. Baldassano CF et al. Rethinking the treatment paradigm for bipolar depression: the importance of long-term management. CNS Spectr 2004; 9:11–18.
6. National Institute for Health and Clinical Excellence. Bipolar disorder. The management of bipolar disorder in adults, children and adolescents, in primary and secondary care. Clinical Guidance 38. http://www.nice.org.uk. 2006.
7. Geddes JR et al. Long-term lithium therapy for bipolar disorder: systematic review and meta-analysis of randomized controlled trials. Am J Psychiatry 2004; 161:217–22.
8. Yatham LN et al. Bipolar depression: criteria for treatment selection, definition of refractoriness, and treatment options. Bipolar Disord 2003; 5:85–97.
9. Calabrese JR et al. A placebo-controlled 18-month trial of lamotrigine and lithium maintenance treatment in recently depressed patients with bipolar I disorder. J Clin Psychiatry 2003; 64:1013–24.
10. Prien RF et al. Lithium carbonate and imipramine in prevention of affective episodes. A comparison in recurrent affective illness. Arch Gen Psychiatry 1973; 29:420–5.
11. Goodwin FK et al. Suicide risk in bipolar disorder during treatment with lithium and divalproex. JAMA 2003; 290:1467–73.
12. Kessing LV et al. Suicide risk in patients treated with lithium. Arch Gen Psychiatry 2005; 62:860–6.
13. Montgomery SA et al. Pharmacotherapy of depression and mixed states in bipolar disorder. J Affect Disord 2000; 59 Suppl 1:S39–56.
14. Calabrese JR et al. International Consensus Group on Bipolar I Depression Treatment Guidelines. J Clin Psychiatry 2004; 65:571–9.
15. Nemeroff CB et al. Double-blind, placebo-controlled comparison of imipramine and paroxetine in the treatment of bipolar depression. Am J Psychiatry 2001; 158:906–12.
16. Vieta E et al. A randomized trial comparing paroxetine and venlafaxine in the treatment of bipolar depressed patients taking mood stabilizers. J Clin Psychiatry 2002; 63:508–12.
17. Young LT et al. Double-blind comparison of addition of a second mood stabilizer versus an antidepressant to an initial mood stabilizer for treatment of patients with bipolar depression. Am J Psychiatry 2000; 157:124–6.
18. Fawcett JA. Lithium combinations in acute and maintenance treatment of unipolar and bipolar depression. J Clin Psychiatry 2003; 64 Suppl 5:32–7.
19. Altshuler L et al. The impact of antidepressant discontinuation versus antidepressant continuation on 1-year risk for relapse of bipolar depression: a retrospective chart review. J Clin Psychiatry 2001; 62:612–16.
20. Erfurth A et al. Bupropion as add-on strategy in difficult-to-treat bipolar depressive patients. Neuropsychobiology 2002; 45 Suppl 1:33–6.
21. Sachs GS et al. Effectiveness of adjunctive antidepressant treatment for bipolar depression. N Engl J Med 2007; 356:1711–22.
22. Goldberg JF et al. Adjunctive antidepressant use and symptomatic recovery among bipolar depressed patients with concomitant manic symptoms: findings from the STEP-BD. Am J Psychiatry 2007; 164:1348–55.
23. Post RM et al. Mood switch in bipolar depression: comparison of adjunctive venlafaxine, bupropion and sertraline. Br J Psychiatry 2006; 189:124–31.
24. Leverich GS et al. Risk of switch in mood polarity to hypomania or mania in patients with bipolar depression during acute and continuation trials of venlafaxine, sertraline, and bupropion as adjuncts to mood stabilizers. Am J Psychiatry 2006; 163:232–9.
25. Salvi V et al. The use of antidepressants in bipolar disorder. J Clin Psychiatry 2008; 69:1307–18.
26. Altshuler LL et al. Impact of antidepressant continuation after acute positive or partial treatment response for bipolar depression: a blinded, randomized study. J Clin Psychiatry 2009; 70:450–7.
27. Baldassano CF et al. What drugs are best for bipolar depression? Ann Clin Psychiatry 2003; 15:225–32.
28. Calabrese JR et al. A double-blind placebo-controlled study of lamotrigine monotherapy in outpatients with bipolar I depression. Lamictal 602 Study Group. J Clin Psychiatry 1999; 60:79–88.
29. Bowden CL et al. Lamotrigine in the treatment of bipolar depression. Eur Neuropsychopharmacol 1999; 9 Suppl 4:S113–17.
30. Marangell LB et al. Lamotrigine treatment of bipolar disorder: data from the first 500 patients in STEP-BD. Bipolar Disord 2004; 6:139–43.
31. Schaffer A et al. Randomized, double-blind pilot trial comparing lamotrigine versus citalopram for the treatment of bipolar depression. J Affect Disord 2006; 96:95–9.
32. Bowden CL et al. Impact of lamotrigine and lithium on weight in obese and nonobese patients with bipolar I disorder. Am J Psychiatry 2006; 163: 1199–201.
33. Suppes T et al. A single blind comparison of lithium and lamotrigine for the treatment of bipolar II depression. J Affect Disord 2008; 111:334–43.
34. Geddes JR et al. Lamotrigine for treatment of bipolar depression: independent meta-analysis and meta-regression of individual patient data from five randomised trials. Br J Psychiatry 2009; 194:4–9.
35. Calabrese JR et al. Lamotrigine in the acute treatment of bipolar depression: results of five double-blind, placebo-controlled clinical trials. Bipolar Disord 2008; 10:323–33.
36. van der Loos ML et al. Efficacy and safety of lamotrigine as add-on treatment to lithium in bipolar depression: a multicenter, double-blind, placebo-controlled trial. J Clin Psychiatry 2009; 70:223–31.
37. Newport DJ et al. Lamotrigine in bipolar disorder: efficacy during pregnancy. Bipolar Disord 2008; 10:432–6.
38. Tohen M et al. Efficacy of olanzapine and olanzapine-fluoxetine combination in the treatment of bipolar I depression. Arch Gen Psychiatry 2003; 60:1079–88.
39. Brown EB et al. A 7-week, randomized, double-blind trial of olanzapine/fluoxetine combination versus lamotrigine in the treatment of bipolar I depression. J Clin Psychiatry 2006; 67:1025–33.
40. Corya SA et al. A 24-week open-label extension study of olanzapine-fluoxetine combination and olanzapine monotherapy in the treatment of bipolar depression. J Clin Psychiatry 2006; 67:798–806.
41. Dube S et al. Onset of antidepressant effect of olanzapine and olanzapine/fluoxetine combination in bipolar depression. Bipolar Disord 2007; 9:618–27.
42. Calabrese JR et al. A randomized, double-blind, placebo-controlled trial of quetiapine in the treatment of bipolar I or II depression. Am J Psychiatry 2005; 162:1351–60.
43. Thase ME et al. Efficacy of quetiapine monotherapy in bipolar I and II depression: a double-blind, placebo-controlled study (the BOLDER II study). J Clin Psychopharmacol 2006; 26:600–9.
44. Hirschfeld RM et al. Quetiapine in the treatment of anxiety in patients with bipolar I or II depression: a secondary analysis from a randomized, double-blind, placebo-controlled study. J Clin Psychiatry 2006; 67:355–62.
45. Milev R et al. Add-on quetiapine for bipolar depression: a 12-month open-label trial. Can J Psychiatry 2006; 51:523–30.
46. Weisler RH et al. Efficacy of quetiapine monotherapy for the treatment of depressive episodes in bipolar I disorder: a post hoc analysis of combined results from 2 double-blind, randomized, placebo-controlled studies. J Clin Psychiatry 2008; 69:769–82.
47. Vieta E et al. Efficacy and safety of quetiapine in combination with lithium or divalproex for maintenance of patients with bipolar I disorder (international trial 126). J Affect Disord 2008; 109:251–63.
48. Suppes T et al. Maintenance treatment for patients with bipolar I disorder: results from a north american study of quetiapine in combination with lithium or divalproex (trial 127). Am J Psychiatry 2009; 166:476–88.
49. Nolen WA et al. Quetiapine or lithium versus placebo for maintenance treatment of bipolar I disorder after stabilization on quetiapine. 2008. Poster presented at 17th European Congress of Psychiatry, 24–28 January 2008, Lisbon, Portugal.

Bipolar disorder

149

50. Young AH et al. A double-blind, placebo-controlled study with acute and continuation phase of quetiapine in adults with bipolar depression (EMBOLDEN I). 2008. Poster presented at the 3rd Biennial Conference of the International Society of Bipolar Disorders, 27–28 January 2008, Delhi, India.

51. McElroy S et al. A double-blind placebo-controlled study with acute and continuation phase of quetiapine in adults with bipolar depression (EMBOLDEN II). 2008. Poster presented at the 3rd Biennial Conference of the International Society for Bipolar Disorders, 27–28 January 2008, Delhi, India.

52. Goodwin G. Evidence-based guidelines for treating bipolar disorder: revised second edition – recommendations from the British Association for Psychopharmacology. J Psychopharmacol 2009; 23:346–88.

53. Goldberg JF et al. Preliminary randomized, double-blind, placebo-controlled trial of pramipexole added to mood stabilizers for treatment-resistant bipolar depression. Am J Psychiatry 2004; 161:564–6.

54. Zarate CA Jr et al. Pramipexole for bipolar II depression: a placebo-controlled proof of concept study. Biol Psychiatry 2004; 56:54–60.

55. Goodwin GM et al. The British Association for Psychopharmacology guidelines for treatment of bipolar disorder: a summary. J Psychopharmacol 2003; 17:3–6.

56. Goodwin GM. Evidence-based guidelines for treating bipolar disorder: recommendations from the British Association for Psychopharmacology. J Psychopharmacol 2003; 17:149–73.

57. Davis LL et al. Divalproex in the treatment of bipolar depression: a placebo-controlled study. J Affect Disord 2005; 85:259–66.

58. Ghaemi SN et al. Divalproex in the treatment of acute bipolar depression: a preliminary double-blind, randomized, placebo-controlled pilot study. J Clin Psychiatry 2007; 68:1840–4.

59. Dilsaver SC et al. Treatment of bipolar depression with carbamazepine: results of an open study. Biol Psychiatry 1996; 40:935–937.

60. Amsterdam JD et al. Short-term fluoxetine monotherapy for bipolar type II or bipolar NOS major depression – low manic switch rate. Bipolar Disord 2004; 6:75–81.

61. Amsterdam JD et al. Efficacy and safety of fluoxetine in treating bipolar II major depressive episode. J Clin Psychopharmacol 1998; 18:435–40.

62. Amsterdam J. Efficacy and safety of venlafaxine in the treatment of bipolar II major depressive episode. J Clin Psychopharmacol 1998; 18:414–17.

63. Amsterdam JD et al. Venlafaxine monotherapy in women with bipolar II and unipolar major depression. J Affect Disord 2000; 59:225–9.

64. Silverstone T. Moclobemide vs. imipramine in bipolar depression: a multicentre double-blind clinical trial. Acta Psychiatr Scand 2001; 104:104–9.

65. Ghaemi SN et al. Antidepressant treatment in bipolar versus unipolar depression. Am J Psychiatry 2004; 161:163–5.

66. Post RM et al. A re-evaluation of the role of antidepressants in the treatment of bipolar depression: data from the Stanley Foundation Bipolar Network. Bipolar Disord 2003; 5:396–406.

67. Amsterdam JD et al. Comparison of fluoxetine, olanzapine, and combined fluoxetine plus olanzapine initial therapy of bipolar type I and type II major depression – lack of manic induction. J Affect Disord 2005; 87:121–30.

68. Amsterdam JD et al. Fluoxetine monotherapy of bipolar type II and bipolar NOS major depression: a double-blind, placebo-substitution, continuation study. Int Clin Psychopharmacol 2005; 20:257–64.

69. Ketter TA et al. Adjunctive aripiprazole in treatment-resistant bipolar depression. Ann Clin Psychiatry 2006; 18:169–72.

70. Mazza M et al. Beneficial acute antidepressant effects of aripiprazole as an adjunctive treatment or monotherapy in bipolar patients unresponsive to mood stabilizers: results from a 16-week open-label trial. Expert Opin Pharmacother 2008; 9:3145–9.

71. Wang PW et al. Gabapentin augmentation therapy in bipolar depression. Bipolar Disord 2002; 4:296–301.

72. Ashton H et al. GABA-ergic drugs: exit stage left, enter stage right. J Psychopharmacol 2003; 17:174–8.

73. Chengappa KN et al. Inositol as an add-on treatment for bipolar depression. Bipolar Disord 2000; 2:47–55.

74. Frye MA et al. A placebo-controlled evaluation of adjunctive modafinil in the treatment of bipolar depression. Am J Psychiatry 2007; 164:1242–9.

75. Singh J et al. Case report: Successful riluzole augmentation therapy in treatment-resistant bipolar depression following the development of rash with lamotrigine. Psychopharmacology 2004; 173:227–8.

76. Bauer M. Thyroid hormone augmentation with levothyroxine in bipolar depression. Bipolar Disord 2002; 4 Suppl 1:109–10.

77. Young AH et al. Improvements in neurocognitive function and mood following adjunctive treatment with mifepristone (RU-486) in bipolar disorder. Neuropsychopharmacology 2004; 29:1538–45.

78. Ghaemi SN et al. An open prospective study of zonisamide in acute bipolar depression. J Clin Psychopharmacol 2006; 26:385–8.

79. Anand A et al. A preliminary open-label study of zonisamide treatment for bipolar depression in 10 patients. J Clin Psychiatry 2005;66:195–8.

Further reading

Fountoulakis KN et al. Treatment of bipolar depression: an update. J Affect Disord 2008; 109:21–34.

Goodwin GM et al. ECNP consensus meeting. Bipolar depression. Nice, March 2007. Eur Neuropsychopharmacol 2008; 18:535–49.

Nierenberg AA. An analysis of the efficacy of treatments for bipolar depression. J Clin Psychiatry 2008; 69 Suppl 5:4–8.

Thase ME. Quetiapine monotherapy for bipolar depression. Neuropsychiatr Dis Treat 2008;4:11–21.

Rapid-cycling bipolar affective disorder

Rapid-cycling is usually defined as bipolar disorder in which four or more episodes of (hypo) mania or depression occur in a 12-month period. It is generally held to be less responsive to drug treatment than non-rapid-cycling bipolar illness[1,2] and entails considerable depressive morbidity and suicide risk[3]. The following table outlines a treatment strategy for rapid-cycling based on rather limited data and very few direct comparisons of drugs[4]. This strategy is broadly in line with UK NICE guidelines[5] which suggest a combination of lithium and valproate as first-line treatment and (somewhat bizarrely) lithium alone 'as second-line treatment'.

In practice, response to treatment is sometimes idiosyncratic: individuals sometimes show significant response only to one or two drugs. Spontaneous or treatment-related remissions occur in around a third of rapid-cyclers[6]. Non-drug methods may also be considered[7,8].

Table		
Step	*Suggested treatment*	*References*
Step 1	Withdraw antidepressants	9–11
Step 2	Evaluate possible precipitants (e.g. alcohol, thyroid dysfunction, external stressors)	2,11
Step 3	Optimise mood-stabiliser treatment Consider combining mood-stabilisers, e.g. lithium + valproate Lithium may be relatively less effective but this is not certain[12]	13–17
Step 4	Consider other (usually adjunct) treatment options: (alphabetical order) Aripiprazole (15–30 mg/day) Clozapine (usual doses) Lamotrigine (up to 225 mg/day) Levetiracetam (up to 2000 mg/day) Nimodipine (180 mg/day) Olanzapine (usual doses) Quetiapine (300–600 mg/day) Risperidone (up to 6 mg/day) Thyroxine (150–400 µg/day)] Topiramate (up to 300 mg/day) Choice of drug is determined by patient factors – few comparative efficacy data to guide choice. Quetiapine probably has best supporting data and may be considered treatment of choice at this stage.	13,18–33

References

1. Calabrese JR et al. Current research on rapid cycling bipolar disorder and its treatment. J Affect Disord 2001; 67:241–55.
2. Kupka RW et al. Rapid and non-rapid cycling bipolar disorder: a meta-analysis of clinical studies. J Clin Psychiatry 2003; 64:1483–94.
3. Coryell W et al. The long-term course of rapid-cycling bipolar disorder. Arch Gen Psychiatry 2003; 60:914–20.
4. Tondo L et al. Rapid-cycling bipolar disorder: effects of long-term treatments. Acta Psychiatr Scand 2003; 108:4–14.
5. National Institute for Health and Clinical Excellence. Bipolar disorder. The management of bipolar disorder in adults, children and adolescents, in primary and secondary care. Clinical Guidance 38. http://www.nice.org.uk. 2006.
6. Koukopoulos A et al. Duration and stability of the rapid-cycling course: a long-term personal follow-up of 109 patients. J Affect Disord 2003; 73:75–85.
7. Dell'Osso B et al. Augmentative transcranial magnetic stimulation (TMS) combined with brain navigation in drug-resistant rapid cycling bipolar depression: A case report of acute and maintenance efficacy. World J Biol Psychiatry 2008; Epub ahead of print. DOI: 10.1080/15622970701806192.
8. Marangell LB et al. A 1-year pilot study of vagus nerve stimulation in treatment-resistant rapid-cycling bipolar disorder. J Clin Psychiatry 2008; 69:183–9.
9. Wehr TA et al. Can antidepressants cause mania and worsen the course of affective illness? Am J Psychiatry 1987; 144:1403–11.
10. Altshuler LL et al. Antidepressant-induced mania and cycle acceleration: a controversy revisited. Am J Psychiatry 1995; 152:1130–8.
11. American Psychiatric Association. Practice guideline for the treatment of patients with bipolar disorder. Am J Psychiatry 2002; 159 Suppl 4:1–50.
12. Calabrese JR et al. A 20-month, double-blind, maintenance trial of lithium versus divalproex in rapid-cycling bipolar disorder. Am J Psychiatry 2005; 162:2152–61.
13. Sanger TM et al. Olanzapine in the acute treatment of bipolar I disorder with a history of rapid cycling. J Affect Disord 2003; 73:155–61.
14. Taylor DM et al. Treatment options for rapid-cycling bipolar affective disorder. Psychiatr Bull 1996; 20:601–3.
15. Kemp DE et al. A 6-month, double-blind, maintenance trial of lithium monotherapy versus the combination of lithium and divalproex for rapid-cycling bipolar disorder and co-occurring substance abuse or dependence. J Clin Psychiatry 2009; 70:113–21.
16. da Rocha FF et al. Addition of lamotrigine to valproic acid: a successful outcome in a case of rapid-cycling bipolar affective disorder. Prog Neuropsychopharmacol Biol Psychiatry 2007; 31:1548–9.
17. Woo YS et al. Lamotrigine added to valproate successfully treated a case of ultra-rapid cycling bipolar disorder. Psychiatry Clin Neurosci 2007; 61:130–1.
18. Calabrese JR et al. Clozapine prophylaxis in rapid cycling bipolar disorder. J Clin Psychopharmacol 1991; 11:396–7.
19. Vieta E et al. Quetiapine in the treatment of rapid cycling bipolar disorder. Bipolar Disord 2002; 4:335–40.
20. Goodnick PJ. Nimodipine treatment of rapid cycling bipolar disorder. J Clin Psychiatry 1995; 56:330.
21. Pazzaglia PJ et al. Preliminary controlled trial of nimodipine in ultra-rapid cycling affective dysregulation. Psychiatry Res 1993; 49:257–72.
22. Bauer MS et al. Rapid cycling bipolar affective disorder. Arch Gen Psychiatry 1990; 47:435–40.
23. Fatemi SH et al. Lamotrigine in rapid-cycling bipolar disorder. J Clin Psychiatry 1997; 58:522–7.
24. Calabrese JR et al. A double-blind, placebo-controlled, prophylaxis study of lamotrigine in rapid-cycling bipolar disorder. Lamictal 614 Study Group. J Clin Psychiatry 2000; 61:841–50.
25. Braunig P et al. Levetiracetam in the treatment of rapid cycling bipolar disorder. J Psychopharmacol 2003; 17:239–41.
26. Vieta E et al. Treatment of refractory rapid cycling bipolar disorder with risperidone. J Clin Psychopharmacol 1998; 18:172–4.
27. Jacobsen FM. Risperidone in the treatment of affective illness and obsessive-compulsive disorder. J Clin Psychiatry 1995; 56:423–9.
28. Chen CK et al. Combination treatment of clozapine and topiramate in resistant rapid-cycling bipolar disorder. Clin Neuropharmacol 2005; 28:136–8.
29. Goldberg JF et al. Effectiveness of quetiapine in rapid cycling bipolar disorder: a preliminary study. J Affect Disord 2008; 105:305–10.
30. Vieta E et al. Quetiapine monotherapy in the treatment of patients with bipolar I or II depression and a rapid-cycling disease course: a randomized, double-blind, placebo-controlled study. Bipolar Disord 2007; 9:413–25.
31. Langosch JM et al. Efficacy of quetiapine monotherapy in rapid-cycling bipolar disorder in comparison with sodium valproate. J Clin Psychopharmacol 2008; 28:555–60.
32. Suppes T et al. Efficacy and safety of aripiprazole in subpopulations with acute manic or mixed episodes of bipolar I disorder. J Affect Disord 2008; 107:145–54.
33. Muzina DJ et al. Aripiprazole monotherapy in patients with rapid-cycling bipolar I disorder: an analysis from a long-term, double-blind, placebo-controlled study. Int J Clin Pract 2008; 62:679–87.

Prophylaxis in bipolar disorder

NICE recommends that a mood-stabiliser should be prescribed as prophylaxis:

* after a single manic episode that was associated with significant risk and adverse consequences or
* in the case of bipolar I illness, after two or more acute episodes or
* in the case of bipolar II illness, if there is significant functional impairment, frequent episodes or significant risk of suicide[1].

Note that residual symptoms after an acute episode are a strong predictor of recurrence[2]. Most evidence supports the efficacy of lithium[3–6]. Carbamazepine is somewhat less effective[4] and the long-term efficacy of valproate is uncertain[7–9], although it probably protects against relapse both into depression and mania[10]. Lithium has the advantage of an accepted anti-suicidal effect[11–13] but perhaps relative to other mood-stabilisers, the disadvantage of a worsened outcome following abrupt discontinuation[14–17].Conventional antipsychotics have traditionally been used and are perceived to be effective although the objective evidence base is, again, weak[18,19].

Evidence supports the efficacy of some second-generation antipsychotics particularly olanzapine[1,8], quetiapine[20,21] and aripiprazole[22]. Whether atypicals are more effective than typicals or are truly associated with a reduced overall side-effect burden remains untested.

NICE recommend[1]

* Lithium, olanzapine or valproate as first-line prophylactic agents (quetiapine can now be added to this list)
* Treatment for at least 2 years (longer in high-risk patients)
* Antidepressants (SSRIs are preferred) may be used in combination with a mood-stabiliser to treat acute episodes of depression but should not be routinely used for prophylaxis
* Chronic or recurrent depression may be treated with an SSRI or CBT in combination with a mood-stabiliser or quetiapine or lamotrigine
* Combined lithium and valproate for the prophylaxis of rapid cycling illness.

*Note that valproate is teratogenic and should not be routinely used in women of childbearing age (see Pregnancy section, Chapter 7).

A significant proportion of patients with bipolar illness fail to be treated adequately with a single mood-stabiliser, so combinations of mood-stabilisers[23,24] or a mood-stabiliser and an antipsychotic[24,25] are commonly used. Also, there is evidence that where combination treatments are effective in mania, then continuation with the same combination provides optimal prophylaxis[25]. The use of polypharmacy needs to be balanced against the likely increased side-effect burden. Combinations of two from lithium, olanzapine and valproate are recommend by NICE[1]. Carbamazepine is considered to be third line. Lamotrigine may be useful in bipolar II disorder[1] and seems to prevent recurrence of depression[26]. The patient's views about 'acceptable risk' of recurrence versus 'acceptable side-effect burden' are paramount.

References

1.   National Institute for Health and Clinical Excellence. Bipolar disorder. The Management of bipolar disorder in adults, children and adolescents, in primary and secondary care. Clinical Guidance 38. http://www.nice.org.uk. 2006.
2.   Perlis RH et al. Predictors of recurrence in bipolar disorder: primary outcomes from the Systematic Treatment Enhancement Program for Bipolar Disorder (STEP-BD). Am J Psychiatry 2006; 163:217–24.
3.   Geddes JR et al. Long-term lithium therapy for bipolar disorder: systematic review and meta-analysis of randomized controlled trials. Am J Psychiatry 2004; 161:217–22.
4.   Hartong EG et al. Prophylactic efficacy of lithium versus carbamazepine in treatment-naive bipolar patients. J Clin Psychiatry 2003; 64:144–51.
5.   Young AH et al. Lithium in mood disorders: increasing evidence base, declining use? Br J Psychiatry 2007; 191:474–6.
6.   Biel MG et al. Continuation versus discontinuation of lithium in recurrent bipolar illness: a naturalistic study. Bipolar Disord 2007; 9:435–42.
7.   Bowden CL et al. A randomized, placebo-controlled 12-month trial of divalproex and lithium in treatment of outpatients with bipolar I disorder. Divalproex Maintenance Study Group. Arch Gen Psychiatry 2000; 57:481–9.
8.   Tohen M et al. Olanzapine versus divalproex sodium for the treatment of acute mania and maintenance of remission: a 47-week study. Am J Psychiatry 2003; 160:1263–71.
9.   Macritchie KA et al. Valproic acid, valproate and divalproex in the maintenance treatment of bipolar disorder. Cochrane Database Syst Rev 2001;CD003196.
10. Smith LA et al. Effectiveness of mood stabilizers and antipsychotics in the maintenance phase of bipolar disorder: a systematic review of randomized controlled trials. Bipolar Disord 2007; 9:394–412.
11. Cipriani A et al. Lithium in the prevention of suicidal behavior and all-cause mortality in patients with mood disorders: a systematic review of randomized trials. Am J Psychiatry 2005; 162:1805–19.
12. Kessing LV et al. Suicide risk in patients treated with lithium. Arch Gen Psychiatry 2005; 62:860–6.
13. Young AH et al. Lithium in maintenance therapy for bipolar disorder. J Psychopharmacol 2006; 20:17–22.
14. Mander AJ et al. Rapid recurrence of mania following abrupt discontinuation of lithium. Lancet 1988; 2:15–17.
15. Faedda GL et al. Outcome after rapid vs gradual discontinuation of lithium treatment in bipolar disorders. Arch Gen Psychiatry 1993; 50:448–55.
16. Macritchie KA et al. Does 'rebound mania' occur after stopping carbamazepine? A pilot study. J Psychopharmacol 2000; 14:266–8.
17. Franks MA et al. Bouncing back: is the bipolar rebound phenomenon peculiar to lithium? A retrospective naturalistic study. J Psychopharmacol 2008; 22:452–6.
18. Gao K et al. Typical and atypical antipsychotics in bipolar depression. J Clin Psychiatry 2005; 66:1376–85.
19. Hellewell JS. A review of the evidence for the use of antipsychotics in the maintenance treatment of bipolar disorders. J Psychopharmacol 2006; 20:39–45.
20. Vieta E et al. Efficacy and safety of quetiapine in combination with lithium or divalproex for maintenance of patients with bipolar I disorder (international trial 126). J Affect Disord 2008; 109:251–63.
21. Suppes T et al. Maintenance treatment for patients with bipolar I disorder: results from a north american study of quetiapine in combination with lithium or divalproex (trial 127). Am J Psychiatry 2009; 166:476–488.
22. Keck PE Jr et al. Aripiprazole monotherapy for maintenance therapy in bipolar I disorder: a 100-week, double-blind study versus placebo. J Clin Psychiatry 2007; 68:1480–91.
23. Freeman MP et al. Mood stabilizer combinations: a review of safety and efficacy. Am J Psychiatry 1998; 155:12–21.
24. Muzina DJ et al. Maintenance therapies in bipolar disorder: focus on randomized controlled trials. Aust N Z J Psychiatry 2005; 39:652–61.
25. Tohen M et al. Relapse prevention in bipolar I disorder: 18-month comparison of olanzapine plus mood stabiliser v. mood stabiliser alone. Br J Psychiatry 2004; 184:337–45.
26. Bowden CL et al. A placebo-controlled 18-month trial of lamotrigine and lithium maintenance treatment in recently manic or hypomanic patients with bipolar I disorder. Arch Gen Psychiatry 2003; 60:392–400.

Further reading

Sachs GS. Decision tree for the treatment of bipolar disorder. J Clin Psychiatry 2003; 64:35–40.

chapter 4

Depression and anxiety

Antidepressants

Effectiveness

The *severity* of depression at which antidepressants show consistent benefits over placebo is poorly defined. In general, the more severe the symptoms, the greater the benefit[1,2]. Antidepressants are normally recommended as first-line treatment in patients whose depression is of at least moderate severity. Of this patient group, approximately 20% will recover with no treatment at all, 30% will respond to placebo and 50% will respond to antidepressant drug treatment[3]. This gives a NNT of 3 for antidepressant over true no-treatment control and an NNT of 5 for antidepressant over placebo. Note though that response in clinical trials is generally defined as a 50% reduction in depression rating scale scores, a somewhat arbitrary dichotomy, and that change measured using continuous scales tends to show a relatively small mean difference between active treatment and placebo.

In patients with sub-syndromal depression it is difficult to separate the response rate to antidepressants from that to placebo; antidepressant treatment is not indicated unless the patient has a history of severe depression (where less severe symptoms may indicate the onset of another episode), or if symptoms persist. Patients with dysthymia (symptom *duration* of at least 2 years) benefit from antidepressant treatment; the minimum duration of symptoms associated with benefit is unknown. In other patients, the side effects associated with antidepressant treatment may outweigh any small benefit seen.

Onset of action

It is widely held that antidepressants do not exert their effects for 2–4 weeks. This is a myth. All antidepressants show a pattern of response where the rate of improvement is highest during weeks 1–2 and lowest during weeks 4–6. Statistical separation from placebo is seen at 2–4 weeks in single trials (hence the idea of a lag effect) but after only 1–2 weeks in (statistically more powerful) meta-analyses[4,5]. Thus where large numbers of patients are treated and detailed rating scales are used an antidepressant effect is evident at 1 week. In practice using simple observations, an antidepressant effect in an individual is often seen by 2 weeks. It follows that in individuals where no antidepressant effect is evident after 2 weeks' treatment, a change in dose or drug may be indicated.

Choice of antidepressant and relative side effects

Selective serotonin re-uptake inhibitors (SSRIs) are well tolerated compared with the older tricyclic antidepressants (TCAs) and mono-amine oxidase inhibitors (MAOIs), and are generally recommended as first-line pharmacological treatment for depression[1]. There is no evidence of any clinically meaningful difference in efficacy between SSRIs, although side-effect profiles differ. For example, paroxetine has been associated with more weight gain and a higher incidence of sexual dysfunction, and sertraline with a higher incidence of diarrhoea than other SSRIs[6]. Newer dual re-uptake inhibitors such as venlafaxine and duloxetine tend to be tolerated less well than SSRIs but better than TCAs. With all drugs there is marked inter-individual variation in tolerability which is not easily predicted by knowledge of a drug's likely adverse effects. A flexible approach is usually required to find the right drug for a particular patient.

As well as headache and GI symptoms, SSRIs as a class are associated with a range of other side effects including sexual dysfunction (see relevant section), hyponatraemia (see section on hyponatraemia) and GI bleeds (see section on SSRIs and bleeding). TCAs have a number of adverse cardiovascular effects (hypotension, tachycardia and QTc prolongation), and are particularly toxic in overdose[7] (see section on overdose). MAOIs have the potential to interact with tyramine-containing foods to cause hypertensive crisis. All antidepressant drugs can cause discontinuation symptoms with short half-life drugs being most problematic in this respect (see section on discontinuation). See following pages for a summary of the clinically relevant side effects of available antidepressant drugs.

Drug interactions

Some SSRIs are potent inhibitors of individual or multiple hepatic cytochrome P450 (CYP) pathways and the magnitude of these effects is dose-related. A number of clinically significant drug interactions can therefore be predicted. For example fluvoxamine is a potent inhibitor of CYP1A2 which can result in increased theophylline serum levels, and fluoxetine is a potent inhibitor of CYP2D6 which can result in increased seizure risk with clozapine.

Antidepressants can also cause pharmacodynamic interactions. For example, the cardiotoxicity of TCAs may be exacerbated by drugs such as diuretics that can cause electrolyte disturbances. A summary of clinically relevant drug interactions with antidepressants can be found later in this chapter.

Potential pharmacokinetic and pharmacodynamic interactions between antidepressants have to be considered when switching from one antidepressant to another (see section on switching antidepressants).

Suicidality

Antidepressant treatment has been associated with an increased risk of suicidal thoughts and acts, particularly in adolescents and young adults[8] leading to the recommendation that patients should be warned of this potential adverse effect during the early weeks of treatment and know how to seek help if required. All antidepressants have been implicated, including those that are marketed for an indication other than depression (e.g. atomoxetine). It should be noted that; (1) although the relative risk may be elevated above placebo rates in some patient groups, the absolute risk remains very small, and; (2) the most effective way to prevent suicidal thoughts and acts is to treat depression, and antidepressant drugs are the most effective treatment currently available[3]. For the most part, suicidality is greatly reduced by the use of antidepressants[9-11].

Duration of treatment

Antidepressants relieve the symptoms of depression but do not treat the underlying cause. They should therefore be taken for 6–9 months after recovery from a single episode (to cover the assumed duration of most single untreated episodes). In those patients who have had multiple episodes, there is evidence of benefit from maintenance treatment for at least 2 years; no upper duration of treatment has been identified. There are few data on which to base recommendations about the duration of treatment of augmentation regimens.

Next step treatments

Approximately a third of patients do not respond to the first antidepressant that is prescribed. Options in this group include dose escalation, switching to a different drug and a number of augmentation strategies. The lessons from STAR*D are that a small proportion of non-responders will respond with each treatment change, but that effect sizes are modest and there is no clear difference in effectiveness between strategies. (See section on refractory depression.)

Use of antidepressants in anxiety spectrum disorders

Antidepressants are first-line treatments in a number of anxiety spectrum disorders. See section on anxiety.

References

1. National Institute for Health and Clinical Excellence. Depression (amended) management of depression in primary and secondary care. 2007. http://www.nice.org.uk.
2. Kirsch I et al. Initial severity and antidepressant benefits: a meta-analysis of data submitted to the Food and Drug Administration. PLoS Med 2008; 5:e45.
3. Anderson IM et al. Evidence-based guidelines for treating depressive disorders with antidepressants: a revision of the 2000 British Association for Psychopharmacology guidelines. J Psychopharmacol 2008; 22:343–96.
4. Taylor MJ et al. Early onset of selective serotonin reuptake inhibitor antidepressant action: systematic review and meta-analysis. Arch Gen Psychiatry 2006; 63:1217–23.
5. Papakostas GI et al. A meta-analysis of early sustained response rates between antidepressants and placebo for the treatment of major depressive disorder. J Clin Psychopharmacol 2006; 26:56–60.
6. Gartlehner G et al. Comparative benefits and harms of second-generation antidepressants: background paper for the American College of Physicians. Ann Intern Med 2008; 149:734–50.
7. Flanagan RJ. Fatal toxicity of drugs used in psychiatry. Hum Psychopharmacol 2008; 23 Suppl 1:43–51.
8. Friedman RA et al. Expanding the black box – depression, antidepressants, and the risk of suicide. N Engl J Med 2007; 356:2343–6.
9. Simon GE et al. Suicide risk during antidepressant treatment. Am J Psychiatry 2006; 163:41–7.
10. Mulder RT et al. Antidepressant treatment is associated with a reduction in suicidal ideation and suicide attempts. Acta Psychiatr Scand 2008; 118:116–22.
11. Tondo L et al. Suicidal status during antidepressant treatment in 789 Sardinian patients with major affective disorder. Acta Psychiatr Scand 2008; 118:106–15.

Antidepressant drugs – tricyclics*

Tricyclic	Licensed indication	Licensed doses (elderly doses not included)	Main adverse effects	Major interactions	Approx. half-life (h)	Cost (£)
Amitriptyline	Depression Nocturnal enuresis in children	30–200 mg/day 7–10 yr: 10–20 mg 11–16 yr: 25–50 mg at night for maximum of 3 months	Sedation, often with hangover; postural hypotension; tachycardia/ arrhythmia; dry mouth, blurred vision, constipation, urinary retention	SSRIs (except citalopram), phenothiazines, cimetidine – ↑ plasma levels of TCAs alcohol, antimuscarinics, antipsychotics, MAOIs	9–25 18–96 Active metabolite (nortriptyline)	0.04/50 mg
Clomipramine	Depression Phobic and obsessional states Adjunctive treatment of cataplexy associated with narcolepsy	10–250 mg/day 10–150 mg/day 10–75 mg/day	As for amitriptyline	As for amitriptyline	12–36 36 Active metabolite (desmethyl-clomipramine)	0.13/50 mg
Dosulepin (dothiepin)	Depression	75–225 mg/day	As for amitriptyline	As for amitriptyline	14–45 22–60 Active metabolite (desmethyldosulepin)	0.06/75 mg

Drug	Indication	Dose			Half-life (h)	Cost
Doxepin	Depression	10–300 mg/day (up to 100 mg as a single dose)	As for amitriptyline	As for amitriptyline	8–24 33–80 Active metabolite (desmethyldoxepin)	0.20/50 mg
Imipramine	Depression Nocturnal enuresis in children	10–200 mg/day (up to 100 mg as a single dose; up to 300 mg in hospital patients) 7 yr: 25 mg 8–11 yr: 25–50 mg >11 yr: 50–75 mg at night for maximum of 3 months	As for amitriptyline but less sedative	As for amitriptyline	~19 12–36 Active metabolite (desipramine)	0.04/25 mg
Lofepramine	Depression	140–210 mg/day	As for amitriptyline but less sedative/anticholinergic/cardiotoxic Constipation common	As for amitriptyline	1.5–6? 12–24 Active metabolite (desipramine)	0.31/70 mg
Nortriptyline	Depression Nocturnal enuresis in children	30–150 mg/day 7 yr: 10 mg 8–11 yrs: 10–20 mg >11 yr: 25–35 mg at night for max. 3 months	As for amitriptyline but less sedative/anticholinergic/hypotensive Constipation may be problematic	As for amitriptyline	15–39	0.21/25 mg
Trimipramine	Depression	30–300 mg/day	As for amitriptyline but more sedative	As for amitriptyline Safer with MAOIs than other tricyclics	7–23 ~23	0.27/50 mg

*For full details refer to the manufacturer's information.

Depression & anxiety

Antidepressant drugs – SSRIs*

SSRI	Licensed indication	Licensed doses (elderly doses not included)	Main adverse effects	Major interactions	Approx. half-life (h)	Cost (£)
Citalopram	Depression – treatment of the initial phase and as maintenance therapy against potential relapse or recurrence	20–60 mg/day Use lowest dose – evidence for higher doses poor	Nausea, vomiting, dyspepsia, abdominal pain, diarrhoea, rash, sweating, agitation, anxiety, headache, insomnia, tremor, sexual dysfunction (male and female), hyponatraemia, cutaneous bleeding disorders	Not a potent inhibitor of most cytochrome enzymes Avoid – MAOIs Avoid – St John's Wort Caution with alcohol (although no inter-action seen) NSAIDs/tryptophan/warfarin	~33 Has weak active metabolites	0.04/20 mg (generic available – price may vary) Drops 0.67/16 mg/8 drops (= 20 mg tablet)
	Panic disorder ± agoraphobia	10 mg for 1 week, increasing up to 60 mg/day	Discontinuation symptoms may occur			

Escitalopram	Depression	10–20 mg/day	As for citalopram	As for citalopram	~30 Has weak active metabolites	0.53/10 mg
	Panic disorder ± agoraphobia	5 mg/day for 1 week, increasing up to 20 mg/day				
	Social anxiety	10–20 mg/day				
	Generalised anxiety disorder	10–20 mg/day				
	OCD	10–20 mg/day				
Fluoxetine	Depression	20 mg/day	As for citalopram but insomnia and agitation possibly more common	Inhibits CYP2D6, CYP3A4. Increases plasma levels of some antipsychotics/ some benzos/ carbamazepine/ ciclosporin/phenytoin/ tricyclics	4–6 days 4–16 days Active metabolite (norfluoxetine)	0.03/20 mg (generic – price may vary)
	OCD	20–60 mg/day	Rash may occur more frequently	MAOIs – never Avoid: selegiline/ St John's wort		
	Bulimia nervosa	60 mg/day	May alter insulin requirements	Caution – alcohol (although no interaction seen)/ NSAIDs/tryptophan/ warfarin		Liquid 0.95/20 mg/5 ml
	Higher doses possible – see SPC	(up to 60 mg/day)				

(Cont.)

SSRI	Licensed indication	Licensed doses (elderly doses not included)	Main adverse effects	Major interactions	Approx. half-life (h)	Cost (£)
Fluvoxamine	Depression	100–300 mg/day bd if >150 mg	As for citalopram but nausea more common	Inhibits CYP1A2/2C9/3A4 Increases plasma levels of some benzos/ carbamazepine/ ciclosporin/ methadone/olanzapine/ clozapine/phenytoin/ propranolol/ theophylline/some tricyclics/warfarin MAOIs – never Caution: alcohol/ lithium/NSAIDs/St John's wort/ tryptophan/warfarin	17–22	0.28/100 mg
	OCD	100–300 mg/day (start at 50 mg/day) bd if >150 mg				
Paroxetine	Depression	20–50 mg/day Use lowest dose – evidence for higher doses poor	As for citalopram but antimuscarinic effects and sedation more common Extrapyramidal symptoms more common, but rare Discontinuation symptoms common – withdraw slowly	Potent inhibitor of CYP2D6 Increases plasma level of some antipsychotics/ tricyclics MAOIs – never Avoid: St John's wort Caution: alcohol/ lithium/NSAIDs/ tryptophan/warfarin	~24 (non-linear kinetics)	0.10/20 mg (generic – price may vary)
	OCD	20–60 mg/day				
	Panic disorder ± agoraphobia	10–60 mg/day				Liquid 0.63/20 mg/ 10 ml
	Social phobia/social anxiety disorders	20–50 mg/day				
	PTSD	20–50 mg/day				
	Generalised anxiety disorder	20–50 mg/day				

Sertraline	Depression ± anxiety and prevention of relapse or recurrence of depression ± anxiety	50–200 mg/day Use 50–100 mg – evidence for higher doses poor	As for citalopram	Inhibits CYP2D6 (more likely to occur at doses ≥100 mg/day). Increases plasma levels of some antipsychotics/tricyclics Avoid: St John's wort Caution: alcohol (although no interaction seen)/lithium/NSAIDs/tryptophan/warfarin	~26	0.06/100 mg generic – price may vary
	OCD (under specialist supervision in children)	50–200 mg/day (adults) 6–12 yr: 25–50 mg/day			Has a weak active metabolite	
		13–17 yr: 50–200 mg/day may be increased in steps of 50 mg at intervals of 1 week				
	PTSD in women	25–200 mg/day				

*For full details refer to the manufacturer's information.

Antidepressant drugs – MAOIs*

MAOI	Licensed indication	Licensed doses (elderly doses not included)	Main adverse effects	Major interactions	Approx. half-life (h)	Cost (£)
Isocarboxazid	Depression	30 mg/day in single or divided doses (increased after 4 weeks if necessary to max 60 mg/day for 4–6 weeks) then reduce to usual maintenance dose 10–20 mg/day (but up to 40 mg/day may be required)	Postural hypotension, dizziness, drowsiness, insomnia, headaches, oedema, anticholinergic adverse effects, nervousness, paraesthesia, weight gain, hepatotoxicity, leucopenia, hypertensive crisis	Tyramine in food, sympathomimetics, alcohol, opioids, antidepressants, levadopa, 5HT1 agonists (buspirone)	36	0.81/10 mg
Phenelzine	Depression	15 mg tds–q.i.d. (hospital patients: max. 30 mg tds) Consider reducing to lowest possible maintenance dose	As for isocarboxazid but more postural hypotension, less hepatotoxicity	As for isocarboxazid. Probably safest of MAOIs and is the one that should be used if combinations are considered	~1 (effects on MAO are irreversible)	0.20/15 mg

| Tranylcypromine | Depression | 10 mg bd
Doses >30 mg/day under close supervision only

Usual maintenance:
10 mg/day
Last dose no later than 3 pm | As for isocarboxazid but insomnia, nervousness, hypertensive crisis more common than with other MAOIs; hepatotoxicity less common than phenelzine
Mild dependence as amphetamine-like structure | As for isocarboxazid but interactions more severe

Never use in combination therapy with other antidepressants | 2.5 | 1.08/10 mg |
| Moclobemide (Reversible inhibitor of MAO-A) | Depression

Social phobia | 150–600 mg/day (bd after food)

300–600 mg/day (bd after food) | Sleep disturbances, nausea, agitation, confusion | Tyramine interactions rare and mild but possible if high doses (>600 mg/day) used or if large quantities of tyramine ingested
CNS excitation/depression with dextromethorphan/pethidine

Avoid: clomipramine/levodopa/selegiline/sympathomimetics/SSRIs

Caution with fentanyl/morphine/tricyclics

Cimetidine – use half-dose of moclobemide | 2–4 | 0.25/150 mg |

*For full details refer to the manufacturer's information and BNF.

Antidepressant drugs – others*

Antidepressant	Licensed indication	Licensed doses (elderly doses not included)	Main adverse effects	Major interactions	Approx. half-life (h)	Cost (£)
Duloxetine	Depression (and other non-psychiatric indications) GAD	60–120 mg/day Limited data to support advantage of doses above 60 mg/day 30 mg/day increasing to 60 mg or 120 mg	Nausea, insomnia, headache, dizziness, dry mouth, somnolence, constipation, anorexia. Small increases in heart rate and blood pressure including hypertensive crisis	Metabolised by CYP1A2 and CYP2D6. Inhibitor of CYP2D6 Caution with drugs acting on either enzyme MAOIs – avoid Caution: alcohol (although no interaction seen)	12 (metabolites inactive)	0.99/60 mg
Mianserin	Depression – particularly where sedation required	30–90 mg/day	Sedation, rash; rarely: blood dyscrasia, jaundice, arthralgia No anticholinergic effects Sexual dysfunction uncommon Low cardiotoxicity	Other sedatives, alcohol MAOIs: avoid Effect on hepatic enzymes unclear, so caution is required	10–20 2-desmethyl-mianserin is major metabolite (?activity)	0.40/30 mg

Drug	Indication	Dose	Side effects	Metabolism/Interactions	Half-life	Cost/formulation
Mirtazapine	Depression	15–45 mg/day	Increased appetite, weight gain, drowsiness, oedema, dizziness, headache, blood dyscrasia. Nausea/sexual dysfunction relatively uncommon	Minimal effect on CYP2D6/1A2/3A4 Caution: alcohol/sedatives	20–40 / 25 Active metabolite (demethyl-mirtazapine)	0.10/30 mg (generic available – price may vary)
Reboxetine	Depression – acute and maintenance	4–6 mg bd	Insomnia, sweating, dizziness, dry mouth, constipation, nausea, tachycardia, urinary hesitancy, headache Erectile dysfunction may occur rarely	Metabolised by CYP3A4 – avoid drugs inhibiting this enzyme (e.g. erythromycin ketoconazole). Minimal effect on CYP2D6/3A4 MAOIs: avoid No interaction with alcohol	13	0.32/4 mg
Trazodone	Depression ± anxiety / Anxiety	150–300 mg/day (up to 600 mg/day in hospitalised patients) bd dosing above 300 mg/day / 75–300 mg/day	Sedation, dizziness, headache, nausea, vomiting, tremor, postural hypotension, tachycardia, priapism Not anticholinergic, less cardiotoxic than tricyclics	Caution: sedatives/alcohol/other antidepressants/digoxin/phenytoin MAOIs: avoid	5–13 (biphasic) / 4–9 Active metabolite (mCPP)	0.13/100 mg / Liquid 1.11/ 100 mg/10 ml

(Cont.)

Antidepressant	Licensed indication	Licensed doses (elderly doses not included)	Main adverse effects	Major interactions	Approx. half-life (h)	Cost (£)
Venlafaxine	Depression ± anxiety and prevention of relapse or recurrence of depression	75–375 mg/day (bd) with food 75–225 mg XL/day (od) with food	Nausea, insomnia, dry mouth, somnolence, dizziness, sweating, nervousness, headache, sexual dysfunction, constipation	Metabolised by CYP2D6/3A4– caution with drugs known to inhibit both isozymes Minimal inhibitory effects on CYP2D6	5 11 Active metabolite (O-desmethyl-venlafaxine)	0.70/75 mg 0.41/75 mg XL (generic available – prices may vary)
	Generalised anxiety disorder (XL prep only)	75 mg XL/day (discontinue if no response after 8 weeks)	Elevation of blood pressure at higher doses. Avoid if at risk of arrhythmia. Discontinuation symptoms common – withdraw slowly	No effects on CYP1A2/2C9/3A4 MAOIs: avoid Caution: alcohol (although no interaction seen)/cimetidine/clozapine/warfarin		

*For full details refer to the manufacturer's information.

Agomelatine

Agomelatine is an M_1/M_2 melatonin agonist and $5HT_{2C}$ antagonist[1]. Melatonin-like effects appear to promote sleep whereas $5HT_{2C}$ antagonism provokes release of dopamine and norepinephrine in the frontal cortex[2,3]. Serotonin levels appear not to be affected[3].

There is good evidence that agomelatine is more effective than placebo and as effective as active comparators (venlafaxine, paroxetine) in major depression[4–7]. Agomelatine also seems effective in severe depression[8] and in the prevention of depressive relapse[9]. There is evidence that agomelatine is effective in GAD[10]. Agomelatine-related adverse effects occur at a similar frequency to placebo[11]. Sexual adverse effects are rare and certainly much less frequent than with serotonergic antidepressants[12,13]. Discontinuation symptoms seem not to occur[14]. Agomelatine improves subjective sleep quality[15] and normalises sleep–wake rhythm in depressed subjects[16,17].

The place of agomelatine in the treatment of depression has yet to be established. It received European marketing authorisation in February 2009. Its licence[18] states that liver function tests should be performed in all patients at initiation of treatment and then at around 6, 12 and 24 weeks.

References

1. Zupancic M et al. Agomelatine. A preliminary review of a new antidepressant. CNS Drugs 2006; 20:981–92.
2. Millan MJ et al. The novel melatonin agonist agomelatine (S20098) is an antagonist at 5-hydroxytryptamine2C receptors, blockade of which enhances the activity of frontocortical dopaminergic and adrenergic pathways. J Pharmacol Exp Ther 2003; 306:954–64.
3. Hamon M et al. Agomelatine, a novel pharmcological approach to treating depression. Eur Neuropsychopharmacol 2007; 16 Suppl 4:S337–8.
4. Kennedy SH et al. Placebo-controlled trial of agomelatine in the treatment of major depressive disorder. Eur Neuropsychopharmacol 2006; 16:93–100.
5. Montgomery SA et al. Antidepressant efficacy of agomelatine in major depressive disorder: meta-analysis of three pivotal studies. Eur Neuropsychopharmacol 2006; 16 Suppl 4:S319.
6. Kennedy SH et al. Antidepressant efficacy of agomelatine 25–50 mg versus venlafaxine 75–150 mg: two randomized, double-blind studies. Eur Neuropsychopharmacol 2006; 16 Suppl 4:S319.
7. Olie JP et al. Efficacy of agomelatine, a MT1/MT2 receptor agonist with 5-HT2C antagonistic properties, in major depressive disorder. Int J Neuropsychopharmacol 2007; 10:661–73.
8. Montgomery SA et al. Severe depression and antidepressants: focus on a pooled analysis of placebo-controlled studies on agomelatine. Int Clin Psychopharmacol 2007; 22:283–91.
9. Goodwin G et al. Long-term efficacy of agomelatine, a novel antidepressant, in the prevention of relapse in out-patients with major depressive disorder. Eur Neuropsychopharmacol 2007; 17 Suppl 4:S361–2.
10. Stein DJ et al. Efficacy of agomelatine in generalized anxiety disorder: a randomized, double-blind, placebo-controlled study. J Clin Psychopharmacol 2008; 28:561–6.
11. Dolder CR et al. Agomelatine treatment of major depressive disorder. Annal Pharmacotherapy 2008; 42:1822–31.
12. Kennedy SH et al. A double-blind comparison of sexual functioning, antidepressant efficacy, and tolerability between agomelatine and venlafaxine XR. J Clin Psychopharmacol 2008; 28:329–33.
13. Rouillon F. Efficacy and tolerance profile of agomelatine and practical use in depressed patients. Int Clin Psychopharmacol 2006; 21 Suppl 1:S31–5.
14. Montgomery SA et al. Absence of discontinuation symptoms with agomelatine and occurrence of discontinuation symptoms with paroxetine: a randomized, double-blind, placebo-controlled discontinuation study. Int Clin Psychopharmacol 2004; 19:271–80.
15. Lemoine P et al. Improvement in subjective sleep in major depressive disorder with a novel antidepressant, agomelatine: randomized, double-blind comparison with venlafaxine. J Clin Psychiatry 2007; 68:1723–32.
16. Quera Salva MA et al. Major depressive disorder, sleep EEG and agomelatine: an open-label study. Int J Neuropsychopharmacol 2007; 10:691–6.
17. Guilleminault C et al. Impact of the melatonergic antidepressant agomelatine on sleep–wake rhythms of depressed patients. Eur Neuropsychopharmacol 2006; 16 Suppl 4:S317–18.
18. European Medicines Agency. Summary of Product Characteristics. Valdoxan. 2009. http://www.emea.europa.eu/

Depression & anxiety

Treatment of affective illness

Depression

Basic principles of prescribing in depression

- Discuss with the patient choice of drug and utility/availability of other, non-pharmacological treatments
- Discuss with the patient likely outcomes, such as gradual relief from depressive symptoms over several weeks
- Prescribe a dose of antidepressant (after titration, if necessary) that is likely to be effective
- For a single episode, continue treatment for at least 6–9 months after resolution of symptoms (multiple episodes may require longer)
- Withdraw antidepressants gradually; always inform patients of the risk and nature of discontinuation symptoms

---

Official guidance on the treatment of depression

NICE guidelines[1] – a summary
- Antidepressants are not recommended as first-line treatment in recent-onset, mild depression – active monitoring, individual guided self-help, CBT or exercise are preferred
- Antidepressants are recommended for the treatment of moderate to severe depression and for dysthymia
- When an antidepressant is prescribed, a generic SSRI is recommended
- All patients should be informed about the withdrawal (discontinuation) effects of antidepressants
- For severe depression, a combination of an antidepressant and CBT is recommended
- For treatment-resistant depression recommended strategies include augmentation with lithium, an antipsychotic or a second antidepressant
- Patients with two prior episodes and functional impairment should be treated for at least 2 years
- The use of ECT is supported in severe and treatment-resistant depression.

MHRA/CSM Expert Working Group on SSRIs[2] – a summary
- Use the lowest possible dose
- Monitor closely in early stages for restlessness, agitation and suicidality. This is particularly important in young people (<30 years)
- Doses should be tapered gradually on stopping
- Venlafaxine use was originally restricted but this guidance has now been reversed (venlafaxine is probably not cardiotoxic)[3,4], but has a less favourable profile in overdose than SSRIs.

References

1. National Institute for Health and Clinical Excellence. Depression: the treatment and management of depression in adults (update). In Press. 2009. http://www.nice.org.uk/
2. Committee on Safety of Medicines. Report of the CSM expert working group on the safety of selective serotonin reuptake inhibitor antidepressants. 2004. http://www.mhra.gov.uk
3. Taylor D et al. Volte-face on venlafaxine – reasons and reflections. J Psychopharmacol 2006; 20:597–601.
4. Medicines and Healthcare Products Regulatory Agency. Venlafaxine (Efexor) Summary of Basis for Regulatory Position. http://www.mhra.gov.uk. 2006.

Depression & anxiety

Drug treatment of depression

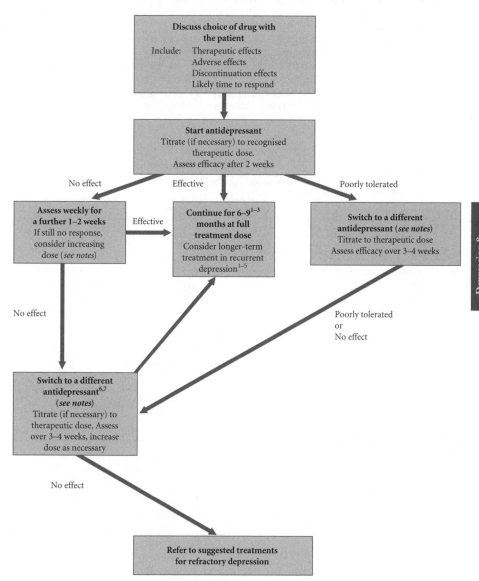

Depression &
anxiety

Notes
- Tools such as the Montgomery–Asberg Depression Rating Scale[8] and the Hamilton Depression Rating Scale[9] are recommended to assess drug effect.
- Switching between drug classes in cases of poor tolerability is not clearly supported by published studies but has a strong theoretical basis. In cases of non-response, there is some

evidence that switching within a drug class is effective[7,10–13], but switching between classes is, in practice, the most common option and is supported by some analyses[14].

- There is minimal evidence to support increasing the dose of SSRIs in depression[15]. Slightly better evidence suggests that increasing the dose of venlafaxine, escitalopram and tricyclics may be helpful[2].
- Switch treatments early (e.g. after a week or two) if adverse effects intolerable or if no improvement *at all* is seen by 3–4 weeks. Opinions on when to switch vary somewhat but it is clear that antidepressants have a fairly prompt onset of action[16–18] and that non-response at 2–6 weeks is a good predictor of overall non-response[19–21]. The absence of any improvement at all at 3–4 weeks should normally provoke a change in treatment (BAP guidelines suggest 4 weeks[2]). If there is some improvement at this time, continue and assess for a further 2–3 weeks.

References

1. American Psychiatric Association. Practice guideline for the treatment of patients with major depressive disorder (revision). Am J Psychiatry 2000; 157:1–45.
2. Anderson IM et al. Evidence-based guidelines for treating depressive disorders with antidepressants: a revision of the 2000 British Association for Psychopharmacology guidelines. J Psychopharmacol 2008; 22:343–96.
3. Crismon ML et al. The Texas Medication Algorithm Project: report of the Texas Consensus Conference Panel on Medication Treatment of Major Depressive Disorder. J Clin Psychiatry 1999; 60:142–56.
4. Kocsis JH et al. Maintenance therapy for chronic depression. A controlled clinical trial of desipramine. Arch Gen Psychiatry 1996; 53:769–74.
5. Dekker J et al. The use of antidepressants after recovery from depression. Euro J Psychiatry 2000; 14:207–12.
6. Nelson JC. Treatment of antidepressant nonresponders: augmentation or switch? J Clin Psychiatry 1998; 59 Suppl 15:35–41.
7. Joffe RT. Substitution therapy in patients with major depression. CNS Drugs 1999; 11:175–80.
8. Montgomery SA et al. A new depression scale designed to be sensitive to change. Br J Psychiatry 1979; 134:382–9.
9. Hamilton M. Development of a rating scale for primary depressive illness. Br J Soc Clin Psychol 1967; 6:278–96.
10. Thase ME et al. Citalopram treatment of fluoxetine nonresponders. J Clin Psychiatry 2001; 62:683–7.
11. Rush AJ et al. Bupropion-SR, sertraline, or venlafaxine-XR after failure of SSRIs for depression. N Engl J Med 2006; 354:1231–42.
12. Ruhe HG et al. Switching antidepressants after a first selective serotonin reuptake inhibitor in major depressive disorder: a systematic review. J Clin Psychiatry 2006; 67:1836–55.
13. Brent D et al. Switching to another SSRI or to venlafaxine with or without cognitive behavioral therapy for adolescents with SSRI-resistant depression: The TORDIA Randomized Controlled Trial. JAMA 2008; 299:901–13.
14. Papakostas GI et al. Treatment of SSRI-resistant depression: a meta-analysis comparing within- versus across-class switches. Biol Psychiatry 2008; 63:699–704.
15. Adli M et al. Is dose escalation of antidepressants a rational strategy after a medium-dose treatment has failed? A systematic review. Eur Arch Psychiatry Clin Neurosci 2005; 255:387–400.
16. Papakostas GI et al. A meta-analysis of early sustained response rates between antidepressants and placebo for the treatment of major depressive disorder. J Clin Psychopharmacol 2006; 26:56–60.
17. Taylor MJ et al. Early onset of selective serotonin reuptake inhibitor antidepressant action: systematic review and meta-analysis. Arch Gen Psychiatry 2006; 63:1217–23.
18. Posternak MA et al. Is there a delay in the antidepressant effect? A meta-analysis. J Clin Psychiatry 2005; 66:148–58.
19. Szegedi A et al. Early improvement in the first 2 weeks as a predictor of treatment outcome in patients with major depressive disorder: a meta-analysis including 6562 patients. J Clin Psychiatry 2009; 70:344–353.
20. Baldwin DS et al. How long should a trial of escitalopram treatment be in patients with major depressive disorder, generalised anxiety disorder or social anxiety disorder? An exploration of the randomised controlled trial database. Hum Psychopharmacol 2009; 24:269–275.
21. Nierenberg AA et al. Early nonresponse to fluoxetine as a predictor of poor 8-week outcome. Am J Psychiatry 1995; 152:1500–3.

Further reading

Barbui C et al. Amitriptyline v. the rest: still the leading antidepressant after 40 years of randomised controlled trials. Br J Psychiatry 2001; 178:129–44.
Cipriani A et al. Comparative efficacy and acceptability of 12 new-generation antidepressants: a multiple-treatments meta-analysis. Lancet 2009; 373:746–758.
Smith D et al. Efficacy and tolerability of venlafaxine compared with selective serotonin reuptake inhibitors and other antidepressants: a meta-analysis. Br J Psychiatry 2002; 180:396–404.
Trivedi MH et al. Clinical results for patients with major depressive disorder in the Texas Medication Algorithm Project. Arch Gen Psychiatry 2004; 61:669–80.

Recognised minimum effective doses – antidepressants

Tricyclics	
Tricyclics	Unclear; at least 75–100 mg/day[1], possibly 125 mg/day[2]
Lofepramine	140 mg/day[3]
SSRIs	
Citalopram	20 mg/day[4]
Escitalopram	10 mg/day[5]
Fluoxetine	20 mg/day[6]
Fluvoxamine	50 mg/day[7]
Paroxetine	20 mg/day[8]
Sertraline	50 mg/day[9]
Others	
Agomelatine	25 mg/day[10]
Duloxetine	60 mg/day[11,12]
Mirtazapine	30 mg/day[13]
Moclobemide	300 mg/[14]
Reboxetine	8 mg/day[15]
Trazodone	150 mg/day[16]
Venlafaxine	75 mg/day[17]

Depression & anxiety

References

1. Furukawa TA et al. Meta-analysis of effects and side effects of low dosage tricyclic antidepressants in depression: systematic review. BMJ 2002; 325:991.
2. Donoghue J et al. Suboptimal use of antidepressants in the treatment of depression. CNS Drugs 2000; 13:365–8.
3. Lancaster SG et al. Lofepramine. A review of its pharmacodynamic and pharmacokinetic properties, and therapeutic efficacy in depressive illness. Drugs 1989; 37:123–40.
4. Montgomery SA et al. The optimal dosing regimen for citalopram – a meta-analysis of nine placebo-controlled studies. Int Clin Psychopharmacol 1994; 9 Suppl 1:35–40.
5. Burke WJ et al. Fixed-dose trial of the single isomer SSRI escitalopram in depressed outpatients. J Clin Psychiatry 2002; 63:331–6.
6. Altamura AC et al. The evidence for 20 mg a day of fluoxetine as the optimal dose in the treatment of depression. Br J Psychiatry Suppl 1988; 109–112.
7. Walczak DD et al. The oral dose–effect relationship for fluvoxamine: a fixed-dose comparison against placebo in depressed outpatients. Ann Clin Psychiatry 1996; 8:139–51.
8. Dunner DL et al. Optimal dose regimen for paroxetine. J Clin Psychiatry 1992; 53 Suppl:21–6.
9. Moon CAL et al. A double-blind comparison of sertraline and clomipramine in the treatment of major depressive disorder and associative anxiety in general practice. J Psychopharmacol 1994; 8:171–6.
10. Loo H et al. Determination of the dose of agomelatine, a melatoninergic agonist and selective 5-HT(2C) antagonist, in the treatment of major depressive disorder: a placebo-controlled dose range study. Int Clin Psychopharmacol 2002; 17:239–47.
11. Goldstein DJ et al. Duloxetine in the treatment of depression: a double-blind placebo-controlled comparison with paroxetine. J Clin Psychopharmacol 2004; 24:389–99.
12. Detke MJ et al. Duloxetine, 60 mg once daily, for major depressive disorder: a randomized double-blind placebo-controlled trial. J Clin Psychiatry 2002; 63:308–15.
13. van Moffaert M et al. Mirtazapine is more effective than trazodone: a double-blind controlled study in hospitalized patients with major depression. Int Clin Psychopharmacol 1995; 10:3–9.
14. Priest RG et al. Moclobemide in the treatment of depression. Rev Contemp Pharmacother 1994; 5:35–43.
15. Schatzberg AF. Clinical efficacy of reboxetine in major depression. J Clin Psychiatry 2000; 61 Suppl 10:31–8.
16. Brogden RN et al. Trazodone: a review of its pharmacological properties and therapeutic use in depression and anxiety. Drugs 1981; 21:401–29.
17. Feighner JP et al. Efficacy of once-daily venlafaxine extended release (XR) for symptoms of anxiety in depressed outpatients. J Affect Disord 1998; 47:55–62.

Antidepressant prophylaxis

First episode

A single episode of depression should be treated for at least 6–9 months after full remission[1]. If antidepressant therapy is stopped immediately on recovery, 50% of patients experience a return of their depressive symptoms within 3–6 months[1,2].

Recurrent depression

Of those patients who have one episode of major depression, 50–85% will go on to have a second episode, and 80–90% of those who have a second episode, will go on to have a third[3]. Many factors are known to increase the risk of recurrence, including a family history of depression, recurrent dysthymia, concurrent non-affective psychiatric illness, female gender, long episode duration, degree of treatment resistance[1], chronic medical illness and social factors (e.g. lack of confiding relationships and psychosocial stressors). Some prescription drugs may precipitate depression[4,5].

The figure below outlines the risk of recurrence for multiple-episode patients: those recruited to the study had already experienced at least three episodes of depression, with 3 years or less between episodes[6,7]. People with depression are at increased risk of cardiovascular disease[8]. Suicide mortality is significantly increased over population norms.

A meta-analysis of antidepressant continuation studies[9] concluded that continuing treatment with antidepressants reduces the odds of depressive relapse by around two-thirds, which is approximately equal to halving the absolute risk. The risk of relapse is greatest in the first few months after discontinuation; this holds true irrespective of the duration of prior treatment[10]. Benefits persist at 36 months and beyond and seem to be similar across heterogeneous patient groups (first episode, multiple episode and chronic), although none of the studies included first-episode patients only. Specific studies in first-episode patients are required to confirm that treatment beyond 6–9 months confers additional benefit in this patient group. Most data are for adults.

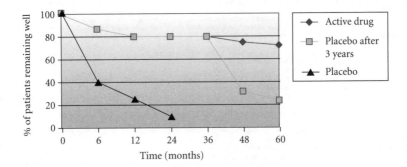

An RCT of maintenance treatment in elderly patients, many of whom were first episode, found continuation treatment with antidepressants to be beneficial over 2 years with a similar effect size to that seen in adults[11]. One small RCT (n = 22) demonstrated benefit from prophylactic antidepressants in adolescents[12].

Many patients who might benefit from maintenance treatment with antidepressants do not receive them[13].

NICE recommends that[14]:

- Patients who have had two or more episodes of depression in the recent past, and who have experienced significant functional impairment during these episodes, should be advised to continue antidepressants for at least 2 years.
- Patients on maintenance treatment should be re-evaluated, taking into account age, co-morbid conditions and other risk factors in the decision to continue maintenance treatment beyond 2 years.

Dose for prophylaxis

Adults should receive the same dose as used for acute treatment[1]. There is some evidence to support the use of lower doses in elderly patients: dosulepin 75 mg/day offers effective prophylaxis[15]. There is no evidence to support the use of lower than standard doses of SSRIs[16].

Relapse rates after ECT are similar to those after stopping antidepressants[17]. Antidepressant prophylaxis will be required, ideally with a different drug from the one that failed to get the patient well in the first instance, although good data in this area are lacking.

Lithium also has some efficacy in the prophylaxis of unipolar depression; efficacy relative to antidepressants is unknown[18]. NICE recommends that lithium should not be used as the sole prophylactic drug[14]. There is some support for the use of a combination of lithium and nortriptyline[19].

Maintenance treatment with lithium protects against suicide[1].

Key points that patients should know

- A single episode of depression should be treated for at least 6–9 months after remission.
- The risk of recurrence of depressive illness is high and increases with each episode.
- Those who have had multiple episodes may require treatment for many years.
- The chances of staying well are greatly increased by taking antidepressants.
- Antidepressants are:
  - effective
  - not addictive
  - not known to lose their efficacy over time
  - not known to cause new long-term side effects.
- Medication needs to be continued at the treatment dose. If side effects are intolerable, it may be possible to find a more suitable alternative.
- If patients decide to stop their medication, this must not be done suddenly, as this may lead to unpleasant discontinuation effects (see section in this chapter). The medication needs to be reduced slowly under the supervision of a doctor.

Depression & anxiety

References

1. Anderson IM et al. Evidence-based guidelines for treating depressive disorders with antidepressants: a revision of the 2000 British Association for Psychopharmacology guidelines. J Psychopharmacol 2008; 22:343–396.
2. Reimherr FW et al. Optimal length of continuation therapy in depression: a prospective assessment during long-term fluoxetine treatment. Am J Psychiatry 1998; 155:1247–53.
3. Forshall S et al. Maintenance pharmacotherapy of unipolar depression. Psychiatr Bull 1999; 23:370–3.
4. National Institute for Health and Clinical Excellence. The treatment and management of depression in adults with chronic physical health problems (partial update of CG23). 2009. http://www.nice.org.uk/
5. Patten SB et al. Drug-induced depression. Psychother Psychosom 1997; 66:63–73.
6. Frank E et al. Three-year outcomes for maintenance therapies in recurrent depression. Arch Gen Psychiatry 1990; 47:1093–9.
7. Kupfer DJ et al. Five-year outcome for maintenance therapies in recurrent depression. Arch Gen Psychiatry 1992; 49:769–73.
8. Taylor D. Antidepressant drugs and cardiovascular pathology: a clinical overview of effectiveness and safety. Acta Psychiatr Scand 2008; 118:434–442.
9. Geddes JR et al. Relapse prevention with antidepressant drug treatment in depressive disorders: a systematic review. Lancet 2003; 361:653–61.
10. Keller MB et al. The Prevention of Recurrent Episodes of Depression with Venlafaxine for Two Years (PREVENT) Study: Outcomes from the 2-year and combined maintenance phases. J Clin Psychiatry 2007; 68:1246–56.
11. Reynolds CF, III et al. Maintenance treatment of major depression in old age. N Engl J Med 2006; 354:1130–8.
12. Cheung A et al. Maintenance study for adolescent depression. J Child Adolesc Psychopharmacol 2008; 18:389–94.
13. Holma IA et al. Maintenance pharmacotherapy for recurrent major depressive disorder: 5-year follow-up study. Br J Psychiatry 2008; 193:163–4.
14. National Institute for Clinical Excellence. Depression: the treatment and management of depression in adults (update). 2009. http://www.nice.org.uk/
15. Old Age Depression Interest Group. How long should the elderly take antidepressants? A double-blind placebo-controlled study of continuation/prophylaxis therapy with dothiepin. Br J Psychiatry 1993; 162:175–82.
16. Franchini L et al. Dose–response efficacy of paroxetine in preventing depressive recurrences: a randomized, double-blind study. J Clin Psychiatry 1998; 59:229–32.
17. Nobler MS, Sackeim HA. Refractory depression and electroconvulsive therapy. In: Nolen WA, Zohar J, Roose SP, editors. Refractory Depression: current strategies and future directions. Chichester: John Wiley & Sons Ltd; 1994. 69–81.
18. Cipriani A et al. Lithium versus antidepressants in the long-term treatment of unipolar affective disorder. Cochrane Database Syst Rev 2006; CD003492.
19. Sackeim HA et al. Continuation pharmacotherapy in the prevention of relapse following electroconvulsive therapy: a randomized controlled trial. JAMA 2001; 285:1299–307.

Further reading

Jackson GA et al. Psychiatrist's attitudes to maintenance drug treatment in depression. Psychiatr Bull 1999; 23:74–7.

Treatment of refractory depression – first choice

Refractory depression is difficult to treat successfully and outcomes are poor[1] especially if evidence-based protocols are not followed[2]. The evidence base has been substantially improved by publication of results of the STAR-D programme (Sequenced Treatment Alternatives to Relieve Depression). This was a pragmatic effectiveness study which used remission of symptoms as its main outcome. At stage 1[3], 2786 subjects received citalopram (mean dose 41.8 mg/day) for 14 weeks; remission was seen in 28% (response (50% reduction in symptoms score) 47%). Subjects who failed to remit were entered into the continued study of sequential treatments[4–8]. Remission rates are given in the table below. Very few statistically significant differences were noted from this point on. At stage 3[7], T_3 was found to be significantly better tolerated than lithium. At stage 4[8], tranylcypromine was less effective and less well tolerated than the mirtazapine/venlafaxine combination. Overall, remission rates, as can be seen, were worryingly low, although it should be noted that the patient cohort consisted of subjects with long histories of recurrent depression.

STAR-D shows that the treatment of refractory depression requires a flexible approach and that response to a particular treatment option is not readily predicted by pharmacology or previous treatments. The programme has established bupropion and buspirone augmentation as worthwhile options and resurrected from obscurity the use of T_3 augmentation and of nortriptyline.

Figure Remission rates in STAR-D

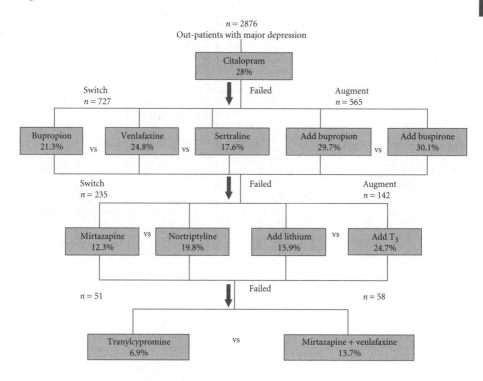

177

Table Refractory depression – first choice: commonly used treatments generally well supported by published literature (no preference implied by order)

Treatment	Advantages	Disadvantages	Refs
Add lithium Aim for plasma level of 0.4–1.0 mmol/L	• Well established • Effective in around half of cases • Well supported in the literature • Recommended by NICE	• Sometimes poorly tolerated at higher plasma levels • Potentially toxic (NICE recommend ECG) • Usually needs specialist referral • Plasma monitoring is essential	7,9–11
ECT	• Well established • Effective • Well supported in the literature	• Poor reputation in public domain • Necessitates general anaesthetic • Needs specialist referral • Usually reserved for last-line treatment • Usually combined with other treatments	12–14
Add tri-iodothyronine (20–50 μg/day) Higher doses have been safely used	• Usually well tolerated • Good literature support (including by STAR-D)	• TFT monitoring required • Usually needs specialist referral • Some negative studies	7,15–19
Combine olanzapine and fluoxetine (12.5 mg + 50 mg daily)	• Well researched • Usually well tolerated • Olanzapine + TCA may also be effective	• Expensive • Risk of weight gain • Limited clinical experience in UK	20–25
Add quetiapine (300–600 mg/day) to SSRI/SNRI	• Developing evidence base • Usually well tolerated • Plausible explanation for antidepressant effect	• Hypotension, sedation, constipation can be problematic	26–30
Add risperidone (0.5–2 mg/day) to antidepressant	• Developing evidence base • Usually well tolerated	• Hypotension • Hyperprolactinaemia	31–35
Add aripiprazole (5–20 mg/day) to antidepressant	• Developing evidence base (including good RCT) • Usually well tolerated	• Akathisia and restlessness common	36–42

Table Refractory depression – first choice: commonly used treatments generally well supported by published literature (no preference implied by order) (Cont.)

Treatment	Advantages	Disadvantages	Refs
SSRI + bupropion up to 400 mg/day	• Supported by STAR-D • Well tolerated	• Not licensed for depression in the UK	5,43–47
SSRI or venlafaxine + mianserin (30 mg/day) or mirtazapine (30–45 mg/day)	• Recommended by NICE • Usually well tolerated • Reasonable literature support • Becoming more widely used	• Risk of serotonin syndrome (inform patient) • Risk of blood dyscrasia with mianserin	8,48–50

Note: Data relating to augmentation or switching strategies in refractory depression are poor by evidence-based standards[51,52]. Recommendations are therefore partly based on clinical experience and expert consensus. Always consider non-drug approaches (e.g. CBT).

References

1. Dunner DL et al. Prospective, long-term, multicenter study of the naturalistic outcomes of patients with treatment-resistant depression. J Clin Psychiatry 2006; 67:688–95.
2. Trivedi MH et al. Clinical results for patients with major depressive disorder in the Texas Medication Algorithm Project. Arch Gen Psychiatry 2004; 61:669–80.
3. Trivedi MH et al. Evaluation of outcomes with citalopram for depression using measurement-based care in STAR*D: implications for clinical practice. Am J Psychiatry 2006; 163:28–40.
4. Rush AJ et al. Bupropion-SR, sertraline, or venlafaxine-XR after failure of SSRIs for depression. N Engl J Med 2006; 354:1231–42.
5. Trivedi MH et al. Medication augmentation after the failure of SSRIs for depression. N Engl J Med 2006; 354:1243–52.
6. Fava M et al. A comparison of mirtazapine and nortriptyline following two consecutive failed medication treatments for depressed outpatients: a STAR*D report. Am J Psychiatry 2006; 163:1161–72.
7. Nierenberg AA et al. A comparison of lithium and T(3) augmentation following two failed medication treatments for depression: a STAR*D report. Am J Psychiatry 2006; 163:1519–30.
8. McGrath PJ et al. Tranylcypromine versus venlafaxine plus mirtazapine following three failed antidepressant medication trials for depression: a STAR*D report. Am J Psychiatry 2006; 163:1531–41.
9. Fava M et al. Lithium and tricyclic augmentation of fluoxetine treatment for resistant major depression: a double-blind, controlled study. Am J Psychiatry 1994; 151:1372–4.
10. Dinan TG. Lithium augmentation in sertraline-resistant depression: a preliminary dose–response study. Acta Psychiatr Scand 1993; 88:300–1.
11. Bauer M et al. Lithium augmentation in treatment-resistant depression: meta-analysis of placebo-controlled studies. J Clin Psychopharmacol 1999; 19:427–34.
12. Folkerts HW et al. Electroconvulsive therapy vs. paroxetine in treatment-resistant depression – a randomized study. Acta Psychiatr Scand 1997; 96:334–42.
13. Gonzalez-Pinto A et al. Efficacy and safety of venlafaxine-ECT combination in treatment-resistant depression. J Neuropsychiatry Clin Neurosci 2002; 14:206–9.
14. Eranti S et al. A randomized, controlled trial with 6-month follow-up of repetitive transcranial magnetic stimulation and electroconvulsive therapy for severe depression. Am J Psychiatry 2007; 164:73–81.
15. Joffe RT et al. A comparison of triiodothyronine and thyroxine in the potentiation of tricyclic antidepressants. Psychiatry Res 1990; 32:241–51.
16. Anderson IM. Drug treatment of depression: reflections on the evidence. Adv Psychiatr Treat 2003; 9:11–20.
17. Iosifescu DV et al. An open study of triiodothyronine augmentation of selective serotonin reuptake inhibitors in treatment-resistant major depressive disorder. J Clin Psychiatry 2005; 66:1038–42.
18. Abraham G et al. T3 augmentation of SSRI resistant depression. J Affect Disord 2006; 91:211–15.
19. Kelly TF et al. Long term augmentation with T3 in refractory major depression. J Affect Disord 2009; 115:230–3.
20. Dube S et al. Meta-analysis of olanzapine/fluoxetine use in treatment-resistant depression. 2002. Poster presented at: 15th European College of Neuropsychopharmacology, 5–9 October 2002, Barcelona, Spain.
21. Corya SA et al. Long-term antidepressant efficacy and safety of olanzapine/fluoxetine combination: a 76-week open-label study. J Clin Psychiatry 2003; 64:1349–56.
22. Corya S et al. Safety meta-analysis of olanzapine/fluoxetine combination versus fluoxetine. 2002. Poster presented at: 15th European College of Neuropsychopharmacology, 5–9 October 2002, Barcelona, Spain.
23. Shelton RC et al. Olanzapine/fluoxetine combination for treatment-resistant depression: a controlled study of SSRI and nortriptyline resistance. J Clin Psychiatry 2005; 66:1289–97.
24. Corya SA et al. A randomized, double-blind comparison of olanzapine/fluoxetine combination, olanzapine, fluoxetine, and venlafaxine in treatment-resistant depression. Depress Anxiety 2006; 23:364–72.
25. Takahashi H et al. Augmentation with olanzapine in TCA-refractory depression with melancholic features: a consecutive case series. Hum Psychopharmacol 2008; 23:217–20.
26. Anderson IM et al. Efficacy, safety and tolerability of quetiapine augmentation in treatment resistant depression: an open-label, pilot study. J Affect Disord 2009;Epub ahead of print. Doi:10.1016/j.jad.2008.12.010.
27. Jensen NH et al. N-desalkylquetiapine, a potent norepinephrine reuptake inhibitor and partial 5-HT1A agonist, as a putative mediator of quetiapine's antidepressant activity. Neuropsychopharmacology 2008; 33:2303–12.
28. Sagud M et al. Quetiapine augmentation in treatment-resistant depression: a naturalistic study. Psychopharmacology 2006; 187:511–14.

29. Mattingly G et al. NR250: quetiapine combination for treatment-resistant depression. 2006. Poster presented at 150th Annual Meeting of the American Psychiatric Association, 20–25 May 2006, Toronto, Canada.

30. Doree JP et al. NR725: comparison of quetiapine vs lithium in treatment of resistant depression. 2004. Poster presented at 157th Annual Meeting of the American Psychiatric Association, 1–6 May 2004, New York, USA.

31. Yoshimura R et al. Addition of risperidone to sertraline improves sertraline-resistant refractory depression without influencing plasma concentrations of sertraline and desmethylsertraline. Hum Psychopharmacol 2008; 23:707–13.

32. Mahmoud RA et al. Risperidone for treatment-refractory major depressive disorder: a randomized trial. Ann Intern Med 2007; 147:593–602.

33. Ostroff RB et al. Risperidone augmentation of selective serotonin reuptake inhibitors in major depression. J Clin Psychiatry 1999; 60:256–9.

34. Rapaport MH et al. Effects of risperidone augmentation in patients with treatment-resistant depression: Results of open-label treatment followed by double-blind continuation. Neuropsychopharmacology 2006; 31:2505–13.

35. Stoll AL et al. Tranylcypromine plus risperidone for treatment-refractory major depression. J Clin Psychopharmacol 2000; 20:495–6.

36. Marcus RN et al. The efficacy and safety of aripiprazole as adjunctive therapy in major depressive disorder: a second multicenter, randomized, double-blind, placebo-controlled study. J Clin Psychopharmacol 2008; 28:156–65.

37. Sokolski KN. Adjunctive aripiprazole for bupropion-resistant major depression. Ann Pharmacother 2008; 42:1124–9.

38. Hellerstein DJ et al. Aripiprazole as an adjunctive treatment for refractory unipolar depression. Prog Neuropsychopharmacol Biol Psychiatry 2008; 32:744–50.

39. Simon JS et al. Aripiprazole augmentation of antidepressants for the treatment of partially responding and nonresponding patients with major depressive disorder. J Clin Psychiatry 2005; 66:1216–20.

40. Papakostas GI et al. Aripiprazole augmentation of selective serotonin reuptake inhibitors for treatment-resistant major depressive disorder. J Clin Psychiatry 2005; 66:1326–30.

41. Patkar AA et al. An open-label, rater-blinded, augmentation study of aripiprazole in treatment-resistant depression. Prim Care Companion J Clin Psychiatry 2006; 8:82–7.

42. Berman RM et al. The efficacy and safety of aripiprazole as adjunctive therapy in major depressive disorder: a multicenter, randomized, double-blind, placebo-controlled study. J Clin Psychiatry 2007; 68:843–53.

43. Zisook S et al. Use of bupropion in combination with serotonin reuptake inhibitors. Biol Psychiatry 2006; 59:203–10.

44. Fatemi SH et al. Venlafaxine and bupropion combination therapy in a case of treatment-resistant depression. Ann Pharmacother 1999; 33:701–3.

45. Pierre JM et al. Bupropion–tranylcypromine combination for treatment-refractory depression. J Clin Psychiatry 2000; 61:450–1.

46. Lam RW et al. Citalopram and bupropion-SR: combining versus switching in patients with treatment-resistant depression. J Clin Psychiatry 2004; 65:337–40.

47. Papakostas GI et al. The combination of duloxetine and bupropion for treatment-resistant major depressive disorder. Depress Anxiety 2006; 23:178–81.

48. Carpenter LL et al. A double-blind, placebo-controlled study of antidepressant augmentation with mirtazapine. Biol Psychiatry 2002; 51:183–8.

49. Carpenter LL et al. Mirtazapine augmentation in the treatment of refractory depression. J Clin Psychiatry 1999; 60:45–9.

50. Ferreri M et al. Benefits from mianserin augmentation of fluoxetine in patients with major depression non-responders to fluoxetine alone. Acta Psychiatr Scand 2001; 103:66–72.

51. Lam RW et al. Combining antidepressants for treatment-resistant depression: a review. J Clin Psychiatry 2002; 63:685–93.

52. Stimpson N et al. Randomised controlled trials investigating pharmacological and psychological interventions for treatment-refractory depression. Systematic review. Br J Psychiatry 2002; 181:284–94.

Depression & anxiety

Treatment of refractory depression – second choice

Table Second choice: less commonly used, variably supported by published evaluations (no preference implied by order)

Treatment	Advantages	Disadvantages	Refs
Add lamotrigine (aim for 200 mg/day but lower doses may be effective)	• Reasonably well researched • Quite widely used • Probably more robust data for bipolar depression	• Slow titration • Risk of rash • Appropriate dosing unclear	1–5
Add pindolol (5 mg t.d.s. or 7.5 mg once daily)	• Well tolerated • Can be initiated in primary care • Reasonably well researched (but combined with SSRIs, trazodone, venlafaxine only)	• Data mainly relate to acceleration of response • Refractory data contradictory – some negative studies • Appropriate dosing unclear; higher doses may be more effective	6–10
SSRI + buspirone up to 60 mg/day	• Supported by STAR-D	• Higher doses required poorly tolerated (dizziness common)	11–14
Venlafaxine (>200 mg/day)	• Usually well tolerated • Can be initiated in primary care • Recommended by NICE • Supported by STAR-D	• Limited support in literature • Nausea and vomiting more common • Discontinuation reactions common • Blood pressure monitoring essential	15–18

Depression & anxiety

References

1. Calabrese JR et al. A double-blind placebo-controlled study of lamotrigine monotherapy in outpatients with bipolar I depression. Lamictal 602 Study Group. J Clin Psychiatry 1999; 60:79–88.
2. Maltese TM. Adjunctive lamotrigine treatment for major depression. Am J Psychiatry 1999; 156:1833.
3. Normann C et al. Lamotrigine as adjunct to paroxetine in acute depression: a placebo-controlled, double-blind study. J Clin Psychiatry 2002; 63:337–44.
4. Barbee JG et al. Lamotrigine as an augmentation agent in treatment-resistant depression. J Clin Psychiatry 2002; 63:737–41.
5. Barbosa L et al. A double-blind, randomized, placebo-controlled trial of augmentation with lamotrigine or placebo in patients concomitantly treated with fluoxetine for resistant major depressive episodes. J Clin Psychiatry 2003; 64:403–7.
6. Rabiner EA et al. Pindolol augmentation of selective serotonin reuptake inhibitors: PET evidence that the dose used in clinical trials is too low. Am J Psychiatry 2001; 158:2080–2.
7. McAskill R et al. Pindolol augmentation of antidepressant therapy. Br J Psychiatry 1998; 173:203–8.
8. Rasanen P et al. Mitchell B. Balter Award – 1998. Pindolol and major affective disorders: a three-year follow-up study of 30,485 patients. J Clin Psychopharmacol 1999; 19:297–302.
9. Perry EB et al. Pindolol augmentation in depressed patients resistant to selective serotonin reuptake inhibitors: a double-blind, randomized, controlled trial. J Clin Psychiatry 2004; 65:238–43.
10. Sokolski KN et al. Once-daily high-dose pindolol for SSRI-refractory depression. Psychiatry Res 2004; 125:81–6.
11. Trivedi MH et al. Medication augmentation after the failure of SSRIs for depression. N Engl J Med 2006; 354:1243–52.
12. Bakish D. Fluoxetine potentiation by buspirone: three case histories. Can J Psychiatry 1991; 36:749–50.
13. Onder E et al. Faster response in depressive patients treated with fluoxetine alone than in combination with buspirone. J Affect Disord 2003; 76:223–7.
14. Appelberg BG et al. Patients with severe depression may benefit from buspirone augmentation of selective serotonin reuptake inhibitors: results from a placebo-controlled, randomized, double-blind, placebo wash-in study. J Clin Psychiatry 2001; 62:448–52.
15. Poirier MF et al. Venlafaxine and paroxetine in treatment-resistant depression. Double-blind, randomised comparison. Br J Psychiatry 1999; 175:12–16.
16. Nierenberg AA et al. Venlafaxine for treatment-resistant unipolar depression. J Clin Psychopharmacol 1994; 14:419–23.
17. Smith D et al. Efficacy and tolerability of venlafaxine compared with selective serotonin reuptake inhibitors and other antidepressants: a meta-analysis. Br J Psychiatry 2002; 180:396–404.
18. Rush AJ et al. Bupropion-SR, sertraline, or venlafaxine-XR after failure of SSRIs for depression. N Engl J Med 2006; 354:1231–42.

Treatment of refractory depression – other reported treatments

Table Other reported treatments (alphabetical order – no preference implied). Prescribers *must* familiarise themselves with the primary literature before using these strategies.

Treatment	Comments	References
Add amantadine (up to 300 mg/day)	Limited data	1
Add carbergoline 2 mg/day	Very limited data	2
Add clonazepam 0.5–1.0 mg/day	Use of benzodiazepines is widespread but not well supported	3
Add mecamylamine (up to 10 mg/day)	One pilot study of 21 patients	4
Add metyrapone 1000 mg/day	Data relate to non-refractory illness	5
Add tryptophan 2–3 g tds	Long history of successful use	6–9
Add yohimbine (up to 30 mg/day)	Data relate to non-refractory illness	10
Add zinc (25 mg Zn^+/day)	One RCT (n = 60) showed good results in refractory illness	11
Add ziprasidone (up to 160 mg/day)	Reasonably well supported	12
Combine MAOI and TCA, e.g. trimipramine and phenelzine	Long history of successful use, but great care needed	13,14
Dexamethasone 3–4 mg/day	Use for 4 days only. Limited data	15,16
Ketoconazole 400–800 mg/day	Rarely used. Risk of hepatotoxicity	17
Modafinil 100–400 mg/day	Data mainly relate to non-refractory illness. Usually added to antidepressant treatment. May worsen anxiety (see section on stimulants in depression)	18–21
Nemifitide (40–240 mg/day SC)	One pilot study in 25 patients	22
Nortriptyline ± lithium	Re-emergent treatment option	23–26

(Cont.)

Table Other reported treatments (alphabetical order – no preference implied). (Cont.)

Treatment	Comments	References
Oestrogens (various regimens)	Limited data	27
Omega-3-triglycerides EPA 1000–2000 mg/day	Developing database. Usually added to antidepressant treatment	28–30
Pramipexole 0.125–5 mg/day	Few data in refractory unipolar depression	31
Riluzole 100–200 mg/day	Very limited data. Costly	32
S-adenosyl-L-methionine 400 mg/day IM; 1600 mg/day oral	Limited data in refractory depression	33,34
SSRI + TCA	Formerly widely used	35
rTMS	Extensive database	36–40
TCA – high dose	Formerly widely used	41
Testosterone gel	Effective in those with low testosterone levels	42
Vagus nerve stimulation	Developing database	43–46
Venlafaxine – very high dose (up to 600 mg/day)	Cardiac monitoring essential	47
Venlafaxine + IV clomipramine	Cardiac monitoring essential	48

Depression & anxiety

References

1. Stryjer R et al. Amantadine as augmentation therapy in the management of treatment-resistant depression. Int Clin Psychopharmacol 2003; 18:93–6.
2. Takahashi H et al. Addition of a dopamine agonist, cabergoline, to a serotonin-noradrenalin reuptake inhibitor, milnacipran as a therapeutic option in the treatment of refractory depression: two case reports. Clin Neuropharmacol 2003; 26:230–2.
3. Smith WT et al. Short-term augmentation of fluoxetine with clonazepam in the treatment of depression: a double-blind study. Am J Psychiatry 1998; 155:1339–45.
4. George TP et al. Nicotinic antagonist augmentation of selective serotonin reuptake inhibitor-refractory major depressive disorder: a preliminary study. J Clin Psychopharmacol 2008; 28:340–4.
5. Jahn H et al. Metyrapone as additive treatment in major depression: a double-blind and placebo-controlled trial. Arch Gen Psychiatry 2004; 61:1235–44.
6. Angst J et al. The treatment of depression with L-5-hydroxytryptophan versus imipramine. Results of two open and one double-blind study. Arch Psychiatr Nervenkr 1977; 224:175–86.
7. Alino JJ et al. 5-Hydroxytryptophan (5-HTP) and a MAOI (nialamide) in the treatment of depressions. A double-blind controlled study. Int Pharmacopsychiatry 1976; 11:8–15.
8. Hale AS et al. Clomipramine, tryptophan and lithium in combination for resistant endogenous depression: seven case studies. Br J Psychiatry 1987; 151:213–17.
9. Young SN. Use of tryptophan in combination with other antidepressant treatments: a review. J Psychiatry Neurosci 1991; 16:241–6.
10. Sanacora G et al. Addition of the alpha2-antagonist yohimbine to fluoxetine: effects on rate of antidepressant response. Neuropsychopharmacology 2004; 29:1166–71.
11. Siwek M et al. Zinc supplementation augments efficacy of imipramine in treatment resistant patients: a double blind, placebo-controlled study. J Affect Disord 2009; Epub ahead of print. Doi:10.1016/j.jad.2009.02.014.
12. Papakostas GI et al. Ziprasidone augmentation of selective serotonin reuptake inhibitors (SSRIs) for SSRI-resistant major depressive disorder. J Clin Psychiatry 2004; 65:217–21.
13. White K et al. The combined use of MAOIs and tricyclics. J Clin Psychiatry 1984; 45:67–9.
14. Kennedy N et al. Treatment and response in refractory depression: results from a specialist affective disorders service. J Affect Disord 2004; 81:49–53.
15. Dinan TG et al. Dexamethasone augmentation in treatment-resistant depression. Acta Psychiatr Scand 1997; 95:58–61.
16. Bodani M et al. The use of dexamethasone in elderly patients with antidepressant-resistant depressive illness. J Psychopharmacol 1999; 13:196–7.
17. Wolkowitz OM et al. Antiglucocorticoid treatment of depression: double-blind ketoconazole. Biol Psychiatry 1999; 45:1070–4.
18. DeBattista C et al. A prospective trial of modafinil as an adjunctive treatment of major depression. J Clin Psychopharmacol 2004; 24:87–90.
19. Ninan PT et al. Adjunctive modafinil at initiation of treatment with a selective serotonin reuptake inhibitor enhances the degree and onset of therapeutic effects in patients with major depressive disorder and fatigue. J Clin Psychiatry 2004; 65:414–20.
20. Menza MA et al. Modafinil augmentation of antidepressant treatment in depression. J Clin Psychiatry 2000; 61:378–81.
21. Taneja I et al. A randomized, double-blind, crossover trial of modafinil on mood. J Clin Psychopharmacol 2007; 27:76–8.
22. Feighner JP et al. Clinical effect of nemifitide, a novel pentapeptide antidepressant, in the treatment of severely depressed refractory patients. Int Clin Psychopharmacol 2008; 23:29–35.
23. Nierenberg AA et al. Nortriptyline for treatment-resistant depression. J Clin Psychiatry 2003; 64:35–9.

24. Nierenberg AA et al. Lithium augmentation of nortriptyline for subjects resistant to multiple antidepressants. J Clin Psychopharmacol 2003; 23:92–5.

25. Fava M et al. A comparison of mirtazapine and nortriptyline following two consecutive failed medication treatments for depressed outpatients: a STAR*D report. Am J Psychiatry 2006; 163:1161–72.

26. Shelton RC et al. Olanzapine/fluoxetine combination for treatment-resistant depression: a controlled study of SSRI and nortriptyline resistance. J Clin Psychiatry 2005; 66:1289–97.

27. Stahl SM. Basic psychopharmacology of antidepressants, part 2: Oestrogen as an adjunct to antidepressant treatment. J Clin Psychiatry 1998; 59 Suppl 4:15–24.

28. Peet M et al. A dose-ranging exploratory study of the effects of ethyl-eicosapentaenoate in patients with persistent schizophrenic symptoms. J Psychiatr Res 2002; 36:7–18.

29. Su KP et al. Omega-3 fatty acids as a psychotherapeutic agent for a pregnant schizophrenic patient. Eur Neuropsychopharmacol 2001; 11:295–9.

30. Nemets B et al. Addition of omega-3 fatty acid to maintenance medication treatment for recurrent unipolar depressive disorder. Am J Psychiatry 2002; 159:477–9.

31. Whiskey E et al. Pramipexole in unipolar and bipolar depression. Psychiatr Bull 2004; 28:438–40.

32. Zarate CA Jr et al. An open-label trial of riluzole in patients with treatment-resistant major depression. Am J Psychiatry 2004; 161:171–4.

33. Pancheri P et al. A double-blind, randomized parallel-group, efficacy and safety study of intramuscular S-adenosyl-L-methionine 1,4-butanedisulphonate (SAMe) versus imipramine in patients with major depressive disorder. Int J Neuropsychopharmacol 2002; 5:287–94.

34. Alpert JE et al. S-adenosyl-L-methionine (SAMe) as an adjunct for resistant major depressive disorder: an open trial following partial or nonresponse to selective serotonin reuptake inhibitors or venlafaxine. J Clin Psychopharmacol 2004; 24:661–4.

35. Taylor D. Selective serotonin reuptake inhibitors and tricyclic antidepressants in combination – interactions and therapeutic uses. Br J Psychiatry 1995; 167:575–80.

36. Huang CC et al. An open trial of daily left prefrontal cortex repetitive transcranial magnetic stimulation for treating medication-resistant depression. Eur Psychiatry 2004; 19:523–4.

37. Su TP et al. Add-on rTMS for medication-resistant depression: a randomized, double-blind, sham-controlled trial in Chinese patients. J Clin Psychiatry 2005; 66:930–7.

38. Fitzgerald PB et al. A randomized trial of low-frequency right-prefrontal-cortex transcranial magnetic stimulation as augmentation in treatment-resistant major depression. Int J Neuropsychopharmacol 2006; 9:655–66.

39. Fitzgerald PB et al. A randomized, controlled trial of sequential bilateral repetitive transcranial magnetic stimulation for treatment-resistant depression. Am J Psychiatry 2006; 163:88–94.

40. Murphy DN et al. Transcranial direct current stimulation as a therapeutic tool for the treatment of major depression: insights from past and recent clinical studies. Curr Opin Psychiatry 2009; 22:306–11.

41. Malhi GS et al. Management of resistant depression. Int J Psychiatry Clin Pract 1997; 1:269–276.

42. Pope HG Jr et al. Testosterone gel supplementation for men with refractory depression: a randomized, placebo-controlled trial. Am J Psychiatry 2003; 160:105–11.

43. Matthews K et al. Vagus nerve stimulation and refractory depression: please can you switch me on doctor? Br J Psychiatry 2003; 183:181–3.

44. George MS et al. Vagus nerve stimulation for the treatment of depression and other neuropsychiatric disorders. Expert Rev Neurother 2007; 7:63–74.

45. Corcoran CD et al. Vagus nerve stimulation in chronic treatment-resistant depression: preliminary findings of an open-label study. Br J Psychiatry 2006; 189:282–3.

46. Nemeroff CB et al. VNS therapy in treatment-resistant depression: clinical evidence and putative neurobiological mechanisms. Neuropsychopharmacology 2006; 31:1345–55.

47. Harrison CL et al. Tolerability of high-dose venlafaxine in depressed patients. J Psychopharmacol 2004; 18:200–4.

48. Fountoulakis KN et al. Combined oral venlafaxine and intravenous clomipramine-A: successful temporary response in a patient with extremely refractory depression. Can J Psychiatry 2004; 49:73–4.

Further reading

Fekadu A et al. What happens to patients with treatment-resistant depression? A systematic review of medium to long term outcome studies. J Affect Disord 2009; 116:4–11.

Depression & anxiety

Psychotic depression

Depressed patients who have psychotic symptoms are generally more severely unwell than those who do not have psychotic symptoms[1]. Combined treatment with an antidepressant and an antipsychotic is often recommended first line[2], but the data underpinning this practice are not strong[3,4].

A combination of an antidepressant and antipsychotic is more effective than an antipsychotic alone but it is not clear if it more effective than an antidepressant alone[3]. When given in adequate doses, TCAs are probably more effective than newer antidepressants in the treatment of psychotic depression[3,5].

There are few studies of newer antidepressants and atypical antipsychotics, either alone or in combination, specifically for psychotic depression. A large RCT showed response rates of 64% for combined olanzapine and fluoxetine compared to 35% for olanzapine alone and 28% for placebo[6]. There was no fluoxetine-alone group. Small open studies have found quetiapine[7], aripiprazole[8] and amisulpride[9] augmentation of an antidepressant to be effective and relatively well tolerated, but again there were no data available for antidepressant treatment alone. In clinical practice, only a small proportion of patients with psychotic depression receive an antipsychotic drug[10], perhaps reflecting clinicians' uncertainty regarding the risk–benefit ratio of this treatment strategy.

Long-term outcome is generally poorer for psychotic than non-psychotic depression[11,12]. Patients with psychotic depression may also have a poorer response to combined pharmacological and psychological treatment than those with non-psychotic depression[13].

Psychotic depression is one of the indications for ECT. Not only is ECT effective, it may also be more protective against relapse in psychotic depression than in non-psychotic depression[14]. One small RCT demonstrated superiority of maintenance ECT plus nortriptyline over nortriptyline alone at 2 years[15].

Novel approaches being developed include those based on antiglucocorticoid strategies; one small open study found rapid effects of the glucocorticoid receptor antagonist mifepristone[16], although these findings have been criticised[17]. There is an anecdotal report of the successful use of methylphenidate in a patient who did not respond to robust doses of an antidepressant and antipsychotic combined[18].

There is no specific indication for other therapies or augmentation strategies in psychotic depression over and above that for resistant depression or psychosis described elsewhere.

References

1. Gaudiano BA et al. Depressive symptom profiles and severity patterns in outpatients with psychotic vs nonpsychotic major depression. Compr Psychiatry 2008; 49:421–9.
2. Anderson IM et al. Evidence-based guidelines for treating depressive disorders with antidepressants: a revision of the 2000 British Association for Psychopharmacology guidelines. J Psychopharmacol 2008; 22:343–96.
3. Wijkstra JAAP et al. Pharmacological treatment for unipolar psychotic depression: Systematic review and meta-analysis. Br J Psychiatry 2006; 188:410–15.
4. Mulsant BH et al. A double-blind randomized comparison of nortriptyline plus perphenazine versus nortriptyline plus placebo in the treatment of psychotic depression in late life. J Clin Psychiatry 2001; 62:597–604.
5. Birkenhager TK et al. Efficacy of imipramine in psychotic versus nonpsychotic depression. J Clin Psychopharmacol 2008; 28:166–70.
6. Rothschild AJ et al. A double-blind, randomized study of olanzapine and olanzapine/fluoxetine combination for major depression with psychotic features. J Clin Psychopharmacol 2004; 24:365–73.
7. Konstantinidis A et al. Quetiapine in combination with citalopram in patients with unipolar psychotic depression. Prog Neuropsychopharmacol Biol Psychiatry 2007; 31:242–7.
8. Matthews JD et al. An open study of aripiprazole and escitalopram for psychotic major depressive disorder. J Clin Psychopharmacol 2009; 29:73–6.

9. Politis AM et al. Combination therapy with amisulpride and antidepressants: clinical observations in case series of elderly patients with psychotic depression. Prog Neuropsychopharmacol Biol Psychiatry 2008; 32:1227–30.
10. Andreescu C et al. Persisting low use of antipsychotics in the treatment of major depressive disorder with psychotic features. J Clin Psychiatry 2007; 68:194–200.
11. Flint AJ et al. Two-year outcome of psychotic depression in late life. Am J Psychiatry 1998; 155:178–83.
12. Maj M et al. Phenomenology and prognostic significance of delusions in major depressive disorder: a 10-year prospective follow-up study. J Clin Psychiatry 2007; 68:1411–17.
13. Gaudiano BA et al. Differential response to combined treatment in patients with psychotic versus nonpsychotic major depression. J Nerv Ment Dis 2005; 193:625–8.
14. Birkenhager TK et al. One-year outcome of psychotic depression after successful electroconvulsive therapy. J ECT 2005; 21:221–6.
15. Navarro V et al. Continuation/maintenance treatment with nortriptyline versus combined nortriptyline and ECT in late-life psychotic depression: a two-year randomized study. Am J Geriatr Psychiatry 2008; 16:498–505.
16. Belanoff JK et al. An open label trial of C-1073 (mifepristone) for psychotic major depression. Biol Psychiatry 2002; 52:386–392.
17. Rubin RT. Dr. Rubin replies (Letter). Am J Psychiatry 2004; 161:1722.
18. Huang CC et al. Adjunctive use of methylphenidate in the treatment of psychotic unipolar depression. Clin Neuropharmacol 2008; 31:245–7.

Further reading

Keller J et al. Current issues in the classification of psychotic major depression. Schizophr Bull 2007; 33:877–85.
Tyrka AR et al. Psychotic major depression: a benefit-risk assessment of treatment options. Drug Saf 2006; 29:491–508.

Depression & anxiety

Electroconvulsive therapy (ECT) and psychotropics

The table below summarises the effect of various psychotropics on seizure duration during ECT. Note that there are few well-controlled studies in this area and so recommendations should be viewed with this in mind. Note also that choice of anaesthetic agent profoundly affects seizure duration[1-5].

Drug	Effect on ECT seizure duration	Comments[6-10]
Benzodiazepines	Reduced	All may raise seizure threshold and so should be avoided where possible. Many are long-acting and may need to be discontinued some days before ECT. Benzodiazepines may also complicate anaesthesia If sedation is required, consider hydroxyzine. If benzodiazepine use is very long term and essential, continue and use higher stimulus
SSRIs[11-15]	Minimal effect; small increase possible	Generally considered safe to use during ECT. Beware complex pharmacokinetic interactions with anaesthetic agents
Venlafaxine[16]	Minimal effect at standard doses	Limited data suggest no effect on seizure duration but possibility of increased risk of asystole with doses above 300 mg/day. Clearly epileptogenic in higher doses. ECG advised
Duloxetine[17]	Not known	One case report suggests duloxetine does not complicate ECT
TCAs[12,13]	Possibly increased	Few data relevant to ECT but many TCAs lower seizure threshold. TCAs are associated with arrhythmia following ECT and should be avoided in elderly patients and those with cardiac disease. In others, it is preferable to continue TCA treatment during ECT. Close monitoring is essential. Beware hypotension and risk of prolonged seizures
MAOIs[18]	Minimal effect	Data relating to ECT very limited but long history of ECT use during MAOI therapy MAOIs probably do not affect seizure duration but interactions with sympathomimetics occasionally used in anaesthesia are possible and may lead to hypertensive crisis MAOIs may be continued during ECT but the anaesthetist must be informed. Beware hypotension

Depression & anxiety

187

(Cont.)		
Drug	*Effect on ECT seizure duration*	*Comments[6–10]*
Lithium[19–21]	Possibly increased	Conflicting data on lithium and ECT. The combination may be more likely to lead to delirium and confusion, and some authorities suggest discontinuing lithium 48 hours before ECT. In the UK, ECT is often used during lithium therapy but starting with a low stimulus and with very close monitoring. The combination is generally well tolerated
		Note that lithium potentiates the effects of non-depolarising neuromuscular blockers such as suxamethonium
Antipsychotics[22–25]	Variable – increased with phenothiazines and clozapine Others – no obvious effect reported	Few published data but widely used. Phenothiazines and clozapine are perhaps most likely to prolong seizures, and some suggest withdrawal before ECT. However, safe concurrent use has been reported. ECT and antipsychotics appear generally to be a safe combination. Few data on aripiprazole, but it too appears to be safe
Anticonvulsants[26,27]	Reduced	If used as a mood-stabiliser, continue but be prepared to use higher energy stimulus (not always required). If used for epilepsy, their effect is to normalise seizure threshold. Interactions are possible. Valproate may prolong the effect of thiopental; carbamazepine may inhibit neuromuscular blockade. Lamotrigine is reported to cause no problems
Barbiturates	Reduced	All barbiturates reduce seizure duration in ECT but are widely used as sedative anaesthetic agents
		Thiopental and methohexital may be associated with cardiac arrhythmia

For drugs known to lower seizure threshold, treatment is best begun with a low-energy stimulus (50 mC). Staff should be alerted to the possibility of prolonged seizures and IV diazepam should be available. With drugs known to elevate seizure threshold, higher stimuli may, of course, be required. Methods are available to lower seizure threshold or prolong seizures[28], but discussion of these is beyond the scope of this book.

ECT frequently causes confusion and disorientation; more rarely, it causes delirium. Close observation is essential. Very limited data support the use of thiamine (200 mg daily) in reducing post-ECT confusion[29]. Donepezil has been shown to improve recovery time post ECT (and appears to be safe)[30]. Ibuprofen may be used to prevent headache[31].

References

1. Avramov MN et al. The comparative effects of methohexital, propofol, and etomidate for electroconvulsive therapy. Anesth Analg 1995; 81:596–602.
2. Stadtland C et al. A switch from propofol to etomidate during an ECT course increases EEG and motor seizure duration. J ECT 2002; 18:22–5.
3. Gazdag G et al. Etomidate versus propofol for electroconvulsive therapy in patients with schizophrenia. J ECT 2004; 20:225–9.
4. Conca A et al. Etomidate vs. thiopentone in electroconvulsive therapy. An interdisciplinary challenge for anesthesiology and psychiatry. Pharmacopsychiatry 2003; 36:94–7.
5. Rasmussen KG et al. Seizure length with sevoflurane and thiopental for induction of general anesthesia in electroconvulsive therapy: a randomized double-blind trial. J ECT 2006; 22:240–2.
6. Curran S, Freeman CP. ECT and drugs. In: Freeman CP, editor. The ECT Handbook – The Second Report of the Royal College of Psychiatrists' Special Committee on ECT. Dorchester: Henry Ling Ltd; 1995.
7. Kellner CH et al. ECT–drug interactions: a review. Psychopharmacol Bull 1991; 27:595–609.
8. Welch CA. Electroconvulsive therapy. In: Ciraulo DA, Shader RI, Greenblatt DJ, editors. Drug Interactions in Psychiatry. 2nd ed. Baltimore: Williams and Wilkins; 1995; 399–414.
9. Naguib M et al. Interactions between psychotropics, anaesthetics and electroconvulsive therapy: implications for drug choice and patient management. CNS Drugs 2002; 16:229–47.
10. Maidment I. The interaction between psychiatric medicines and ECT. Hosp Pharm 1997; 4:102–5.
11. Masdrakis VG et al. The safety of the electroconvulsive therapy-escitalopram combination. J ECT 2008; 24:289–91.
12. Dursun SM et al. Effects of antidepressant treatments on first-ECT seizure duration in depression. Prog Neuropsychopharmacol Biol Psychiatry 2001; 25:437–43.
13. Baghai TC et al. The influence of concomitant antidepressant medication on safety, tolerability and clinical effectiveness of electroconvulsive therapy. World J Biol Psychiatry 2006; 7:82–90.
14. Jarvis MR et al. Novel antidepressants and maintenance electroconvulsive therapy: a review. Ann Clin Psychiatry 1992; 4:275–84.
15. Papakostas YG et al. Administration of citalopram before ECT: seizure duration and hormone responses. J ECT 2000; 16:356–60.
16. Gonzalez-Pinto A et al. Efficacy and safety of venlafaxine–ECT combination in treatment-resistant depression. J Neuropsychiatry Clin Neurosci 2002; 14:206–9.
17. Hanretta AT et al. Combined use of ECT with duloxetine and olanzapine: a case report. J ECT 2006; 22:139–41.
18. Dolenc TJ et al. Electroconvulsive therapy in patients taking monoamine oxidase inhibitors. J ECT 2004; 20:258–61.
19. Jha AK et al. Negative interaction between lithium and electroconvulsive therapy – a case-control study. Br J Psychiatry 1996; 168:241–3.
20. Rucker J et al. A case of prolonged seizure after ECT in a patient treated with clomipramine, lithium, L-tryptophan, quetiapine, and thyroxine for major depression. J ECT 2008; 24:272–4.
21. Dolenc TJ et al. The safety of electroconvulsive therapy and lithium in combination: a case series and review of the literature. J ECT 2005; 21:165–70.
22. Havaki-Kontaxaki BJ et al. Concurrent administration of clozapine and electroconvulsive therapy in clozapine-resistant schizophrenia. Clin Neuropharmacol 2006; 29:52–6.
23. Nothdurfter C et al. The influence of concomitant neuroleptic medication on safety, tolerability and clinical effectiveness of electroconvulsive therapy. World J Biol Psychiatry 2006; 7:162–70.
24. Gazdag G et al. The impact of neuroleptic medication on seizure threshold and duration in electroconvulsive therapy. Ideggyogy Sz 2004; 57:385–90.
25. Masdrakis VG et al. The safety of the electroconvulsive therapy-aripiprazole combination: four case reports. J ECT 2008; 24:236–8.
26. Penland HR et al. Combined use of lamotrigine and electroconvulsive therapy in bipolar depression: a case series. J ECT 2006; 22:142–7.
27. Zarate CA Jr et al. Combined valproate or carbamazepine and electroconvulsive therapy. Ann Clin Psychiatry 1997; 9:19–25.
28. Datto C et al. Augmentation of seizure induction in electroconvulsive therapy: a clinical reappraisal. J ECT 2002; 18:118–25.
29. Linton CR et al. Using thiamine to reduce post-ECT confusion. Int J Geriatr Psychiatry 2002; 17:189–92.
30. Prakash J et al. Therapeutic and prophylactic utility of the memory-enhancing drug donepezil hydrochloride on cognition of patients undergoing electroconvulsive therapy: a randomized controlled trial. J ECT 2006; 22:163–8.
31. Leung M et al. Pretreatment with ibuprofen to prevent electroconvulsive therapy-induced headache. J Clin Psychiatry 2003; 64:551–3.

Further reading

National Institute for Clinical Excellence. The clinical effectiveness and cost effectiveness of electroconvulsive therapy (ECT) for depressive illness, schizophrenia, catatonia and mania. Technology Appraisal 59, April 2003.
Patra KK et al. Implications of herbal alternative medicine for electroconvulsive therapy. J ECT 2004; 20:186–94.

Depression & anxiety

Stimulants in depression

Psychostimulants reduce fatigue, promote wakefulness and are mood elevating (as distinct from antidepressant). Amphetamines have been used as treatments for depression since the 1930s[1] and more recently modafinil has been evaluated as an adjunct to standard antidepressants[2]. Amphetamines are now rarely used in depression because of their propensity for the development of tolerance and dependence. Prolonged use of high doses is associated with paranoid psychosis[3]. Methylphenidate is now more widely used but may have similar shortcomings. Modafinil seems not to induce tolerance, dependence or psychosis but lacks the euphoric effects of amphetamines.

Psychostimulants differ importantly from standard antidepressants in that their effects are usually seen within a few hours. Amphetamines and methylphenidate may thus be useful where a prompt effect is required and where dependence would not be problematic (e.g. in depression associated with terminal illness). Their use might also be justified in severe, prolonged depression unresponsive to standard treatments (e.g. in those considered for psychosurgery). Modafinil might justifiably be used as an adjunct to antidepressants in a wider range of patients and as a specific treatment for hypersomnia and fatigue.

The table below outlines support (or the absence of it) for the use of psychostimulants in various clinical situations. Generally speaking, data relating to stimulants in depression are poor and inconclusive[4,5]. Careful consideration should be given to the use of any psychostimulant in depression since their short- and long-term safety has not been clearly established. Inclusion of individual drugs in the table below should not in itself be considered a recommendation for their use.

Table Stimulants in depression

Clinical use	Regimens evaluated	Comments	Recommendations
Monotherapy in uncomplicated depression	Modafinil 100–200 mg a day[6,7]	Case reports only – efficacy unproven	Standard antidepressants preferred. Avoid psychostimulants as monotherapy in uncomplicated depression
	Methylphenidate 20–40 mg a day[8,9]	Minimal efficacy	
	Dexamphetamine 20 mg a day[8]	Minimal efficacy	
Adjunctive therapy to accelerate response	SSRI + methylphenidate 10–20 mg a day[10,11]	No clear effect on time to response	Data very limited. Psychostimulants not recommended
	Tricyclic + methylphenidate 5–15 mg a day[12]	Single open-label trial suggests faster response	
Adjunctive treatment of depression with fatigue and hypersomnia	SSRI + modafinil 200 mg/day[13,14]	Beneficial effect only on hypersomnia. Modafinil may induce suicidal ideation	Avoid modafinil in this patient group

Table Stimulants in depression (Cont.)

Clinical use	Regimens evaluated	Comments	Recommendations
Adjunctive therapy in refractory depression	SSRI + modafinil 100–400 mg a day[15–20] MAOI + dexamfetamine 7.5–40 mg a day[21]	Effect mainly on fatigue and daytime sleepiness Support by single case series	Data limited. Only modafinil can be recommended and only for specific symptoms
Adjunctive treatment in bipolar depression	Mood-stabiliser and/or antidepressants + modafinil 100–200 mg/day[22]	Significantly superior to placebo. No evidence of switching to mania	Possible treatment option where other standard treatments fail
Monotherapy in late-stage terminal cancer	Methylphenidate 5–30 mg a day[23–27] Dexamfetamine 2.5–20 mg a day[28,29]	Case series and open prospective studies Beneficial effects seen on mood, fatigue and pain	Useful treatment options in those expected to live only for a few weeks. Best reserved for hospices and other specialist units
Monotherapy for depression in the very old	Methylphenidate 1.25–20 mg a day[30,31]	Use supported by two placebo-controlled studies. Rapid effect observed on mood and activity	Recommended only where patients fail to tolerate standard antidepressants or where contra-indications apply
Monotherapy in post-stroke depression	Methylphenidate 5–40 mg a day[32–34] Modafinil 100 mg/day[35]	Variable support but including a placebo-controlled trial[32]. Effect on mood evident after a few days Single case report	Standard antidepressants preferred. Further investigation required: stimulants may improve cognition and motor function
Monotherapy in depression secondary to medical illness	Methylphenidate 5–20 mg/day[36] Dexamfetamine 2.5–30 mg/day[37,38]	Limited data	Psychostimulants now not appropriate therapy. Standard antidepressant preferred
Monotherapy in depression and fatigue associated with HIV	Dexamfetamine 2.5–40 mg/day[39,40]	Supported by one good, controlled study[40] Beneficial effect on mood and fatigue	Possible treatment option where fatigue is not responsive to standard antidepressants

Depression & anxiety

191

References

1. Satel SL et al. Stimulants in the treatment of depression: a critical overview. J Clin Psychiatry 1989; 50:241–9.
2. Menza MA et al. Modafinil augmentation of antidepressant treatment in depression. J Clin Psychiatry 2000; 61:378–81.
3. Warneke L. Psychostimulants in psychiatry. Can J Psychiatry 1990; 35:3–10.
4. Candy M et al. Psychostimulants for depression. Cochrane Database Syst Rev 2008; CD006722.
5. Hardy SE. Methylphenidate for the treatment of depressive symptoms, including fatigue and apathy, in medically ill older adults and terminally ill adults. Am J Geriatr Pharmacother 2009; 7:34–59.
6. Lundt L. Modafinil treatment in patients with measonal affective disorder/winter depression: An open-label pilot study. J Affect Disord 2004; 81:173–8.
7. Kaufman KR et al. Modafinil monotherapy in depression. Eur Psychiatry 2002; 17:167–9.
8. Little KY. d-Amphetamine versus methylphenidate effects in depressed inpatients. J Clin Psychiatry 1993; 54:349–55.
9. Robin AA et al. A controlled trial of methylphenidate (ritalin) in the treatment of depressive states. J Neurol Neurosurg Psychiatry 1958; 21:55–7.
10. Lavretsky H et al. Combined treatment with methylphenidate and citalopram for accelerated response in the elderly: An open trial. J Clin Psychiatry 2003; 64:1410–14.
11. Postolache TT et al. Early augmentation of sertraline with methylphenidate. J Clin Psychiatry 1999; 60:123–4.
12. Gwirtsman HE et al. The antidepressant response to tricyclics in major depressives is accelerated with adjunctive use of methylphenidate. Psychopharmacol Bull 1994; 30:157–64.
13. Dunlop BW et al. Coadministration of modafinil and a selective serotonin reuptake inhibitor from the initiation of treatment of major depressive disorder with fatigue and sleepiness: a double-blind, placebo-controlled study. J Clin Psychopharmacol 2007; 27:614–19.
14. Fava M et al. Modafinil augmentation of selective serotonin reuptake inhibitor therapy in MDD partial responders with persistent fatigue and sleepiness. Ann Clin Psychiatry 2007; 19:153–9.
15. DeBattista C et al. Adjunct modafinil for the short-term treatment of fatigue and sleepiness in patients with major depressive disorder: A preliminary double-blind, placebo-controlled study. J Clin Psychiatry 2003; 64:1057–64.
16. Fava M et al. A multicenter, placebo-controlled study of modafinil augmentation in partial responders to selective serotonin reuptake inhibitors with persistent fatigue and sleepiness. J Clin Psychiatry 2005; 66:85–93.
17. Rasmussen NA et al. Modafinil augmentation in depressed patients with partial response to antidepressants: A pilot study on self-reported symptoms covered by the major depression inventory (MDI) and the symptom checklist (SCL-92). Nord J Psychiatry 2005; 59:173–8.
18. DeBattista C et al. A prospective trial of modafinil as an adjunctive treatment of major depression. J Clin Psychopharmacol 2004; 24:87–90.
19. Markovitz PJ et al. An open-label trial of modafinil augmentation in patients with partial response to antidepressant therapy. J Clin Psychopharmacol 2003; 23:207–9.
20. Ravindran AV et al. Osmotic-release oral system methylphenidate augmentation of antidepressant monotherapy in major depressive disorder: results of a double-blind, randomized, placebo-controlled trial. J Clin Psychiatry 2008; 69:87–94.
21. Fawcett J et al. CNS stimulant potentiation of monoamine oxidase inhibitors in treatment refractory depression. J Clin Psychopharmacol 1991; 11:127–32.
22. Frye MA et al. A placebo-controlled evaluation of adjunctive modafinil in the treatment of bipolar depression. Am J Psychiatry 2007; 164:1242–9.
23. Fernandez F et al. Methylphenidate for depressive disorders in cancer patients. Psychosomatics 1987; 28:455–61.
24. Macleod AD. Methylphenidate in terminal depression. J Pain Symptom Manage 1998; 16:193–8.
25. Homsi J et al. Methylphenidate for depression in hospice practice. Am J Hosp Palliat Care 2000; 17:393–8.
26. Sarhill N et al. Methylphenidate for fatigue in advanced cancer: A prospective open-label pilot study. Am J Hosp Palliat Care 2001; 18:187–92.
27. Homsi J et al. A phase II study of methylphenidate for depression in advanced cancer. Am J Hosp Palliat Care 2001; 18:403–7.
28. Burns MM et al. Dextroamphetamine treatment for depression in terminally ill patients. Psychosomatics 1994; 35:80–3.
29. Olin J et al. Psychostimulants for depression in hospitalized cancer patients. Psychosomatics 1996; 37:57–62.
30. Kaplitz SE. Withdrawn, apathetic geriatric patients responsive to methylphenidate. J Am Geriatr Soc 1975; 23:271–6.
31. Wallace AE et al. Double-blind, placebo-controlled trial of methylphenidate in older, depressed, medically ill patients. Am J Psychiatry 1995; 152:929–31.
32. Grade C et al. Methylphenidate in early poststroke recovery: A double-blind, placebo-controlled study. Arch Phys Med Rehabil 1998; 79:1047–50.
33. Lazarus LW et al. Efficacy and side effects of methylphenidate for poststroke depression. J Clin Psychiatry 1992; 53:447–9.
34. Lingam VR et al. Methylphenidate in treating poststroke depression. J Clin Psychiatry 1988; 49:151–3.
35. Sugden SG et al. Modafinil monotherapy in poststroke depression. Psychosomatics 2004; 45:80–1.
36. Rosenberg PB et al. Methylphenidate in depressed medically ill patients. J Clin Psychiatry 1991; 52:263–7.
37. Woods SW et al. Psychostimulant treatment of depressive disorders secondary to medical illness. J Clin Psychiatry 1986; 47:12–15.
38. Kaufmann MW et al. The use of d-amphetamine in medically ill depressed patients. J Clin Psychiatry 1982; 43:463–4.
39. Wagner GJ et al. Dexamphetamine as a treatment for depression and low energy in AIDS patients: A pilot study. J Psychosom Res 1997; 42:407–11.
40. Wagner GJ et al. Effects of dextroamphetamine on depression and fatigue in men with HIV: A double-blind, placebo-controlled trial. J Clin Psychiatry 2000; 61:436–40.

Antidepressant-induced hyponatraemia

Most antidepressants have been associated with hyponatraemia; the onset is usually within 30 days of starting treatment[1] and is probably not dose-related[1,2]. The mechanism of this adverse effect is probably the syndrome of inappropriate secretion of antidiuretic hormone (SIADH); serotonin is thought to be involved in the regulation of ADH release. Hyponatraemia is a potentially serious adverse effect of antidepressants that demands careful monitoring, particularly in those patients at greatest risk (see table below).

Table Risk factors[1,3,4]
Old age
Female sex
Low body weight
Low baseline sodium concentration
Some drug treatments (e.g. diuretics, NSAIDs, carbamazepine, cancer chemotherapy)
Reduced renal function (especially acute and chronic renal failure)
Medical co-morbidity (e.g. hypothyroidism, diabetes, COPD, hypertension, head injury, CVA, various cancers)
Warm weather (summer)

Antidepressants

No antidepressant has been shown *not* to be associated with hyponatraemia and most have a reported association[5]. It has been suggested that serotonergic drugs are relatively more likely to cause hyponatraemia[6,7], although this is disputed[8]. None of the newer serotonergic drugs are free of this effect – cases of hyponatraemia have been described with mirtazapine[9–11], escitalopram[12,13] and duloxetine[2]. Noradrenergic antidepressants are clearly linked to hyponatraemia[14–18] but there are notably few reports linking MAOIs to hyponatraemia[19,20].

Monitoring

All patients taking antidepressants should be observed for signs of hyponatraemia (dizziness, nausea, lethargy, confusion, cramps, seizures). Serum sodium should be determined (at baseline and 2 and 4 weeks, and then 3-monthly[21]) for those at high risk of drug-induced hyponatraemia. The high-risk factors are as follows:

- extreme old age (>80 years)
- history of hyponatraemia
- co-therapy with other drugs known to be associated with hyponatraemia (as above)
- reduced renal function (GFR <50 ml/min)
- medical co-morbidity (as above).

Note that hyponatraemia is common in elderly patients so monitoring is essential[22,23].

Treatment[24]

It may be possible to manage mild hyponatraemia with fluid restriction[4]. Some suggest increasing sodium intake[2], although this is likely to be impractical. If symptoms persist, the antidepressant should be discontinued.

- The normal range for serum sodium is 136–145 mmol/L.
- If serum sodium is >125 mmol/L – monitor sodium daily until normal. Symptoms include headache, nausea, vomiting, muscle cramps, restlessness, lethargy, confusion and disorientation. Consider withdrawing the offending antidepressant.
- If serum sodium is <125 mmol/L – refer to specialist medical care. There is an increased risk of life-threatening symptoms such as seizures, coma and respiratory arrest. The antidepressant should be discontinued immediately. (Note risk of discontinuation symptoms which may complicate the clinical picture.)

Restarting treatment

- For those who develop hyponatraemia with an SSRI, there are many case reports of recurrent hyponatraemia on rechallenge with the same, or a different SSRI, and relatively fewer with an antidepressant from another class[9,25]. There are also case reports of successful rechallenge[1].
- Prescribe a drug from a different class. Consider noradrenergic drugs such as reboxetine and lofepramine or an MAOI such as moclobemide. Begin with a low dose, increasing slowly, and monitor closely. If hyponatraemia recurs and continued antidepressant use is essential, consider water restriction and/or careful use of demeclocycline (see BNF).
- Consider ECT.

Other psychotropics

Carbamazepine has a well-known association with SIADH. Note also that antipsychotic use has been linked to hyponatraemia[26-28] (see section in Chapter 2).

References

1. Egger C et al. A review on hyponatremia associated with SSRIs, reboxetine and venlafaxine. Int J Psychiatry Clin Pract 2006; 10:17–26.
2. Kruger S et al. Duloxetine and hyponatremia: a report of 5 cases. J Clin Psychopharmacol 2007; 27:101–4.
3. Jacob S et al. Hyponatremia associated with selective serotonin-reuptake inhibitors in older adults. Ann Pharmacother 2006; 40:1618–22.
4. Roxanas M et al. Venlafaxine hyponatraemia: incidence, mechanism and management. Aust N Z J Psychiatry 2007; 41:411–18.
5. Thomas A et al. Hyponatraemia and the syndrome of inappropriate antidiuretic hormone secretion associated with drug therapy in psychiatric patients. CNS Drugs 1995; 5:357–69.
6. Movig KL et al. Serotonergic antidepressants associated with an increased risk for hyponatraemia in the elderly. Eur J Clin Pharmacol 2002; 58:143–8.
7. Movig KL et al. Association between antidepressant drug use and hyponatraemia: a case-control study. Br J Clin Pharmacol 2002; 53:363–9.
8. Kirby D et al. Hyponatraemia and selective serotonin re-uptake inhibitors in elderly patients. Int J Geriatr Psychiatry 2001; 16:484–93.
9. Bavbek N et al. Recurrent hyponatremia associated with citalopram and mirtazapine. Am J Kidney Dis 2006; 48:e61–2.
10. Ladino M et al. Mirtazapine-induced hyponatremia in an elderly hospice patient. J Palliat Med 2006; 9:258–60.
11. Cheah CY et al. Mirtazapine associated with profound hyponatremia: two case reports. Am J Geriatr Pharmacother 2008; 6:91–5.
12. Grover S et al. Escitalopram-associated hyponatremia. Psychiatry Clin Neurosci 2007; 61:132–3.
13. Covyeou JA et al. Hyponatremia associated with escitalopram. N Engl J Med 2007; 356:94–5.
14. O'Sullivan D et al. Hyponatraemia and lofepramine. Br J Psychiatry 1987; 150:720–1.
15. Wylie KR et al. Lofepramine-induced hyponatraemia. Br J Psychiatry 1989; 154:419–20.
16. Ranieri P et al. Reboxetine and hyponatremia. N Engl J Med 2000; 342:215–16.
17. Miller MG. Tricyclics as a possible cause of hyponatremia in psychiatric patients. Am J Psychiatry 1989; 146:807.
18. Colgate R. Hyponatraemia and inappropriate secretion of antidiuretic hormone associated with the use of imipramine. Br J Psychiatry 1993; 163:819–22.
19. Mercier S et al. Severe hyponatremia induced by moclobemide (in French). Therapie 1997; 52:82–3.
20. Peterson JC et al. Inappropriate antidiuretic hormone secondary to a monamine oxidase inhibitor. JAMA 1978; 239:1422–3.
21. Arinzon ZH et al. Delayed recurrent SIADH associated with SSRIs. Ann Pharmacother 2002; 36:1175–7.
22. Fabian TJ et al. Paroxetine-induced hyponatremia in older adults: a 12-week prospective study. Arch Intern Med 2004; 164:327–32.
23. Fabian TJ et al. Paroxetine-induced hyponatremia in the elderly due to the syndrome of inappropriate secretion of antidiuretic hormone (SIADH). J Geriatr Psychiatry Neurol 2003; 16:160–4.
24. Sharma H et al. Antidepressant-induced hyponatraemia in the aged. Avoidance and management strategies. Drugs Aging 1996; 8:430–5.
25. Dirks AC et al. Recurrent hyponatremia after substitution of citalopram with duloxetine. J Clin Psychopharmacol 2007; 27:313.
26. Ohsawa H et al. An epidemiological study on hyponatremia in psychiatric patients in mental hospitals in Nara Prefecture. Jpn J Psychiatry Neurol 1992; 46:883–9.
27. Leadbetter RA et al. Differential effects of neuroleptic and clozapine on polydipsia and intermittent hyponatremia. J Clin Psychiatry 1994; 55 Suppl B: 110–13.
28. Collins A et al. SIADH induced by two atypical antipsychotics. Int J Geriatr Psychiatry 2000; 15:282–3.

Post-stroke depression

Depression is a common problem seen in at least 30–40% of survivors of stroke[1,2]. Post-stroke depression also slows functional rehabilitation[3]. Antidepressants may be beneficial not only by reducing depressive symptoms but also by allowing faster rehabilitation[4].

Prophylaxis
The high incidence of depression after stroke makes prophylaxis worthy of consideration. Pooled data suggest a robust prophylactic effect for antidepressants[5]. Nortriptyline, fluoxetine, escitalopram and sertraline appear to prevent post-stroke depression[6–9]. Mirtazapine may both protect against depressive episodes and treat them[10]. Mianserin seems ineffective[11]. Amitriptyline is effective in treating central post-stroke pain[12].

Treatment
Treatment is complicated by medical co-morbidity and by the potential for interaction with other co-prescribed drugs (especially warfarin – see below). Contra-indication to antidepressant treatment is more likely with tricyclics than with SSRIs[13]. Fluoxetine[14,15], citalopram[16] and nortriptyline[17,18] are probably the most studied[19] and seem to be effective and safe. SSRIs and nortriptyline are widely recommended for post-stroke depression. Reboxetine may also be effective and well tolerated[20]. Despite fears, SSRIs seem not to increase risk of stroke[21], although some doubt remains[22]. (Stroke can be embolic or haemorrhagic – SSRIs may protect against the former and provoke the latter.) Antidepressants are clearly effective in post-stroke depression[23] and treatment should not usually be withheld.

Post-stroke depression – recommended drugs

SSRIs*
Mirtazapine**
Nortriptyline

*If the patient is also taking warfarin, suggest citalopram (probably lowest interaction potential[24]). Where SSRIs are given in any anticoagulated or aspirin-treated patient, consideration should be given to the prescription of a proton-pump inhibitor for gastric protection.
**Mirtazapine has a small effect on INR.

Depression & anxiety

References

1. Gainotti G et al. Relation between depression after stroke, antidepressant therapy, and functional recovery. J Neurol Neurosurg Psychiatry 2001; 71:258–61.
2. Hayee MA et al. Depression after stroke-analysis of 297 stroke patients. Bangladesh Med Res Counc Bull 2001; 27:96–102.
3. Paolucci S et al. Post-stroke depression, antidepressant treatment and rehabilitation results. A case-control study. Cerebrovasc Dis 2001; 12:264–71.
4. Gainotti G et al. Determinants and consequences of post-stroke depression. Curr Opin Neurol 2002; 15:85–9.
5. Chen Y et al. Antidepressant prophylaxis for poststroke depression: a meta-analysis. Int Clin Psychopharmacol 2007; 22:159–66.
6. Narushima K et al. Preventing poststroke depression: a 12-week double-blind randomized treatment trial and 21-month follow-up. J Nerv Ment Dis 2002; 190:296–303.
7. Rasmussen A et al. A double-blind, placebo-controlled study of sertraline in the prevention of depression in stroke patients. Psychosomatics 2003; 44:216–21.
8. Robinson RG et al. Escitalopram and problem-solving therapy for prevention of poststroke depression: a randomized controlled trial. JAMA 2008; 299:2391–400.
9. Almeida OP et al. Preventing depression after stroke: results from a randomized placebo-controlled trial. J Clin Psychiatry 2006; 67:1104–9.
10. Niedermaier N et al. Prevention and treatment of poststroke depression with mirtazapine in patients with acute stroke. J Clin Psychiatry 2004; 65:1619–23.
11. Palomaki H et al. Prevention of poststroke depression: 1 year randomised placebo controlled double blind trial of mianserin with 6 month follow up after therapy. J Neurol Neurosurg Psychiatry 1999; 66:490–4.
12. Lampl C et al. Amitriptyline in the prophylaxis of central poststroke pain. Preliminary results of 39 patients in a placebo-controlled, long-term study. Stroke 2002; 33:3030–2.
13. Cole MG et al. Feasibility and effectiveness of treatments for post-stroke depression in elderly inpatients: systematic review. J Geriatr Psychiatry Neurol 2001; 14:37–41.
14. Wiart L et al. Fluoxetine in early poststroke depression: a double-blind placebo-controlled study. Stroke 2000; 31:1829–32.
15. Choi-Kwon S et al. Fluoxetine improves the quality of life in patients with poststroke emotional disturbances. Cerebrovasc Dis 2008; 26:266–71.
16. Andersen G et al. Effective treatment of poststroke depression with the selective serotonin reuptake inhibitor citalopram. Stroke 1994; 25:1099–104.
17. Robinson RG et al. Nortriptyline versus fluoxetine in the treatment of depression and in short-term recovery after stroke: a placebo-controlled, double-blind study. Am J Psychiatry 2000; 157:351–9.
18. Zhang Wh et al. Nortriptyline protects mitochondria and reduces cerebral ischemia/hypoxia injury. Stroke 2008; 39:455–62.
19. Starkstein SE et al. Antidepressant therapy in post-stroke depression. Expert Opin Pharmacother 2008; 9:1291–8.
20. Rampello L et al. An evaluation of efficacy and safety of reboxetine in elderly patients affected by "retarded" post-stroke depression. A random, placebo-controlled study. Arch Gerontol Geriatr 2005; 40:275–85.
21. Bak S et al. Selective serotonin reuptake inhibitors and the risk of stroke: a population-based case-control study. Stroke 2002; 33:1465–73.
22. Ramasubbu R. SSRI treatment-associated stroke: causality assessment in two cases. Ann Pharmacother 2004; 38:1197–201.
23. Chen Y et al. Treatment effects of antidepressants in patients with post-stroke depression: a meta-analysis. Ann Pharmacother 2006; 40:2115–22.
24. Sayal KS et al. Psychotropic interactions with warfarin. Acta Psychiatr Scand 2000; 102:250–5.

SSRIs and bleeding

Serotonin is released from platelets in response to vascular injury and promotes vasoconstriction and morphological changes in platelets that lead to aggregation[1]. Serotonin alone is a relatively weak platelet aggregator. Selective serotonin reuptake inhibitors (SSRIs) inhibit the serotonin transporter which is responsible for the uptake of serotonin into platelets. It might thus be predicted that SSRIs will deplete platelet serotonin leading to a reduced ability to form clots and a subsequent increase in the risk of bleeding.

Several database studies have found that patients who take SSRIs are at significantly increased risk of being admitted to hospital with an upper gastrointestinal (GI) bleed compared with age- and sex-matched controls[2,3–5]. This association holds when age, gender, and the effects of other drugs such as aspirin and non-steroidal anti-inflammatory drugs (NSAIDs) are controlled for. Co-prescription of low-dose aspirin at least doubles the risk of GI bleeding associated with SSRIs alone and co-prescription of NSAIDs approximately quadruples risk[6]. The elderly and those with a history of GI bleeding are at greatest risk[4,5,7]. The risk may be greatest with SSRIs that have a high affinity for the serotonin transporter[5]. Risk decreases to the same level as controls in past users of SSRIs indicating that bleeding is likely to be associated with treatment rather than some inherent characteristic of the patients being treated[3].

The excess risk of bleeding is not confined to upper GI bleeds. The risk of lower GI bleeds may also be increased[8] and an increased risk of uterine bleeding has also been reported[9]. One study[10] found that patients prescribed SSRIs who underwent orthopaedic surgery had an almost four-fold risk of requiring a blood transfusion. This equated to one additional patient requiring transfusion for every 10 SSRI patients undergoing surgery and was double the risk of patients who were taking NSAIDs alone. It should be noted in this context that treatment with SSRIs has been associated with a 2.4-fold increase in the risk of hip fracture[11] and a 2-fold increase of fracture in old age[12]. The combination of advanced age, SSRI treatment, orthopaedic surgery and NSAIDs clearly presents a very high risk. However, there does not seem to be an increased risk of bleeding in patients who undergo coronary artery bypass surgery[13]. Similarly the risk of post-partum haemorrhage does not seem to be increased[14]. SSRIs should be used cautiously in patients with cirrhosis or other risk factors for internal bleeding[15].

It is likely that SSRIs are responsible for an additional three episodes of bleeding in every 1000 patient years of treatment over the normal background incidence[3,9] but this figure masks large variations in risk. For example 1 in 85 patients with a history of GI bleed will have a further bleed attributable to treatment with a SSRI[7]. One database study suggests that gastro-protective drugs (PPIs) decrease the risk of GI bleeds associated with SSRIs (alone or in combination with NSAIDs) although not quite to control levels[4].

Some studies have been prompted by the hypothesis that the increased risk of upper GI bleeds associated with SSRIs may be balanced by a decreased risk of embolic events. One database study failed to find a reduction in the risk of a first myocardial infarction in SSRI-treated patients compared with controls[16], while another[17] found a reduction in the risk of being admitted to hospital with a first MI in smokers on SSRIs. The effect size in the second study was large: approximately 1 in 10 hospitalisations were avoided in SSRI-treated patients[17]. This is similar to the effect size of other antiplatelet therapies such as aspirin[18].

In patients who take warfarin, SSRIs increase the risk of a non-GI bleed almost two-fold (similar to the effect size of NSAIDs) but do not seem to increase the risk of a GI bleed[19]. In keeping with

Depression & anxiety

these findings, SSRI use in anticoagulated patients being treated for acute coronary syndromes may decrease the risk of minor cardiac events at the expense of an increased risk of a minor bleed[20].

Three large database studies have failed to find a reduction in the risk of an ischaemic stroke (or increase in the risk of haemorrhagic stroke) in SSRI users[21-23].

Summary

SSRIs increase the risk of bleeding in:

* Patients with haemostatic defects, including those that are drug-induced (e.g. by warfarin or antiplatelet drugs). Bleeds may not be confined to the GI tract
* Patients who take drugs that cause GI injury (e.g. NSAIDs or steroids)
* The very old and those with a history of GI bleeding; this is a high-risk group

In high-risk patients, gastro-protective drugs such as PPIs may reduce the risk of GI bleeding substantially (but do not eliminate it completely)

References

1. Skop BP et al. Potential vascular and bleeding complications of treatment with selective serotonin reuptake inhibitors. Psychosomatics 1996; 37:12–16.
2. de Abajo FJ et al. Association between selective serotonin reuptake inhibitors and upper gastrointestinal bleeding: population based case-control study. BMJ 1999; 319:1106–9.
3. Dalton SO et al. Use of selective serotonin reuptake inhibitors and risk of upper gastrointestinal tract bleeding: a population-based cohort study. Arch Intern Med 2003; 163:59–64.
4. de Abajo FJ et al. Risk of upper gastrointestinal tract bleeding associated with selective serotonin reuptake inhibitors and venlafaxine therapy: interaction with nonsteroidal anti-inflammatory drugs and effect of acid-suppressing agents. Arch Gen Psychiatry 2008; 65:795–803.
5. Lewis JD et al. Moderate and high affinity serotonin reuptake inhibitors increase the risk of upper gastrointestinal toxicity. Pharmacoepidemiol Drug Saf 2008; 17:328–35.
6. Paton C et al. SSRIs and gastrointestinal bleeding. BMJ 2005; 331:529–30.
7. van Walraven C et al. Inhibition of serotonin reuptake by antidepressants and upper gastrointestinal bleeding in elderly patients: retrospective cohort study. BMJ 2001; 323:655–8.
8. Wessinger S et al. Increased use of selective serotonin reuptake inhibitors in patients admitted with gastrointestinal haemorrhage: a multicentre retrospective analysis. Aliment Pharmacol Ther 2006; 23:937–44.
9. Meijer WE et al. Association of risk of abnormal bleeding with degree of serotonin reuptake inhibition by antidepressants. Arch Intern Med 2004; 164:2367–70.
10. Movig KL et al. Relationship of serotonergic antidepressants and need for blood transfusion in orthopedic surgical patients. Arch Intern Med 2003; 163:2354–8.
11. Liu B et al. Use of selective serotonin-reuptake inhibitors of tricyclic antidepressants and risk of hip fractures in elderly people. Lancet 1998; 351:1303–7.
12. Richards JB et al. Effect of selective serotonin reuptake inhibitors on the risk of fracture. Arch Intern Med 2007; 167:188–94.
13. Andreasen JJ et al. Effect of selective serotonin reuptake inhibitors on requirement for allogeneic red blood cell transfusion following coronary artery bypass surgery. Am J Cardiovasc Drugs 2006; 6:243–50.
14. Salkeld E et al. The risk of postpartum hemorrhage with selective serotonin reuptake inhibitors and other antidepressants. J Clin Psychopharmacol 2008; 28:230–4.
15. Weinrieb RM et al. A critical review of selective serotonin reuptake inhibitor-associated bleeding: balancing the risk of treating hepatitis C-infected patients. J Clin Psychiatry 2003; 64:1502–10.
16. Meier CR et al. Use of selective serotonin reuptake inhibitors and risk of developing first-time acute myocardial infarction. Br J Clin Pharmacol 2001; 52:179–84.
17. Sauer WH et al. Selective serotonin reuptake inhibitors and myocardial infarction. Circulation 2001; 104:1894–8.
18. Antiplatelet Trialists' Collaboration. Collaborative overview of randomised trials of antiplatelet therapy – I: Prevention of death, myocardial infarction, and stroke by prolonged antiplatelet therapy in various categories of patients. BMJ 1994; 308:81–106.
19. Schalekamp T et al. Increased bleeding risk with concurrent use of selective serotonin reuptake inhibitors and coumarins. Arch Intern Med 2008; 168:180–5.
20. Ziegelstein RC et al. Selective serotonin reuptake inhibitor use by patients with acute coronary syndromes. Am J Med 2007; 120:525–30.
21. Bak S et al. Selective serotonin reuptake inhibitors and the risk of stroke: a population-based case-control study. Stroke 2002; 33:1465–73.
22. Barbui C et al. Past use of selective serotonin reuptake inhibitors and the risk of cerebrovascular events in the elderly. Int Clin Psychopharmacol 2005; 20:169–71.
23. Kharofa J et al. Selective serotonin reuptake inhibitors and risk of hemorrhagic stroke. Stroke 2007; 38:3049–51.

Further reading

Dalton SO et al. SSRIs and upper gastrointestinal bleeding: what is known and how should it influence prescribing? CNS Drugs 2006; 20:143–51.

Depression & anxiety

Antidepressants and diabetes mellitus

Depression and diabetes

There is an established link between diabetes and depression[1]. Prevalence rates of co-morbid depressive symptoms in diabetic patients have been reported to range from 9–60% depending on the screening method used and a diagnosis of diabetes is linked to an increased likelihood of anti-depressant prescription[2,3]. Having diabetes doubles the odds of co-morbid depression[4]. Patients with depression and diabetes have a high number of cardiovascular risk factors and increased mortality[5,6]. The presence of depression has a negative impact on metabolic control and likewise poor metabolic control may worsen depression[7]. Considering all of the above, the treatment of co-morbid depression in patients with diabetes is of vital importance and drug choice should take into account likely effects on metabolic control (see table).

Table	Effect of antidepressants on glucose homeostasis and weight
Antidepressant class	**Effect on glucose homeostasis and weight**
SSRIs[8–14]	• Studies indicate that SSRIs have a favourable effect on diabetic parameters in patients with type II diabetes. Insulin requirements may be decreased • Fluoxetine has been associated with improvement in HbA_{1c} levels, reduced insulin requirements, weight loss and enhanced insulin sensitivity. Its effect on insulin sensitivity is independent of its effect on weight loss. It may also enhance sympathetic responses to hyperglycaemia • Controversial evidence that long term (greater than 2 years) SSRIs may increase the risk of diabetes
TCAs[14–17]	• TCAs are associated with increased appetite, weight gain and hyperglycaemia • Nortriptyline improved depression but worsened glycaemic control in diabetic patients in one study. Overall improvement in depression had a beneficial effect on HbA_{1c}. Clomipramine reported to precipitate diabetes • Long-term use of TCAs may increase risk of diabetes
MAOIs[18,19]	• Irreversible MAOIs have a tendency to cause extreme hypoglycaemic episodes and weight gain • No known effects with moclobemide
SNRIs[16,20]	• SNRIs do not appear to disrupt glycaemic control and have minimal impact on weight • Studies of duloxetine in the treatment of diabetic neuropathy show that it has little influence on glycaemic control. No data in depression and diabetes • Limited data on venlafaxine
Mirtazapine, reboxetine and trazodone[2,21]	• Mirtazapine is associated with weight gain but little is known about its effect in diabetes • Mirtazapine does not appear to impair glucose tolerance in non-diabetic depressed patients • No data with trazodone and reboxetine

Depression & anxiety

Table	Recommendations
• All patients with a diagnosis of depression should be screened for diabetes	

Table	In those who are diabetic
• Use SSRIs first line; most data support fluoxetine • SNRIs are also likely to be safe but there are fewer supporting data • Avoid TCAs and MAOIs if possible due to their effects on weight and glucose homeostasis • Monitor blood glucose carefully when antidepressant treatment is initiated, when the dose is changed and after discontinuation	

References

1. Katon WJ. The comorbidity of diabetes mellitus and depression. Am J Med 2008; 121 Suppl 2:S8–15.
2. Musselman DL et al. Relationship of depression to diabetes types 1 and 2: epidemiology, biology, and treatment. Biol Psychiatry 2003; 54:317–29.
3. Knol MJ et al. Antidepressant use before and after initiation of diabetes mellitus treatment. Diabetologia 2009; 52:425–32.
4. Anderson RJ et al. The prevalence of comorbid depression in adults with diabetes: a meta-analysis. Diabetes Care 2001; 24:1069–78.
5. Katon WJ et al. Cardiac risk factors in patients with diabetes mellitus and major depression. J Gen Intern Med 2004; 19:1192–9.
6. Katon WJ et al. The association of comorbid depression with mortality in patients with type 2 diabetes. Diabetes Care 2005; 28:2668–72.
7. Lustman PJ et al. Depression in diabetic patients: the relationship between mood and glycemic control. J Diabetes Complications 2005; 19:113–22.
8. Maheux P et al. Fluoxetine improves insulin sensitivity in obese patients with non-insulin-dependent diabetes mellitus independently of weight loss. Int J Obes Relat Metab Disord 1997; 21:97–102.
9. Gulseren L et al. Comparison of fluoxetine and paroxetine in type II diabetes mellitus patients. Arch Med Res 2005; 36:159–65.
10. Lustman PJ et al. Sertraline for prevention of depression recurrence in diabetes mellitus: a randomized, double-blind, placebo-controlled trial. Arch Gen Psychiatry 2006; 63:521–9.
11. Gray DS et al. A randomized double-blind clinical trial of fluoxetine in obese diabetics. Int J Obes Relat Metab Disord 1992; 16 Suppl 4:S67–72.
12. Knol MJ et al. Influence of antidepressants on glycaemic control in patients with diabetes mellitus. Pharmacoepidemiol Drug Saf 2008; 17:577–86.
13. Briscoe VJ et al. Effects of a selective serotonin reuptake inhibitor, fluoxetine, on counterregulatory responses to hypoglycemia in healthy individuals. Diabetes 2008; 57:2453–60.
14. Andersohn F et al. Long-term use of antidepressants for depressive disorders and the risk of diabetes mellitus. Am J Psychiatry 2009; 166:591–598.
15. Lustman PJ et al. Effects of nortriptyline on depression and glycemic control in diabetes: results of a double-blind, placebo-controlled trial. Psychosom Med 1997; 59:241–50.
16. McIntyre RS et al. The effect of antidepressants on glucose homeostasis and insulin sensitivity: synthesis and mechanisms. Expert Opin Drug Saf 2006; 5:157–68.
17. Mumoli N et al. Clomipramine-induced diabetes. Ann Intern Med 2008; 149:595–6.
18. Goodnick PJ. Use of antidepressants in treatment of comorbid diabetes mellitus and depression as well as in diabetic neuropathy. Ann Clin Psychiatry 2001; 13:31–41.
19. McIntyre RS et al. Mood and psychotic disorders and type 2 diabetes: a metabolic triad. Can J Diab 2005; 29:122–32.
20. Raskin J et al. Duloxetine versus routine care in the long-term management of diabetic peripheral neuropathic pain. J Palliat Med 2006; 9:29–40.
21. Himmerich H et al. Changes in weight and glucose tolerance during treatment with mirtazapine. Diabetes Care 2006; 29:170.

Treatment of depression in the elderly

The prevalence of most physical illnesses increases with age. Many physical problems such as cardiovascular disease, chronic pain and Parkinson's disease are associated with a high risk of depressive illness[1]. The morbidity and mortality associated with depression are increased, as the elderly are more physically frail and therefore more likely to suffer serious consequences from self-neglect (e.g. life-threatening dehydration or hypothermia) and immobility (e.g. venous stasis). Almost 20% of completed suicides occur in the elderly[2].

In common with placebo-controlled studies in younger adults, at least some adequately powered studies in elderly patients have failed to find 'active' antidepressants to be more effective than placebo[3,4], although it is commonly perceived that the elderly may take longer to respond to antidepressants than younger adults[5]. It may however be possible to identify non-responders as early as 4 weeks into treatment[6]. Two studies have found that elderly people who had recovered from an episode of depression and had received antidepressants for 2 years, 60% relapsed within 2 years if antidepressant treatment was withdrawn[7,8]. This finding held true for first-episode patients. Lower doses of antidepressants may be effective as prophylaxis. Dothiepin (dosulepin) 75 mg/day has been shown to be effective in this regard[9]. Note that NICE recommend that dosulepin should not be used as it is particularly cardiotoxic in overdose[10]. There is no evidence to suggest that the response to antidepressants is reduced in the physically ill[11], although outcome in the elderly in general is often suboptimal[12,13].

There is no ideal antidepressant. All are associated with problems. SSRIs are generally better tolerated than TCAs[14]; they do, however, increase the risk of GI and other bleeds, particularly in the very elderly and those with established risk factors such as a history of bleeds or treatment with a NSAID, steroid or warfarin (see section on SSRIs and bleeding). The elderly are also particularly prone to develop hyponatraemia with SSRIs (see section on hyponatraemia), as well as postural hypotension and falls. Ultimately, choice is determined by the individual clinical circumstances of each patient, particularly physical co-morbidity and concomitant medication (both prescribed and 'over the counter').

References

1. Katona C et al. Impact of screening old people with physical illness for depression? Lancet 2000; 356:91–92.
2. Cattell H et al. One hundred cases of suicide in elderly people. Br J Psychiatry 1995; 166:451–7.
3. Schatzberg A et al. A double-blind, placebo-controlled study of venlafaxine and fluoxetine in geriatric outpatients with major depression. Am J Geriatr Psychiatry 2006; 14:361–70.
4. Wilson K et al. Antidepressant versus placebo for depressed elderly. Cochrane Database Syst Rev 2001;CD000561.
5. Paykel ES et al. Residual symptoms after partial remission: an important outcome in depression. Psychol Med 1995; 25:1171–80.
6. Mulsant BH et al. What is the optimal duration of a short-term antidepressant trial when treating geriatric depression? J Clin Psychopharmacol 2006; 26:113–20.
7. Flint AJ et al. Recurrence of first-episode geriatric depression after discontinuation of maintenance antidepressants. Am J Psychiatry 1999; 156:943–5.
8. Reynolds CF III et al. Maintenance treatment of major depression in old age. N Engl J Med 2006; 354:1130–8.
9. Old Age Depression Interest Group. How long should the elderly take antidepressants? A double-blind placebo-controlled study of continuation/prophylaxis therapy with dothiepin. Br J Psychiatry 1993; 162:175–82.
10. National Institute for Clinical Excellence. Depression: the treatment and management of depression in adults (update). 2009. http://www.nice.org.uk/
11. Evans M et al. Placebo-controlled treatment trial of depression in elderly physically ill patients. Int J Geriatr Psychiatry 1997; 12:817–24.
12. Heeren TJ et al. Treatment, outcome and predictors of response in elderly depressed in-patients. Br J Psychiatry 1997; 170:436–40.
13. Tuma TA. Outcome of hospital-treated depression at 4.5 years. An elderly and a younger adult cohort compared. Br J Psychiatry 2000; 176:224–8.
14. Mottram P et al. Antidepressants for depressed elderly. Cochrane Database Syst Rev 2006; CD003491.
15. Draper B et al. Tolerability of selective serotonin reuptake inhibitors: issues relevant to the elderly. Drugs Aging 2008; 25:501–19.
16. Bose A et al. Escitalopram in the acute treatment of depressed patients aged 60 years or older. Am J Geriatr Psychiatry 2008; 16:14–20.
17. Raskin J et al. Safety and tolerability of duloxetine at 60 mg once daily in elderly patients with major depressive disorder. J Clin Psychopharmacol 2008; 28:32–8.
18. Johnson EM et al. Cardiovascular changes associated with venlafaxine in the treatment of late-life depression. Am J Geriatr Psychiatry 2006; 14: 796–802.

Further reading

Juurlink DN et al. The risk of suicide with selective serotonin reuptake inhibitors in the elderly. Am J Psychiatry 2006; 163:813–21.
National Service Framework for Older People. London: Department of Health (a whole supplement dedicated to the use of medicines in older people), 2001.
Pacher P et al. Selective serotonin reuptake inhibitor antidepressants increase the risk of falls and hip fractures in elderly people by inhibiting cardio-vascular ion channels. Med Hypotheses 2001; 57:469–71.
Spina E et al. Clinically significant drug interactions with antidepressants in the elderly. Drugs Aging 2002; 19:299–320.
Van der Wurff FB et al. Electroconvulsive therapy for the depressed elderly. Cochrane Database Syst Rev 2003;CD003593.

Depression & anxiety

Table   Antidepressants and the elderly

	Anticholinergic side-effect (urinary retention, dry mouth, blurred vision, constipation)	Postural hypotension	Sedation
Older tricyclics[15]	Variable: moderate with nortriptyline, imipramine and dosulepin (dothiepin) Marked with others	All can cause postural hypotension Dosage titration is required	Variable: from minimal with imipramine to profound with trimipramine
Lofepramine	Moderate, although constipation/sweating can be severe	Can be a problem but generally better tolerated than the older tricyclics	Minimal
SSRIs[15,16]	Dry mouth can be a problem with paroxetine	Much less of a problem, but an increased risk of falls is documented with SSRIs	Can be a problem with paroxetine and fluvoxamine Unlikely with the other SSRIs
Others[17,18]	Minimal with mirtazapine and venlafaxine Can be rarely a problem with reboxetine Duloxetine – few effects	Venlafaxine can cause hypotension at lower doses, but it can increase BP at higher doses, as can duloxetine	Mirtazapine, mianserin and trazodone are sedative Duloxetine – neutral effects

Further reading

Pinquart M et al. Treatments for later-life depressive conditions: a meta-analytic comparison of pharmaco-therapy and psychotherapy.

Depression & anxiety

Weight gain	Safety in overdose	Other side-effects	Drug interactions
All tricyclics can cause weight gain	Dosulepin and amitriptyline are the most toxic (seizures and cardiac arrhythmia)	Seizures, anticholinergic-induced cognitive impairment Increased risk of bleeds with serotonergic drugs	Mainly pharmacodynamic: increased sedation with benzodiazepines, increased hypotension with diuretics, increased constipation with other anti-cholinergic drugs, etc.
Few data, but lack of spontaneous reports may indicate less potential than the older tricyclics	Relatively safe	Raised LFTs	
Paroxetine and possibly citalopram may cause weight gain Others are weight-neutral	Safe with the possible exception of citalopram one minor metabolite can cause significant QTc prolongation	GI effects and headaches, hyponatraemia, increased risk of bleeds in the elderly, orofacial dyskinesia with paroxetine	Fluvoxamine, fluoxetine and paroxetine are potent inhibitors of several hepatic cytochrome enzymes. Sertraline is safer and citalopram and escitalopram are safest
Greatest problem is with mirtazapine, although the elderly are not particularly prone	Venlafaxine is more toxic in overdose than SSRIs, but safer than TCAs Others are relatively safe	Insomnia and hypokalaemia with reboxetine Nausea with venlafaxine Weight loss and nausea with duloxetine	Duloxetine inhibits CYP2D6 Moclobemide and venlafaxine inhibit CYP450 enzymes. Check for potential interactions Reboxetine is safe

Depression & anxiety

Am J Psychiatry 2006; 163:1493–501.

Cardiac effects of antidepressants

Drug	Heart rate	Blood pressure	QTc
Tricyclics[1–4]	Increase in heart rate	Postural hypotension	Prolongation of QTc interval
Lofepramine[1,5]	Modest increase in heart rate	Less decrease in postural blood pressure compared with other TCAs	Can possibly prolong QTc interval at higher doses
MAOIs[1,6]	Decrease in heart rate	Postural hypotension Risk of hypertensive crisis	Unclear but may shorten QTc interval
Fluoxetine[7–10]	Small decrease in mean heart rate	Minimal effect on blood pressure	No effect on QTc interval
Paroxetine[11,12]	Small decrease in mean heart rate	Minimal effect on blood pressure	No effect on QTc interval
Sertraline[13–16]	Minimal effect on heart rate	Minimal effect on blood pressure	No effect on QTc interval
Citalopram[17–20] (assume same for escitalopram)	Small decrease in heart rate	Slight drop in systolic blood pressure	No effect on QTc interval in normal doses. Prolongation in overdose
Fluvoxamine[21]	Minimal effect on heart rate	Small drops in systolic blood pressure	No significant effect on QTc
Venlafaxine[22–26]	Marginally increased	Some increase in postural blood pressure. At higher doses increase in blood pressure	Possible prolongation in overdose
Duloxetine[26–29]	Slight increase	Important effect (see SPC). Caution in hypertension	No effect on QTc
Mirtazapine[30,31]	Minimal effect on heart rate	Minimal effect on blood pressure	No effect on QTc
Reboxetine[32–34]	Significant increase in heart rate	Marginal increase in both systolic and diastolic blood pressure. Postural decrease at higher doses	No effect on QTc
Moclobemide[35–37]	Marginal decrease in heart rate	Minimal effect on blood pressure. Isolated cases of hypertensive episodes	No effect on QTc interval in normal doses. Prolongation in overdose
Trazodone[1,38,39]	Decrease in heart rate more common, although increase can also occur	Can cause significant postural hypotension	Can prolong QTc interval
Agomelatine[40]	No changes reported	No changes reported	No effect on ECG noted

SSRIs are generally recommended in cardiac disease but beware cytochrome-medicated interactions with co-administered depression worsens prognosis in cardiovascular diesase[43]. Treatment of depression with SSRIs should not therefore be CBT may be ineffective in this respect[44]. Note that the anti-platelet effect of SSRIs may have adverse consequences too:

Arrhythmia	Conduction disturbance	Licensed restrictions post-MI	Comments
Class I anti-arrhythmic activity. Ventricular arrhythmia common in overdose. Torsade de Pointes reported	Slows cardiac conduction – blocks cardiac Na/K channels	CI in patients with recent MI	TCAs affect cardiac contractility. Some TCAs linked to ischaemic heart disease and sudden cardiac death. Avoid in coronary artery disease
May occur at higher doses, but rare	Unclear	CI in patients with recent MI	Less cardiotoxic than other TCAs. Reasons unclear
May cause arrhythmia and decrease LVF	No clear effect on cardiac conduction	Use with caution in patients with cardiovascular disease	
None	None	Caution. Clinical experience is limited	Evidence of safety post MI
None	None	General caution in cardiac patients	Probably safe post MI
None	None	None – drug of choice	Safe post MI and in heart failure
Torsade de Pointes reported, mainly in overdose	None	Caution	Minor metabolite which may ↑QTc interval. Evidence of safety in coronary artery disease
None	None	Caution	Limited changes in ECG have been observed
Rare reports of cardiac arrhythmia in overdose	Rare reports of conduction abnormalities	Has not been evaluated in post-MI patients. Avoid	Evidence for arrhythmogenic potential is slim, but avoid in coronary disease
None	None	Caution in patients with recent MI	Limited clinical experience
None	None	Caution in patients with recent MI	Evidence of safety post MI
Rhythm abnormalities may occur	Atrial and ventricular ectopic beats, especially in the elderly	Caution in patient with cardiac disease	Probably best avoided in coronary disease
None	None	None	Possibly arrhythmogenic in overdose
Rhythm abnormalities may occur	Unclear	Care in patients with severe cardiac disease	May be arrhythmogenic in patients with pre-existing cardiac disease
No arrhythmia reported	Unclear	See SPC	Limited data

cardiac drugs. Mirtazapine is a suitable alternative[31]. SSRIs may protect against myocardial infarction[41,42], and untreated withheld post-MI. Protective effects of treatment of depression post-MI appear to relate to antidepressant administration. upper GI bleeding is more common in those taking SSRIs[45].

References

1. Warrington SJ et al. The cardiovascular effects of antidepressants. Psychol Med Monogr Suppl 1989; 16:i–40.
2. Hippisley-Cox J et al. Antidepressants as risk factor for ischaemic heart disease: case-control study in primary care. BMJ 2001; 323:666–9.
3. Whyte IM et al. Relative toxicity of venlafaxine and selective serotonin reuptake inhibitors in overdose compared to tricyclic antidepressants. QJM 2003; 96:369–74.
4. van NC et al. Psychotropic drugs associated with corrected QT interval prolongation. J Clin Psychopharmacol 2009; 29:9–15.
5. Stern H et al. Cardiovascular effects of single doses of the antidepressants amitriptyline and lofepramine in healthy subjects. Pharmacopsychiatry 1985; 18:272–7.
6. Waring WS et al. Acute myocarditis after massive phenelzine overdose. Eur J Clin Pharmacol 2007; 63:1007–9.
7. Fisch C. Effect of fluoxetine on the electrocardiogram. J Clin Psychiatry 1985; 46:42–4.
8. Ellison JM et al. Fluoxetine-induced bradycardia and syncope in two patients. J Clin Psychiatry 1990; 51:385–6.
9. Roose SP et al. Cardiovascular effects of fluoxetine in depressed patients with heart disease. Am J Psychiatry 1998; 155:660–5.
10. Strik JJ et al. Efficacy and safety of fluoxetine in the treatment of patients with major depression after first myocardial infarction: findings from a double-blind, placebo-controlled trial. Psychosom Med 2000; 62:783–9.
11. Kuhs H et al. Cardiovascular effects of paroxetine. Psychopharmacology 1990; 102:379–82.
12. Roose SP et al. Comparison of paroxetine and nortriptyline in depressed patients with ischemic heart disease. JAMA 1998; 279:287–91.
13. Shapiro PA et al. An open-label preliminary trial of sertraline for treatment of major depression after acute myocardial infarction (the SADHAT Trial). Sertraline Anti-Depressant Heart Attack Trial. Am Heart J 1999; 137:1100–6.
14. Glassman AH et al. Sertraline treatment of major depression in patients with acute MI or unstable angina. JAMA 2002; 288:701–9.
15. Winkler D et al. Trazodone-induced cardiac arrhythmias: a report of two cases. Hum Psychopharmacol 2006; 21:61–2.
16. Jiang W et al. Safety and efficacy of sertraline for depression in patients with CHF (SADHART-CHF): a randomized, double-blind, placebo-controlled trial of sertraline for major depression with congestive heart failure. Am Heart J 2008; 156:437–44.
17. Rasmussen SL et al. Cardiac safety of citalopram: prospective trials and retrospective analyses. J Clin Psychopharmacol 1999; 19:407–15.
18. Catalano G et al. QTc interval prolongation associated with citalopram overdose: a case report and literature review. Clin Neuropharmacol 2001; 24:158–62.
19. Lesperance F et al. Effects of citalopram and interpersonal psychotherapy on depression in patients with coronary artery disease: the Canadian Cardiac Randomized Evaluation of Antidepressant and Psychotherapy Efficacy (CREATE) trial. JAMA 2007; 297:367–79.
20. Astrom-Lilja C et al. Drug-induced torsades de pointes: a review of the Swedish pharmacovigilance database. Pharmacoepidemiol Drug Saf 2008; 17:587–92.
21. Strik JJ et al. Cardiac side-effects of two selective serotonin reuptake inhibitors in middle-aged and elderly depressed patients. Int Clin Psychopharmacol 1998; 13:263–7.
22. Wyeth Pharmaceuticals. Summary of Product Characteristics. Exefor. 2009. http://emc.medicines.org.uk/
23. Khawaja IS et al. Cardiovascular effects of selective serotonin reuptake inhibitors and other novel antidepressants. Heart Dis 2003; 5:153–60.
24. Letsas K et al. QT interval prolongation associated with venlafaxine administration. Int J Cardiol 2006; 109:116–17.
25. Taylor D et al. Volte-face on venlafaxine – reasons and reflections. J Psychopharmacol 2006; 20:597–601.
26. Colucci VJ et al. Heart failure worsening and exacerbation after venlafaxine and duloxetine therapy. Ann Pharmacother 2008; 42:882–7.
27. Sharma A et al. Pharmacokinetics and safety of duloxetine, a dual-serotonin and norepinephrine reuptake inhibitor. J Clin Pharmacol 2000; 40:161–7.
28. Schatzberg AF. Efficacy and tolerability of duloxetine, a novel dual reuptake inhibitor, in the treatment of major depressive disorder. J Clin Psychiatry 2003; 64 Suppl 13:30–7.
29. Detke MJ et al. Duloxetine, 60 mg once daily, for major depressive disorder: a randomized double-blind placebo-controlled trial. J Clin Psychiatry 2002; 63:308–15.
30. Montgomery SA. Safety of mirtazapine: a review. Int Clin Psychopharmacol 1995; 10 Suppl 4:37–45.
31. Honig A et al. Treatment of post-myocardial infarction depressive disorder: a randomized, placebo-controlled trial with mirtazapine. Psychosom Med 2007; 69:606–13.
32. Mucci M. Reboxetine: a review of antidepressant tolerability. J Psychopharmacol 1997; 11:S33–7.
33. Holm KJ et al. Reboxetine : a review of its use in depression. CNS Drugs 1999; 12:65–83.
34. Fleishaker JC et al. Lack of effect of reboxetine on cardiac repolarization. Clin Pharmacol Ther 2001; 70:261–9.
35. Moll E et al. Safety and efficacy during long-term treatment with moclobemide. Clin Neuropharmacol 1994; 17 Suppl 1:S74–87.
36. Hilton S et al. Moclobemide safety: monitoring a newly developed product in the 1990s. J Clin Psychopharmacol 1995; 15:76S–83S.
37. Downes MA et al. QTc abnormalities in deliberate self-poisoning with moclobemide. Intern Med J 2005; 35:388–91.
38. Service JA et al. QT Prolongation and delayed atrioventricular conduction caused by acute ingestion of trazodone. Clin Toxicol (Phila) 2008; 46:71–3.
39. Dattilo PB et al. Prolonged QT associated with an overdose of trazodone. J Clin Psychiatry 2007; 68:1309–10.
40. Dolder CR et al. Agomelatine treatment of major depressive disorder. The Annals of Pharmacotherapy 2008; 42:1822–31.
41. Sauer WH et al. Selective serotonin reuptake inhibitors and myocardial infarction. Circulation 2001; 104:1894–8.
42. Sauer WH et al. Effect of antidepressants and their relative affinity for the serotonin transporter on the risk of myocardial infarction. Circulation 2003; 108:32–6.
43. Davies SJ et al. Treatment of anxiety and depressive disorders in patients with cardiovascular disease. BMJ 2004; 328:939–43.
44. Berkman LF et al. Effects of treating depression and low perceived social support on clinical events after myocardial infarction: the Enhancing Recovery in Coronary Heart Disease Patients (ENRICHD) Randomized Trial. JAMA 2003; 289:3106–16.
45. Dalton SO et al. Use of selective serotonin reuptake inhibitors and risk of upper gastrointestinal tract bleeding: a population-based cohort study. Arch Intern Med 2003; 163:59–64.

Further reading

Alvarez W et al. Safety of antidepressant drugs in the patient with cardiac disease. A review of the literature. Pharmacotherapy 2003; 23:754–71.
Roose SP. Treatment of depression in patients with heart disease. Biol Psychiatry 2003; 54:262–8.
Taylor D. Antidepressant drugs and cardiovascular pathology: a clinical overview of effectiveness and safety. Acta Psychiatr Scand 2008; 118:434–42.
Von Kanel R. Platelet hyperactivity in clinical depression and the beneficial effect of antidepressant drug treatment: how strong is the evidence? Acta Psychiatr Scand 2004; 110:163–77.

Antidepressant-induced arrhythmia

Depression confers an increased of risk of cardiovascular disease[1] and sudden cardiac death[2] perhaps because of platelet activation[3], decreased heart rate variability[4], reduced physical activity[5] and/or other factors.

Tricyclic antidepressants (TCAs) have established arrhythmogenic activity, which arises as a result of potent blockade of cardiac sodium channels and variable activity at potassium channels[6]. ECG changes produced include PR, QRS and QT prolongation and the Brugada syndrome[7]. In patients taking tricyclics, ECG monitoring is a more accurate and useful measure of toxicity than plasma level monitoring. Lofepramine, for reasons unknown, seems to lack the arrhythmogenicity of other TCAs.

There is limited evidence that venlafaxine is a sodium channel antagonist[8] and a weak antagonist at hERG potassium channels. Arrhythmia is a rare occurrence even after massive overdose[9–11] and ECG changes no more common than with SSRIs[12]. No ECG changes are seen in therapeutic dosing[13]. Moclobemide[14], citalopram[15,16], bupropion (amfebutamone)[17], trazodone[18,19] and sertraline[20], amongst others[1], have been reported to prolong the QTc interval in overdose but the clinical consequences of this are uncertain. QT changes are not usually seen at normal clinical doses[21]. There is clear evidence for the safety of sertraline[22] and mirtazapine[23] (and to a lesser extent, citalopram[23], fluoxetine[24] and bupropion[25]) in subjects at risk of arrhythmia due to recent myocardial infarction. Another study supports the safety of citalopram in patients with coronary artery disease[26] (although citalopram is strongly linked to a risk of torsades de pointes[27]).

Relative cardiotoxicity of antidepressants is difficult to establish with any precision. Yellow Card (ADROIT) data suggest that all marketed antidepressants are associated with arrhythmia (ranging from clinically insignificant to life-threatening) and sudden cardiac death. For a substantial proportion of drugs these figures are more likely to reflect coincidence rather than causation. The Fatal Toxicity Index (FTI) may provide some means for comparison. This is a measure of the number of overdose deaths per million (FP10) prescriptions issued. FTI figures suggest high toxicity for tricyclic drugs (especially dosulepin but not lofepramine), medium toxicity for venlafaxine and moclobemide, and low toxicity for SSRIs, mirtazapine and reboxetine[28–32]. However, FTI does not necessarily reflect only cardiotoxicity (antidepressants variously cause serotonin syndrome, seizures and coma) and is, in any case, open to other influences. This is best evidenced in the change in FTI over time. A good example here is nortriptyline, the FTI of which has been estimated at 0.6[16] and 39.2[12] and several values in between[28,29,31]. This change probably reflects changes in the type of patient prescribed nortriptyline. There is good evidence that venlafaxine is relatively more often prescribed to patients with more severe depression and who are relatively more likely to attempt suicide[33,34]. This is likely to inflate venlafaxine's FTI and erroneously suggest greater inherent toxicity. On the other hand, drugs with consistently low FTIs can probably be assumed to have very low risk of arrhythmias.

Depression & anxiety

Summary

- Sertraline is recommended post-MI, but other SSRIs and mirtazapine are also likely to be safe
- Bupropion, citalopram, moclobemide, lofepramine and venlafaxine should be used with caution or avoided in those at risk of serious arrhythmia (those with heart failure, left ventricular hypertrophy, previous arrhythmia or MI). An ECG should be performed at baseline and 1 week after every increase in dose
- TCAs (with the exception of lofepramine) are best avoided completely in patients at risk of serious arrhythmia. If use of a TCA cannot be avoided, an ECG should be performed at baseline, 1 week after each increase in dose and periodically throughout treatment. Frequency will be determined by the stability of the cardiac disorder and the TCA (and dose) being used; advice from cardiology should be sought
- The arrhythmogenic potential of TCAs and other antidepressants is dose-related. Consideration should be given to ECG monitoring of all patients prescribed doses towards the top of the licensed range and those who are prescribed other drugs that through pharmacokinetic (e.g. fluoxetine) or pharmacodynamic (e.g. diuretics) mechanisms may add to the risk posed by the TCA

References

1. Taylor D. Antidepressant drugs and cardiovascular pathology: a clinical overview of effectiveness and safety. Acta Psychiatr Scand 2008; 118:434–42.
2. Whang W et al. Depression and risk of sudden cardiac death and coronary heart disease in women: results from the Nurses' Health Study. J Am Coll Cardiol 2009; 53:950–8.
3. Ziegelstein RC et al. Platelet function in patients with major depression. Intern Med J 2009; 39:38–43.
4. Glassman AH et al. Heart rate variability in acute coronary syndrome patients with major depression: influence of sertraline and mood improvement. Arch Gen Psychiatry 2007; 64:1025–31.
5. Whooley MA et al. Depressive symptoms, health behaviors, and risk of cardiovascular events in patients with coronary heart disease. JAMA 2008; 300:2379–88.
6. Thanacoody HK et al. Tricyclic antidepressant poisoning: cardiovascular toxicity. Toxicol Rev 2005; 24:205–14.
7. Sicouri S et al. Sudden cardiac death secondary to antidepressant and antipsychotic drugs. Expert Opin Drug Saf 2008; 7:181–94.
8. Khalifa M et al. Mechanism of sodium channel block by venlafaxine in guinea pig ventricular myocytes. J Pharmacol Exp Ther 1999; 291:280–4.
9. Colbridge MG et al. Venlafaxine in overdose – expereince of the National Poisons Information Service (London centre). J Toxicol Clin Toxicol 1999; 37:383.
10. Blythe D et al. Cardiovascular and neurological toxicity of venlafaxine. Hum Exp Toxicol 1999; 18:309–13.
11. Combes A et al. Conduction disturbances associated with venlafaxine. Ann Intern Med 2001; 134:166–7.
12. Whyte IM et al. Relative toxicity of venlafaxine and selective serotonin reuptake inhibitors in overdose compared to tricyclic antidepressants. QJM 2003; 96:369–74.
13. Feighner JP. Cardiovascular safety in depressed patients: focus on venlafaxine. J Clin Psychiatry 1995; 56:574–9.
14. Downes MA et al. QTc abnormalities in deliberate self-poisoning with moclobemide. Intern Med J 2005; 35:388–91.
15. Kelly CA et al. Comparative toxicity of citalopram and the newer antidepressants after overdose. J Toxicol Clin Toxicol 2004; 42:67–71.
16. Grundemar L et al. Symptoms and signs of severe citalopram overdose. Lancet 1997; 349:1602.
17. Isbister GK et al. Bupropion overdose: QTc prolongation and its clinical significance. Ann Pharmacother 2003; 37:999–1002.
18. Service JA et al. QT Prolongation and delayed atrioventricular conduction caused by acute ingestion of trazodone. Clin Toxicol (Phila) 2008; 46:71–3.
19. Dattilo PB et al. Prolonged QT associated with an overdose of trazodone. J Clin Psychiatry 2007; 68:1309–10.
20. de Boer RA et al. QT interval prolongation after sertraline overdose: a case report. BMC Emerg Med 2005; 5:5.
21. van NC et al. Psychotropic drugs associated with corrected QT interval prolongation. J Clin Psychopharmacol 2009; 29:9–15.
22. Glassman AH et al. Sertraline treatment of major depression in patients with acute MI or unstable angina. JAMA 2002; 288:701–9.
23. van Melle JP et al. Effects of antidepressant treatment following myocardial infarction. Br J Psychiatry 2007; 190:460–6.
24. Strik JJ et al. Efficacy and safety of fluoxetine in the treatment of patients with major depression after first myocardial infarction: findings from a double-blind, placebo-controlled trial. Psychosom Med 2000; 62:783–9.
25. Rigotti NA et al. Bupropion for smokers hospitalized with acute cardiovascular disease. Am J Med 2006; 119:1080–7.
26. Lesperance F et al. Effects of citalopram and interpersonal psychotherapy on depression in patients with coronary artery disease: the Canadian Cardiac Randomized Evaluation of Antidepressant and Psychotherapy Efficacy (CREATE) trial. JAMA 2007; 297:367–79.
27. Astrom-Lilja C et al. Drug-induced torsades de pointes: a review of the Swedish pharmacovigilance database. Pharmacoepidemiol Drug Saf 2008; 17:587–92.
28. Crome P. The toxicity of drugs used for suicide. Acta Psychiatr Scand Suppl 1993; 371:33–7.
29. Cheeta S et al. Antidepressant-related deaths and antidepressant prescriptions in England and Wales, 1998–2000. Br J Psychiatry 2004; 184:41–7.
30. Buckley NA et al. Fatal toxicity of serotoninergic and other antidepressant drugs: analysis of United Kingdom mortality data. BMJ 2002; 325:1332–3.
31. Buckley NA et al. Greater toxicity in overdose of dothiepin than of other tricyclic antidepressants. Lancet 1994; 343:159–62.
32. Morgan O et al. Fatal toxicity of antidepressants in England and Wales, 1993–2002. Health Stat Q 2004; 18–24.
33. Egberts ACG et al. Channeling of three newly introduced antidepressants to patients not responding satisfactorily to previous treatment. J Clin Psychopharmacol 1997; 17:149–55.
34. Mines D et al. Prevalence of risk factors for suicide in patients prescribed venlafaxine, fluoxetine, and citalopram. Pharmacoepidemiol Drug Saf 2005; 14:367–72.

Depression & anxiety

Antidepressants and sexual dysfunction

Primary sexual disorders are common, although reliable normative data are lacking[1]. Reported prevalence rates vary depending on the method of data collection (low numbers with spontaneous reports, increasing with confidential questionnaires and further still with direct questioning)[1,2]. Physical illness, psychiatric illness, substance misuse and prescribed drug treatment can all cause sexual dysfunction[1,2]. Baseline sexual functioning should be determined, if possible (questionnaires may be useful), because sexual function can affect quality of life and compliance (sexual dysfunction is one of the major causes of treatment dropout[3]). Complaints of sexual dysfunction may also indicate progression or inadequate treatment of underlying medical or psychiatric conditions. It may also be the result of drug treatment and intervention may greatly improve quality of life[4].

Effects of depression

Both depression and the drugs used to treat it can cause disorders of desire, arousal and orgasm. The precise nature of the sexual dysfunction may indicate whether depression or treatment is the more likely cause. For example, 40–50% of people with depression report diminished libido and problems regarding sexual arousal in the month before diagnosis, compared with only 15–20% who experience orgasm problems before taking an antidepressant[5]. In general, the prevalence and severity of sexual dysfunction increases with the severity of depression[6]. In some patients reporting sexual dysfunction before or at diagnosis, sexual functioning improves on treatment with antidepressants[7]. In any cohort of people with depression there will be some who do not have sexual dysfunction and some, but not all, will develop sexual dysfunction on antidepressants. Amongst those presenting with sexual dysfunction, some will see an improvement, some no change and some a worsening when taking an antidepressant[8].

Effects of antidepressant drugs

Antidepressants can cause sedation, hormonal changes, disturbance of cholinergic/adrenergic balance, peripheral alpha-adrenergic antagonism, inhibition of nitric oxide and increased serotonin neurotransmission, all of which can result in sexual dysfunction[9]. Sexual dysfunction has been reported as a side effect of all antidepressants, although rates vary (see table below). The overall impact of antidepressants on sexual function is likely to be dose-dependent. Individual susceptibility also varies and may be at least partially genetically determined[10]. All effects are reversible.

Not all of the sexual side effects of antidepressants are undesirable[1]: serotonergic antidepressants including clomipramine are effective in the treatment of premature ejaculation[11] and may also be beneficial in paraphilias.

Sexual side effects can be minimised by careful selection of the antidepressant drug – see following table.

Table Sexual adverse effects of antidepressant drugs

Drug	Approximate prevalence	Type of problem
Tricyclics[12–15]	30%	Decreased libido, erectile dysfunction, delayed orgasm, impaired ejaculation. Prevalence of delayed orgasm with clomipramine may be at least double that with other TCAs. Painful ejaculation reported rarely
Trazodone[3,16–18]	Unknown	Impaired ejaculation and both increases and decreases in libido reported. Used in some cases to promote erection. Priapism occurs in approximately 0.01%
MAOIs[3,19]	40%	Similar to TCAs, although prevalence may be higher[1]. Moclobemide much less likely to cause problems than older MAOIs (4% v 40%)
SSRIs[3,20–23]	60–70%	Affects all phases of the sexual response; decreased libido and delayed orgasm most commonly reported[24]. Paroxetine is associated with more erectile dysfunction and decreased vaginal lubrication than the other SSRIs. Difficult to determine relative prevalence but there is evidence that ejaculatory delay is worse with paroxetine than citalopram[25] Penile and vaginal anaesthesia have been reported rarely with fluoxetine and other SSRIs[26]. Painful ejaculation reported rarely[27] as is priapism[28]
Venlafaxine[3]	70%	Decreased libido and delayed orgasm common. Erectile dysfunction less common. Rare reports of painful ejaculation[27] and priapism[28]
Mirtazapine[3,21]	25%	Decreased libido and delayed orgasm possible. Erectile dysfunction and absence of orgasm less common
Reboxetine[29]	5–10%	Various abnormalities of orgasmic function
Duloxetine[30]	46%	Any sexual dysfunction with a score ≥5 on the ASEX scale, with a statistical significance seen for the specific item 'ease of orgasm' in male patients

Treatment

A thorough assessment is essential to exclude physical causes such as diabetes and cardiovascular disease, and psychological and relationship difficulties. Spontaneous remission occurs in approximately 10% of cases and partial remission in a further 11%[3]. If this does not happen, the dose may be reduced or the antidepressant discontinued where appropriate.

Drug 'holidays' or delayed dosing may be used[31] as can dose reduction. This approach is problematic as the patient may relapse or experience antidepressant discontinuation symptoms. More logical is a switch to a different drug that is less likely to cause the specific sexual problem experienced (see table above). Note that amfebutamone (bupropion – not licensed for depression in UK) may have the lowest risk of sexual dysfunction[32,33], among newer antidepressants. It is widely used in the USA as a first-line antidepressant with minimal risk of sexual side effects, and as an adjunct (antidote) in patients with SSRI-induced sexual dysfunction[34]. Preliminary data support the reduction of sexual side effects in patients treated with duloxetine when mirtazapine is added[35].

Selegiline transdermal patches (licensed for the treatment of depression in the USA) seem to be associated with a low risk of sexual side-effects[36]. Agomelatine seems not to cause sexual adverse effects (see section on agomelatine).

Adjunctive or 'antidote' drugs may also be used (see section in this chapter for further information).

Sildenafil is more effective than placebo at improving erectile function in men[37], and in improving sexual function in women taking SSRIs[38].

A Cochrane review of the 'strategies for managing sexual dysfunction induced by antidepressant medication' found that the addition of sildenafil, tadalafil or bupropion may improve sexual function but that other augmentation strategies did not[39].

References

1. Baldwin DS et al. Effects of antidepressant drugs on sexual function. Int J Psychiatry Clin Pract 1997; 1:47–58.
2. Pollack MH et al. Genitourinary and sexual adverse effects of psychotropic medication. Int J Psychiatry Med 1992; 22:305–27.
3. Montejo AL et al. Incidence of sexual dysfunction associated with antidepressant agents: a prospective multicenter study of 1022 outpatients. Spanish Working Group for the Study of Psychotropic-Related Sexual Dysfunction. J Clin Psychiatry 2001; 62 Suppl 3:10–21.
4. Segraves RT. Effects of psychotropic drugs on human erection and ejaculation. Arch Gen Psychiatry 1989; 46:275–84.
5. Kennedy SH et al. Sexual dysfunction before antidepressant therapy in major depression. J Affect Disord 1999; 56:201–8.
6. Cheng JY et al. Depressive symptomatology and male sexual functions in late life. J Affect Disord 2007; 104:225–9.
7. Saiz-Ruiz J et al. Assessment of sexual functioning in depressed patients treated with mirtazapine: a naturalistic 6-month study. Hum Psychopharmacol 2005; 20:435–40.
8. Werneke U et al. Antidepressants and sexual dysfunction. Acta Psychiatr Scand 2006; 114:384–97.
9. Clayton AH. Recognition and assessment of sexual dysfunction associated with depression. J Clin Psychiatry 2001; 62 Suppl 3:5–9.
10. Bishop JR et al. Serotonin 2A -1438 G/A and G-protein Beta3 subunit C825T polymorphisms in patients with depression and SSRI-associated sexual side-effects. Neuropsychopharmacology 2006; 31:2281–8.
11. Waldinger MD. Premature ejaculation: definition and drug treatment. Drugs 2007; 67:547–68.
12. Harrison WM et al. Effects of antidepressant medication on sexual function: a controlled study. J Clin Psychopharmacol 1986; 6:144–9.
13. Beaumont G. Sexual side-effects of clomipramine (Anafranil). J Int Med Res 1977; 5:37–44.
14. Rickels K et al. Nefazodone: aspects of efficacy. J Clin Psychiatry 1995; 56 Suppl 6:43–6.
15. Sovner R. Anorgasmia associated with imipramine but not desipramine: case report. J Clin Psychiatry 1983; 44:345–6.
16. Gartrell N. Increased libido in women receiving trazodone. Am J Psychiatry 1986; 143:781–2.
17. Sullivan G. Increased libido in three men treated with trazodone. J Clin Psychiatry 1988; 49:202–3.
18. Thompson JW, Jr. et al. Psychotropic medication and priapism: a comprehensive review. J Clin Psychiatry 1990; 51:430–3.
19. Lesko LM et al. Three cases of female anorgasmia associated with MAOIs. Am J Psychiatry 1982; 139:1353–4.
20. Herman JB et al. Fluoxetine-induced sexual dysfunction. J Clin Psychiatry 1990; 51:25–7.
21. Gelenberg AJ et al. Mirtazapine substitution in SSRI-induced sexual dysfunction. J Clin Psychiatry 2000; 61:356–60.
22. Jacobsen FM. Fluoxetine-induced sexual dysfunction and an open trial of yohimbine. J Clin Psychiatry 1992; 53:119–22.
23. Lauerma H. Successful treatment of citalopram-induced anorgasmia by cyproheptadine. Acta Psychiatr Scand 1996; 93:69–70.
24. Demyttenaere K et al. Review: Bupropion and SSRI-induced side effects. J Psychopharmacol 2008; 22:792–804.
25. Waldinger MD et al. SSRIs and ejaculation: a double-blind, randomized, fixed-dose study with paroxetine and citalopram. J Clin Psychopharmacol 2001; 21:556–60.
26. Praharaj SK. Serotonin reuptake inhibitor induced sensory disturbances. Br J Clin Pharmacol 2004; 58:673–4.
27. Ilie CP et al. Painful ejaculation. BJU Int 2007; 99:1335–9.
28. Tran QT et al. Priapism, ecstasy, and marijuana: is there a connection? Adv Urol 2008; doi:10.1155/2008/193694.
29. Haberfellner EM. Sexual dysfunction caused by reboxetine. Pharmacopsychiatry 2002; 35:77–8.
30. Delgado PL et al. Sexual functioning assessed in 4 double-blind placebo- and paroxetine-controlled trials of duloxetine for major depressive disorder. J Clin Psychiatry 2005; 66:686–92.
31. Rothschild AJ. Selective serotonin reuptake inhibitor-induced sexual dysfunction: efficacy of a drug holiday. Am J Psychiatry 1995; 152:1514–16.
32. Clayton AH et al. Prevalence of sexual dysfunction among newer antidepressants. J Clin Psychiatry 2002; 63:357–66.
33. Clayton AH et al. Bupropion extended release compared with escitalopram: effects on sexual functioning and antidepressant efficacy in 2 randomized, double-blind, placebo-controlled studies. J Clin Psychiatry 2006; 67:736–46.
34. Balon R et al. Survey of treatment practices for sexual dysfunction(s) associated with anti-depressants. J Sex Marital Ther 2008; 34:353–65.
35. Ravindran LN et al. Combining mirtazapine and duloxetine in treatment-resistant depression improves outcomes and sexual function. J Clin Psychopharmacol 2008; 28:107–8.
36. Clayton AH et al. Symptoms of sexual dysfunction in patients treated for major depressive disorder: a meta-analysis comparing selegiline transdermal system and placebo using a patient-rated scale. J Clin Psychiatry 2007; 68:1860–6.
37. Fava M et al. Efficacy and safety of sildenafil in men with serotonergic antidepressant-associated erectile dysfunction: results from a randomized, double-blind, placebo-controlled trial. J Clin Psychiatry 2006; 67:240–6.
38. Nurnberg HG et al. Sildenafil treatment of women with antidepressant-associated sexual dysfunction: a randomized controlled trial. JAMA 2008; 300:395–404.
39. Rudkin L et al. Strategies for managing sexual dysfunction induced by antidepressant medication. Cochrane Database Syst Rev 2004;CD003382.

Depression & anxiety

Further reading

Fava M et al. Sexual functioning and SSRIs. J Clin Psychiatry 2002; 63 (Suppl 5):13–16.

Antidepressants and hyperprolactinaemia

Prolactin release is controlled by endogenous dopamine but is also indirectly modulated by serotonin via stimulation of $5HT_{1C}$ and $5HT_2$ receptors[1,2]. Increased plasma prolactin (with or without symptoms) is very occasionally seen with antidepressant use. Where antidepressant-induced hyperprolactinaemia does occur, rises in prolactin are usually small and short-lived and so symptoms are very rare. Routine monitoring of prolactin is not recommended but where symptoms suggest the possibility of hyperprolactinaemia then measurement of plasma prolactin is essential. Where symptomatic hyperprolactinaemia is confirmed, a switch to mirtazapine is recommended (see below).

Some details of associations between antidepressants and increased prolactin are given in the table below.

Table Reported associations between antidepressants and increased prolactin

Drug/group	Prospective studies	Case reports/series
Tricyclics	Small mean changes seen in some studies[3,4] but no changes in others[3,5]	Symptomatic hyperprolactinaemia reported with dosulepin[6] and clomipramine[7,8]
MAOIs	Small mean changes observed with phenelzine[3] and tranylcypromine[9]	None
SSRIs	Prospective studies largely show no change in prolactin[10–12]. Some evidence from prescription event monitoring that SSRIs are associated with higher risk of non-puerperal lactation[13]	Galactorrhoea reported with fluoxetine[14] and paroxetine[15]
SNRIs	Clear association observed between venlafaxine and prolactin elevation[16]	Galactorrhoea reported with venlafaxine[17] and duloxetine[18]
Reboxetine	Small, transient elevation of prolactin observed after reboxetine administration[19]	None
Mirtazapine	Strong evidence that mirtazapine has no effect on prolactin[20–22]	None
Bupropion	Single doses of up to 100 mg seem not to affect prolactin[23]	None

References

1. Emiliano AB et al. From galactorrhea to osteopenia: rethinking serotonin–prolactin interactions. Neuropsychopharmacology 2004; 29:833–46.
2. Rittenhouse PA et al. Neurons in the hypothalamic paraventricular nucleus mediate the serotonergic stimulation of prolactin secretion via 5-HT1c/2 receptors. Endocrinology 1993; 133:661–7.
3. Meltzer HY et al. Effect of antidepressants on neuroendocrine axis in humans. Adv Biochem Psychopharmacol 1982; 32:303–16.
4. Fava GA et al. Prolactin, cortisol, and antidepressant treatment. Am J Psychiatry 1988; 145:358–60.
5. Meltzer HY et al. Lack of effect of tricyclic antidepressants on serum prolactin levels. Psychopharmacology (Berl) 1977; 51:185–7.
6. Gadd EM et al. Antidepressants and galactorrhoea. Int Clin Psychopharmacol 1987; 2:361–3.
7. Anand VS. Clomipramine-induced galactorrhoea and amenorrhoea. Br J Psychiatry 1985; 147:87–8.
8. Fowlie S et al. Hyperprolactinaemia and nonpuerperal lactation associated with clomipramine. Scott Med J 1987; 32:52.
9. Price LH et al. Effects of tranylcypromine treatment on neuroendocrine, behavioral, and autonomic responses to tryptophan in depressed patients. Life Sci 1985; 37:809–18.
10. Sagud M et al. Effects of sertraline treatment on plasma cortisol, prolactin and thyroid hormones in female depressed patients. Neuropsychobiology 2002; 45:139–43.
11. Schlosser R et al. Effects of subchronic paroxetine administration on night-time endocrinological profiles in healthy male volunteers. Psychoneuroendocrinology 2000; 25:377–88.
12. Nadeem HS et al. Comparison of the effects of citalopram and escitalopram on 5-Ht-mediated neuroendocrine responses. Neuropsychopharmacology 2004; 29:1699–703.
13. Egberts AC et al. Non-puerperal lactation associated with antidepressant drug use. Br J Clin Pharmacol 1997; 44:277–81.
14. Peterson MC. Reversible galactorrhea and prolactin elevation related to fluoxetine. Mayo Clin Proc 2001; 76:215–16.
15. Morrison J et al. Galactorrhea induced by paroxetine. Can J Psychiatry 2001; 46:88–9.
16. Daffner-Bugia C et al. The neuroendocrine effects of venlafaxine in healthy subjects. Hum Psychopharmacol 1996; 11:1–9.
17. Sternbach H. Venlafaxine-induced galactorrhea. J Clin Psychopharmacol 2003; 23:109–10.
18. Ashton AK et al. Hyperprolactinemia and galactorrhea induced by serotonin and norepinephrine reuptake inhibiting antidepressants. Am J Psychiatry 2007; 164:1121–2.
19. Schule C et al. Reboxetine acutely stimulates cortisol, ACTH, growth hormone and prolactin secretion in healthy male subjects. Psychoneuroendocrinology 2004; 29:185–200.
20. Laakmann G et al. Effects of mirtazapine on growth hormone, prolactin, and cortisol secretion in healthy male subjects. Psychoneuroendocrinology 1999; 24:769–84.
21. Laakmann G et al. Mirtazapine: an inhibitor of cortisol secretion that does not influence growth hormone and prolactin secretion. J Clin Psychopharmacol 2000; 20:101–3.
22. Schule C et al. The influence of mirtazapine on anterior pituitary hormone secretion in healthy male subjects. Psychopharmacology (Berl) 2002; 163: 95–101.
23. Whiteman PD et al. Bupropion fails to affect plasma prolactin and growth hormone in normal subjects. Br J Clin Pharmacol 1982; 13:745.

Antidepressants – swapping and stopping

General guidelines
- All antidepressants have the potential to cause withdrawal phenomena[1]. When taken continuously *for 6 weeks or longer*, antidepressants should not be stopped abruptly unless a serious adverse event has occurred (e.g. cardiac arrhythmia with a tricyclic). (See section on discontinuation.)
- Although abrupt cessation is generally not recommended, slow tapering may not reduce the incidence or severity of discontinuation reactions[2]. Some patients may therefore prefer abrupt cessation and a shorter discontinuation syndrome.
- When changing from one antidepressant to another, abrupt withdrawal should usually be avoided. Cross-tapering is preferred, in which the dose of the ineffective or poorly tolerated drug is slowly reduced while the new drug is slowly introduced.

Example		*Week 1*	*Week 2*	*Week 3*	*Week 4*
Withdrawing dosulepin	150 mg OD	100 mg OD	50 mg OD	25 mg OD	Nil
Introducing citalopram	Nil	10 mg OD	10 mg OD	20 mg OD	20 mg OD

- The speed of cross-tapering is best judged by monitoring patient tolerability. No clear guidelines are available, so caution is required.
- Note that the co-administration of some antidepressants, even when cross-tapering, is absolutely contra-indicated. In other cases, theoretical risks or lack of experience preclude recommending cross-tapering.
- In some cases cross-tapering may not be considered necessary. An example is when switching from one SSRI to another: their effects are so similar that administration of the second drug is likely to ameliorate withdrawal effects of the first. In fact, the use of fluoxetine has been advocated as an abrupt switch treatment for SSRI discontinuation symptoms[3]. Abrupt cessation may also be acceptable when switching to a drug with a similar, but not identical, mode of action[4]. Thus, in some cases, abruptly stopping one antidepressant and starting another antidepressant at the usual dose may not only be well tolerated, but may also reduce the risk of discontinuation symptoms.
- Potential dangers of simultaneously administering two antidepressants include pharmacodynamic interactions (serotonin syndrome[5-8], hypotension, drowsiness) and pharmacokinetic interactions (e.g. elevation of tricyclic plasma levels by some SSRIs).

Serotonin syndrome – symptoms[5,6]	
Increasing severity	Restlessness Diaphoresis Tremor Shivering Myoclonus Confusion Convulsions Death

- The advice given in the following table should be treated with caution and patients should be very carefully monitored when switching.
- At the time of writing, no information is available on methods for switching to or from agomelatine[9]. Until information becomes available, it is recommended that prior antidepressants are stopped completely before starting agomelatine. Agomelatine should also be stopped completely before beginning another antidepressant. Given agomelatine's mode of action (melatonin agonism; $5HT_{2C}$ antagonism), it is not expected to mitigate discontinuation reactions of other antidepressants.

References

1. Taylor D et al. Antidepressant withdrawal symptoms-telephone calls to a national medication helpline. J Affect Disord 2006; 95:129–33.
2. Tint A et al. The effect of rate of antidepressant tapering on the incidence of discontinuation symptoms: a randomised study. J Psychopharmacol 2008; 22:330–2.
3. Benazzi F. Fluoxetine for the treatment of SSRI discontinuation syndrome. Int J Neuropsychopharmacol 2008; 11:725–6.
4. Perahia DG et al. Switching to duloxetine from selective serotonin reuptake inhibitor antidepressants: a multicenter trial comparing 2 switching techniques. J Clin Psychiatry 2008; 69:95–105.
5. Sternbach H. The serotonin syndrome. Am J Psychiatry 1991; 148:705–13.
6. Mir S et al. Serotonin syndrome. Psychiatr Bull 1999; 23:742–7.
7. Pan JJ et al. Serotonin syndrome induced by low-dose venlafaxine. Ann Pharmacother 2003; 37:209–11.
8. Houlihan DJ. Serotonin syndrome resulting from coadministration of tramadol, venlafaxine, and mirtazapine. Ann Pharmacother 2004; 38:411–13.
9. Dolder CR et al. Agomelatine treatment of major depressive disorder. The Annals of Pharmacotherapy 2008; 42:1822–31.

Depression & anxiety

215

Table Antidepressants – swapping and stopping*

To / From	MAOIs-hydrazines	Tranyl-cypromine[a]	Tricyclics	Citalopram/escitalopram	Fluoxetine	Paroxetine
MAOIs-hydrazines	Withdraw and wait for 2 weeks	Withdraw and wait for 2 weeks	Withdraw and wait for 2 weeks	Withdraw and wait for 2 weeks	Withdraw and wait for 2 weeks	Withdraw and wait for 2 weeks
Tranyl-cypromine	Withdraw and wait for 2 weeks		Withdraw and wait for 2 weeks	Withdraw and wait for 2 weeks	Withdraw and wait for 2 weeks	Withdraw and wait for 2 weeks
Tricyclics	Withdraw and wait for 1 week	Withdraw and wait for 1 week	Cross-taper cautiously	Halve dose and add citalopram, then slow withdrawal[c]	Halve dose and add fluoxetine, then slow withdrawal[c]	Halve dose and add paroxetine, then slow withdrawal[c]
Citalopram/escitalopram	Withdraw and wait for 1 week	Withdraw and wait for 1 week	Cross-taper cautiously[c]		Withdraw, then start fluoxetine at 10 mg/day	Withdraw, and start paroxetine at 10 mg/day
Paroxetine	Withdraw and wait for 2 weeks	Withdraw and wait for 1 week	Cross-taper cautiously with very low dose of tricyclic[c]	Withdraw and start citalopram	Withdraw, then start fluoxetine	
Fluoxetine[d]	Withdraw and wait 5–6 weeks	Withdraw and wait 5–6 weeks	Stop fluoxetine. Wait 4–7 days. Start tricyclic at very low dose and increase very slowly	Stop fluoxetine. Wait 4–7 days. Start citalopram at 10 mg/day and increase slowly		Stop fluoxetine. Wait 4–7 days, then start paroxetine 10 mg/day

*Note: Advice given in this table is partly derived from manufacturers' information and partly theoretical. Caution is required in every instance.

Sertraline	Trazodone	Moclobemide	Reboxetine	Venlafaxine	Mirtazapine	Duloxetine
Withdraw and wait for 2 weeks	Withdraw and wait for 2 weeks	Withdraw and wait for 2 weeks[b]	Withdraw and wait for 2 weeks	Withdraw and wait for 2 weeks	Withdraw and wait for 2 weeks	Withdraw and wait for 2 weeks
Withdraw and wait for 2 weeks	Withdraw and wait for 2 weeks	Withdraw and wait for 2 weeks[b]	Withdraw and wait for 2 weeks	Withdraw and wait for 2 weeks	Withdraw and wait for 2 weeks	Withdraw and wait for 2 weeks
Halve dose and add sertraline, then slow with-drawal[c]	Halve dose and add trazodone, then slow withdrawal	Withdraw and wait at least 1 week	Cross-taper cautiously	Cross-taper cautiously, starting with venlafaxine 37.5 mg/day	Cross-taper cautiously	Cross-taper cautiously, start at 60 mg alt die. Increase slowly
Withdraw, and start sertraline at 25 mg/day	Withdraw before starting titration of trazodone	Withdraw and wait at least 1 week	Cross-taper cautiously	Cross-taper cautiously. Start venlafaxine 37.5 mg/day and increase very slowly	Cross-taper cautiously	Abrupt switch possible. Start at 60 mg/day
Withdraw and start sertraline at 25 mg/day	Withdraw before starting titration of trazodone	Withdraw and wait for 1 week	Cross-taper cautiously	Cross-taper cautiously. Start venlafaxine 37.5 mg/day and increase very slowly	Cross-taper cautiously	Abrupt switch possible. Start at 60 mg/day
Stop fluoxetine. Wait 4–7 days, then start sertraline 25 mg/day	Stop fluoxetine. Wait 4–7 days then start low-dose trazodone	Withdraw and wait at least 5 weeks	Withdraw. Start reboxetine at 2 mg bd and increase cautiously	Withdraw. Start venlafaxine at 37.5 mg/day. Increase very slowly	Withdraw, wait 4–7 days and start mirtazapine cautiously	Abrupt switch possible. Start at 60 mg/day

Table Antidepressants – swapping and stopping* (Cont.)

To From	MAOIs-hydrazines	Tranyl-cypromine[a]	Tricyclics	Citalopram/escitalopram	Fluoxetine	Paroxetine
Sertraline	Withdraw and wait for 2 weeks[b]	Withdraw and wait for 2 weeks	Cross-taper cautiously with very low dose of tricyclic[c]	Withdraw, then start citalopram	Withdraw, then start fluoxetine	Withdraw, then start paroxetine
Trazodone	Withdraw and wait at least 1 week	Withdraw and wait at least 1 week	Cross- taper cautiously with very low dose of tricyclic	Withdraw, then start citalopram	Withdraw, then start fluoxetine	Withdraw, then start paroxetine
Moclobemide	Withdraw and wait 24 hours	Withdraw and wait 24 hours	Withdraw and wait 24 hours	Withdraw and wait 24 hours	Withdraw and wait 24 hours	Withdraw and wait 24 hours
Reboxetine	Withdraw and wait at least 1 week	Withdraw and wait at least 1 week	Cross-taper cautiously	Cross-taper cautiously	Cross-taper cautiously	Cross-taper cautiously
Venlafaxine	Withdraw and wait at least 1 week	Withdraw and wait at least 1 week	Cross-taper cautiously with very low dose of tricyclic[c]	Cross-taper cautiously. Start with 10 mg/day	Cross-taper cautiously. Start with 20 mg every other day	Cross-taper cautiously. Start with 10 mg/day
Mirtazapine	Withdraw and wait for 1 week	Withdraw and wait for 1 week	Withdraw, then start tricyclic	Withdraw, then start citalopram	Withdraw, then start fluoxetine	Withdraw, then start paroxetine
Duloxetine	Withdraw and wait at least 5 days	Withdraw and wait at least 5 days	Cross-taper cautiously with very low dose of tricyclic	Withdraw, then start citalopram	Withdraw, then start fluoxetine	Withdraw, then start paroxetine
Stopping[e]	Reduce over 4 weeks	Reduce over 4 weeks	Reduce over 4 weeks	Reduce over 4 weeks	At 20mg/ day, just stop At 40mg/day, reduce over 2 weeks	Reduce over 4 weeks or longer, if necessary[f]

Notes

[a] SPC for tranylcypromine suggests at least 1-week gap between cessation of prior drug and starting tranylcypromine.

[b] Abrupt switching is possible but not recommended.

[c] Do not co-administer clomipramine and SSRIs or venlafaxine. Withdraw clomipramine before starting.

[d] Beware: interactions with fluoxetine may still occur for 5 weeks after stopping fluoxetine because of its long half-life.

[e] See general guidelines at beginning of this section.

[f] Withdrawal effects seem to be more pronounced. Slow withdrawal over 1–3 months may be necessary. Some patients may prefer abrupt withdrawal (to shorten overall duration of discontinuation effects).

Sertraline	Trazodone	Moclobemide	Reboxetine	Venlafaxine	Mirtazapine	Duloxetine
	Withdraw before starting trazodone	Withdraw and wait at least 2 weeks	Cross-taper cautiously	Cross-taper cautiously. Start venlafaxine at 37.5 mg/day	Cross-taper cautiously	Abrupt switch possible. Start at 60 mg/day
Withdraw, then start sertraline		Withdraw and wait at least 1 week	Withdraw, start reboxetine at 2 mg bd and increase cautiously	Cross-taper cautiously. Start venlafaxine at 37.5 mg/day	Cross-taper cautiously	Withdraw, start at 60 mg alt die. Increase slowly
Withdraw and wait 24 hours	Withdraw and wait 24 hours		Withdraw and wait 24 hours	Withdraw and wait 24 hours	Withdraw and wait 24 hours	Withdraw and wait 24 hours
Cross-taper cautiously	Cross-taper cautiously	Withdraw and wait at least 1 week		Cross-taper cautiously	Cross-taper cautiously	Cross-taper cautiously
Cross-taper cautiously. Start with 25 mg/day	Cross-taper cautiously	Withdraw and wait at least 1 week	Cross-taper cautiously		Cross-taper cautiously	Withdraw, start at 60 mg alt die. Increase slowly
Withdraw, then start sertraline	Withdraw, then start trazodone	Withdraw and wait 1 week	Withdraw. then start reboxetine	Cross-taper cautiously		Withdraw, start at 60 mg alt die. Increase slowly
Withdraw, then start sertraline	Withdraw, then start trazodone	Withdraw and wait 1 week	Cross-taper cautiously	Withdraw, then start venlafaxine	Withdraw, then start mirtazapine	
Reduce over 4 weeks	Reduce over 4 weeks	Reduce over 4 weeks	Reduce over 4 weeks	Reduce over 4 weeks or longer, if necessary[f]	Reduce over 4 weeks	Reduce over 4 weeks

Depression & anxiety

219

Antidepressant discontinuation symptoms

What are discontinuation symptoms?

The term 'discontinuation symptoms' is used to describe symptoms experienced on stopping prescribed drugs that are not drugs of dependence. There is an important semantic difference between 'discontinuation' and 'withdrawal' symptoms – the latter implies addiction; the former does not. While this distinction is important for precise medical terminology, it may be irrelevant to patient experience. Discontinuation symptoms may occur after stopping many drugs, including antidepressants, and can sometimes be explained in the context of 'receptor rebound'[1,2] – e.g. an antidepressant with potent anticholinergic side effects may be associated with diarrhoea on discontinuation.

Discontinuation symptoms may be entirely new or similar to some of the original symptoms of the illness, and so cannot be attributed to other causes. They can be broadly divided into six categories; affective (e.g. irritability); gastrointestinal (e.g. nausea); neuromotor (e.g. ataxia); vasomotor (e.g. diaphoresis); neurosensory (e.g. paraesthesia) and; other neurological (e.g. increase dreaming)[2]. Discontinuation symptoms are experienced by at least a third of patients[3–5] and are seen to some extent with all antidepressants[6].

The onset is usually within 5 days of stopping treatment (depending on the half-life of the antidepressant) or occasionally during taper or after missed doses[7,8] (short-half-life drugs only). Symptoms can vary in form and intensity and occur in any combination. They are usually mild and self-limiting, but can occasionally be severe and prolonged. The perception of symptom severity is probably made worse by the absence of forewarnings. Some symptoms are more likely with individual drugs (see below table). Symptoms can be quantified using the discontinuation-emergent signs and symptoms (DESS) scale[4].

Table	Antidepressant discontinuation symptoms		
	MAOIs	*TCAs*	*SSRIs and related*
Symptoms	*Common* Agitation, irritability, ataxia, movement disorders, insomnia, somnolence, vivid dreams, cognitive impairment, slowed speech, pressured speech	*Common* Flu-like symptoms (chills, myalgia, excessive sweating, headache, nausea), insomnia, excessive dreaming	*Common* Flu-like symptoms, 'shock-like' sensations, dizziness exacerbated by movement, insomnia, excessive (vivid) dreaming, irritability, crying spells
	Occasionally Hallucinations, paranoid delusions	*Occasionally* Movement disorders, mania, cardiac arrhythmia	*Occasionally* Movement disorders, problems with concentration and memory
Drugs most commonly associated with discontinuation symptoms	All Tranylcypromine is partly metabolised to amfetamine and is therefore associated with a true 'withdrawal syndrome'	Amitriptyline Imipramine	Paroxetine Venlafaxine
Early data from one RCT suggest that agomelatine is associated with low, if any, risk of discontinuation symptoms[9].			

Depression & anxiety

Clinical relevance[10]

The symptoms of a discontinuation reaction may be mistaken for a relapse of illness or the emergence of a new physical illness[11] leading to unnecessary investigations or reintroduction of the antidepressant. Symptoms may be severe enough to interfere with daily functioning and those who have experienced discontinuation symptoms may reason (perhaps appropriately) that antidepressants are 'addictive' and not wish to accept treatment. There is also evidence of emergent suicidal thoughts on discontinuation with paroxetine[12]

Who is most at risk?[11,13,14]

Although anyone can experience discontinuation symptoms, the risk is increased in those prescribed short-half-life drugs[4,7,15–17] (e.g. paroxetine, venlafaxine), particularly if they do not take them regularly. Two-thirds of patients prescribed antidepressants may skip a few doses from time to time[18], and many patients stop their antidepressant abruptly[3]. The risk is also increased in those who have been taking antidepressants for 8 weeks or longer[19], those who have developed anxiety symptoms at the start of antidepressant therapy (particularly with SSRIs), those receiving other centrally acting medication (e.g. antihypertensives, antihistamines, antipsychotics), children and adolescents, and those who have experienced discontinuation symptoms before.

Antidepressant discontinuation symptoms are common in neonates born to woman taking antidepressants. See pregnancy section in Chapter 7.

How to avoid[11,13,15]

Generally, antidepressant therapy should be discontinued over at least a 4-week period (this is not required with fluoxetine)[7]. The shorter the half-life of the drug, the more important that this rule is followed. The end of the taper may need to be slower, as symptoms may not appear until the reduction in the total daily dosage of the antidepressant is (proportionately) substantial. Patients receiving MAOIs may need to be tapered over a longer period. Tranylcypromine may be particularly difficult to stop. At-risk patients (see above) may need a slower taper.

Many people suffer symptoms despite slow withdrawal and even if they have received adequate education regarding discontinuation symptoms[12,17]. For these patients the option of abrupt withdrawal should be discussed. Some may prefer to face a week or two of intense symptoms rather than months of less severe discontinuation syndrome.

How to treat[10,11]

There are few systematic studies in this area. Treatment is pragmatic. If symptoms are mild, reassure the patient that these symptoms are common after discontinuing an antidepressant and will pass in a few days. If symptoms are severe, reintroduce the original antidepressant (or another with a longer half-life from the same class) and taper gradually while monitoring for symptoms.

Some evidence supports the use of anticholinergic agents in tricyclic withdrawal[20] and fluoxetine for symptoms associated with stopping clomipramine[21] or venlafaxine[22] – fluoxetine, having a longer plasma half-life, seems to be associated with a lower incidence of discontinuation symptoms than other similar drugs[23].

Key points that patients should know

*   Antidepressants are not addictive (a survey of nearly 2000 people across the UK conducted in 1997 found that 74% thought that antidepressants were addictive[24]). It is important to dispel this myth. In order for a drug to be addictive it must also fulfil certain other criteria including tolerance, escalating use, etc. This should be discussed. Note, however, that this semantic and categorical distinction may be lost on many people.

- Patients should be informed that they may experience discontinuation symptoms (and the most likely symptoms associated with the drug that they are taking) when they stop their antidepressant.
- Antidepressants should not be stopped abruptly. The dose should be tapered over at least 4 weeks. Fluoxetine is an exception to this rule[7]. Abrupt cessation may be necessary in those suffering symptoms on prolonged taper.
- Discontinuation symptoms may occur after missed doses if the antidepressant prescribed has a short half-life. A very few patients may experience pre-dose discontinuation symptoms which provoke the taking of the antidepressant at an earlier time each day.

References

1. Blier P et al. Physiologic mechanisms underlying the antidepressant discontinuation syndrome. J Clin Psychiatry 2006; 67 Suppl 4:8–13.
2. Delgado PL. Monoamine depletion studies: implications for antidepressant discontinuation syndrome. J Clin Psychiatry 2006; 67 Suppl 4:22–6.
3. van Geffen EC et al. Discontinuation symptoms in users of selective serotonin reuptake inhibitors in clinical practice: tapering versus abrupt discontinuation. Eur J Clin Pharmacol 2005; 61:303–7.
4. Fava M. Prospective studies of adverse events related to antidepressant discontinuation. J Clin Psychiatry 2006; 67 Suppl 4:14–21.
5. Perahia DG et al. Symptoms following abrupt discontinuation of duloxetine treatment in patients with major depressive disorder. J Affect Disord 2005; 89:207–12.
6. Taylor D et al. Antidepressant withdrawal symptoms-telephone calls to a national medication helpline. J Affect Disord 2006; 95:129–33.
7. Rosenbaum JF et al. Selective serotonin reuptake inhibitor discontinuation syndrome: a randomized clinical trial. Biol Psychiatry 1998; 44:77–87.
8. Michelson D et al. Interruption of selective serotonin reuptake inhibitor treatment. Double-blind, placebo-controlled trial. Br J Psychiatry 2000; 176:363–8.
9. Montgomery SA et al. Absence of discontinuation symptoms with agomelatine and occurrence of discontinuation symptoms with paroxetine: a randomized, double-blind, placebo-controlled discontinuation study. Int Clin Psychopharmacol 2004; 19:271–80.
10. Lejoyeux M et al. Antidepressant withdrawal syndrome: recognition, prevention and management. CNS Drugs 1996; 5:278–92.
11. Haddad PM. Antidepressant discontinuation syndromes. Drug Saf 2001; 24:183–97.
12. Tint A et al. The effect of rate of antidepressant tapering on the incidence of discontinuation symptoms: a randomised study. J Psychopharmacol 2008; 22:330–2.
13. Lejoyeux M et al. Antidepressant withdrawal syndrome: recognition, prevention and management. CNS Drugs 1996; 5:278–92.
14. Anon. Antidepressant discontinuation syndrome: update on serotonin reuptake inhibitors. J Clin Psychiatry 1997; 58 (Suppl 7):3–40.
15. Sir A et al. Randomized trial of sertraline versus venlafaxine XR in major depression: efficacy and discontinuation symptoms. J Clin Psychiatry 2005; 66:1312–20.
16. Baldwin DS et al. A double-blind, randomized, parallel-group, flexible-dose study to evaluate the tolerability, efficacy and effects of treatment discontinuation with escitalopram and paroxetine in patients with major depressive disorder. Int Clin Psychopharmacol 2006; 21:159–69.
17. Fava GA et al. Effects of gradual discontinuation of selective serotonin reuptake inhibitors in panic disorder with agoraphobia. Int J Neuropsychopharmacol 2007; 10:835–8.
18. Meijer WE et al. Spontaneous lapses in dosing during chronic treatment with selective serotonin reuptake inhibitors. Br J Psychiatry 2001; 179:519–22.
19. Kramer JC et al. Withdrawal symptoms following dicontinuation of imipramine therapy. Am J Psychiatry 1961; 118:549–50.
20. Dilsaver SC et al. Antidepressant withdrawal symptoms treated with anticholinergic agents. Am J Psychiatry 1983; 140:249–51.
21. Benazzi F. Fluoxetine for clomipramine withdrawal symptoms. Am J Psychiatry 1999; 156:661–2.
22. Giakas WJ et al. Intractable withdrawal from venlafaxine treated with fluoxetine. Psychiatr Ann 1997; 27:85–93.
23. Coupland NJ et al. Serotonin reuptake inhibitor withdrawal. J Clin Psychopharmacol 1996; 16:356–62.
24. Paykel ES et al. Changes in public attitudes to depression during the Defeat Depression Campaign. Br J Psychiatry 1998; 173:519–22.

Further reading

Blier P et al. Physiologic mechanisms underlying the antidepressant discontinuation syndrome. J Clin Psychiatry 2006; 67 Suppl 4:8–13.
Haddad PM et al. Recognising and managing antidepressant discontinuation symptoms. Adv Psychiatr Treat 2007; 13:447–57.
Schatzberg AF et al. Antidepressant discontinuation syndrome: consensus panel recommendations for clinical management and additional research. J Clin Psychiatry 2006; 67 Suppl 4:27–30.
Shelton RC. The nature of the discontinuation syndrome associated with antidepressant drugs. J Clin Psychiatry 2006; 67 Suppl 4:3–7.

St John's Wort

St John's Wort (SJW) is the popular name for the plant *Hypericum perforatum*. It contains a combination of at least ten different components, including hypericins, flavonoids and xanthons[1]. Preparations of SJW are often unstandardised and this has complicated the interpretation of clinical trials.

The active ingredient(s) and mechanism(s) of action of SJW are unclear. Constituents of SJW may inhibit MAO[2], inhibit the re-uptake of norepinephrine and serotonin[3], up-regulate serotonin receptors[3] and decrease serotonin receptor expression[4].

Some preparations of SJW have been granted a traditional herbal registration certificate; note that this is based on traditional use rather than proven efficacy and tolerability. SJW is licensed in Germany for the treatment of depression.

Evidence for SJW in the treatment of depression
A number of trials have been published that examined the efficacy of SJW in the treatment of depression. They have been extensively reviewed[5–7] and most authors conclude[4,9] that SJW is likely to be effective in the treatment of dysthymia[8] and mild-to-moderate depression. Cochrane concludes that SJW is more effective than placebo in the treatment of mild–moderate depression, and is as effective as, and better tolerated than, standard antidepressants[7]. Studies concluded in German-speaking countries showed more favourable results than studies concluded elsewhere. Efficacy in severe depression remains uncertain[7].

It should be noted that:

- The active component of SJW for treating depression has not yet been determined. The trials used different preparations of SJW which were standardised according to their total content of hypericins. However, evidence suggests that hypericins alone do not treat depression[10].
- Published studies are generally acute treatment studies. There are fewer data to support the effectiveness of SJW in the medium term[11] or for prophylaxis[12].

On balance, SJW should not be prescribed: we lack understanding of what the active ingredient is or what constitutes a therapeutic dose. Most preparations of SJW are unlicensed.

Adverse effects
SJW appears to be well tolerated. Pooled data from 35 RCTS show that drop-out rates and adverse effects were less than with older antidepressants, slightly less than SSRIs and similar to placebo[13]. The most common, if infrequent, side effects are dry mouth, nausea, constipation, fatigue, dizziness, headache and restlessness[14–17]. In addition, SJW contains a red pigment that can cause photosensitivity reactions[18]. It has been suggested that hypericin may be phototoxic to the retina, and contribute to the early development of macular degeneration[19]. SJW may also share the propensity of SSRIs to increase the risk of bleeding; a case report describes prolonged epistaxis after nasal insertion of SJW[20]. In common with other antidepressant drugs, SJW has been known to precipitate hypomania in people with bipolar affective disorder[21].

Drug interactions
SJW is an inducer of intestinal and hepatic CYP3A4, CYP2C and intestinal p-glycoprotein[22–24]; hyperforin is responsible for this effect[25]. The hyperforin content of SJW preparations varies 50-fold, which will result in a different propensity for drug interactions between brands. CYP3A4 activity returns to normal approximately 7 days after SJW is discontinued[26].

Studies have shown that SJW significantly reduces plasma concentrations of digoxin and indinavir[27,28] (a drug used in the treatment of HIV). According to a number of case reports, SJW has lowered the plasma concentrations of theophylline, cyclosporin, warfarin, gliclazide, atorvastatin and the combined oral contraceptive pill and has led to treatment failure[24,29,30]. There is a theoretical risk that SJW may interact with some anticonvulsant drugs[31]. Serotonin syndrome has been reported when SJW was taken together with sertraline, paroxetine, nefazodone and the triptans[31,32] (a group of serotonin agonists used to treat migraine). SJW should not be taken with any drugs that have a predominantly serotonergic action.

Key points that patients should know

- Evidence suggests that SJW may be effective in the treatment of mild-to-moderate depression, but we do not know enough about how much should be taken or what the side effects are. There is less evidence of benefit in severe depression.
- Most preparations of SJW are unlicensed.
- SJW can interact with other medicines, resulting in serious side effects. Some important drugs may be metabolised more rapidly and therefore become ineffective with serious consequences (e.g. increased viral load in HIV, failure of oral contraceptives leading to unwanted pregnancy, reduced anticoagulant effect with warfarin leading to thrombosis).
- The symptoms of depression can sometimes be caused by other physical or mental illness. It is important that these possible causes are investigated.
- It is always best to consult the doctor if any herbal or natural remedy is being taken or the patient is thinking of taking one.

Many people regard herbal remedies as 'natural' and therefore harmless[33]. Many are not aware of the potential of such remedies for causing side effects or interacting with other drugs. A large study from Germany (n = 588), where SJW is a licensed antidepressant, found that for every prescription written for SJW, one person purchased SJW without seeking the advice of a doctor[34]. Many of these people had severe or persistent depression and few told their doctor that they took SJW. A small US study (n = 22) found that people tend to take SJW because it is easy to obtain alternative medicines and also because they perceive herbal medicines as being purer and safer than prescription medicines. Few would discuss this medication with their conventional health-care provider[17]. Clinicians need to be proactive in asking patients if they use such treatments and try to dispel the myth that natural is the same as safe.

References

1. Linde K et al. St John's wort for depression: meta-analysis of randomised controlled trials. Br J Psychiatry 2005; 186:99–107.
2. Cott JM. In vitro receptor binding and enzyme inhibition by *Hypericum perforatum* extract. Pharmacopsychiatry 1997; 30 Suppl 2:108–12.
3. Muller WE et al. Effects of *Hypericum* extract (LI 160) in biochemical models of antidepressant activity. Pharmacopsychiatry 1997; 30 Suppl 2:102–7.
4. Kasper S et al. Superior efficacy of St John's wort extract WS 5570 compared to placebo in patients with major depression: a randomized, double-blind, placebo-controlled, multi-center trial [ISRCTN77277298]. BMC Med 2006; 4:14.
5. Linde K et al. St John's wort for depression: meta-analysis of randomised controlled trials. Br J Psychiatry 2005; 186:99–107.
6. National Institute of Clinical Excellence. Depression: management of depression in primary and secondary care – clinical guidance. http://www.nice.org.uk. 2004.
7. Linde K et al. St John's Wort for major depression. Cochrane Database Syst Rev 2008;CD000448.
8. Randlov C et al. The efficacy of St. John's Wort in patients with minor depressive symptoms or dysthymia – a double-blind placebo-controlled study. Phytomedicine 2006; 13:215–21.
9. Kasper S et al. Efficacy of St. John's wort extract WS 5570 in acute treatment of mild depression: a reanalysis of data from controlled clinical trials. Eur Arch Psychiatry Clin Neurosci 2008; 258:59–63.
10. Teufel-Mayer R et al. Effects of long-term administration of *Hypericum* extracts on the affinity and density of the central serotonergic 5-HT1 A and 5-HT2 A receptors. Pharmacopsychiatry 1997; 30 Suppl 2:113–16.
11. Anghelescu IG et al. Comparison of *Hypericum* extract WS 5570 and paroxetine in ongoing treatment after recovery from an episode of moderate to severe depression: results from a randomized multicenter study. Pharmacopsychiatry 2006; 39:213–19.
12. Kasper S et al. Continuation and long-term maintenance treatment with Hypericum extract WS 5570 after recovery from an acute episode of moderate depression – a double-blind, randomized, placebo controlled long-term trial. Eur Neuropsychopharmacol 2008; 18:803–13.
13. Knuppel L et al. Adverse effects of St. John's Wort: a systematic review. J Clin Psychiatry 2004; 65:1470–9.
14. Volz HP. Controlled clinical trials of *Hypericum* extracts in depressed patients – an overview. Pharmacopsychiatry 1997; 30 Suppl 2:72–6.
15. Gaster B et al. St John's Wort for depression: a systematic review. Arch Intern Med 2000; 160:152–6.
16. Woelk H. Comparison of St John's Wort and imipramine for treating depression: randomised controlled trial. BMJ 2000; 321:536–9.
17. Wagner PJ et al. Taking the edge off: why patients choose St. John's Wort. J Fam Pract 1999; 48:615–19.
18. Bove GM. Acute neuropathy after exposure to sun in a patient treated with St John's Wort. Lancet 1998; 352:1121–2.

19. Wielgus AR et al. Phototoxicity in human retinal pigment epithelial cells promoted by hypericin, a component of St. John's wort. Photochem Photobiol 2007; 83:706–13.
20. Crampsey DP et al. Nasal insertion of St John's wort: an unusual cause of epistaxis. J Laryngol Otol 2007; 121:279–80.
21. Nierenberg AA et al. Mania associated with St. John's wort. Biol Psychiatry 1999; 46:1707–8.
22. Singh YN. Potential for interaction of kava and St. John's wort with drugs. J Ethnopharmacol 2005; 100:108–13.
23. Ernst E. Second thoughts about safety of St John's wort. Lancet 1999; 354:2014–16.
24. Xu H et al. Effects of St John's wort and CYP2C9 genotype on the pharmacokinetics and pharmacodynamics of gliclazide. Br J Pharmacol 2008; 153:1579–86.
25. Madabushi R et al. Hyperforin in St. John's wort drug interactions. Eur J Clin Pharmacol 2006; 62:225–33.
26. Imai H et al. The recovery time-course of CYP3A after induction by St John's wort administration. Br J Clin Pharmacol 2008; 65:701–7.
27. Johne A et al. Pharmacokinetic interaction of digoxin with an herbal extract from St John's wort (*Hypericum perforatum*). Clin Pharmacol Ther 1999; 66:338–45.
28. Piscitelli SC et al. Indinavir concentrations and St John's wort. Lancet 2000; 355:547–8.
29. Ernst E. Second thoughts about safety of St John's wort. Lancet 1999; 354:2014–16.
30. Andren L et al. Interaction between a commercially available St. John's wort product (Movina) and atorvastatin in patients with hypercholesterolemia. Eur J Clin Pharmacol 2007; 63:913–16.
31. Anon. Reminder: St John's wort (*Hypericum perforatum*) interactions. Curr Prob Pharmacovigilance 2000; 26:6.
32. Lantz MS et al. St. John's wort and antidepressant drug interactions in the elderly. J Geriatr Psychiatry Neurol 1999; 12:7–10.
33. Barnes J et al. Different standards for reporting ADRs to herbal remedies and conventional OTC medicines: face-to-face interviews with 515 users of herbal remedies. Br J Clin Pharmacol 1998; 45:496–500.
34. Linden M et al. Self medication with St. John's wort in depressive disorders: an observational study in community pharmacies. J Affect Disord 2008; 107:205–10.

Further reading

Mills E et al. Interaction of St John's Wort with conventional drugs: systematic review of clinical trials. BMJ 2004; 329:27–30.
Werneke U et al. How effective is St John's Wort? The evidence revisited. J Clin Psychiatry 2004; 65:611–617.

Depression & anxiety

Drug interactions with antidepressants

Drugs can interact with each other in two different ways:

- Pharmacokinetic interactions, where one drug interferes with the absorption, distribution, metabolism or elimination of another drug. This may result in subtherapeutic effect or toxicity. The largest group of pharmacokinetic interactions involves drugs that inhibit or induce hepatic CYP450 enzymes (see the table opposite). Other enzyme systems include FMO[1] and UGT[2]. While both of these latter enzyme systems are involved in the metabolism of psychotropic drugs, the potential for drugs to inhibit or induce these enzyme systems has been poorly studied.

  The clinical consequences of pharmacokinetic interactions in an individual patient can be difficult to predict. The following factors affect outcome of interactions: the degree of enzyme inhibition or induction, the pharmacokinetic properties of the affected drug and other co-administered drugs, the relationship between plasma level and pharmacodynamic effect for the affected drug, and patient-specific factors such as variability in the role of primary and secondary metabolic pathways and the presence of co-morbid physical illness[3].

- Pharmacodynamic interactions, where the effects of one drug are altered by another drug via physiological mechanisms such as direct competition at receptor sites (e.g. dopamine agonists with dopamine blockers negate any therapeutic effect), augmentation of the same neurotransmitter pathway (e.g. fluoxetine with tramadol can lead to serotonin syndrome) or an effect on the physiological functioning of an organ/organ system in different ways (e.g. two different antiarrhythmic drugs). Most of these interactions can be easily predicted by a sound knowledge of pharmacology. An up-to-date list of important interactions can be found at the back of the BNF.

Pharmacodynamic interactions
Tricyclic antidepressants[4,5]:

- are H$_1$ blockers (sedative). This effect can be exacerbated by other sedative drugs or alcohol. Beware respiratory depression
- are anticholinergic (dry mouth, blurred vision, constipation). This effect can be exacerbated by other anticholinergic drugs such as antihistamines or antipsychotics. Beware cognitive impairment and GI obstruction
- are adrenergic α_1 blockers (postural hypotension). This effect can be exacerbated by other drugs that block α_1-receptors and by antihypertensive drugs in general. Epinephrine in combination with α_1-blockers can lead to hypertension
- are arrhythmogenic. Caution is required with other drugs that can alter cardiac conduction directly (e.g. antiarrhythmics or phenothiazines) or indirectly through a potential to cause electrolyte disturbance (e.g. diuretics)
- lower the seizure threshold. Caution is required with other proconvulsive drugs (e.g. antipsychotics) and particularly if the patient is being treated for epilepsy (higher doses of anticonvulsants may be required)
- may be serotonergic (e.g. amitriptyline, clomipramine). There is the potential for these drugs to interact with other serotonergic drugs (e.g. tramadol, SSRIs, selegiline) to cause serotonin syndrome.

(Cont.)

Table Pharmacokinetic interactions[6-11]

p4501A2 *Genetic polymorphism* *Ultra-rapid metabolisers occur*	p4502C *5–10% of* *Caucasians poor* *metabolisers*	p4502D6 *3–5% of* *Caucasians poor* *metabolisers*	p4503A *60% p450* *content*
Induced by: cigarette smoke charcoal cooking carbamazepine omeprazole phenobarbitone phenytoin	*Induced by:* phenytoin rifampicin	*Induced by:* carbamazepine phenytoin	*Induced by:* carbamazepine phenytoin prednisolone rifampicin
Inhibited by: cimetidine ciprofloxacin erythromycin fluvoxamine paroxetine	*Inhibited by:* cimetidine fluoxetine fluvoxamine sertraline	*Inhibited by:* chlorpromazine duloxetine fluoxetine fluphenazine haloperidol paroxetine sertraline (?) tricyclics	*Inhibited by:* erythromycin norfluoxetine fluvoxamine ketoconazole paroxetine sertraline (?) tricyclics
Metabolises: agomelatine caffeine clozapine haloperidol mirtazapine olanzapine theophylline tricyclics warfarin	*Metabolises:* agomelatine diazepam omeprazole phenytoin tolbutamide tricyclics warfarin	*Metabolises:* clozapine codeine donepezil haloperidol phenothiazines risperidone TCA-secondary amines tramadol trazodone venlafaxine	*Metabolises:* benzodiazepines calcium blockers carbamazepine cimetidine clozapine codeine donepezil erythromycin galantamine methadone mirtazapine risperidone steroids terfenadine tricyclics valproate venlafaxine Z-hypnotics

Depression & anxiety

(Cont.)

SSRIs[7,12,13]:

- increase serotonergic neurotransmission. The main concern is serotonin syndrome
- inhibit platelet aggregation and increase the risk of bleeding, particularly of the upper GI tract. This effect is exacerbated by aspirin and NSAIDs (see section on SSRIs and bleeding).

MAOIs[14]:

- prevent the destruction of monoamine neurotransmitters. Sympathomimetic and dopamin-ergic drugs can lead to monoamine overload and hypertensive crisis. Pethidine and fermented foods can have the same effect
- can interact with serotonergic drugs to cause serotonin syndrome.

Avoid/minimise problems by:

- avoiding antidepressant polypharmacy
- avoiding the co-prescription of other drugs with a similar pharmacology but not marketed as antidepressants (e.g. bupropion, sibutramine)
- knowing your pharmacology (most interactions can be easily predicted).

References

1. Cashman JR. Human flavin-containing monooxygenase: substrate specificity and role in drug metabolism. Curr Drug Metab 2000; 1:181–91.
2. Anderson GD. A mechanistic approach to antiepileptic drug interactions. Ann Pharmacother 1998; 32:554–63.
3. Devane CL. Antidepressant-drug interactions are potentially but rarely clinically significant. Neuropsychopharmacology 2006; 31:1594–1604.
4. British Medical Association and Royal Pharmaceutical Society of Great Britain. British National Formulary. 57th edition. London: BMJ Group and RPS Publishing; 2009.
5. Watsky EJ et al. Psychotropic drug interactions. Hosp Community Psychiatry 1991; 42:247–56.
6. Lin JH et al. Inhibition and induction of cytochrome P450 and the clinical implications. Clin Pharmacokinet 1998; 35:361–90.
7. Mitchell PB. Drug interactions of clinical significance with selective serotonin reuptake inhibitors. Drug Saf 1997; 17:390–406.
8. Richelson E. Pharmacokinetic interactions of antidepressants. J Clin Psychiatry 1998; 59 Suppl 10:22–6.
9. Greenblatt DJ et al. Drug interactions with newer antidepressants: role of human cytochromes P450. J Clin Psychiatry 1998; 59 Suppl 15:19–27.
10. Taylor D. Pharmacokinetic interactions involving clozapine. Br J Psychiatry 1997; 171:109–12.
11. Dolder CR et al. Agomelatine treatment of major depressive disorder. Ann Pharmacotherapy 2008; 42:1822–31.
12. Edwards JG et al. Systematic review and guide to selection of selective serotonin reuptake inhibitors. Drugs 1999; 57:507–33.
13. Loke YK et al. Meta-analysis: gastrointestinal bleeding due to interaction between selective serotonin uptake inhibitors and non-steroidal anti-inflammatory drugs. Aliment Pharmacol Ther 2008; 27:31–40.
14. Livingston MG et al. Monoamine oxidase inhibitors. An update on drug interactions. Drug Saf 1996; 14:219–27.

Antidepressants: relative adverse effects – a rough guide

Drug	Sedation	Hypotension	Anticholi-nergic effects	Forms available
Tricyclics				
Amitriptyline	+++	+++	+++	tabs, liq
Clomipramine	++	+++	++	tabs/caps, liq
Dosulepin	+++	+++	++	tabs, caps
Doxepin	+++	++	+++	caps
Imipramine	++	+++	+++	tabs, liq
Lofepramine	+	+	+	tabs, liq
Nortriptyline	+	++	+	tabs
Trimipramine	+++	+++	++	tabs, caps
Other antidepressants				
Agomelatine	+	–	–	tabs
Duloxetine	+/–	–	–	caps
Mianserin	++	–	–	tabs
Mirtazapine	+++	+/–	+	tabs, soluble tabs, liq
Reboxetine	+	–	+	tabs
Trazodone	+++	++	–	caps, tabs, liq
Venlafaxine	+/–	–	+/–	tabs, caps
Selective serotonin reuptake inhibitors (SSRIs)				
Citalopram	+/–	–	–	tabs, liq
Escitalopram	+/–	–	–	tabs, liq
Fluoxetine	–	–	–	caps, liq
Fluvoxamine	+	–	–	tabs
Paroxetine	+	–	+	tabs, liq
Sertraline	–	–	–	tabs
Monoamine oxidase inhibitors (MAOIs)				
Isocarboxazid	+	++	++	tabs
Phenelzine	+	+	+	tabs
Tranylcypromine	–	+	+	tabs
Reversible inhibitor of monoamine oxidase A (RIMA)				
Moclobemide	–	–	–	tabs
Key: +++ High incidence/severity ++ Moderate + Low – Very low/none				

Depression & anxiety

229

Antidepressants – alternative routes of administration

In rare cases, patients may be unable or unwilling to take antidepressants orally, and alternative treatments including psychological interventions and electroconvulsive therapy (ECT) are either impractical or contra-indicated.

One such scenario is depression in the medically ill[1], particularly in those who have undergone surgical resection procedures affecting the gastrointestinal tract. Where the intragastric (IG) route is used to deliver nutrition, antidepressants can usually be crushed and administered with food. If an intrajejunal (IJ) tube is used then more care is required because of changes in pharmacokinetics; there are few data on the exact site of absorption for the majority of antidepressants. In clinical practice it is often assumed (perhaps wrongly) that administration via the IJ route is likely to result in the same absorption characteristics as via the oral or IG route.

Very few non-oral formulations are available as commercial products. Most formulations do not have UK licences and may be very difficult to obtain, being available only through pharmaceutical importers or from Specials manufacturers. In addition, the use of these preparations beyond their licence or in an absence of a licence usually means that accountability for adverse effects lies with the prescriber. As a consequence, non-oral administration of antidepressants should be undertaken only when absolutely necessary.

Alternative antidepressant delivery methods

Sublingual
There are a small number of case reports supporting the effectiveness of fluoxetine liquid used sublingually in depressed, medically compromised patients[2]. In these reports doses of up to 60 mg a day produced plasma fluoxetine and norfluoxetine levels towards the lower end of the proposed therapeutic range[2].

Intravenous and intramuscular injections
The only SSRI available both as an intravenous and oral formulation is citalopram. When used, IV citalopram has been shown to be effective in the treatment of depression[3]. The IV preparation appears to be well-tolerated with the most common adverse events being nausea, headache, tremor and somnolence; similar to oral administration[4,5]. Mirtazapine is also available as an intravenous preparation. It has been administered by slow infusion at a dose of 15 mg a day for 14 days in two studies and was well tolerated in depressed patients[6,7].

Amitriptyline is available as both an IV and IM injection and both routes have been used in the treatment of post-operative pain and depression. The concentration of the IM preparation (10 mg/ml) necessitates a high-volume injection to achieve antidepressant doses; this clearly discourages its use[8]. Clomipramine is also available as an IV formulation. Pulse-loading doses of intravenous clomipramine have been shown to produce a larger more rapid decrease in obsessive-compulsive disorder symptoms compared with oral doses[9,10]. The potential for serious cardiac side effects when using any tricyclic antidepressant intravenously necessitates monitoring of pulse, blood pressure and ECG.

It has been suggested that intravenous administration of antidepressants has several advantages over the oral route, notably the avoidance of the first-pass effect, leading to higher drug plasma levels[9,11], and perhaps greater response as has been reported with clomipramine. Some authors claim a greater or more rapid improvement is generally seen[11,12], however negative reports also exist[3,12,13]. Note that the placebo effect associated with IV administration is known to be large[14]. Note also that calculating the correct parenteral dose of antidepressants is difficult given the variable first-pass effect to which oral drugs are usually subjected. Parenteral doses can be expected to be much lower than oral doses and give the same effect.

Transdermal

Oral selegiline at doses greater than 20 mg/day may be an effective antidepressant, but enzyme selectivity is lost at these doses, necessitating a tyramine-restricted diet[15,16]. Selegiline can be administered transdermally; this route bypasses first-pass metabolism, thereby providing a higher, more sustained, plasma concentration of selegiline while being relatively sparing of the gastrointestinal MAO-A system[17,18]; there seems to be no need for tyramine restriction when the lower-dose patch (6 mg/24 h) is used and there have been no reports of hypertensive reactions even with the higher-dose patch. However, because safety experience with the higher doses (9 mg/24 h and 12 mg/24 h) is more limited, it is recommended that patients using these patches should avoid very high tyramine content food substances[19].

When administered transdermally, application site reactions and insomnia are the two most commonly reported adverse effects; both are dose-related, usually mild or moderate in intensity and do not lead to dropout from treatment[19,20].

Rectal

The rectal mucosa lacks the extensive villi and microvilli of other parts of the gastrointestinal tract, limiting its surface area. Therefore rectal agents need to be in a formulation that maximises the extent of contact the active ingredient will have with the mucosa. There are no readily available antidepressant suppositories, but extemporaneous preparation is possible. For example, amitriptyline (in cocoa butter) suppositories have been manufactured by a hospital pharmacy and administered in a dose of 50 mg twice daily with some subjective success[21,22]. Doxepin capsules have been administered via the rectal route directly in the treatment of cancer-related pain (without a special formulation) and produced plasma concentrations within the supposed therapeutic range[23]. Similarly it has been reported that extemporaneously manufactured imipramine and clomipramine suppositories produced plasma levels comparable with the oral route of administration[24]. Trazodone has also been successfully administered in a suppository formulation post-operatively for a patient who was stable on the oral formulation prior to surgery[22,23].

Table Antidepressants – alternative routes

Drug name and route	Dosing information	Manufacturer	Notes
Sublingual fluoxetine	Doses up to 60 mg a day	Use liquid fluoxetine preparation	Plasma levels may be slightly lower compared with oral dosing
Intravenous amitriptyline	25–100 mg given in 250 ml NaCl 0.9% by slow infusion over 120 minutes	Contact local importer	Adverse effects tend to be dose-related and are largely similar to the oral formulation. At higher doses drowsiness and dizziness occur. Bradycardia may occur with doses around 100 mg
Intravenous clomipramine	25 mg/2 ml injection. Doses from 25 mg to 250 mg in 500 ml NaCl 0.9% by slow infusion over 90 minutes	Novartis Defiante	The most common reported side effects are similar to the oral formulation, which included nausea, sweating, restlessness, flushing, drowsiness, fatigue, abdominal distress and nervousness
Intravenous citalopram	40 mg/ml injection. Doses from 20 to 40 mg in 250 ml NaCl 0.9% or glucose 5%. Doses up to 80 mg have been used for OCD. Rate of infusion is 20 mg per hour	Lundbeck	The most commonly reported side effects are nausea, headache, tremor and somnolence similar to adverse effects of the oral preparation
Intravenous mirtazapine	6 mg/2 ml infusion solution. 15 mg/5 ml infusion solution. Dose 15 mg in glucose 5% over 60 minutes	Contact local importer	The most common reported side effects are nausea, sedation and dizziness similar to side effects of the oral preparation
Intramuscular preparations-amitriptyline	Amitriptyline 10 mg/mL Elavil®	Zeneca	IM preparations are very rarely used because of the requirement of a high volume. Many preparations have been discontinued
Topical selegiline	6 mg/24 h, 9 mg/24 h, 12 mg/24 h	Bristol Myers Squib	The 6 mg/24 h dose does not require a tyramine-restricted diet. At higher doses, although no hypertensive crisis reactions have been reported, the manufacturer recommends avoiding high-tyramine-content food substances. Application site reactions and insomnia are the most common reported side effects

Table Antidepressants – alternative routes (Cont.)

Drug name and route	Dosing information	Manufacturer	Notes
Rectal amitriptyline	Doses up to 50 mg bd	Suppositories have been manufactured by pharmacies or manufacturing departments	Very little information on rectal administration. Largely in the form of case reports
Rectal clomipramine	No detailed information available		
Rectal imipramine	No detailed information available		
Rectal doxepin	No detailed information available	Capsules have been used rectally	
Rectal trazodone	No detailed information available	Suppositories have been manufactured by pharmacies or manufacturing departments	Trazodone in the rectal formulation has been used for post-operative or cancer pain control rather than antidepressant activity

References

1. Cipriani A et al. Metareview on short-term effectiveness and safety of antidepressants for depression: an evidence-based approach to inform clinical practice. Can J Psychiatry 2007; 52:553–62.
2. Maltese TM. Adjunctive lamotrigine treatment for major depression (Letter). Am J Psychiatry 1999; 156:1833.
3. Baumann P et al. A double-blind double-dummy study of citalopram comparing infusion versus oral administration. J Affect Disord 1998; 49:203–10.
4. Guelfi JD et al. Efficacy of intravenous citalopram compared with oral citalopram for severe depression. Safety and efficacy data from a double-blind, double-dummy trial. J Affect Disord 2000; 58:201–9.
5. Kasper S et al. Intravenous antidepressant treatment: focus on citalopram. Eur Arch Psychiatry Clin Neurosci 2002; 252:105–9.
6. Konstantinidis A et al. Intravenous mirtazapine in the treatment of depressed inpatients. Eur Neuropsychopharmacol 2002; 12:57–60.
7. Muhlbacher M et al. Intravenous mirtazapine is safe and effective in the treatment of depressed inpatients. Neuropsychobiology 2006; 53:83–7.
8. RX List. Elavil (amitriptyline HCI). http://www.rxlist.com. 2008.
9. Deisenhammer EA et al. Intravenous versus oral administration of amitriptyline in patients with major depression. J Clin Psychopharmacol 2000; 20:417–22.
10. Koran LM et al. Pulse loading versus gradual dosing of intravenous clomipramine in obsessive-compulsive disorder. Eur Neuropsychopharmacol 1998; 8:121–6.
11. Koran LM et al. Rapid benefit of intravenous pulse loading of clomipramine in obsessive-compulsive disorder. Am J Psychiatry 1997; 154:396–401.
12. Svestka J et al. [Citalopram (Seropram) in tablet and infusion forms in the treatment of major depression]. Cesk Psychiatr 1993; 89:331–9.
13. Pollock BG et al. Acute antidepressant effect following pulse loading with intravenous and oral clomipramine. Arch Gen Psychiatry 1989; 46:29–35.
14. Sallee FR et al. Pulse intravenous clomipramine for depressed adolescents: double-blind, controlled trial. Am J Psychiatry 1997; 154:668–73.
15. Sunderland T et al. High-dose selegiline in treatment-resistant older depressive patients. Arch Gen Psychiatry 1994; 51:607–15.
16. Mann JJ et al. A controlled study of the antidepressant efficacy and side effects of (-)-deprenyl. A selective monoamine oxidase inhibitor. Arch Gen Psychiatry 1989; 46:45–50.
17. Wecker L et al. Transdermal selegiline: targeted effects on monoamine oxidases in the brain. Biol Psychiatry 2003; 54:1099–1104.
18. Azzaro AJ et al. Pharmacokinetics and absolute bioavailability of selegiline following treatment of healthy subjects with the selegiline transdermal system (6 mg/24 h): a comparison with oral selegiline capsules. J Clin Pharmacol 2007; 47:1256–67.
19. Amsterdam JD et al. Selegiline transdermal system in the prevention of relapse of major depressive disorder: a 52-week, double-blind, placebo-substitution, parallel-group clinical trial. J Clin Psychopharmacol 2006; 26:579–86.
20. Robinson DS et al. The selegiline transdermal system in major depressive disorder: a systematic review of safety and tolerability. J Affect Disord 2008; 105:15–23.
21. Adams S. Amitriptyline suppositories. N Engl J Med 1982; 306:996.
22. Mirassou MM. Rectal antidepressant medication in the treatment of depression. J Clin Psychiatry 1998; 59:29.
23. Storey P et al. Rectal doxepin and carbamazepine therapy in patients with cancer. N Engl J Med 1992; 327:1318–19.
24. Chaumeil JC et al. Formulation of suppositories containing imipramine and clomipramine chlorhydrates. Drug Dev Ind Pharm 1988; 15–17:2225–39.

Depression & anxiety

Anxiety spectrum disorders

Anxiety is a normal emotion that is experienced by everyone at some time. Symptoms can be psychological, physical, or a mixture of both. Intervention is required when symptoms become disabling.

There are several disorders within the overall spectrum of anxiety disorders, each with its own characteristic symptoms. These are outlined briefly in the table on the following pages. Anxiety disorders can occur on their own, be co-morbid with other psychiatric disorders (particularly depression), be a consequence of physical illness such as thyrotoxicosis or be drug-induced (e.g. by caffeine). Co-morbidity with other psychiatric disorders is very common.

Anxiety spectrum disorders tend to be chronic and treatment is often only partially successful. Note that people with anxiety disorders may be particularly prone to side effects[1]. High initial doses in particular may be poorly tolerated.

Benzodiazepines

Benzodiazepines provide rapid symptomatic relief from acute anxiety states[2]. All guidelines and consensus statements recommend that this group of drugs should only be used to treat anxiety that is severe, disabling, or subjecting the individual to extreme distress. Because of their potential to cause physical dependence and withdrawal symptoms, these drugs should be used at the lowest effective dose for the shortest period of time (maximum 4 weeks), while medium/long-term treatment strategies are put in place. For the majority of patients these recommendations are sensible and should be adhered to. A very small number of patients with severely disabling anxiety may benefit from long-term treatment with a benzodiazepine and these patients should not be denied treatment[3]. Benzodiazepines are known to be over-prescribed in the long term for both treatment of anxiety[4] and depression[5]; usually in place of more appropriate treatment.

NICE recommends that benzodiazepines should not be used to treat panic disorder[6]. They should be used with care in post-traumatic stress disorder (PTSD)[7].

SSRI – dose and duration of treatment

When used to treat generalised anxiety disorder (GAD), SSRIs should initially be prescribed at half the normal starting dose for the treatment of depression and the dose titrated upwards into the normal antidepressant dosage range as tolerated (initial worsening of anxiety may be seen when treatment is started[8]). Response is usually seen within 6 weeks and continues to increase over time[9]. The optimal duration of treatment has not been determined but should be at least one year[10]. Effective treatment of GAD may prevent the development of major depression[10].

When used to treat panic disorder, the same starting dose and dosage titration as in GAD should be used. Doses of clomipramine[11], citalopram[12] and sertraline[13] towards the bottom of the antidepressant range give the best balance between efficacy and side effects, whereas higher doses of paroxetine (40 mg and above) may be required[14]. Higher doses may be effective when standard doses have failed. Onset of action may be as long as 6 weeks. Women may respond better to SSRIs than men[15]. There is some evidence that augmentation with clonazepam leads to a more rapid response (but not a greater magnitude of response overall)[14,16]. The optimal duration of treatment is unknown, but should be at least 8 months[17]; a large naturalistic study showed convincing evidence of benefit for at least 3 years[18]. Less than 50% are likely to remain well after medication is withdrawn[19].

Lower starting doses are also required in post-traumatic stress disorder (PTSD), with high doses (e.g. fluoxetine 60 mg) often being required for full effect. Response is usually seen within 8 weeks, but can take up to 12 weeks[19]. Treatment should be continued for at least 6 months and probably longer[20,21].

Although the doses of SSRIs licensed for the treatment of obsessive-compulsive disorder (OCD) are higher than those licensed for the treatment of depression (e.g. fluoxetine 60 mg, paroxetine

40–60 mg), lower (standard antidepressant) doses may be effective, particularly for maintenance treatment[22]. Initial response is usually slower to emerge than in depression (can take 10–12 weeks). The relapse rate in those who continue treatment for 2 years is half that of those who stop treatment after initial response (25–40% vs 80%)[23]. In most people with OCD, the condition is persistent and symptom severity fluctuates over time[24].

Body dysmorphic disorder (BDD) should be treated initially with CBT. If symptoms are moderate–severe, adding an SSRI may improve outcome[25]. Buspirone may usefully augment the SSRI[25].

Standard antidepressant starting doses are well tolerated in social phobia[26–28], and dosage titration may benefit some patients but is not always required. Response is usually seen within 8 weeks and treatment should be continued for at least a year and probably longer[29].

All patients treated with SSRIs should be monitored for the development of akathisia, increased anxiety and the emergence of suicidal ideation; the risk is thought to be greatest in those <30 years, those with co-morbid depression and those already known to be at higher risk of suicide[25].

SSRIs should not be stopped abruptly, as patients with anxiety spectrum disorders are particularly sensitive to discontinuation symptoms (see section on discontinuation). The dose should be reduced as slowly as tolerated over several weeks to months.

Psychological approaches

There is good evidence to support the efficacy of some psychological interventions in anxiety spectrum disorders. Examples include exposure therapy in OCD and social phobia. Initial drug therapy may be required to help the patient become more receptive to psychological input. Some studies suggest that optimal outcome is achieved by combining psychological and drug therapies[6,30], but negative studies also exist[31,32].

A discussion of the evidence base for psychological interventions is outside the scope of these guidelines. Further information can be found at www.doh.gov.uk[33]. It is recognised that for many patients psychological therapies are an appropriate first-line treatment, and indeed this is supported by NICE[6].

Summary of NICE guidelines for the treatment of generalised anxiety disorder, panic disorder[6] and OCD[25]

- Psychological therapy is more effective than pharmacological therapy and should be used as first line where possible. Details of the types of therapy recommended and their duration can be found in the NICE guidelines.
- Pharmacological therapy is also effective. Most evidence supports the use of the SSRIs.

Panic disorder
- Benzodiazepines should not be used.
- A SSRI should be used as first line. If SSRIs are contra-indicated or there is no response, imipramine or clomipramine can be used.
- Self-help (based on CBT principles) should be encouraged.

Generalised anxiety disorder
- Benzodiazepines should not be used beyond 2–4 weeks.
- A SSRI should be used as first line.
- Self-help (based on CBT principles) should be encouraged.

OCD (where there is moderate or severe functional impairment)
- Use an SSRI or intensive CBT.
- Combine the SSRI and CBT if response to single strategy is suboptimal.
- Use clomipramine if SSRIs fail.
- If response is still suboptimal, add an antipsychotic or combine clomipramine and citalopram.

Table

	Generalised anxiety disorder[6–10,34–46]	Panic disorder[1,12–14, 16,17,19,31,32,47–55]
Clinical presentation	• Irrational worries • Motor tension • Hypervigilance • Somatic symptoms (e.g. hyperventilation, tachycardia and sweating)	• Sudden unpredictable episodes of severe anxiety • Shortness of breath • Fear of suffocation/dying • Urgent desire to flee
Emergency management	Benzodiazepines (normally for short-term use only: max. 2–4 weeks, but see ref. 3)	Benzodiazepines (have a rapid effect, although panic symptoms return quickly if the drug is withdrawn) NICE do *not* recommend benzodiazepines
First-line drug treatment. Treatment of anxiety may prevent the subsequent development of depression[10]	• SSRIs (although may initially exacerbate symptoms. A lower starting is often required) • Mirtazapine • Venlafaxine • Pregabalin • Duloxetine	• SSRIs (therapeutic effect can be delayed and patients can experience an initial exacerbation of panic symptoms)
Other treatments (less well tolerated or weaker evidence base)	• Buspirone (has a delayed onset of action) • Hydroxyzine • β-Blockers (useful for somatic symptoms, particularly tachycardia) • Some TCAs (e.g. imipramine, clomipramine) • MAOIs	• MAOIs • Mirtazapine • Some TCAs (e.g. imipramine, clomipramine) • Valproate • Venlafaxine
More experimental	• Tiagabine • Riluzole	• Gabapentin • Inositol • Pindolol (as augmentation)
Non-drug treatments See www.doh.org.uk and NICE[6]	• Reassurance • Anxiety management, including relaxation training drug and exposure therapy • CBT	• CBT • Anxiety management, including relaxation, training • Combined drug and psychological therapy not consistently better than pharmacological treatment alone

Post-traumatic stress disorder[1,20,22,56–68]	Obsessive compulsive disorder[23,69–82]	Social phobia[27–29,83–87]
• History of a traumatic life event (as perceived by the sufferer) • Emotional numbness or detachment • Intrusive flashbacks or vivid dreams • Disabling fear of re-exposure, causing avoidance of perceived similar situations	• Obsessional thinking (e.g. constantly thinking that the door has been left unlocked) • Compulsive behaviour (e.g. constantly going back to check)	• Extreme fear of social situations (e.g. eating in public or public speaking) • Fear of humiliation or embarrassment • Avoidant behaviour (e.g. never eating in restaurants) • Anxious anticipation (e.g. feeling sick on entering a restaurant)
Not usually appropriate	Not usually appropriate	Benzodiazepines (have a rapid effect and may be useful on a PRN basis)
• SSRIs	• SSRIs • Clomipramine	• SSRIs
• Antipsychotics (as augmentation) • Mirtazapine • MAOIs • Serotonergic TCAs • Venlafaxine	• Antipsychotics as antidepressant augmentation; effect most marked when added to low dose SSRIs • Clonazepam (benzodiazepines in general are mainly useful in reducing associated anxiety; only careful short-term use supported by NICE) • Citalopram augmentation of clomipramine • Mirtazapine augmentation of SSRI (supported by NICE)	• Buspirone (adjunct to SSRIs only) • Clonazepam (as augmentation) • Moclobemide • Propranolol (performance anxiety only) • Venlafaxine • Valproate
• Carbamazepine • Clonidine • Lamotrigine • Prazosin (for nightmares) • Phenytoin • Tiagabine • Valproate	• Duloxetine/venlafaxine (not recommended by NICE) • Buspirone • Clomipramine (IV pulse loading) • Anti-androgen treatment	• Levetiracetam
• Debriefing should be available if desired • Counselling • Anxiety management • CBT, especially for avoidance behaviours or intrusive images	• Exposure therapy • Behavioural therapy • CBT • Combined drug and psychological therapy may be the most effective option • Surgery	• CBT • Exposure therapy (combined drug and exposure therapy may be the more effective)

Depression & anxiety

References

1. Nash JR et al. Pharmacotherapy of anxiety. Handb Exp Pharmacol 2005; 469–501.
2. Martin JL et al. Benzodiazepines in generalized anxiety disorder: heterogeneity of outcomes based on a systematic review and meta-analysis of clinical trials. J Psychopharmacol 2007; 21:774–82.
3. Royal College of Psychiatrist. Benzodiazepines: risks, benefits or dependence. A re-evaluation. Council Report 59. http://www.rcpsych.ac.uk/. 1997.
4. Benitez CI et al. Use of benzodiazepines and selective serotonin reuptake inhibitors in middle-aged and older adults with anxiety disorders: a longitudinal and prospective study. Am J Geriatr Psychiatry 2008; 16:5–13.
5. Demyttenaere K et al. Clinical factors influencing the prescription of antidepressants and benzodiazepines: results from the European study of the epidemiology of mental disorders (ESEMeD). J Affect Disord 2008; 110:84–93.
6. National Institute for Health and Clinical Excellence. Anxiety (amended). Management of anxiety (panic disorder, with or without agoraphobia, and generalised anxiety disorder) in adults in primary, secondary and community care. Clinical Guidance 22. Amended April 2007. 2007. http://www.nice.org.uk
7. Davidson JR. Use of benzodiazepines in social anxiety disorder, generalized anxiety disorder, and posttraumatic stress disorder. J Clin Psychiatry 2004; 65 Suppl 5:29–33.
8. Scott A et al. Antidepressant drugs in the treatment of anxiety disorders. Adv Psychiatr Treat 2001; 7:275–82.
9. Ballenger JC. Remission rates in patients with anxiety disorders treated with paroxetine. J Clin Psychiatry 2004; 65:1696–707.
10. Davidson J et al. A psychopharmacological treatment algorithm for generalised anxiety disorder (GAD). J Psychopharmacol 2008; Epub ahead of print. 10.1177/0269881108096505.
11. Goodwin RD et al. Psychopharmacologic treatment of generalized anxiety disorder and the risk of major depression. Am J Psychiatry 2002; 159:1935–7.
12. Caillard V et al. Comparative effects of low and high doses of clomipramine and placebo in panic disorder: a double-blind controlled study. French University Antidepressant Group. Acta Psychiatr Scand 1999; 99:51–8.
13. Wade AG et al. The effect of citalopram in panic disorder. Br J Psychiatry 1997; 170:549–553.
14. Londborg PD et al. Sertraline in the treatment of panic disorder. A multi-site, double-blind, placebo-controlled, fixed-dose investigation. Br J Psychiatry 1998; 173:54–60.
15. Clayton AH et al. Sex differences in clinical presentation and response in panic disorder: pooled data from sertraline treatment studies. Arch Womens Ment Health 2006; 9:151–7.
16. Pollack MH et al. Combined paroxetine and clonazepam treatment strategies compared to paroxetine monotherapy for panic disorder. J Psychopharmacol 2003; 17:276–82.
17. Rickels K et al. Panic disorder: long-term pharmacotherapy and discontinuation. J Clin Psychopharmacol 1998; 18:12S–18S.
18. Choy Y et al. Three-year medication prophylaxis in panic disorder: to continue or discontinue? A naturalistic study. Compr Psychiatry 2007; 48:419–25.
19. Michelson D et al. Continuing treatment of panic disorder after acute response: randomised, placebo-controlled trial with fluoxetine. The Fluoxetine Panic Disorder Study Group. Br J Psychiatry 1999; 174:213–18.
20. Davidson JR et al. Efficacy of sertraline in preventing relapse of posttraumatic stress disorder: results of a 28-week double-blind, placebo-controlled study. Am J Psychiatry 2001; 158:1974–81.
21. Stein DJ et al. Pharmacotherapy for post traumatic stress disorder (PTSD). Cochrane Database Syst Rev 2006; CD002795.
22. Martenyi F et al. Fluoxetine v. placebo in prevention of relapse in post-traumatic stress disorder. Br J Psychiatry 2002; 181:315–20.
23. The Expert Consensus Panel for obsessive-compulsive disorder. Treatment of obsessive-compulsive disorder. J Clin Psychiatry 1997; 58 Suppl 4:2–72.
24. Catapano F et al. Obsessive-compulsive disorder: a 3-year prospective follow-up study of patients treated with serotonin reuptake inhibitors OCD follow-up study. J Psychiatr Res 2006; 40:502–10.
25. National Institute for Clinical Excellence. Obsessive-compulsive disorder: Information for the public. Clinical Guidance 31. http://www.nice.org.uk. 2005.
26. Greist JH et al. Efficacy and tolerability of serotonin transport inhibitors in obsessive-compulsive disorder. A meta-analysis. Arch Gen Psychiatry 1995; 52:53–60.
27. Liebowitz MR et al. A randomized, double-blind, fixed-dose comparison of paroxetine and placebo in the treatment of generalized social anxiety disorder. J Clin Psychiatry 2002; 63:66–74.
28. Blomhoff S et al. Randomised controlled general practice trial of sertraline, exposure therapy and combined treatment in generalised social phobia. Br J Psychiatry 2001; 179:23–30.
29. Hood SD, Nutt DJ. Psychopharmacological treatments: an overview. In: Crozier R, Alden E, editors. International Handbook of Social Anxiety. Oxford: John Wiley and Sons Ltd; 2001.
30. National Institute of Clinical Excellence. Anxiety: management of anxiety (panic disorder, with or without agoraphobia, and generalised anxiety disorder) in adults in primary, secondary and community care. http://www.nice.org.uk. 2004.
31. van Apeldoorn FJ et al. Is a combined therapy more effective than either CBT or SSRI alone? Results of a multicenter trial on panic disorder with or without agoraphobia. Acta Psychiatr Scand 2008; 117:260–70.
32. Marcus SM et al. A comparison of medication side effect reports by panic disorder patients with and without concomitant cognitive behavior therapy. Am J Psychiatry 2007; 164:273–5.
33. Department of Health. Treatment choice in psychological therapies and counselling: Evidence based clinical practice guideline. http://www.dh.gov.uk/, 2001.
34. Rickels K et al. Antidepressants for the treatment of generalized anxiety disorder. A placebo-controlled comparison of imipramine, trazodone, and diazepam. Arch Gen Psychiatry 1993; 50:884–95.
35. Lader M et al. A multicentre double-blind comparison of hydroxyzine, buspirone and placebo in patients with generalized anxiety disorder. Psychopharmacology 1998; 139:402–6.
36. Kapczinski F et al. Antidepressants for generalized anxiety disorder. Cochrane Database Syst Rev 2003; CD003592.
37. Rickels K et al. Paroxetine treatment of generalized anxiety disorder: a double-blind, placebo-controlled study. Am J Psychiatry 2003; 160:749–56.
38. Allgulander C et al. Efficacy of sertraline in a 12-week trial for generalized anxiety disorder. Am J Psychiatry 2004; 161:1642–9.
39. Lenox-Smith AJ et al. A double-blind, randomised, placebo controlled study of venlafaxine XL in patients with generalised anxiety disorder in primary care. Br J Gen Pract 2003; 53:772–7.
40. Rosenthal M. Tiagabine for the treatment of generalized anxiety disorder: a randomized, open-label, clinical trial with paroxetine as a positive control. J Clin Psychiatry 2003; 64:1245–9.
41. Baldwin DS et al. Escitalopram and paroxetine in the treatment of generalised anxiety disorder: randomised, placebo-controlled, double-blind study. Br J Psychiatry 2006; 189:264–72.
42. Pande AC et al. Pregabalin in generalized anxiety disorder: a placebo-controlled trial. Am J Psychiatry 2003; 160:533–40.
43. Rickels K et al. Remission of generalized anxiety disorder: a review of the paroxetine clinical trials database. J Clin Psychiatry 2006; 67:41–7.
44. Mathew SJ et al. Open-label trial of riluzole in generalized anxiety disorder. Am J Psychiatry 2005; 162:2379–81.
45. Schuurmans J et al. A randomized, controlled trial of the effectiveness of cognitive-behavioral therapy and sertraline versus a waitlist control group for anxiety disorders in older adults. Am J Geriatr Psychiatry 2006; 14:255–63.
46. Chessick CA et al. Azapirones for generalized anxiety disorder. Cochrane Database Syst Rev 2006; 3:CD006115.

47. Versiani M et al. Reboxetine, a unique selective NRI, prevents relapse and recurrence in long-term treatment of major depressive disorder. J Clin Psychiatry 1999; 60:400–6.
48. Bakker A et al. SSRIs vs. TCAs in the treatment of panic disorder: a meta-analysis. Acta Psychiatr Scand 2002; 106:163–7.
49. Benjamin J et al. Double-blind, placebo-controlled, crossover trial of inositol treatment for panic disorder. Am J Psychiatry 1995; 152:1084–6.
50. Otto MW et al. An effect-size analysis of the relative efficacy and tolerability of serotonin selective reuptake inhibitors for panic disorder. Am J Psychiatry 2001; 158:1989–92.
51. Sheehan DV et al. Efficacy and tolerability of controlled-release paroxetine in the treatment of panic disorder. J Clin Psychiatry 2005; 66:34–40.
52. Bradwejn J et al. Venlafaxine extended-release capsules in panic disorder: flexible-dose, double-blind, placebo-controlled study. Br J Psychiatry 2005; 187:352–9.
53. Pollack M et al. A randomized controlled trial of venlafaxine ER and paroxetine in the treatment of outpatients with panic disorder. Psychopharmacology (Berl) 2007; 194:233–42.
54. Ferguson JM et al. Relapse prevention of panic disorder in adult outpatient responders to treatment with venlafaxine extended release. J Clin Psychiatry 2007; 68:58–68.
55. Buch S et al. Successful use of phenelzine in treatment-resistant panic disorder. J Clin Psychiatry 2007; 68:335–6.
56. Connor KM et al. Fluoxetine in post-traumatic stress disorder. Randomised, double-blind study. Br J Psychiatry 1999; 175:17–22.
57. Taylor FB. Tiagabine for posttraumatic stress disorder: a case series of 7 women. J Clin Psychiatry 2003; 64:1421–5.
58. Pivac N et al. Olanzapine versus fluphenazine in an open trial in patients with psychotic combat-related post-traumatic stress disorder. Psychopharmacology 2004; 175:451–6.
59. Filteau MJ et al. Quetiapine reduces flashbacks in chronic posttraumatic stress disorder. Can J Psychiatry 2003; 48:282–3.
60. Jakovljevic M et al. Olanzapine in the treatment-resistant, combat-related PTSD – a series of case reports. Acta Psychiatr Scand 2003; 107:394–6.
61. Otte C et al. Valproate monotherapy in the treatment of civilian patients with non-combat-related posttraumatic stress disorder: an open-label study. J Clin Psychopharmacol 2004; 24:106–8.
62. Davidson JR et al. Mirtazapine vs. placebo in posttraumatic stress disorder: a pilot trial. Biol Psychiatry 2003; 53:188–91.
63. Bremner DJ et al. Treatment of posttraumatic stress disorder with phenytoin: an open-label pilot study. J Clin Psychiatry 2004; 65:1559–64.
64. Schoenfeld FB et al. Current concepts in pharmacotherapy for posttraumatic stress disorder. Psychiatr Serv 2004; 55:519–31.
65. Cooper J et al. Pharmacotherapy for posttraumatic stress disorder: empirical review and clinical recommendations. Aust N Z J Psychiatry 2005; 39:674–82.
66. Davidson J et al. Treatment of posttraumatic stress disorder with venlafaxine extended release: a 6-month randomized controlled trial. Arch Gen Psychiatry 2006; 63:1158–65.
67. Raskind MA et al. A parallel group placebo controlled study of prazosin for trauma nightmares and sleep disturbance in combat veterans with post-traumatic stress disorder. Biol Psychiatry 2007; 61:928–34.
68. Padala PR et al. Risperidone monotherapy for post-traumatic stress disorder related to sexual assault and domestic abuse in women. Int Clin Psychopharmacol 2006; 21:275–80.
69. Koran LM et al. Rapid benefit of intravenous pulse loading of clomipramine in obsessive-compulsive disorder. Am J Psychiatry 1997; 154:396–401.
70. Maina G et al. Antipsychotic augmentation for treatment resistant obsessive-compulsive disorder: what if antipsychotic is discontinued? Int Clin Psychopharmacol 2003; 18:23–8.
71. Pallanti S et al. Response acceleration with mirtazapine augmentation of citalopram in obsessive-compulsive disorder patients without comorbid depression: a pilot study. J Clin Psychiatry 2004; 65:1394–9.
72. Hollander E et al. Venlafaxine in treatment-resistant obsessive-compulsive disorder. J Clin Psychiatry 2003; 64:546–50.
73. Dell'Osso B et al. Serotonin-norepinephrine reuptake inhibitors in the treatment of obsessive-compulsive disorder: A critical review. J Clin Psychiatry 2006; 67:600–10.
74. Sousa MB et al. A randomized clinical trial of cognitive-behavioral group therapy and sertraline in the treatment of obsessive-compulsive disorder. J Clin Psychiatry 2006; 67:1133–9.
75. Eriksson T. Anti-androgenic treatment of obsessive-compulsive disorder: an open-label clinical trial of the long-acting gonadotropin-releasing hormone analogue triptorelin. Int Clin Psychopharmacol 2007; 22:57–61.
76. Soomro GM et al. Selective serotonin re-uptake inhibitors (SSRIs) versus placebo for obsessive compulsive disorder (OCD). Cochrane Database Syst Rev 2008;CD001765.
77. Skapinakis P et al. Antipsychotic augmentation of serotonergic antidepressants in treatment-resistant obsessive-compulsive disorder: a meta-analysis of the randomized controlled trials. Eur Neuropsychopharmacol 2007; 17:79–93.
78. Dell'Osso B et al. Switching from serotonin reuptake inhibitors to duloxetine in patients with resistant obsessive compulsive disorder: a case series. J Psychopharmacol 2008; 22:210–13.
79. Ruck C et al. Capsulotomy for obsessive-compulsive disorder: long-term follow-up of 25 patients. Arch Gen Psychiatry 2008; 65:914–21.
80. Fineberg NA et al. Escitalopram prevents relapse of obsessive-compulsive disorder. Eur Neuropsychopharmacol 2007; 17:430–9.
81. Storch EA et al. Aripiprazole augmentation of incomplete treatment response in an adolescent male with obsessive-compulsive disorder. Depress Anxiety 2008; 25:172–4.
82. Denys D et al. Quetiapine addition in obsessive-compulsive disorder: is treatment outcome affected by type and dose of serotonin reuptake inhibitors? Biol Psychiatry 2007; 61:412–14.
83. Blanco C et al. Pharmacological treatment of social anxiety disorder: a meta-analysis. Depress Anxiety 2003; 18:29–40.
84. Stein MB et al. Efficacy of low and higher dose extended-release venlafaxine in generalized social anxiety disorder: a 6-month randomized controlled trial. Psychopharmacology 2005; 177:280–4.
85. Aarre TF. Phenelzine efficacy in refractory social anxiety disorder: a case series. Nord J Psychiatry 2003; 57:313–15.
86. Simon NM et al. An open-label study of levetiracetam for the treatment of social anxiety disorder. J Clin Psychiatry 2004; 65:1219–22.
87. Kinrys G et al. Valproic acid for the treatment of social anxiety disorder. Int Clin Psychopharmacol 2003; 18:169–72.

Further reading

Baldwin DS et al. Evidence-based guidelines for the pharmacological treatment of anxiety disorders: recommendations from the British Association for Psychopharmacology. J Psychopharmacol 2005; 19:567–96.
de Quervain DJ et al. Glucocorticoids for the treatment of post-traumatic stress disorder and phobias: a novel therapeutic approach. Eur J Pharmacol 2008; 583:365–71.
Heyman I et al. Obsessive-compulsive disorder. BMJ 2006; 333:424–9.
Hidalgo RB et al. An effect-size analysis of pharmacologic treatments for generalized anxiety disorder. J Psychopharmacol 2007; 21:864–72.

Benzodiazepines

Benzodiazepines are normally divided into two groups depending on their half-life: hypnotics (short half-life) or anxiolytics (long half-life). Although benzodiazepines have a place in the treatment of some forms of epilepsy and severe muscle spasm, and as premedicants in some surgical procedures, the vast majority of prescriptions are written for their hypnotic and anxiolytic effects. Benzodiazepines are also used for rapid tranquillisation (see section in Chapter 7) and, as adjuncts, in the treatment of depression and schizophrenia.

Benzodiazepines are commonly prescribed; a recent European study found that almost 10% of adults had taken a benzodiazepine over the course of a year[1].

Anxiolytic effect

Benzodiazepines reduce pathological anxiety, agitation and tension. Although useful in the short-term management of generalised anxiety disorder[2,3] either alone or to augment SSRIs, benzodiazepines are clearly addictive; many patients continue to take these drugs for years[4] with unknown benefits and many likely harms. Benzodiazepines may be less effective in the short term than hydroxyzine, an antihistamine that is not known to be addictive[5]. If a benzodiazepine is prescribed, this should not routinely be for longer than 1 month. Benzodiazepines have no effect on the course of bereavement[6].

NICE recommends that benzodiazepines should not be routinely used in patients with panic disorder – outcome with CBT or SSRIs is superior[7].

Repeat prescriptions should be avoided in those with major personality problems whose difficulties are unlikely ever to resolve. Benzodiazepines should also be avoided, if possible, in those with a history of substance misuse.

Hypnotic effect

Benzodiazepines inhibit REM sleep and a rebound increase is seen when they are discontinued. There is a debate over the significance of this property[6].

Benzodiazepines are effective hypnotics, at least in the short term. RCTs support the effectiveness of Z hypnotics over a period of at least 6 months[8,9], it is unclear if this holds true for benzodiazepine hypnotics.

Physical causes (pain, dyspnoea, etc.) or substance misuse (most commonly high caffeine consumption) should always be excluded before a hypnotic drug is prescribed. A high proportion of hospitalised patients are prescribed hypnotics[10]. Care should be taken to avoid using hypnotics regularly or for long periods of time.

Be particularly careful to avoid routinely prescribing hypnotics on discharge from hospital, as this may result in iatrogenic dependence.

Use in depression

Benzodiazepines are not a treatment for major depressive illness. The National Service Framework for Mental Health[11] highlights this point by including a requirement that GPs audit the ratio of benzodiazepines to antidepressants prescribed in their practice. NICE found no evidence to support the use of benzodiazepines alongside antidepressants in the initial treatment of depression[12].

Use in psychosis

Benzodiazepines are commonly used for RT, either alone[13,14], or in combination with an antipsychotic; note that a Cochrane review concludes that there is no convincing evidence that combining an antipsychotic and a benzodiazepine offers any advantage over the benzodiazepine alone[15]. A further Cochrane Review concludes that there are no proven benefits of benzodiazepines in people with schizophrenia, outside short-term sedation[16]. A significant minority of patients with established psychotic illness fail to respond adequately to antipsychotics alone, and this can result in benzodiazepines being prescribed on a chronic basis[17]. There is limited evidence that some treatment-resistant patients may benefit from a combination of antipsychotics and benzodiazepines, either by showing a very marked antipsychotic response or by allowing the use of lower-dose antipsychotic regimens.

Side effects

Headaches, confusion, ataxia, dysarthria, blurred vision, gastrointestinal disturbances, jaundice and paradoxical excitement are all possible side effects. A high incidence of reversible psychiatric side effects, specifically loss of memory and depression, led to the withdrawal of triazolam[18]. The use of benzodiazepines has been associated with at least a 50% increase in the risk of hip fracture in the elderly[19,20]. The risk is greatest in the first few days and after 1 month of continuous use. High doses are particularly problematic. This would seem to be a class effect (the risk is not reduced by using short-half-life drugs). Benzodiazepines can cause anterograde amnesia[21] and can adversely affect driving performance[22]. Benzodiazepines can also cause disinhibition; this seems to be more common with short-acting drugs.

Respiratory depression is rare with oral therapy but is possible when the IV route is used. A specific benzodiazepine antagonist, flumazenil, is available. Flumazenil has a much shorter half-life than diazepam, making close observation of the patient essential for several hours after administration.

IV injections can be painful and lead to thrombophlebitis, because of the low water solubility of benzodiazepines, and therefore it is necessary to use solvents in the preparation of injectable forms. Diazepam is available in emulsion form (Diazemuls) to overcome these problems.

Drug interactions

Benzodiazepines do not induce microsomal enzymes and so do not frequently precipitate pharmacokinetic interactions with any other drugs. Most benzodiazepines are metabolised by CYP3A4, which is inhibited by erythromycin, several SSRIs and ketoconazole. It is theoretically possible that co-administration of these drugs will result in higher serum levels of benzodiazepines. Pharmacodynamic interactions (usually increased sedation) can occur. Benzodiazepines are associated with an important interaction with methadone (see Chapter 5).

References

1. Demyttenaere K et al. Clinical factors influencing the prescription of antidepressants and benzodiazepines: results from the European study of the epidemiology of mental disorders (ESEMeD). J Affect Disord 2008; 110:84–93.
2. Martin JL et al. Benzodiazepines in generalized anxiety disorder: heterogeneity of outcomes based on a systematic review and meta-analysis of clinical trials. J Psychopharmacol 2007; 21:774–82.
3. Davidson J et al. A psychopharmacological treatment algorithm for generalised anxiety disorder (GAD). J Psychopharmacol 2008; Epub ahead of print. 10.1177/0269881108096505.
4. Benitez CI et al. Use of benzodiazepines and selective serotonin reuptake inhibitors in middle-aged and older adults with anxiety disorders: a longitudinal and prospective study. Am J Geriatr Psychiatry 2008; 16:5–13.
5. Hidalgo RB et al. An effect-size analysis of pharmacologic treatments for generalized anxiety disorder. J Psychopharmacol 2007; 21:864–72.
6. Vogel GW et al. Drug effects on REM sleep and on endogenous depression. Neurosci Biobehav Rev 1990; 14:49–63.
7. National Institute for Clinical Excellence. Anxiety (amended). Management of anxiety (panic disorder, with or without agoraphobia, and generalised anxiety disorder) in adults in primary, secondary and community care. Clinical Guidance 22. Amended April 2007. 2007. http://www.nice.org.uk
8. Krystal AD et al. Long-term efficacy and safety of zolpidem extended-release 12.5 mg, administered 3 to 7 nights per week for 24 weeks, in patients with chronic primary insomnia: a 6-month, randomized, double-blind, placebo-controlled, parallel-group, multicenter study. Sleep 2008; 31:79–90.

9.   Krystal AD et al. Sustained efficacy of eszopiclone over 6 months of nightly treatment: results of a randomized, double-blind, placebo-controlled study in adults with chronic insomnia. Sleep 2003; 26:793–9.
10.   Mahomed R et al. Prescribing hypnotics in a mental health trust: what consultants say and what they do. Pharm J 2002; 268:657–9.
11.   Department of Health. National Service Framework for Mental Health: Modern Standards and Service Models. http://www.dh.gov.uk/. 1999.
12.   National Institute of Clinical Excellence. Depression: management of depression in primary and secondary care – clinical guidance. http://www.nice.org. uk. 2004.
13.   TREC Collaborative Group. Rapid tranquillisation for agitated patients in emergency psychiatric rooms: a randomised trial of midazolam versus haloperidol plus promethazine. BMJ 2003; 327:708–13.
14.   Alexander J et al. Rapid tranquillisation of violent or agitated patients in a psychiatric emergency setting. Pragmatic randomised trial of intramuscular lorazepam v. haloperidol plus promethazine. Br J Psychiatry 2004; 185:63–9.
15.   Gillies D et al. Benzodiazepines alone or in combination with antipsychotic drugs for acute psychosis. Cochrane Database Syst Rev 2005;CD003079.
16.   Volz A et al. Benzodiazepines for schizophrenia. Cochrane Database Syst Rev 2007;CD006391.
17.   Paton C et al. Benzodiazepines in schizophrenia. Is there a trend towards long-term prescribing? Psychiatr Bull 2000; 24:113–15.
18.   Anon. The sudden withdrawal of triazolam – reasons and consequences. Drug Ther Bull 1991; 29:89–90.
19.   Wang PS et al. Hazardous benzodiazepine regimens in the elderly: effects of half-life, dosage, and duration on risk of hip fracture. Am J Psychiatry 2001; 158:892–98.
20.   Cumming RG et al. Benzodiazepines and risk of hip fractures in older people: a review of the evidence. CNS Drugs 2003; 17:825–37.
21.   Verwey B et al. Memory impairment in those who attempted suicide by benzodiazepine overdose. J Clin Psychiatry 2000; 61:456–9.
22.   Barbone F et al. Association of road-traffic accidents with benzodiazepine use. Lancet 1998; 352:1331–6.

Further reading

Chouinard G. Issues in the clinical use of benzodiazepines: potency, withdrawal, and rebound. J Clin Psychiatry 2004; 65 Suppl 5:7–12.
Royal College of Psychiatrists. Benzodiazepines: risks, benefits and dependence: A re-evaluation. Council Report 59. http://www.rcpsych.ac.uk/ [London]. 1997.

Depression & anxiety

Benzodiazepines and disinhibition

Unexpected increases in aggressive behaviour secondary to drug treatment are usually called disinhibitory or paradoxical reactions. These reactions may be characterised by acute excitement, hyperactivity, increased anxiety, vivid dreams, sexual disinhibition, hostility and rage. It is possible for a drug to have the potential both to decrease and increase aggressive behaviour. Examples include amphetamines, methylphenidate, benzodiazepines and alcohol (note that all are potential drugs of misuse).

How common are disinhibitory reactions with benzodiazepines?

The incidence of disinhibitory reactions varies widely depending on the population studied (see 'Who is at risk?' below). For example, a meta-analysis of benzodiazepine randomised, controlled trials (RCTs) that included many hundreds of patients with a wide range of diagnoses reported an incidence of less than 1% (similar to placebo)[1]; a Norwegian study that reported on 415 cases of 'driving under the influence', in which flunitrazepam was the sole substance implicated, found that 6% could be described as due to disinhibitory reactions[2]. An RCT that recruited patients with panic disorder reported an incidence of 13%[3]; authors of case series (often reporting on use in high-risk patients) reported rates of 10–20%[1]; and an RCT that included patients with borderline personality disorder reported a rate of 58%[4].

Who is at risk?

Those who have learning disability, neurological disorder or CNS degenerative disease[5], are young (child or adolescent) or elderly[5,6], or have a history of aggression/poor impulse control[4,7] are at increased risk of experiencing a disinhibitory reaction. The risk is further increased if the benzodiazepine is a high-potency drug, has a short half-life, is given in a high dose or is administered intravenously (high and rapidly fluctuating plasma levels)[5,8]. Some people may be genetically predisposed[9]. Combinations of risk factors are clearly important: long-acting benzodiazepines may cause disinhibition in high-risk populations such as children[10].

What is the mechanism?[11–13]

Various theories of the mechanism have been proposed: the anxiolytic and amnesic properties of benzodiazepines may lead to a loss of the restraint that governs normal social behaviour, the sedative and amnesic properties of benzodiazepines may lead to a reduced ability to concentrate on the external social cues that guide appropriate behaviour and the benzodiazepine-mediated increases in GABA neurotransmission may lead to a decrease in the restraining influence of the cortex, resulting in untrammelled excitement, anxiety and hostility.

Subjective reports

People who take benzodiazepines rate themselves as being more tolerant and friendly, but respond more to provocation, than placebo-treated patients[14]. People with impulse control problems who take benzodiazepines may self-report feelings of power and overwhelming self-esteem[7]. Psychology rating scales demonstrate increased suggestibility, failure to recognise anger in others and reduced ability to recognise social cues.

Clinical implications

Benzodiazepines are frequently used in rapid tranquillisation and the short-term management of disturbed behaviour. It is important to be aware of their propensity to cause disinhibitory reactions.

Depression & anxiety

Paradoxical/disinhibitory/aggressive outbursts in the context of benzodiazepine use:

- usually occur with high doses of high-potency drugs that are administered parenterally
- are rare in the general population but more frequent in people with impulse control problems or CNS damage and in the very young or very old
- usually occur in response to (very mild) provocation, the exact nature of which is not always obvious to others
- are recognised by others but often not by the sufferer, who often believes that he is friendly and tolerant.

Suspected paradoxical reactions should be clearly documented in the clinical notes. In extreme cases, flumazenil can be used to reverse the reaction. If the benzodiazepine was prescribed to control acute behavioural disturbance, future episodes should be managed with antipsychotic drugs[15] or other non-benzodiazepine sedatives.

References

1. Dietch JT et al. Aggressive dyscontrol in patients treated with benzodiazepines. J Clin Psychiatry 1988; 49:184–8.
2. Bramness JG et al. Flunitrazepam: psychomotor impairment, agitation and paradoxical reactions. Forensic Sci Int 2006; 159:83–91.
3. O'Sullivan GH et al. Safety and side-effects of alprazolam. Controlled study in agoraphobia with panic disorder. Br J Psychiatry 1994; 165:79–86.
4. Gardner DL et al. Alprazolam-induced dyscontrol in borderline personality disorder. Am J Psychiatry 1985; 142:98–100.
5. Bond AJ. Drug-induced behavioural disinhibition incidence, mechanisms and therapeutic implications. CNS Drugs 1998; 9:41–57.
6. Hawkridge SM et al. A risk–benefit assessment of pharmacotherapy for anxiety disorders in children and adolescents. Drug Saf 1998; 19:283–97.
7. Daderman AM et al. Flunitrazepam (Rohypnol) abuse in combination with alcohol causes premeditated, grievous violence in male juvenile offenders. J Am Acad Psychiatry Law 1999; 27:83–99.
8. van der BP et al. Disinhibitory reactions to benzodiazepines: a review. J Oral Maxillofac Surg 1991; 49:519–23.
9. Short TG et al. Paradoxical reactions to benzodiazepines--a genetically determined phenomenon? Anaesth Intensive Care 1987; 15:330–1.
10. Kandemir H et al. Behavioral disinhibition, suicidal ideation, and self-mutilation related to clonazepam. J Child Adolesc Psychopharmacol 2008; 18:409.
11. van der Bijl P et al. Disinhibitory reactions to benzodiazepines: a review. J Oral Maxillofac Surg 1991; 49:519–23.
12. Weisman AM et al. Effects of clorazepate, diazepam, and oxazepam on a laboratory measurement of aggression in men. Int Clin Psychopharmacol 1998; 13:183–8.
13. Blair RJ et al. Selective impairment in the recognition of anger induced by diazepam. Psychopharmacology 1999; 147:335–8.
14. Bond AJ et al. Behavioural aggression in panic disorder after 8 weeks' treatment with alprazolam. J Affect Disord 1995; 35:117–23.
15. Paton C. Benzodiazepines and disinhibition: a review. Psychiatr Bull 2002; 26:460–2.

Depression & anxiety

Benzodiazepines: dependence and detoxification

Benzodiazepines are widely acknowledged as addictive and withdrawal symptoms can occur after 4–6 weeks of continuous use. At least a third of long-term users experience problems on dosage reduction or withdrawal[1]. Short-acting drugs such as lorazepam are associated with more problems on withdrawal than longer-acting drugs such as diazepam[1,2]. To avoid or lessen these problems, good practice dictates that benzodiazepines should not be prescribed as hypnotics or anxiolytics for longer than 4 weeks[3,4]. Intermittent use (i.e. not every day) may also help avoid problems of dependence and tolerance.

Problems on withdrawal[5]

Table	
Physical	*Psychological*
• Stiffness	• Anxiety/insomnia
• Weakness	• Nightmares
• GI disturbance	• Depersonalisation
• Paraesthesia	• Decreased memory and concentration
• Flu-like symptoms	• Delusions and hallucinations
• Visual disturbances	• Depression

In the majority, symptoms last no longer than a few weeks, although a minority experience disabling symptoms for much longer[1,3]. Minimal intervention strategies; for example simply sending the patient a letter advising them to stop taking benzodiazepine[5], increases the odds of successfully stopping three-fold[6]. Continuing support can be required (e.g. psychological therapies or self-help groups).

If clinically indicated and assuming the patient is in agreement, benzodiazepines should be withdrawn as follows.

Confirming use
If benzodiazepines are not prescribed and patients are obtaining their own supply, use should be confirmed by urine screening (a negative urine screen in combination with no signs of benzodiazepine withdrawal, rules out physical dependence). Very short-acting benzodiazepines may not give a positive urine screen despite daily use.

Tolerance test
This will be required if the patient has been obtaining illicit supplies. No benzodiazepines/alcohol should be consumed for 12 hours before the test. A test dose of 10 mg diazepam should be administered (20 mg if consumption of >50 mg daily is claimed or suspected) and the patient observed for 2–3 hours. If there are no signs of sedation, it is generally safe to prescribe the test dose three times a day. Some patients may require much higher doses. Inpatient assessment may be desirable in these cases.

Switching to diazepam
Patients who take short- or intermediate-acting benzodiazepines should be offered an equivalent dose of diazepam (which has a long half-life and therefore provokes less severe withdrawal)[1]. Note that Cochrane are lukewarm about this approach[7]. Approximate 'diazepam equivalent'[1] doses are shown below.

Depression & anxiety

The half-lives of benzodiazepines vary greatly. The degree of sedation that they induce also varies, making it difficult to determine exact equivalents. The above is an approximate guide only. Extra precautions apply in patients with hepatic dysfunction, as diazepam may accumulate to toxic levels. Diazepam substitution may not be appropriate in this group of patients.

Chlordiazepoxide	25 mg
Clonazepam	1–2 mg
Diazepam	10 mg
Lorazepam	1 mg
Lormetazepam	1 mg
Nitrazepam	10 mg
Oxazepam	30 mg
Temazepam	20 mg

Dosage reduction

Systematic reduction strategies are twice as likely to lead to abstinence than simply advising the patient to stop[6]. Although gradual withdrawal is more acceptable to patients than abrupt withdrawal[7], note that there is no evidence to support the differential efficacy of different tapering schedules, either fixed dose or symptom-guided[6]. The following is a suggested taper schedule; some patients may tolerate more rapid reduction and others may require a slower taper.

- Reduce by 10 mg/day every 1–2 weeks, down to a daily dose of 50 mg
- Reduce by 5 mg/day every 1–2 weeks, down to a daily dose of 30 mg
- Reduce by 2 mg/day every 1–2 weeks, down to a daily dose of 20 mg
- Reduce by 1 mg/day every 1–2 weeks until stopped

Usually, no more than 1 week's supply (exact number of tablets) should be issued at any one time.

Anticipating problems[1,5,8]

Problematic withdrawal can be anticipated if previous attempts have been unsuccessful, the patient lacks social support, there is a history of alcohol/polydrug abuse or withdrawal seizures, the patient is elderly, or there is concomitant severe physical/psychiatric disorder or personality disorder. The acceptable rate of withdrawal may inevitably be slower in these patients. Some may never succeed. Risk–benefit analysis may conclude that maintenance treatment with benzodiazepines is appropriate[3]. Some patients may need interventions for underlying disorders masked by benzodiazepine dependence. If the patient is indifferent to withdrawal (i.e. is not motivated to stop), success is unlikely.

Adjunctive treatments

There is some evidence to support the use of antidepressant and mood-stabilising drugs as adjuncts during benzodiazepine withdrawal[1,6,7,9–12]. There is more limited evidence to support the use of pregabalin, even in patients who take very high daily doses of benzodiazepines[13,14]. People with insomnia may benefit from adjunctive treatment with melatonin and those with panic disorder may benefit from CBT during the taper period[6].

References

1. Schweizer E et al. Benzodiazepine dependence and withdrawal: a review of the syndrome and its clinical management. Acta Psychiatr Scand Suppl 1998; 393:95–101.
2. Uhlenhuth EH et al. International study of expert judgment on therapeutic use of benzodiazepines and other psychotherapeutic medications: IV. Therapeutic dose dependence and abuse liability of benzodiazepines in the long-term treatment of anxiety disorders. J Clin Psychopharmacol 1999; 19:23S–9S.
3. Royal College of Psychiatrist. Benzodiazepines: risks, benefits or dependence. A re-evaluation. Council Report 59. http://www.rcpsych.ac.uk/. 1997.
4. Committee on Safety in Medicines. Benzodiazepines, dependence and withdrawl symptoms. Current Problems 1988; 21:1–2.
5. Petursson H. The benzodiazepine withdrawal syndrome. Addiction 1994; 89:1455–9.
6. Voshaar RCO et al. Strategies for discontinuing long-term benzodiazepine use: Meta-analysis. Br J Psychiatry 2006; 189:213–20.
7. Denis C et al. Pharmacological interventions for benzodiazepine mono-dependence management in outpatient settings. Cochrane Database Syst Rev 2006; CD005194.
8. Tyrer P. Risks of dependence on benzodiazepine drugs: the importance of patient selection. BMJ 1989; 298:102–5.
9. Rickels K et al. Imipramine and buspirone in treatment of patients with generalized anxiety disorder who are discontinuing long-term benzodiazepine therapy. Am J Psychiatry 2000; 157:1973–9.
10. Tyrer P et al. A controlled trial of dothiepin and placebo in treating benzodiazepine withdrawal symptoms. Br J Psychiatry 1996; 168:457–61.
11. Schweizer E et al. Carbamazepine treatment in patients discontinuing long-term benzodiazepine therapy. Effects on withdrawal severity and outcome. Arch Gen Psychiatry 1991; 48:448–52.
12. Zitman FG et al. Chronic benzodiazepine use in general practice patients with depression: an evaluation of controlled treatment and taper-off: report on behalf of the Dutch Chronic Benzodiazepine Working Group. Br J Psychiatry 2001; 178:317–24.
13. Oulis P et al. Pregabalin in the discontinuation of long-term benzodiazepines' use. Hum Psychopharmacol 2008; 23:337–40.
14. Oulis P et al. Pregabalin in the discontinuation of long-term benzodiazepine use: a case-series. Int Clin Psychopharmacol 2008; 23:110–12.

Further reading

Heberlein A et al. Neuroendocrine pathways in benzodiazepine dependence: new targets for research and therapy. Hum Psychopharmacol 2008; 23:171–81.
Ahmed M et al. A self-help handout for benzodiazepine discontinuation using cognitive behavioral therapy. Cogn Behav Pract 2008; 15:317–24.

Depression & anxiety

Insomnia

A patient complaining of insomnia may describe one or more of the following symptoms:

- difficulty in falling asleep
- frequent waking during the night
- early-morning wakening
- daytime sleepiness
- a general loss of well-being through the individual's perception of a bad night's sleep.

Insomnia is a common complaint affecting approximately one-third of the UK population in any one year[1]. It is more common in women, in the elderly (some reports suggest 50% of those over 65 years) and in those with medical or psychiatric disorders[2]. Population studies in the UK have found that the prevalence of symptoms of underlying psychiatric illness, particularly depression and anxiety, increases with the severity and chronicity of insomnia[3]. Insomnia that lasts for 1 year or more is an established risk factor for the development of depression[4]. Chronic insomnia rarely remits spontaneously[5].

Before treating insomnia with drugs, consider:

- Is the underlying cause being treated (depression, mania, breathing difficulties, urinary frequency, pain, etc.)?
- Is substance misuse or diet a problem?
- Are other drugs being given at appropriate times (i.e. stimulating drugs in the morning, sedating drugs at night)?
- Are the patient's expectations of sleep realistic (sleep requirements decrease with age)?
- Have all sleep hygiene approaches been tried[1]? (see table below)

Table   Sleep hygiene approaches
• Increase daily exercise (not in the evening)
• Reduce/stop daytime napping
• Reduce caffeine or alcohol intake, especially before bedtime. Avoid caffeine after midday
• Use the bed only for sleeping
• Use anxiety management or relaxation techniques
• Develop a regular routine of rising and retiring at the same time each day, regardless of the amount of sleep taken

Table   Guidelines for prescribing hypnotics[6]
• Use the lowest effective dose
• Use intermittent dosing (alternate nights or less) where possible
• Prescribe for short-term use (no more than 4 weeks) in the majority of cases
• Discontinue slowly
• Be alert for rebound insomnia/withdrawal symptoms
• Advise patients of the interaction with alcohol and other sedating drugs
• Avoid the use of hypnotics in patients with respiratory disease or severe hepatic impairment and in addiction-prone individuals

Short-acting hypnotics are better for patients who have difficulty dropping off to sleep, but tolerance and dependence may develop more quickly[4]. Long-acting hypnotics are more suitable for patients with frequent or early-morning wakening. These drugs may be less likely to cause rebound insomnia and can have next-day anxiolytic action, but next-day sedation and loss of co-ordination are more likely to occur[6]. The risks of treating older people (>60 years) with hypnotics may outweigh the benefits. A meta-analysis has shown the number needed to treat for improved sleep quality was 13 and the number needed to treat for any adverse event was 6[7]. Older patients prescribed hypnotics (especially those with dementia) should be closely monitored to determine if the prescription continues to be justified.

The most widely prescribed hypnotics are the benzodiazepines. Non-benzodiazepine hypnotics such as zopiclone and zolpidem are becoming more widely used but may be just as likely as the benzodiazepines to cause rebound, dependence and neuropsychiatric reactions[8–10]. Zopiclone may impair driving performance more than benzodiazepines[11]. NICE concluded that there is no difference in efficacy between zaleplon, zolpidem and zopiclone and that patients who fail to respond to one drug should not be offered another[12].

A 2 mg CR formulation of melatonin has recently been licensed for the treatment of insomnia in people >55 years old. A meta-analysis supports the efficacy of melatonin in decreasing sleep latency in people with a primary sleep disorder[13], while a second meta-analysis that included studies of people with secondary sleep disorders was essentially negative[14]. Melatonin is not addictive and seems to be well-tolerated; there are concerns that melatonin may worsen seizure control and nocturnal asthma, and may delay gonadal development, but there is little in the way of systematic data to confirm or refute these concerns[15]. Objective tests reveal that melatonin is unlikely to impair driving ability; it does however increase subjective sleepiness[16]. When melatonin is prescribed, a licensed preparation is to be preferred over an unlicensed one where possible; the latter may be food supplements of uncertain quantity[17].

Ramelteon, a highly selective MT_1/MT_2 agonist has been approved for use as a hypnotic in the USA, but is not yet available in the UK. Ramelteon produced significant reductions in latency to persistent sleep and increases in total sleep in a group of patients with chronic primary insomnia[18,19], with no apparent next-day residual effects.

Table Drugs used as hypnotics				
Drug	**Usual therapeutic dose (mg/day)**		**Time until onset (minutes)**	**Duration of action**
	Adult	**Elderly**		
Lormetazepam[†]	0.5–1.5		30–60	Short
Oxazepam[†]	15–30		20–50	Short
Nitrazepam[†]	5–10		20–50	Long
Temazepam*[†]	10–20	Quarter to	30–60	Short
Zaleplon	10	half the	30	Short
Zopiclone	3.75–7.5	adult dose	15–30	Short
Zolpidem	5–10		7–27	Short
Melatonin	2		unclear	Short
Promethazine (not licensed)	25–50		Unclear, but may be 1–2 hours	Long

*Temazepam is a popular drug of misuse. Some of the Controlled Drug Regulations apply to its prescription, supply and administration. Nursing paperwork can be simplified considerably by avoiding the use of this drug.

[†]Changes in Controlled Drug Regulations as of July 2006 mean that benzodiazepines should only be prescribed for a maximum of 28 days at a time.

Over-the-counter remedies for insomnia include valerian–hops combinations and diphenhydramine which may improve sleep to some extent without causing rebound insomnia[20].

Although it is commonly believed that tolerance always develops rapidly to the hypnotic effect of benzodiazepines[12] and zopiclone, there are only limited objective data to support this, and the magnitude of the problem may have been overestimated[5]. Long-term treatment with hypnotics may be beneficial in a very small number of patients. There is a positive 6-month RCT supporting the ongoing efficacy of eszopiclone[21] and another supporting the efficacy of zolpidem[22]. In the latter study, patients who took zolpidem at least three nights each week reported better sleep onset, sleep maintenance and next day functioning. Long-term users of hypnotics however may overestimate the benefits on continuing use: after a period of rebound symptoms immediately after withdrawal, many chronic users will return to the same sleep pattern (drug-free) that they previously associated with hypnotic use[23]. As with all prescribing, the potential benefits and risks of hypnotic drugs have to be considered in the context of the clinical circumstances of each case.

Cognitive behavioural therapy may be more effective than hypnotics in improving sleep in the long term[24]. CBT has been shown to improve sleep quality, reduce hypnotic drug use and improve health-related quality of life among long-term hypnotic users with chronic sleep difficulties[25].

References

1. Hajak G. A comparative assessment of the risks and benefits of zopiclone: a review of 15 years' clinical experience. Drug Saf 1999; 21:457–69.
2. Shapiro CM. ABC of Sleep Disorders. London: BMJ Publishing Group; 1993.
3. Nutt DJ et al. Evaluation of severe insomnia in the general population—implications for the management of insomnia: the UK perspective. J Psychopharmacol 1999; 13:S33–4.
4. Moller HJ. Effectiveness and safety of benzodiazepines. J Clin Psychopharmacol 1999; 19:2S–11S.
5. Nowell PD et al. Benzodiazepines and zolpidem for chronic insomnia: a meta-analysis of treatment efficacy. JAMA 1997; 278:2170–7.
6. Royal College of Psychiatrist. Benzodiazepines: risks, benefits or dependence. A re-evaluation. Council Report 59. http://www.rcpsych.ac.uk/. 1997.
7. Glass J et al. Sedative hypnotics in older people with insomnia: meta-analysis of risks and benefits. BMJ 2005; 331:1169.
8. Sikdar S et al. Zopiclone abuse among polydrug users. Addiction 1996; 91:285–6.
9. Gericke CA et al. Chronic abuse of zolpidem. JAMA 1994; 272:1721–2.
10. Voshaar RC et al. Zolpidem is not superior to temazepam with respect to rebound insomnia: a controlled study. Eur Neuropsychopharmacol 2004; 14:301–6.
11. Barbone F et al. Association of road-traffic accidents with benzodiazepine use. Lancet 1998; 352:1331–6.
12. National Institute of Clinical Excellence. Insomnia – newer hypnotic drugs. Zaleplon, zolpidem and zopiclone for the management of insomnia. Technology Appraisal 77. http://www.nice.org.uk. 2004.
13. Buscemi N et al. The efficacy and safety of exogenous melatonin for primary sleep disorders. A meta-analysis. J Gen Intern Med 2005; 20:1151–8.
14. Buscemi N et al. Efficacy and safety of exogenous melatonin for secondary sleep disorders and sleep disorders accompanying sleep restriction: meta-analysis. Arch Intern Med 2006; 332:385–93.
15. Armour A et al. A randomized, controlled prospective trial of zolpidem and haloperidol for use as sleeping agents in pediatric burn patients. J Burn Care Res 2008; 29:238–47.
16. Suhner A et al. Impact of melatonin on driving performance. J Travel Med 1998; 5:7–13.
17. Medicines and Healthcare Products Regulatory Agency. Restrictions on the import of unlicensed Melatonin products following the grant of a marketing authorisation for Circadin® 2mg tablets. 2008. http://www.mhra.gov.uk
18. Erman M et al. An efficacy, safety, and dose-response study of Ramelteon in patients with chronic primary insomnia. Sleep Med 2006; 7:17–24.
19. Mini L et al. Ramelteon 8 mg/d versus placebo in patients with chronic insomnia: post hoc analysis of a 5-week trial using 50% or greater reduction in latency to persistent sleep as a measure of treatment effect. Clin Ther 2008; 30:1316–23.
20. Morin CM et al. Valerian–hops combination and diphenhydramine for treating insomnia: a randomized placebo-controlled clinical trial. Sleep 2005; 28:1465–71.
21. Krystal AD et al. Sustained efficacy of eszopiclone over 6 months of nightly treatment: results of a randomized, double-blind, placebo-controlled study in adults with chronic insomnia. Sleep 2003; 26:793–9.
22. Krystal AD et al. Long-term efficacy and safety of zolpidem extended-release 12.5 mg, administered 3 to 7 nights per week for 24 weeks, in patients with chronic primary insomnia: a 6-month, randomized, double-blind, placebo-controlled, parallel-group, multicenter study. Sleep 2008; 31:79–90.
23. Poyares D et al. Chronic benzodiazepine usage and withdrawal in insomnia patients. J Psychiatr Res 2004; 38:327–34.
24. Jacobs GD et al. Cognitive behavior therapy and pharmacotherapy for insomnia: a randomized controlled trial and direct comparison. Arch Intern Med 2004; 164:1888–96.
25. Morgan K et al. Psychological treatment for insomnia in the regulation of long-term hypnotic drug use. Health Technol Assess 2004; 8:iii–68.

Further reading

Arendt J et al. Melatonin and its agonists: an update. Br J Psychiatry 2008; 193:267–9.
Arendt J et al. Clinical update: melatonin and sleep disorders. Clin Med 2008; 8:381–3.
Benca RM. Diagnosis and treatment of chronic insomnia: a review. Psychiatr Serv 2005; 56:332–43.
Terzano MG et al. New drugs for insomnia; comparative tolerability of zopiclone, zolpidem and zaleplon. Drug Safety 2003; 26:261–82.

chapter 5

Children and adolescents

Children and adolescents suffer from all the illnesses of adulthood. It is common for psychiatric illness to commence more diffusely, present 'atypically', respond less predictably and be associated with cumulative impairment more subtly. Childhood-onset illness is likely to be at least as severe and functionally disabling as adult-onset illness.

Very few psychotropic drugs are licensed for use in children. This should be carefully explained and informed consent sought from patients and their parents/carers.

Principles of prescribing practice in childhood and adolescence[1]

- **Target symptoms, not diagnoses**
  Diagnosis can be difficult in children and co-morbidity is very common. Treatment should target key symptoms. While a working diagnosis is beneficial to frame expectations and help communication with patients and parents, it should be kept in mind that it may take some time for the illness to evolve.

- **Technical aspects of paediatric prescribing**
  The Medicines Act 1968 and European legislation make provision for doctors to use medicines in an off-label or out-of-licence capacity or to use unlicensed medicines. However, individual prescribers are always responsible for ensuring that there is adequate information to support the quality, efficacy, safety and intended use of a drug before prescribing it. It is recognised that the informed use of unlicensed medicines, or of licensed medicines for unlicensed applications ('off-label' use), is often necessary in paediatric practice. Prescription writing: inclusion of age is a legal requirement in the case of prescription-only medicines for children under 12 years of age, but it is preferable to state the age for all prescriptions for children.

- **Begin with less, go slow and be prepared to end with more**
  In out-patient care, dosage will usually commence lower in mg/kg per day terms than adults and finish higher in mg/kg per day terms, if titrated to a point of maximal response.

- **Multiple medications are often required in the severely ill**
  Monotherapy is ideal. However, childhood-onset illness can be severe and may require treatment with psychosocial approaches in combination with more than one medication[2].

- **Allow time for an adequate trial of treatment**
  Children are generally more ill than their adult counterparts and will often require longer periods of treatment before responding. An adequate trial of treatment for those who have required in-patient care may well take 8 weeks for depression or schizophrenia.

- **Where possible, change one drug at a time**

- **Monitor outcome in more than one setting**
  For symptomatic treatments (such as stimulants for ADHD), bear in mind that the expression of problems may be different across settings (e.g. home and school); a dose titrated against parent reports may be too high for the daytime at school.

- **Patient and family medication education is essential**
  For some child and adolescent psychiatric patients the need for medication will be lifelong. The first experiences with medications are therefore crucial to long-term outcomes and adherence.

References

1. Nunn K, Dey C. The Clinician's Guide to Psychotropic Prescribing in Children and Adolescents. 1 ed. Sydney: Glade Publishing; 2003.
2. Luk E, Reed E. Polypharmacy or Pharmacologically Rich? In: Nunn KP, Dey C, editors. The Clinician's Guide to Psychotropic Prescribing in Children and Adolescents. 2 ed. Sydney: Glade Publishing; 2003. 8–11.

Further reading

For detailed adverse effects of CNS Drugs in Children and Adolescents, see:
BMJ Group and RPS Publishing. Central Nervous System. British National Formulary for Children. London: RPS Publishing; 2008. 209–291.
Martin A, Scahill L, Charney DS, Leckman JF. Pediatric Psychopharmacology: Principles and Practice. New York, USA: Oxford University Press; 2002.
Riddle MA, et al. Introduction: Issues and viewpoints in pediatric psychopharmacology. Int Rev Psychiatry 2008; 20:119–120.

Depression in children and adolescents

Psychological intervention

Psychological treatments should always be considered as first-line treatments for child and adolescent depression. NICE recommends a stepped model of care, with the introduction of medication in association with psychological treatments if there is failure to respond, or if the depression is more severe. Psycho-educational programmes, non-directive supportive therapy, group cognitive behaviour therapy (CBT) and self help are indicated for mild to moderate depression. More specific and/or intensive psychological interventions including CBT, interpersonal psychotherapy and short-term family therapy are recommended for moderate to severe depression.

SSRI treatment

If there is no response to psychological treatment, if psychological forms of therapy are inappropriate, or are simply not available, **fluoxetine**[1-5] is the treatment of choice. Medication should be considered if there is little or no response to psychological treatment after 4–6 sessions. The more severe the depressive episode the more likely it is that pharmacotherapy, in combination with psychological treatment or on its own, should be introduced at an earlier stage in the treatment. The most severe depressive episodes will generally require treatment with antidepressants.

NICE support the use of fluoxetine but only in combination with psychological forms of therapy[1,6]. However this remains a controversial area, with a relatively small evidence base, and clinicians treating depression in young people need to review emerging data and seek advice from specialists if needed. For example, a UK study did not establish the benefits of combined therapy (fluoxetine plus CBT) and has demonstrated that the use of fluoxetine on its own is effective in treating moderate to severe depression[7]. Generally speaking, adolescents can be expected to respond better to antidepressants than younger children, particularly those under 12[5].

Fluoxetine should be administered starting with a low dose of 10 mg daily[1]. Patients and their parents/carers should be well informed about the potential side-effects associated with SSRI treatment and know how to seek help in an emergency. Any pre-existing symptoms which might be interpreted as side-effects (e.g. agitation, anxiety, suicidality) should be noted.

The placebo response rate is high in young people with depression[8]. On average drug and placebo response rates in children and adolescents differ by only 10%[5] and the benefits of active treatment are likely to be marginal; it is estimated that 1 in 6 may benefit[1,5]. There is some evidence to suggest dose increases can improve response[9]. The risk–benefit ratios for the other SSRIs are unfavourable (limited proven efficacy, and increased risk of suicidal thoughts or acts[1,2]). It has been suggested that fluoxetine with its long duration of action may have advantages in relation to poor adolescent compliance[5].

If there is no response to fluoxetine and drug treatment is still considered to be the most favourable option, **an alternative SSRI** may be used cautiously by specialists. The current limited literature suggests some efficacy for sertraline[1,10,11] but one RCT shows it to be inferior to CBT[12]. Citalopram, also recommended by NICE[1], and escitalopram are probably not as effective[3,13,14]. Note that paroxetine and venlafaxine are considered to be unsuitable options[1,3,13].

When prescribing SSRIs it is important that the dose is increased slowly to minimise the risk of treatment-emergent agitation and that patients are monitored closely for the development of treatment-emergent suicidal thoughts and acts. Patients should be seen at least weekly in the early stages of treatment. There is now no doubt that antidepressants increase the risk of suicidal

Children

behaviours in children[15–23]. One RCT which compared CBT with fluoxetine, placebo medication and combined CBT and fluoxetine showed that all treatment arms were effective in reducing suicidal ideation but that the combined treatment of fluoxetine and CBT reduced the risk of suicidal events in contrast to fluoxetine-treated patients who had more suicide related events[22].

Duration of treatment and discontinuation of SSRIs
There is little evidence regarding optimum duration of treatment[24]. Adult guidelines are usually followed (see Chapter 4). At the end of treatment, the antidepressant dose should be tapered slowly to minimise discontinuation symptoms. Ideally this should be done over 6–12 weeks[1]. To consolidate the response to the acute treatment and avoid relapse, treatment with fluoxetine should continue for at least 6 and up to 12 months[25].

Refractory depression and other treatments
There are no clear guidelines for the management of treatment-resistant depression in adolescents[1,26] but there is evidence that adolescents who failed to respond to adequate treatment with one SSRI showed a higher rate of clinical response when switched to another SSRI or venlafaxine when the pharmacotherapy was combined with concurrent CBT. A switch to an SSRI was just as efficacious as a switch to venlafaxine with fewer side effects[27,28]. Augmentation trials in adults and adolescents using bupropion, thyroxine and lamotrigine have shown some positive results[27].

Tricyclic antidepressants are not effective in pre-pubertal children but may have marginal efficacy in adolescents[5,29]. Amitriptyline (up to 200 mg/day), imipramine (up to 300 mg/day) and nortriptyline have all been studied in RCTs. Note that due to more extensive metabolism, young people require higher mg/kg doses than adults. The side-effect burden associated with TCAs may be considerable. Vertigo, orthostatic hypotension, tremor and dry mouth limit tolerability. Tricyclics are also more cardiotoxic in young people than in adults. Baseline and on-treatment ECGs should be performed. Co-prescribing with other drugs known to prolong the QTc interval should be avoided. There is no evidence that adolescents who fail to respond to SSRIs respond to tricyclics. NICE advise against the use of tricyclic antidepressants given the high risk-to-benefit ratio[1]. NICE also advise against the use of St John's Wort in combination with antidepressants or on its own given that little is known about potential interactions and side effects in this age group[1].

Omega-3 fatty acids may be effective in childhood depression but evidence is minimal[30].

Severe depression that is life-threatening or unresponsive to other treatments may respond to ECT[31]. ECT should not be used in children under 12[31]. The effects of ECT on the developing brain are unknown.

Risk of bipolar disorder
Note that up to a third of young people who present with an episode of depression will have a diagnosis of bipolar affective disorder within 5 years. When the presentation is of severe depression, associated with psychosis or rapid mood shifts and worsens on treatment with antidepressants, early bipolar illness should be suspected. Treatment with antidepressants alone is associated with new or worsening rapid cycling in as many as 23% of bipolar patients[32]. Antidepressants increase the risk of adolescents becoming excited or manic during treatment of apparent severe depression[33]. The younger the child, the greater the risk[34]. Early treatment with mood-stabilisers should be considered.

References

1. National Institute for Clinical Excellence. Depression in children and young people: identification and management in primary, community and secondary care. Clinical Guidance 28. http://www.mhra.gov.uk. 2005.
2. Whittington CJ et al. Selective serotonin reuptake inhibitors in childhood depression: systematic review of published versus unpublished data. Lancet 2004; 363:341–1345.
3. Medicines and Healthcare Products Regulatory Agency. Selective serotonin reuptake inhibitors (SSRIs): Overview of regulatory status and CSM advice relating to major depressive disorder (MDD) in children and adolescents including a summary of available safety and efficacy data. http://www.mhra.gov.uk. 2005.
4. Kratochvil CJ et al. Selective serotonin reuptake inhibitors in pediatric depression: is the balance between benefits and risks favorable? J Child Adolesc Psychopharmacol 2006; 16:11–24.
5. Tsapakis EM et al. Efficacy of antidepressants in juvenile depression: meta-analysis. Br J Psychiatry 2008; 193:10–17.
6. March J et al. Fluoxetine, cognitive-behavioral therapy, and their combination for adolescents with depression: Treatment for Adolescents with Depression Study (TADS) randomized controlled trial. JAMA 2004; 292:807–820.
7. Goodyer I et al. Selective serotonin reuptake inhibitors (SSRIs) and routine specialist care with and without cognitive behaviour therapy in adolescents with major depression: randomised controlled trial. BMJ 2007; 335:142.
8. Jureidini JN et al. Efficacy and safety of antidepressants for children and adolescents. BMJ 2004; 328:879–883.
9. Heiligenstein JH et al. Fluoxetine 40–60 mg versus fluoxetine 20 mg in the treatment of children and adolescents with a less-than-complete response to nine-week treatment with fluoxetine 10–20 mg: a pilot study. J Child Adolesc Psychopharmacol 2006; 16:207–217.
10. Donnelly CL et al. Sertraline in children and adolescents with major depressive disorder. J Am Acad Child Adolesc Psychiatry 2006; 45:1162–1170.
11. Rynn M et al. Long-term sertraline treatment of children and adolescents with major depressive disorder. J Child Adolesc Psychopharmacol 2006; 16:103–116.
12. Melvin GA et al. A comparison of cognitive-behavioral therapy, sertraline, and their combination for adolescent depression. J Am Acad Child Adolesc Psychiatry 2006; 45:1151–1161.
13. Wagner KD et al. A double-blind, randomized, placebo-controlled trial of escitalopram in the treatment of pediatric depression. J Am Acad Child Adolesc Psychiatry 2006; 45:280–288.
14. von Knorring AL et al. A randomized, double-blind, placebo-controlled study of citalopram in adolescents with major depressive disorder. J Clin Psychopharmacol 2006; 26:311–315.
15. Martinez C et al. Antidepressant treatment and the risk of fatal and non-fatal self harm in first episode depression: nested case-control study. BMJ 2005; 330:389.
16. Kaizar EE et al. Do antidepressants cause suicidality in children? A Bayesian meta-analysis. Clin Trials 2006; 3:73–90.
17. Mosholder AD et al. Suicidal adverse events in pediatric randomized, controlled clinical trials of antidepressant drugs are associated with active drug treatment: a meta-analysis. J Child Adolesc Psychopharmacol 2006; 16:25–32.
18. Simon GE et al. Suicide risk during antidepressant treatment. Am J Psychiatry 2006; 163:41–47.
19. Olfson M et al. Antidepressant drug therapy and suicide in severely depressed children and adults: A case-control study. Arch Gen Psychiatry 2006; 63:865–872.
20. Hammad TA et al. Suicidality in pediatric patients treated with antidepressant drugs. Arch Gen Psychiatry 2006; 63:332–339.
21. Dubicka B et al. Suicidal behaviour in youths with depression treated with new-generation antidepressants: meta-analysis. Br J Psychiatry 2006; 189:393–398.
22. March J et al. The Treatment for Adolescents with Depression Study (TADS): methods and message at 12 weeks. J Am Acad Child Adolesc Psychiatry 2006; 45:1393–1403.
23. Bridge JA et al. Clinical response and risk for reported suicidal ideation and suicide attempts in pediatric antidepressant treatment: a meta-analysis of randomized controlled trials. JAMA 2007; 297:1683–1696.
24. Kennard BD et al. Relapse and recurrence in pediatric depression. Child Adolesc Psychiatr Clin N Am 2006; 15:1057–1079, xi.
25. Emslie GJ et al. Fluoxetine treatment for prevention of relapse of depression in children and adolescents: a double-blind, placebo-controlled study. J Am Acad Child Adolesc Psychiatry 2004; 43:1397–1405.
26. Birmaher B et al. Practice parameter for the assessment and treatment of children and adolescents with depressive disorders. J Am Acad Child Adolesc Psychiatry 2007; 46:1503–1526.
27. Brent DA et al. Treatment-resistant depression in adolescents: recognition and management. Child Adolesc Psychiatr Clin N Am 2006; 15:1015–1034.
28. Brent D et al. Switching to another SSRI or to venlafaxine with or without cognitive behavioral therapy for adolescents with SSRI-resistant depression: the TORDIA Randomized Controlled Trial. JAMA 2008; 299:901–913.
29. Hazell P et al. Tricyclic drugs for depression in children and adolescents. Cochrane Database Syst Rev 2002;CD002317.
30. Nemets H et al. Omega-3 treatment of childhood depression: a controlled, double-blind pilot study. Am J Psychiatry 2006; 163:1098–1100.
31. McKeough G. Electroconvulsive therapy. In: Nunn KP, Dey C, editors. The Clinician's Guide to Psychotropic Prescribing in Children and Adolescents. 1 ed. Sydney: Glade Publishing; 2003; 358–365.
32. Ghaemi SN et al. Diagnosing bipolar disorder and the effect of antidepressants: a naturalistic study. J Clin Psychiatry 2000; 61:804–808.
33. Baldessarini RJ et al. Risk of mania with antidepressants. Arch Pediatr Adolesc Med 2005; 159:298–299.
34. Martin A et al. Age effects on antidepressant-induced manic conversion. Arch Pediatr Adolesc Med 2004; 158:773–780.

Further reading

Bloch Y et al. Electroconvulsive therapy in adolescents: similarities to and differences from adults. J Am Acad Child Adolesc Psychiatry 2001; 40: 1332–1336.
Fombonne E, Zinck S. Psychopharmacological Treatment of Depression in Children and Adolescents. In: Abela JRZ, Hankin BL, editors. Handbook of Depression in Children and Adolescents. New York: Guilford Press; 2008; 207–223.
Moreno C et al. Antidepressants in child and adolescent depression: where are the bugs? Acta Psychiatr Scand 2007; 115:184–195.

Children

Bipolar illness in children and adolescents

Diagnostic issues

Treatment decisions for bipolar disorder (BAD) in children and adolescents should be informed by a thorough developmental assessment. In this age group, BAD is frequently co-morbid or shows symptom overlap with other child psychiatric disorders, such as attention deficit hyperactivity disorder (ADHD), conduct disorders, and pervasive developmental disorders[1]. These may complicate diagnosis and treatment. Clinicians should be aware that while mood lability is a common and impairing presentation in youth, it should not be equated with bipolar disorder[2,3]. Indeed, a highly controversial broadening of the diagnostic boundaries is thought to have led to the recent dramatic increase in the rates of diagnoses of bipolar disorder in children and adolescents in the USA[4,5]. Common UK clinical practice and guidelines[6] adhere to a more narrow definition of bipolar disorder that insists on the presence of significant elation appearing as part of demarcated episodes of change from baseline functioning.

The evidence base for treatment of bipolar disorder in youth is limited compared with that for the adult disorder. Most trials are open label and there are only a few double blind placebo-controlled trials. Also, most evidence concerns adolescents, rather than children.

Clinical guidance

When treating bipolar illness in children and adolescents clinicians will need to be aware of existing guidelines[6,7] and judiciously extrapolate from the adult literature. Monotherapy and starting doses at the lower end of the therapeutic range should be the default. Previous response, current medication, compliance, family and patient preferences will guide treatment decisions. Structured measurement of symptoms (e.g. Young Mania Rating Scale; YMRS) and impairment (e.g. Clinical Global Impressions; CGI) should be used routinely to evaluate progress and treatment outcome. For presentations with psychosis or severe behavioural disturbance, clinicians should consider the use of an antipsychotic agent as a first line due to its more rapid response compared with lithium. Weight/BMI, glucose, lipid and prolactin levels should be closely monitored. Treatment may be augmented with a mood-stabiliser in partial responders; switch to an alternative antipsychotic should be considered in non-response. Despite the lack of youth-specific data on maintenance therapy, it is reasonable to assume that medication will have to be continued for at least 18 months. This should be discussed with the family and the patient and may influence the choice of the agent used. Drug therapy should be part of a more general package of care that includes reducing psychosocial (e.g. family stress) and biological (e.g. cannabis use) precipitants. Adjunctive family interventions may be helpful in stabilising symptomatology[8] and should be considered. Treatment and monitoring decisions should be made by a specialist.

Specific issues

Bipolar depression is a common clinical challenge whose treatment has not been studied in much detail. Some evidence suggests that lithium[9] and lamotrigine[10] may be effective. Youth may be particularly likely to suffer from antidepressant-induced manic switches[11]. It seems prudent to prescribe antidepressants only in the presence of an antimanic agent[6].

The exact relationship between ADHD and BAD, is part of the ongoing controversy regarding the diagnosis and treatment of BAD in children[12]. This has important treatment implications as stimulant/amphetamine medications used in ADHD could theoretically induce manic states. However, some evidence suggests that stimulants in children with manic symptoms may be well tolerated[13] and that they may be safe and effective to use after mood stabilisation[14]. Caution, a thorough developmental history, and experience with prescribing these drugs are required.

Summary of medicines used in BAD in children

Medication	Comment
Lithium	Open label trials show positive effects in acute treatment[15] and maintenance[16]
	One double-blind placebo-controlled randomised trial showed significant reductions in substance use and clinical ratings in adolescents with BP and co-morbid substance abuse[17]. In a double-blind placebo-controlled maintenance trial, no significant difference in relapse rates was found between lithium and placebo; however, follow up may have been too short[18]
	Adherence to lithium and blood level testing may be difficult in adolescents
	Beware of teratogenicity
	Approved by the FDA
Valproate	Several open-label trials[14,19–22] show valproate to be effective in reducing severity of mania
	No significant differences were found in comparison to lithium or carbamazepine for acute treatment[21] or to lithium for maintenance therapy[23]
	A recent industry-conducted double-blind placebo-controlled multi-site study failed to show efficacy compared with placebo treatment[24]
	Polycystic ovaries and associated infertility are particular concerns when used for adolescent girls and NICE[6] recommends avoiding its use in women of child-bearing age. Use of contraception and folate are essential
Oxcarbazepine	A recent large double-blind placebo-controlled multi-site study did not show significant differences between placebo and oxcarbazepine in reducing mania rating[25]
Carbamazepine	A small open RCT has shown it to be of comparable effect to valproate and lithium[21]
Lamotrigine	An open-label study showed an improvement in CGI and CDRS ratings in bipolar depression compared with baseline[10]
Olanzapine[26–29]	A multi-centre double-blind placebo-controlled industry-conducted study[30] showed olanzapine to be significantly more effective than placebo in YMRS score reduction over a period of 3 weeks. Note the significantly higher weight gain in the treatment group (mean baseline to endpoint weight gain was 3.7 kg for olanzapine versus 0.3 kg for placebo) and the associated significantly increased fasting glucose, total cholesterol, AST, ALT, and uric acid
	Open-label studies suggest olanzapine is effective as monotherapy[27] and as an add on to lithium therapy[26]. An open-label study[28] conducted in children aged 4–6 also showed it to be effective; however, the diagnostic algorithm and outcome measures used for the age group in this study are not universally accepted
Risperidone	Approved by the FDA on the basis of an industry-conducted double-blind randomised placebo-controlled study in children aged 10–17. This showed risperidone to be significantly superior to placebo in reducing YMRS scores from baseline to 3-week follow up[31]
	An open-label study[28] conducted in children aged 4–6 also showed it to be effective; however, the diagnostic algorithm and outcome measures used for the age group in this study are not universally accepted
Quetiapine	Effective as an adjunct to valproate compared with placebo[32] and equally effective as valproate in a double-blind trial[33]
Aripiprazole	Recently approved by the FDA on the basis of a 4-week multi-site double-blind placebo-controlled study of outpatients aged 10–17[34]

Children

References

1. Baroni A et al. Practitioner Review: The assessment of bipolar disorder in children and adolescents. J Child Psychol Psychiat 2009; 50:203–215.
2. Brotman MA et al. Parental diagnoses in youth with narrow phenotype bipolar disorder or severe mood dysregulation. Am J Psychiatry 2007; 164:1238–1241.
3. Stringaris A et al. Mood lability and psychopathology in youth. Psychol Med 2008;1–9.
4. Blader JC et al. Increased rates of bipolar disorder diagnoses among U.S. child, adolescent, and adult inpatients, 1996–2004. Biol Psychiatry 2007; 62:107–114.
5. Moreno C et al. National trends in the outpatient diagnosis and treatment of bipolar disorder in youth. Arch Gen Psychiatry 2007; 64:1032–1039.
6. National Institute for Clinical Excellence. Bipolar disorder. The management of bipolar disorder in adults, children and adolescents, in primary and secondary care. Clinical Guidance 38. http://www.nice.org.uk. 2006.
7. Kowatch RA et al. Treatment guidelines for children and adolescents with bipolar disorder. J Am Acad Child Adolesc Psychiatry 2005; 44:21–235.
8. Miklowitz DJ et al. Family-focused treatment for adolescents with bipolar disorder: results of a 2-year randomized trial. Arch Gen Psychiatry 2008; 65:1053–1061.
9. Patel NC et al. Open-label lithium for the treatment of adolescents with bipolar depression. J Am Acad Child Adolesc Psychiatry 2006; 45:289–297.
10. Chang KD et al. Divalproex monotherapy in the treatment of bipolar offspring with mood and behavioral disorders and at least mild affective symptoms. J Clin Psychiatry 2003; 64:936–942.
11. Baumer FM et al. A pilot study of antidepressant-induced mania in pediatric bipolar disorder: Characteristics, risk factors, and the serotonin transporter gene. Biol Psychiatry 2006; 60:1005–1012.
12. Carlson GA et al. Phenomenology and diagnosis of bipolar disorder in children, adolescents, and adults: complexities and developmental issues. Dev Psychopathol 2006; 18:939–969.
13. Galanter CA et al. Response to methylphenidate in children with attention deficit hyperactivity disorder and manic symptoms in the multimodal treatment study of children with attention deficit hyperactivity disorder titration trial. J Child Adolesc Psychopharmacol 2003; 13:123–136.
14. Scheffer RE et al. Randomized, placebo-controlled trial of mixed amphetamine salts for symptoms of comorbid ADHD in pediatric bipolar disorder after mood stabilization with divalproex sodium. Am J Psychiatry 2005; 162:58–64.
15. Kafantaris V et al. Lithium treatment of acute mania in adolescents: a large open trial. J Am Acad Child Adolesc Psychiatry 2003; 42:1038–1045.
16. Strober M et al. Relapse following discontinuation of lithium maintenance therapy in adolescents with bipolar I illness: a naturalistic study. Am J Psychiatry 1990; 147:457–461.
17. Geller B et al. Double-blind and placebo-controlled study of lithium for adolescent bipolar disorders with secondary substance dependency. J Am Acad Child Adolesc Psychiatry 1998; 37:171–178.
18. Kafantaris V et al. Lithium treatment of acute mania in adolescents: a placebo-controlled discontinuation study. J Am Acad Child Adolesc Psychiatry 2004; 43:984–993.
19. Papatheodorou G et al. The efficacy and safety of divalproex sodium in the treatment of acute mania in adolescents and young adults: an open clinical trial. J Clin Psychopharmacol 1995; 15:110–116.
20. Deltito JA et al. Naturalistic experience with the use of divalproex sodium on an in-patient unit for adolescent psychiatric patients. Acta Psychiatr Scand 1998; 97:236–240.
21. Kowatch RA et al. Effect size of lithium, divalproex sodium, and carbamazepine in children and adolescents with bipolar disorder. J Am Acad Child Adolesc Psychiatry 2000; 39:713–720.
22. Wagner KD et al. An open-label trial of divalproex in children and adolescents with bipolar disorder. J Am Acad Child Adolesc Psychiatry 2002; 41: 1224–1230.
23. Findling RL et al. Double-blind 18-month trial of lithium versus divalproex maintenance treatment in pediatric bipolar disorder. J Am Acad Child Adolesc Psychiatry 2005; 44:409–417.
24. FDA. Memorandum. Depakote ER® (divalproex sodium) for the treatment of bipolar disorder, acute manic or mixed episodes, in children and adolescents aged 10 to 17 yrs. 2008. http://www.fda.gov/.
25. Wagner KD et al. A double-blind, randomized, placebo-controlled trial of oxcarbazepine in the treatment of bipolar disorder in children and adolescents. Am J Psychiatry 2006; 163:1179–1186.
26. Kafantaris V et al. Adjunctive antipsychotic treatment of adolescents with bipolar psychosis. J Am Acad Child Adolesc Psychiatry 2001; 40:1448–1456.
27. Frazier JA et al. A prospective open-label treatment trial of olanzapine monotherapy in children and adolescents with bipolar disorder. J Child Adolesc Psychopharmacol 2001; 11:239–250.
28. Biederman J et al. Open-label, 8-week trial of olanzapine and risperidone for the treatment of bipolar disorder in preschool-age children. Biol Psychiatry 2005; 58:589–594.
29. Fleischhaker C et al. Weight gain associated with clozapine, olanzapine and risperidone in children and adolescents. J Neural Transm 2007; 114:273–280.
30. Tohen M et al. Olanzapine versus placebo in the treatment of adolescents with bipolar mania. Am J Psychiatry 2007; 164:1547–1556.
31. FDA. Memorandum. Recommendation of approvable action for risperidone (Risperdal®) for the treatment of schizophrenia and bipolar I disorder in pediatric patients (response to PWR). 2007. http://www.fda.gov/.
32. Delbello MP et al. A double-blind, randomized, placebo-controlled study of quetiapine as adjunctive treatment for adolescent mania. J Am Acad Child Adolesc Psychiatry 2002; 41:1216–1223.
33. Delbello MP et al. A double-blind randomized pilot study comparing quetiapine and divalproex for adolescent mania. J Am Acad Child Adolesc Psychiatry 2006; 45:305–313.
34. Otsuka Pharmaceutical Development and Commercialization Inc. A phase III trial to test the safety and efficacy of two doses of aripiprazole in child and adolescent patients with bipolar I disorder, manic or mixed episode with or without psychotic features. Clinical Trial NCT00110461. 2009. http://clinicaltrials.gov/.

Anxiety in children and adolescents

Anxiety disorders (including generalised anxiety disorder, separation anxiety, specific phobias, social phobia, post-traumatic stress disorder, selective mutism) are common, affecting 6–20% of children and adolescents[1]. These disorders respond well to cognitive behaviour therapy (CBT) and this is usually the recommended first-line treatment[2,3].

If anxiety is severe and disabling and CBT is inappropriate or has failed, the use of medication should be considered. A large RCT comparing sertraline, CBT and their combination in childhood anxiety disorders, showed that the two monotherapies were equally effective in reducing anxiety at 12 weeks[4]. Combination therapy was significantly more effective than sertraline or CBT alone, and all therapies were significantly better than placebo (improvement: 80.7% for combination therapy (P<0.001); 59.7% for CBT (P<0.001); and 54.9% for sertraline (P<0.001); placebo (23.7%).

The treatment of anxiety in children and adolescents is generally the same as in adults (see Chapter 4). The following additional considerations apply:

- Young people are more likely to develop disinhibition with benzodiazepines than are adults[5]. Care is required.
- Treatment with SSRIs appears to be associated with the development of suicidal thoughts and acts in some young people (more than adults) although this has been mainly shown in depression rather than anxiety[5]. Venlafaxine is considered to be unsuitable for use in the treatment of depression in this age group but is effective in anxiety in children and adolescents[6,7]. Fluoxetine is effective[8,9] and is probably the drug of choice. There are also good-quality RCTs of fluvoxamine and paroxetine in childhood anxiety disorders which demonstrate efficacy[10,11].
- Tricyclic antidepressants are generally poorly tolerated in young people. They are more cardiotoxic than in adults and should be avoided in childhood anxiety disorders.
- Buspirone has been noted by some clinicians to cause disinhibitory reactions and worsen aggression in children. These risks are reduced in adolescents.
- Benzodiazepines are widely used to alleviate acute anxiety in children (e.g. before dental procedures) but are not recommended for longer-term use in anxiety disorders.

References

1. Emslie GJ. Pediatric anxiety – underrecognized and undertreated. N Engl J Med 2008; 359:2835–2836.
2. James A et al. Cognitive behavioural therapy for anxiety disorders in children and adolescents. Cochrane Database Syst Rev 2005;CD004690.
3. Compton SN et al. Cognitive-behavioral psychotherapy for anxiety and depressive disorders in children and adolescents: an evidence-based medicine review. J Am Acad Child Adolesc Psychiatry 2004; 43:930–959.
4. Walkup JT et al. Cognitive behavioral therapy, sertraline, or a combination in childhood anxiety. N Engl J Med 2008; 359:2753–2766.
5. Bridge JA et al. Clinical response and risk for reported suicidal ideation and suicide attempts in pediatric antidepressant treatment: a meta-analysis of randomized controlled trials. JAMA 2007; 297:1683–1696.
6. Rynn MA et al. Efficacy and safety of extended-release venlafaxine in the treatment of generalized anxiety disorder in children and adolescents: two placebo-controlled trials. Am J Psychiatry 2007; 164:290–300.
7. March JS et al. A randomized controlled trial of venlafaxine ER versus placebo in pediatric social anxiety disorder. Biol Psychiatry 2007; 62:1149–1154.
8. Birmaher B et al. Fluoxetine for the treatment of childhood anxiety disorders. J Am Acad Child Adolesc Psychiatry 2003; 42:415–423.
9. Clark DB et al. Fluoxetine for the treatment of childhood anxiety disorders: open-label, long-term extension to a controlled trial. J Am Acad Child Adolesc Psychiatry 2005; 44:1263–1270.
10. The Research Unit on Pediatric Psychopharmacology Anxiety Study Group. Fluvoxamine for the treatment of anxiety disorders in children and adolescents. N Engl J Med 2001; 344:1279–1285.
11. Wagner KD et al. A multicenter, randomized, double-blind, placebo-controlled trial of paroxetine in children and adolescents with social anxiety disorder. Arch Gen Psychiatry 2004; 61:1153–1162.

Children

Obsessive compulsive disorder (OCD) in children and adolescents

The treatment of OCD in children follows the same principles as in adults (see Chapter 4). Cognitive behavioural therapy is effective in this patient group and is treatment of first choice[1,2].

Sertraline[3-5] (from age 6 years) and **fluvoxamine** (from age 8 years) are the selective serotonin reuptake inhibitors (SSRIs) licensed in the UK for the treatment of OCD in young people. There are about 14 high-quality RCTs in paediatric OCD demonstrating efficacy for this group of antidepressants, although not for other types of antidepressants. Fluoxetine, fluvoxamine, paroxetine, citalopram, and sertraline have all been shown to be effective and safe in young people with OCD. Clomipramine remains a useful drug for some individuals, although its side-effect profile (sedation, dry mouth, potential for cardiac side-effects) makes it generally less acceptable, particularly in young people, than SSRIs, which are the first-line medication. All SSRIs appear to be equally effective, although they have different pharmacokinetics and side-effects[4]. In some circumstances SSRIs other than sertraline or fluvoxamine may be prescribed 'off-label' for childhood OCD (see for example below, if the child is also depressed).

Initiation of treatment with medication
Both clomipramine and SSRIs have a delayed onset of action (up to 4 weeks), with the full therapeutic effect not being apparent for as long as 8–12 weeks. It is therefore worth waiting for a response at a moderate therapeutic dose, rather than moving rapidly to high doses, which will increase the likelihood of side-effects. If there is no therapeutic response noticeable on a low dose, or only a partial response, the dose should be increased gradually. It may take several weeks to build up to the therapeutic dose and then the full effects of this may not be evident for several more weeks. In OCD, patients require a trial of an SSRI for at least 12 weeks at the maximum tolerated therapeutic dose. The effective doses needed for OCD in adults seem to be rather higher than those used in depression and this may also be the case in younger people and children.

Prescribing SSRIs in children
There has been recent concern about the use of SSRIs for depression in young people, with meta-analyses suggesting low levels of efficacy and an increase in behavioural activation including suicidal thoughts and behaviours. In contrast, SSRIs appear effective in child and adolescent OCD, with 'numbers needed to treat' (NNT) between 2 to 10, and there is no significant evidence of increased suicidality[5,6]. However, given recent concerns there should be close monitoring for side effects whenever SSRIs are prescribed in youth. The most common side effects of SSRIs in young people are behavioural activation and sometimes appetite suppression or nausea. Fluoxetine is the only recommended SSRI for use in the treatment of *depression* in young people under 18. For children with *OCD and depression*, this should be the chosen SSRI. As for all medications in children, the potential risks of untreated OCD, including a potentially life-long impact on emotional well being, social and educational development need to be weighed against the risks of medication side effects, both acute and long term. Decisions on medication and monitoring are best undertaken by a specialist.

NICE guidelines for the assessment and treatment of OCD

NICE published guidelines in 2005 on the evidence-based treatment options for OCD (and Body Dysmorphic Disorder) for young people and adults. NICE recommends a 'stepped care' model, with increasing intensity of treatment according to clinical severity and complexity[7]. The assessment of the severity and impact of OCD can be aided by the use of the CY-BOCS questionnaire, both at baseline, and as a helpful monitoring tool[8].

The summary treatment algorithm from the NICE guideline is as follows:

Treatment options for children and young people with obsessive compulsive disorder

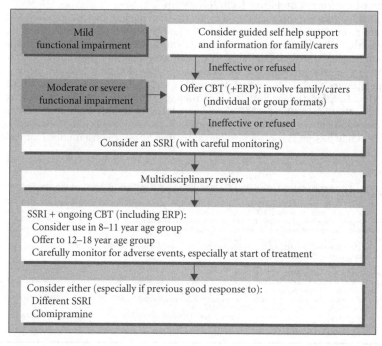

CBT = cognitive behaviour therapy; ERP = exposure and response prevention; SSRI = selective serotonin reuptake inhibitor. (Adapted from NICE guidance[7])
Reprinted with permission[9].

CBT and medication in the treatment of childhood OCD

Medication has occasionally been used as initial treatment where there is no availability of CBT or if the child is unable or unwilling to engage in CBT. Although medication should not be withheld from the child who needs treatment for their OCD, parents and clinicians should be aware of NICE recommendations that all young people with OCD should be offered CBT. Medication may also be indicated in those whose capacity to access CBT is limited by learning disabilities, although every attempt should be made to modify CBT protocols for such children.

The only study that directly compares the efficacy of cognitive behaviour therapy (CBT), sertraline, and their combination, in children and adolescents, concluded that children with OCD should begin treatment with CBT alone or CBT plus an SSRI[2].

Treatment refractory OCD in children

Some children with OCD may fail to respond to an initial SSRI administered for at least 12 weeks at the maximum tolerated dose, in combination with an adequate trial of CBT and ERP. These children should be reassessed, clarifying compliance, and ensuring that co-morbidity is not being missed. These children should usually have additional trials of at least one other SSRI. Following this, if the response is limited, a child should usually be referred to a specialist centre. Trials of clomipramine may be considered and/or augmentation with a low dose of risperidone[9,10]. Often children with more severe or chronic OCD have co-morbidities that can affect the initial response to treatment and long-term prognosis.

Duration of treatment and long-term follow-up

Adult studies have shown that maintenance on long-term medication sustains remission but the risk–benefit ratio of long-term medication is not known for younger people. NICE Guidelines recommend that if a young person has responded to medication, treatment should continue for at least 6 months after remission. Clinical experience suggests that children who have had successful CBT have prolonged remissions and less relapse following discontinuation of medication, but long-term trials are needed. Most people with early-onset OCD should respond to treatment and be able to lead fully functioning lives. It is important that throughout childhood, adolescence and into adult life, the individual with OCD should have access to health-care professionals, treatment opportunities and other support as needed, and NICE recommends that if relapse occurs, people with OCD should be seen as soon as possible rather than be placed on a routine waiting list.

References

1. O'Kearney RT et al. Behavioural and cognitive behavioural therapy for obsessive compulsive disorder in children and adolescents. Cochrane Database Syst Rev 2006;CD004856.
2. Freeman JB et al. Cognitive behavioral treatment for young children with obsessive-compulsive disorder. Biol Psychiatry 2007; 61:337–343.
3. The Pediatric OCD Treatment Study Team (POTS). Cognitive-behavior therapy, sertraline, and their combination for children and adolescents with obsessive-compulsive disorder: the Pediatric OCD Treatment Study (POTS) randomized controlled trial. JAMA 2004; 292:1969–1976.
4. Geller DA et al. Which SSRI? A meta-analysis of pharmacotherapy trials in pediatric obsessive-compulsive disorder. Am J Psychiatry 2003; 160: 1919–1928.
5. March JS et al. Treatment benefit and the risk of suicidality in multicenter, randomized, controlled trials of sertraline in children and adolescents. J Child Adolesc Psychopharmacol 2006; 16:91–102.
6. Bridge JA et al. Clinical response and risk for reported suicidal ideation and suicide attempts in pediatric antidepressant treatment: a meta-analysis of randomized controlled trials. JAMA 2007; 297:1683–1696.
7. National Institute for Clinical Excellence. Obsessive-compulsive disorder: Core interventions in the treatment of obsessive-compulsive disorder and body dysmorphic disorder. Clinical Guidance 31. 2005. http://www.nice.org.uk.
8. Scahill L et al. Children's Yale-Brown Obsessive Compulsive Scale: reliability and validity. J Am Acad Child Adolesc Psychiatry 1997; 36:844–852.
9. Heyman I et al. Obsessive-compulsive disorder. BMJ 2006; 333:424–429.
10. Bloch MH et al. A systematic review: antipsychotic augmentation with treatment refractory obsessive-compulsive disorder. Mol Psychiatry 2006; 11:622–632.

Further reading

Watson HJ et al. Meta-analysis of randomized, controlled treatment trials for pediatric obsessive-compulsive disorder. J Child Psychol Psychiatry 2008; 49:489–498.

Children

Attention deficit hyperactivity disorder (ADHD)

Children

- A diagnosis of ADHD should be made only after a comprehensive assessment by a specialist – usually, a child psychiatrist or a paediatrician with expertise in ADHD[1]. Appropriate psychological, psychosocial and behavioural interventions should be put in place. Drug treatments should be only a part of the overall treatment plan.
- The indication for drug treatment is the presence of impairment resulting from ADHD; in mild to moderate cases the first treatments are usually behaviour therapy and education; medication is indicated as the first line of therapy only in severe cases (e.g. those diagnosed as hyperkinetic disorder), and as second line when psychological approaches have not been successful within a reasonable time (e.g. 8 weeks) or are inappropriate.
- **Methylphenidate** is usually the first choice of drug when a drug is indicated. It is a central nervous stimulant with a large evidence base from trials. Adverse effects include insomnia, anorexia and growth deceleration – which can usually be managed by symptomatic management and/or dose reduction (see table on the following page).
- **Dexamfetamine** is an alternative CNS stimulant; effects and adverse reactions are broadly similar to methylphenidate, but there is much less evidence on efficacy and safety than exists for methylphenidate, and it plays a part in illegal drug taking. Both methylphenidate and dexamfetamine are Controlled Drugs; prescriptions should be written appropriately and for not more than 28 days.
- **Atomoxetine**[2–4] is a suitable first-line alternative. It may be particularly useful for children who do not respond to stimulants or whose medication cannot be administered during the day. It may also be suitable where stimulant diversion is a problem or when 'dopaminergic' adverse effects (such as tics, anxiety and stereotypies) become problematic on stimulants. Parents should be warned of the possibilities of suicidal thinking and liver disease emerging and advised of the possible features that they might notice.
- Third-line drugs include **clonidine**[5] and **tricyclic antidepressants**[6]. Very few children should receive these drugs for ADHD alone. There is some evidence supporting the efficacy of **carbamazepine**[7] and **bupropion**. There is no evidence to support the use of **second-generation antipsychotics**[8] for ADHD symptoms, but risperidone may be helpful in reducing severe coexistent levels of aggression and agitation, especially in those with moderate learning disability[9]. **Modafinil** appears to be effective[10] but has not been compared with standard treatments and its safety is not established.
- Co-morbid psychiatric illness is common in ADHD children. Stimulants are often helpful overall[6] but are unlikely to be appropriate for children who have a psychotic illness and problems with substance misuse should be managed in their own right before considering ADHD treatment[11].
- Once stimulant treatment has been established it is appropriate for repeat prescriptions to be supplied through general practitioners[1].

ADHD – Summary of NICE guidance[12]

- Drug treatment should only be initiated by a specialist and only after comprehensive assessment of mental and physical health and social influences
- Methylphenidate, dexamfetamine and atomoxetine are recommended within their licensed indications
- Methylphenidate is usually first choice, but decision should include consideration of:
  - co-morbid conditions (tics, Tourette's, epilepsy)
  - tolerability and adverse effects
  - convenience of dosing
  - potential for diversion
  - patient/parent preference
- If using methylphenidate, consider modified-release preparations (convenience of single-day dosage, improving adherence, reducing stigma, acceptability to schools); or multiple doses of immediate-release (greater flexibility in controlling timecourse of action, closer initial titration)
- Where more than one agent is considered suitable, the product with the lowest cost should be prescribed

ADHD in adults

Adult ADHD is recognised by both ICD-10 and DSM-IV, and NICE guidance regards the first line of treatment as medication, following the same principles as for drug treatment in children.

- At least 25% of ADHD children will still have symptoms at the age of 30. It is appropriate to **continue treatment started in childhood** in adults whose symptoms remain disabling.
- A new diagnosis of ADHD in an adult should only be made after a comprehensive assessment, including information from other informants and where possible from adults who knew the patient as a child.
- The prevalence of substance misuse and antisocial personality disorder are high in adults whose ADHD was not recognised in childhood[13]. Methylphenidate can be effective in this population[14], but caution is appropriate in prescribing and monitoring.
- **Atomoxetine** is effective[15] and is the only medication licensed for use in adults – and then only when treatment was initiated before the age of 18 years. Monitoring for symptoms of liver dysfunction and suicidal thinking is advised.

References

1. National Institute of Clinical Excellence. Guidance on the use of methylphenidate (Ritalin/Equasym) for attention deficit hyperactivity disorder (ADHD) in childhood. Technology Appraisal 13. http://www.nice.org.uk. 2000.
2. Michelson D et al. Once-daily atomoxetine treatment for children and adolescents with attention deficit hyperactivity disorder: a randomized, placebo-controlled study. Am J Psychiatry 2002; 159:1896–1901.
3. Kratochvil CJ et al. Atomoxetine and methylphenidate treatment in children with ADHD: a prospective, randomized, open-label trial. J Am Acad Child Adolesc Psychiatry 2002; 41:776–784.
4. Weiss M et al. A randomized, placebo-controlled study of once-daily atomoxetine in the school setting in children with ADHD. J Am Acad Child Adolesc Psychiatry 2005; 44:647–655.
5. Connor DF et al. A meta-analysis of clonidine for symptoms of attention-deficit hyperactivity disorder. J Am Acad Child Adolesc Psychiatry 1999; 38:1551–1559.
6. Hazell P. Tricyclic antidepressants in children: is there a rationale for use? CNS Drugs 1996; 5:233–239.
7. Silva RR et al. Carbamazepine use in children and adolescents with features of attention-deficit hyperactivity disorder: a meta-analysis. J Am Acad Child Adolesc Psychiatry 1996; 35:352–358.
8. Einarson TR et al. Novel antipsychotics for patients with attention-deficit hyperactivity disorder: a systematic review. Ottawa: Canadian Coordinating Office for Health Technology Assessment (CCOHTA) 2001;Technology Report No 17.

9. Correia Filho AG et al. Comparison of risperidone and methylphenidate for reducing ADHD symptoms in children and adolescents with moderate mental retardation. J Am Acad Child Adolesc Psychiatry 2005; 44:748–755.
10. Biederman J et al. A comparison of once-daily and divided doses of modafinil in children with attention-deficit/hyperactivity disorder: a randomized, double-blind, and placebo-controlled study. J Clin Psychiatry 2006; 67:727–735.
11. Hutchins P, Hazell P, Nunn K. Attention deficit hyperactivity disorder (ADHD). In: Nunn KP, Dey C, editors. The Clinician's Guide to Psychotropic Prescribing in Children and Adolescents. 1 ed. Sydney: Glade Publishing; 2003; 162–171.
12. National Institute for Clinical Excellence. Methylphenidate, atomoxetine and dexamfetamine for attention deficit hyperactivity disorder (ADHD) in children and adolescents – guidance. Technology Appraisal 98. http://www.nice.org.uk. 2006.
13. Cosgrove PVF. Attention deficit hyperactivity disorder. Primary Care Psychiatry 1997; 3:101–114.
14. Spencer T et al. A double-blind, crossover comparison of methylphenidate and placebo in adults with childhood-onset attention-deficit hyperactivity disorder. Arch Gen Psychiatry 1995; 52:434–443.
15. Spencer T et al. Effectiveness and tolerability of atomoxetine in adults with attention deficit hyperactivity disorder. Am J Psychiatry 1998; 155:693–695.

Further reading

Kutcher S et al. International consensus statement on attention-deficit/hyperactivity disorder (ADHD) and disruptive behaviour disorders (DBDs): clinical implications and treatment practice suggestions. Eur Neuropsychopharmacol 2004; 14:11–28.

National Institute for Clinical Excellence. Attention deficit hyperactivity disorder. Diagnosis and management of ADHD in children, young people and adults. Clinical Guidance 72. 2008. http://www.nice.org.uk/.

Nutt DJ et al. Evidence-based guidelines for management of attention-deficit/hyperactivity disorder in adolescents in transition to adult services and in adults: recommendations from the British Association for Psychopharmacology. J Psychopharmacol 2007; 21:10–41.

Taylor E et al. European clinical guidelines for hyperkinetic disorder – first upgrade. Eur Child Adolesc Psychiatry 2004; 13 Suppl 1:17–30.

Children

Table Prescribing in ADHD – a summary

Medication	Onset and duration of action	Dose	Comment	Recommended monitoring
Methylphenidate immediate release (Ritalin, Equasym)[1,2]	Onset: 20–60 min Duration: 2–4 hours	Initially 5–10 mg daily titrated up to a maximum of 2 mg/kg/day in divided doses using weekly increments of 5–10 mg (maximum 100 mg)	Usually first-line treatment. Generally well tolerated[3] Controlled Drug	BP Pulse Height and weight Monitor for insomnia, mood and appetite change and the development of tics[4]
Methylphenidate sustained release (Concerta XL)[1,2,5–7]	Onset: 30 min–2 hours Duration: 12 hours	Initially 18 mg in the morning, titrated up to a maximum of 54 mg – or after review up to 108 mg in adults. 18 mg Concerta = 15 mg Ritalin	An afternoon dose of Ritalin may be required in some children to optimise treatment Controlled Drug	Discontinue if no benefits seen in 1 month
Also Equasym XL[8,9]	Onset: 20–60 min Duration: 8 hours	Initially 10 mg increasing as necessary to 60 mg once daily (max 100 mg in adults)	Controlled Drug	
Also Medikinet[10]	Onset: 20–60 min Duration up to 8 hours	Dose as Equasym Capsules can be opened and sprinkled[11]	A larger fraction of the drug is available immediately than in other modified-release forms Controlled Drug	

Dexamfetamine immediate release (Dexedrine)[3,12]	Onset: 20–60 min Duration: 3–6 hours	2.5–10 mg daily to start, titrated up to a maximum of 20 mg (occasionally 40 mg) in divided doses using weekly increments of 2.5 mg	Considered to be less well tolerated than methylphenidate[3] Controlled Drug	
Atomoxetine[13,14]	Approximately 4–6 weeks (atomoxetine is a NA reuptake inhibitor)	When switching from a stimulant, continue stimulant for first 4 weeks of therapy For children <70 kg: start with 0.5 mg/kg/day and increase after a minimum of 7 days to 1.2 mg/kg (single or divided doses) and increase up to 1.8 mg/kg/day if necessary For children >70 kg: start with 40 mg and increase after a minimum of 7 days to 80 mg	Efficacy may be a little lower than found for methylphenidate[15]. May be useful where stimulant diversion is a problem[16] Once-daily dosing convenient in school children Not a Controlled Drug	Pulse BP Height Weight

References

1. Wolraich ML et al. Pharmacokinetic considerations in the treatment of attention-deficit hyperactivity disorder with methylphenidate. CNS Drugs 2004; 18:243–250.
2. British Medical Association and Royal Pharmaceutical Society of Great Britain. British National Formulary. 57th edition. London: BMJ Group and RPS Publishing; 2009.
3. Efron D et al. Side effects of methylphenidate and dexamphetamine in children with attention deficit hyperactivity disorder: a double-blind, crossover trial. Pediatrics 1997; 100:662–666.
4. Gadow KD et al. Efficacy of methylphenidate for attention-deficit hyperactivity disorder in children with tic disorder. Arch Gen Psychiatry 1995; 52:444–455.
5. Hoare P et al. 12-month efficacy and safety of OROS MPH in children and adolescents with attention-deficit/hyperactivity disorder switched from MPH. Eur Child Adolesc Psychiatry 2005; 14:305–309.
6. Remschmidt H et al. Symptom control in children and adolescents with attention-deficit/hyperactivity disorder on switching from immediate-release MPH to OROS MPH Results of a 3-week open-label study. Eur Child Adolesc Psychiatry 2005; 14:297–304.
7. Wolraich ML et al. Randomized, controlled trial of OROS methylphenidate once a day in children with attention-deficit/hyperactivity disorder. Pediatrics 2001; 108:883–892.
8. Findling RL et al. Comparison of the clinical efficacy of twice-daily Ritalin and once-daily Equasym XL with placebo in children with Attention Deficit/ Hyperactivity Disorder. Eur Child Adolesc Psychiatry 2006; 15:450–459.
9. Anderson VR et al. Spotlight on Methylphenidate Controlled-Delivery Capsules (Equasym™XL, Metadate CD™) in the treatment of children and adolescents with Attention-Deficit Hyperactivity Disorder. CNS Drugs 2007; 21:173–175.
10. Haessler F et al. A pharmacokinetic study of two modified-release methylphenidate formulations under different food conditions in healthy volunteers. Int J Clin Pharmacol Ther 2008; 46:466–476.
11. Fischer R et al. Bioequivalence of a methylphenidate hydrochloride extended-release preparation: comparison of an intact capsule and an opened capsule sprinkled on applesauce. Int J Clin Pharmacol Ther 2006; 44:135–141.
12. Cyr M et al. Current drug therapy recommendations for the treatment of attention deficit hyperactivity disorder. Drugs 1998; 56:215–223.
13. Kelsey DK et al. Once-daily atomoxetine treatment for children with attention-deficit/hyperactivity disorder, including an assessment of evening and morning behavior: a double-blind, placebo-controlled trial. Pediatrics 2004; 114:e1–e8.
14. Wernicke JF et al. Cardiovascular effects of atomoxetine in children, adolescents, and adults. Drug Saf 2003; 26:729–740.
15. Kratochvil CJ et al. Atomoxetine and methylphenidate treatment in children with ADHD: a prospective, randomized, open-label trial. J Am Acad Child Adolesc Psychiatry 2002; 41:776–784.
16. Heil SH et al. Comparison of the subjective, physiological, and psychomotor effects of atomoxetine and methylphenidate in light drug users. Drug Alcohol Depend 2002; 67:149–156.

Children

Psychosis in children and adolescents

Schizophrenia is rare in children but the incidence increases rapidly in adolescence. Early-onset schizophrenia-spectrum (EOSS) disorder is often chronic and in the majority of cases requires long-term treatment with antipsychotic medication[1].

There have been three major RCTs of first-generation antipsychotics, all of them showing high rates of extrapyramidal side effects (EPS) and significant sedation[1]. Treatment-emergent dyskinesias can also be problematic[2]. First-generation antipsychotics (FGAs) should generally be avoided in children.

There have been a handful of randomised controlled trials of SGAs in EOSS disorder[1,3–7]. Olanzapine, risperidone and aripiprazole have all been shown to be effective in the treatment of acute exacerbations of psychosis, but olanzapine is particularly prone to causing weight gain[1]. In an open-label pilot study quetiapine was found to be less effective than risperidone but with a more favourable side-effect profile[8]. Clozapine is more effective than haloperidol[8] and olanzapine[5]. Ziprasidone should probably be avoided[9,10]. While studies support a lower risk of treatment-emergent EPS with SGAs, this has to be balanced against the risk of significant weight gain and metabolic side effects[1,11,12].

Clozapine seems to be effective in treatment-resistant psychosis in adolescents, although this population may be more prone to neutropenia and seizures than adults[8].

Overall, algorithms for treating psychosis in young people are the same as those for adult patients (see Chapter 2) except that metabolic adverse effects are more common and more intensive monitoring required[13].

References

1. Kumra S et al. Efficacy and tolerability of second-generation antipsychotics in children and adolescents with schizophrenia. Schizophr Bull 2008; 34:60–71.
2. Connor DF et al. Neuroleptic-related dyskinesias in children and adolescents. J Clin Psychiatry 2001; 62:967–974.
3. Sikich L et al. A pilot study of risperidone, olanzapine, and haloperidol in psychotic youth: a double-blind, randomized, 8-week trial. Neuropsychopharmacology 2004; 29:133–145.
4. Kumra S et al. Childhood-onset schizophrenia. A double-blind clozapine-haloperidol comparison. Arch Gen Psychiatry 1996; 53:1090–1097.
5. Shaw P et al. Childhood-onset schizophrenia: A double-blind, randomized clozapine-olanzapine comparison. Arch Gen Psychiatry 2006; 63:721–730.
6. Kumra S et al. Clozapine and "high-dose" olanzapine in refractory early-onset schizophrenia: a 12-week randomized and double-blind comparison. Biol Psychiatry 2008; 63:524–529.
7. Findling RL et al. A multiple-center, randomized, double-blind, placebo-controlled study of oral aripiprazole for treatment of adolescents with schizophrenia. Am J Psychiatry 2008; 165:1432–1441.
8. Kumra S et al. Childhood-onset schizophrenia: an open-label study of olanzapine in adolescents. J Am Acad Child Adolesc Psychiatry 1998; 37: 377–385.
9. Scahill L et al. Sudden death in a patient with Tourette syndrome during a clinical trial of ziprasidone. J Psychopharmacol 2005; 19:205–206.
10. Blair J et al. Electrocardiographic changes in children and adolescents treated with ziprasidone: a prospective study. J Am Acad Child Adolesc Psychiatry 2005; 44:73–79.
11. Theisen FM et al. Prevalence of obesity in adolescent and young adult patients with and without schizophrenia and in relationship to antipsychotic medication. J Psychiatr Res 2001; 35:339–345.
12. Toren P et al. Benefit-risk assessment of atypical antipsychotics in the treatment of schizophrenia and comorbid disorders in children and adolescents. Drug Saf 2004; 27:1135–1156.
13. Patel JK et al. Metabolic profiles of second-generation antipsychotics in early psychosis: findings from the CAFE study. Schizophr Res 2009; 111:9–16.

Further reading

Masi G et al. Children with schizophrenia: clinical picture and pharmacological treatment. CNS Drugs 2006; 20:841–866.

Children

Autism spectrum disorders

Autism spectrum disorders (ASD) are conditions characterised by core deficits in three areas of development; language, social interaction and behaviour (stereotypies and/or restricted and unusual patterns of interests). The autism spectrum comprises autism, Asperger's syndrome and pervasive developmental disorders-not otherwise specified (PDD-NOS) and are categorised under pervasive developmental disorders (PDD) in ICD 10. Rett's syndrome and childhood disintegrative disorder are also categorised under PDD in the ICD, though they are aetiologically distinct, with different characteristics and outcomes from ASD. Therefore we will confine the remainder of this section to discussion of treatments for ASD.

Diagnosis of ASD is now usually relatively straight-forward with a range of well-validated instruments for history taking from parents/guardians and objective assessment of the individual in question. However the heterogeneity of problems seen within the spectrum of these disorders makes detailed clinical assessment of vital importance. Often greatest diagnostic difficulty occurs at the milder end of the spectrum. It is important to evaluate any co-morbid neurodevelopmental, medical and psychiatric disorders that may complicate the symptom profile. These include mental retardation, attention deficit hyperactivity disorder (ADHD), epilepsy, anxiety, obsessive-compulsive and mood disorders, sleep disturbance, self-harm, irritability and aggression towards others.

Pharmacotherapies are commonly used in individuals with ASD as adjuncts to psychological interventions. There are now several published reports describing controlled and open-label clinical trials. These are used to guide current clinical practice. The bulk of the evidence to date is for the efficacy of risperidone, methylphenidate and some selective reuptake inhibitors in the treatment of problem behaviours in ASD. Preliminary controlled trials of sodium valproate, atomoxetine and aripiprazole are promising. There is a potential role for α_2 agonists, cholinergic agents, glutamatergic agents and oxytocin and these require further investigation.

Currently there is no single medication for ASD that alleviates symptoms in all three domains simultaneously. Targeting pharmacological interventions by identifying problem behaviours and the level of impairment these cause is essential. The efficacy and adverse effects associated with pharmacotherapy should be systematically monitored, bearing in mind that individuals with ASD often have impaired communication. Standardised behaviour ratings scales and adverse effect checklists are essential tool in monitoring progress[1].

Pharmacological treatment of core symptoms of ASD
Restricted repetitive behaviours and interests (RRBI) domain
These are an important intervention target to improve overall outcomes in ASD. There is high demand for treatment of this distressing and disruptive core symptom domain.

Serotonin re-uptake inhibitors (SSRIs) have become the most widely prescribed medication to treat RRBIs in paediatric ASD populations. The evidence supporting the effectiveness of SSRIs in ameliorating these symptoms remains limited with the bulk of reports being from single case studies and open-label trials with only a few randomised controlled trials (RCTs) published to date[2-4]. The SSRIs that have been studied include fluoxetine, fluvoxamine, sertraline, citalopram and escitalopram. While side effects have generally been considered to be mild, increased activation and agitation occurred in some subjects. The current available literature reports inconsistent benefit from SSRIs and there remains uncertainty about the optimal dose regimen, which may be lower than those used for treatment of depression in typically developing individuals[5,6]. The mean dose of fluoxetine has been approximately 10 mg per day, starting with 2.5 mg, see table on following page.

Other potential pharmacological treatments include second-generation antipsychotics[7], anticonvulsants[8] and the neuropeptide, oxytocin[9]. Research on risperidone indicates that it is effective in reducing repetitive behaviours in children who have high levels of irritability or aggression[10], though reductions in core repetitive behaviours have been reported[7,11,12].

Social and communication impairment domain

Currently, no drug has been consistently proven to improve the core social and communication impairments in ASD. Risperidone may have a secondary effect through improvement in irritability[13]. Glutamatergic drugs and oxytocin are currently the most promising but clearly much additional work is required in this area[14].

Pharmacological treatment of comorbid problem behaviours in ASD

Inattention, overactivity, and impulsiveness in ASD (symptoms of ADHD)

Children with ASD have high rates of inattention, overactivity, and impulsiveness[15]. Adequate numbers of controlled trials of these symptoms in children with ASD are still lacking. The largest controlled trial to date has been with methylphenidate and conducted by the Research Units on Paediatric Psychopharmacology (RUPP) Autism Network[16,17]. In a retrospective and prospective study of children with ASD, Santosh and colleagues[18] reported positive benefits of treatment with methylphenidate. In general, methylphenidate produces highly variable responses in children with ASD and ADHD symptoms. These responses range from a marked improvement with few side effects through to poor response and/or problematic side effects. However, it is reasonable to proceed with treatment with methylphenidate of ADHD symptoms in ASD. It is advisable to warn parents of the lower likelihood of response and the potential side effects and to proceed with low initial doses (~0.125 mg/kg three times daily) increasing with small increments. Treatment should be stopped immediately if behaviour deteriorates or if there are unacceptable side effects.

Atomoxetine is a relatively new noradrenergic reuptake inhibitor that has been licensed to treat ADHD. There is preliminary evidence from small open-label trials that this is also useful in controlling these symptoms in children with ASD, but large-scale RCTs are awaited[19].

There is some evidence from controlled studies for risperidone and α_2 agonists (clonidine and guanfacine), however there is little or no evidence in favour of SSRIs, venlafaxine, benzodiazepines, or antiepileptic mood-stabilisers[20].

Irritability (aggression, self-injurious behaviour, tantrums)

Second-generation antipsychotics are the first-line pharmacological treatment for children and adolescents with ASD and associated irritability[21,22].

The only *licensed* medication is risperidone[23,24]. Treatment of irritability in adults with ASD is reported in a placebo-controlled trial to respond in a similar way[25]. Though side effects such as weight gain can be problematic, an adverse impact on cognitive performance has not been found after up to 8 weeks treatment[26]. See Medicines and Healthcare Regulatory Agency (MHRA) recommended dosages for risperidone see table on next page.

Other typical antipsychotics, e.g. olanzapine and aripiprazole, are under evaluation. Though the results of on-going research are still awaited, available research suggests that mood-stabilisers and anti-convulsants may not be as effective as atypical psychotics for the treatment of irritability in ASD[27].

Children

Sleep disturbance

Children with ASD have significant sleep problems[28] and there are a range of behavioural and pharmacological treatments available for this group. It is essential to understand the aetiology of the sleep problem before embarking on a course of treatment. Typical sleep problems in this group are sleep-onset insomnia, sleep-maintenance insomnia, and irregularities of the sleep–wake cycle, including early morning awakening.

Melatonin has been shown in several small studies to be beneficial in children with ASD with reductions in sleep latency as well as efficiency. General seizures did not recur in children who were seizure-free nor increase in those with epilepsy[29]. (See section on melatonin.)

Risperidone may benefit sleep difficulties in those with extreme irritability. In the anxious or depressed child, antidepressants may be beneficial. Insomnia due to hyperarousal may benefit from clonidine or clonazepam[30].

Pathologic aggression in children and adolescents

Children and adolescents with psychiatric illness, like adults, may display pathologic aggression (PA) that is destructive, severe, chronic, and unresponsive to psychosocial and psychopharmacological treatment of their underlying condition(s) and psychosocial interventions specifically targeting their aggression. For this subset of young people with persistent aggression, pharmacotherapy may be an appropriate treatment option to optimise their functioning. The most common primary diagnoses include bipolar disorders, autism spectrum disorders, and psychotic illness, and are frequently associated with mental retardation. It is important to understand what drives the aggressive behaviour and to intervene appropriately. This topic is reviewed by Barzman and Findling[31]. In general, the use of pharmacological intervention for PA should only be considered when (1) the underlying condition is adequately treated, (2) any current treatments are not contributing to the PA, and (3) all other treatment options fail to ensure the safety and optimal functioning of the child or young person.

Use of risperidone in children and adolescents

MHRA guidance for risperidone prescribing in children and adolescents

Risperidone is indicated for the treatment of autism in children (aged 5 and over) and adolescents

The dosage of risperidone should be individualised according to the response of the patient

- Dosing should be initiated at 0.25 mg per day for patients <20 kg and 0.5 mg per day for patients ≥ 20 kg
- On Day 4, the dose may be increased by 0.25 mg for patients <20 kg and by 0.5 mg for patients ≥20 kg
- This dose should be maintained and response should be assessed at approximately Day 14
- Only in patients not achieving sufficient clinical response should additional dose increases be considered. Dose increases may proceed at 2-week intervals in increments of 0.25 mg for patients <20 kg or 0.5 mg for patients ≥20 kg

(In clinical studies, the maximum dose studied did not exceed a total daily dose of 1.5 mg in patients <20 kg, 2.5 mg in patients ≥20 kg, or 3.5 mg in patients >45 kg)

Doses of risperidone in paediatric patients with autism spectrum disorders (by total mg/day)				
Weight categories	Days 1–3	Days 4–14+	Increments if dose increases are needed	Dose range
<20 kg	0.25 mg	0.5 mg	+0.25 mg at ≥ 2-week intervals	0.5–1.5 mg
≥20 kg	0.5 mg	1.0 mg	+0.5 mg at ≥ 2-week intervals	1.0–2.5 mg*

*Subjects weighing >45 kg may require higher doses: maximum dose studied was 3.5 mg/day
For prescribers preferring to dose on a mg/kg/day basis the following guidance is provided

Doses of risperidone in paediatric patients with autistic disorder (by mg/kg/day)				
Weight categories	Days 1–3	Days 4–14+	Increments if dose increases are needed	Dose range
All	0.01 mg/kg/day	0.02 mg/kg/day	+0.01 mg/kg/day at ≥2-week intervals	0.02–0.06 mg/kg/ day

General considerations

- Risperidone can be administered once daily or twice daily.
- Patients experiencing somnolence may benefit from a switch in dosing from once daily to either once daily at bedtime or twice daily.
- Once sufficient clinical response has been achieved and maintained, consideration may be given to gradually lowering the dose to achieve the optimal balance of efficacy and safety.
- There is insufficient evidence from controlled trials to indicate how long the patient should be treated.

Adverse effects

Weight gain, somnolence, and hyperglycaemia require monitoring, and the long-term safety of risperidone in children and adolescents with autistic disorder remains to be fully determined.

There is most evidence supporting the use of risperidone in aggressive behaviour[32–34]. There are fewer data for olanzapine, quetiapine, aripiprazole and clozapine. Risperidone can cause significant extrapyramidal side effects (EPS) in young people and like almost all atypical antipsychotics can cause considerable weight gain, metabolic (hyperglycaemia), and hormonal (hyperprolactinaemia) imbalance.

Controlled studies support the use of mood-stabilisers such as lithium[35,36] and sodium valproate[37] as being effective in the treatment of PA in children and adolescents.

There are no controlled trials to date of pharmacological treatments of PA in children younger than 5 years.

Fluoxetine in children and adolescents

When using fluoxetine to treat repetitive behaviours in ASD patients, it has been generally found that much lower doses are required than the therapeutic antidepressant dose. It is advisable to use the liquid preparation and begin at the lowest possible dose, monitoring for side effects. A suitable regimen is outlined in the below table.

Liquid fluoxetine: (as hydrochloride) 20 mg/5 ml

2.5 mg/day a day for 1 week (1 ml syringes available)

Follow with flexible titration schedule based on weight, tolerability, and side effects up to a maximum dose of 0.8 mg/kg/day (0.3 mg/kg for week 2, 0.5 mg/kg/day for week 3, and 0.8 mg/kg/day subsequently). Reduction may be clinically indicated due to reported side effects.

Adverse effects

Monitor for suicidal behaviour, self-harm and hostility, particularly at the beginning of treatment.

Hyponatraemia (possibly due to inappropriate secretion of antidiuretic hormone) has been associated with all types of antidepressants; however, it has been reported more frequently with SSRIs than with other antidepressants. The CSM has advised that hyponatraemia should be considered in all patients who develop drowsiness, confusion, or convulsions while taking an antidepressant. (See section on antidepressant-induced hyponatraemia; Chapter 4)

References

1. Greenhill LL. Assessment of safety in pediatric psychopharmacology. J Am Acad Child Adolesc Psychiatry 2003; 42:625–626.
2. McDougle CJ et al. A double-blind, placebo-controlled study of fluvoxamine in adults with autistic disorder. Arch Gen Psychiatry 1996; 53:1001–1008.
3. Buchsbaum MS et al. Effect of fluoxetine on regional cerebral metabolism in autistic spectrum disorders: a pilot study. Int J Neuropsychopharmacol 2001; 4:119–125.
4. Hollander E et al. A placebo controlled crossover trial of liquid fluoxetine on repetitive behaviors in childhood and adolescent autism. Neuropsychopharmacology 2005; 30:582–589.
5. Aman MG et al. Medication patterns in patients with autism: temporal, regional, and demographic influences. J Child Adolesc Psychopharmacol 2005; 15:116–126.
6. Soorya L et al. Psychopharmacologic interventions for repetitive behaviors in autism spectrum disorders. Child Adolesc Psychiatr Clin N Am 2008; 17:753–771.
7. McDougle CJ et al. Risperidone for the core symptom domains of autism: results from the study by the autism network of the research units on pediatric psychopharmacology. Am J Psychiatry 2005; 162:1142–1148.
8. Hollander E et al. A double-blind placebo-controlled pilot study of olanzapine in childhood/adolescent pervasive developmental disorder. J Child Adolesc Psychopharmacol 2006; 16:541–548.
9. Hollander E et al. Oxytocin infusion reduces repetitive behaviors in adults with autistic and Asperger's disorders. Neuropsychopharmacology 2003; 28:193–198.
10. McDougle CJ et al. A double-blind, placebo-controlled study of risperidone addition in serotonin reuptake inhibitor-refractory obsessive-compulsive disorder. Arch Gen Psychiatry 2000; 57:794–801.
11. McCracken JT et al. Risperidone in children with autism and serious behavioral problems. N Engl J Med 2002; 347:314–321.
12. Arnold LE et al. Parent-defined target symptoms respond to risperidone in RUPP autism study: customer approach to clinical trials. J Am Acad Child Adolesc Psychiatry 2003; 42:1443–1450.
13. Canitano R et al. Risperidone in the treatment of behavioral disorders associated with autism in children and adolescents. Neuropsychiatr Dis Treat 2008; 4:723–730.
14. Posey DJ et al. Developing drugs for core social and communication impairment in autism. Child Adolesc Psychiatr Clin N Am 2008; 17:787–801.
15. Simonoff E et al. Psychiatric disorders in children with autism spectrum disorders: prevalence, comorbidity, and associated factors in a population-derived sample. J Am Acad Child Adolesc Psychiatry 2008; 47:921–929.
16. Research Units on Pediatric Psychopharmacology (RUPP) Autism Network. Randomized, controlled, crossover trial of methylphenidate in pervasive developmental disorders with hyperactivity. Arch Gen Psychiatry 2005; 62:1266–1274.
17. Posey DJ et al. Positive effects of methylphenidate on inattention and hyperactivity in pervasive developmental disorders: an analysis of secondary measures. Biol Psychiatry 2007; 61:538–544.
18. Santosh PJ et al. Impact of comorbid autism spectrum disorders on stimulant response in children with attention deficit hyperactivity disorder: a retrospective and prospective effectiveness study. Child Care Health Dev 2006; 32:575–583.
19. Arnold LE et al. Atomoxetine for hyperactivity in autism spectrum disorders: placebo-controlled crossover pilot trial. J Am Acad Child Adolesc Psychiatry 2006; 45:1196–1205.
20. Aman MG et al. Treatment of inattention, overactivity, and impulsiveness in autism spectrum disorders. Child Adolesc Psychiatr Clin N Am 2008; 17:713–738.
21. McDougle CJ et al. Atypical antipsychotics in children and adolescents with autistic and other pervasive developmental disorders. J Clin Psychiatry 2008; 69 Suppl 4:15–20.

Children

22. Parikh MS et al. Psychopharmacology of aggression in children and adolescents with autism: a critical review of efficacy and tolerability. J Child Adolesc Psychopharmacol 2008; 18:157–178.
23. Jesner OS et al. Risperidone for autism spectrum disorder. Cochrane Database Syst Rev 2007;CD005040.
24. Scahill L et al. Risperidone approved for the treatment of serious behavioral problems in children with autism. J Child Adolesc Psychiatr Nurs 2007; 20:188–190.
25. McDougle CJ et al. A double-blind, placebo-controlled study of risperidone in adults with autistic disorder and other pervasive developmental disorders. Arch Gen Psychiatry 1998; 55:633–641.
26. Aman MG et al. Acute and long-term safety and tolerability of risperidone in children with autism. J Child Adolesc Psychopharmacol 2005; 15: 869–884.
27. Stigler KA et al. Pharmacotherapy of irritability in pervasive developmental disorders. Child Adolesc Psychiatr Clin N Am 2008; 17:739–752.
28. Krakowiak P et al. Sleep problems in children with autism spectrum disorders, developmental delays, and typical development: a population-based study. J Sleep Res 2008; 17:197–206.
29. Andersen IM et al. Melatonin for insomnia in children with autism spectrum disorders. J Child Neurol 2008; 23:482–485.
30. Johnson KP et al. Sleep in children with autism spectrum disorders. Curr Treat Options Neurol 2008; 10:350–359.
31. Barzman DH et al. Pharmacological treatment of pathologic aggression in children. Int Rev Psychiatry 2008; 20:151–157.
32. Aman MG et al. Double-blind, placebo-controlled study of risperidone for the treatment of disruptive behaviors in children with subaverage intelligence. Am J Psychiatry 2002; 159:1337–1346.
33. Snyder R et al. Effects of risperidone on conduct and disruptive behavior disorders in children with subaverage IQs. J Am Acad Child Adolesc Psychiatry 2002; 41:1026–1036.
34. Reyes M et al. A randomized, double-blind, placebo-controlled study of risperidone maintenance treatment in children and adolescents with disruptive behavior disorders. Am J Psychiatry 2006; 163:402–410.
35. Campbell M et al. Lithium in hospitalized aggressive children with conduct disorder: a double-blind and placebo-controlled study. J Am Acad Child Adolesc Psychiatry 1995; 34:445–453.
36. Malone RP et al. A double-blind placebo-controlled study of lithium in hospitalized aggressive children and adolescents with conduct disorder. Arch Gen Psychiatry 2000; 57:649–654.
37. Donovan SJ et al. Divalproex treatment for youth with explosive temper and mood lability: a double-blind, placebo-controlled crossover design. Am J Psychiatry 2000; 157:818–820.

Children

Tics and Tourette syndrome

Transient tics occur in 5–20% of children. Tourette syndrome occurs in about 1% of children and is defined by persistent motor and vocal tics. Eighty per cent of individuals with tics will have outgrown them by adult life. Tics wax and wane over time and are variably exacerbated by external factors such as stress, inactivity and fatigue, depending on the individual. Tics are about 3–4 times more common in boys than girls[1].

Detection and treatment of co-morbidity
Co-morbid OCD, attention deficit hyperactivity disorder, depression, anxiety, and behavioural problems are more prevalent than would be expected by chance, and are often a cause of major impairment in people with tic disorders[2]. These co-morbid conditions are usually treated first before assessing the level of disability caused by the tics.

Education and behavioural treatments
Most people with tics do not require pharmacological treatment; education for the individual with tics, their family and the people they interact with, especially schools, is crucial. Treatment aimed primarily at reducing tics is warranted if they cause distress to the patient or are functionally disabling. There has been a resurgence of interest in behavioural programs[3], with large trials underway.

Studies of **pharmacological interventions** in Tourette syndrome are difficult to interpret for several reasons:

- There is a large inter-individual variation in tic frequency and severity. Small, randomised studies may include patients that are very different at baseline.
- The severity of tics in a given individual varies markedly over time, making it difficult to separate drug effect from natural variation.
- The placebo effect is large.
- The bulk of the literature consists of case reports, case series, open studies and underpowered, randomised studies. Publication bias is also likely to be an issue.
- A high proportion of patients have co-morbid psychiatric illness. It can be difficult to disentangle any direct effect on tics from an effect on the co-morbid illness. This makes it difficult to interpret studies that report improvements in global functioning rather than specific reductions in tics.

Most of the published literature concerns children and adolescents.

Adrenergic α₂ agonists
Clonidine has been shown in open studies to reduce the severity and frequency of tics but in one study this effect did not seem to be convincingly larger that placebo[4]. Other studies have shown more substantial reductions in tics[5–7]. Guanfacine (also an adrenergic α₂ agonist) has been shown to lead to a 30% reduction in tic-rating-scale scores[8]. In the UK, only clonidine is readily available. Therapeutic doses of clonidine are in the order of 3–5 µg/kg, and the dose should be built up gradually. Main side effects are sedation, postural hypotension, and depression. Patients and their families should be informed not to stop clonidine suddenly because of risk of rebound hypertension.

Antipsychotics
Side effects of antipsychotics may outweigh beneficial effects in the treatment of tics and so it is recommended that clonidine is tried first. Antipsychotics may be more effective than clonidine

in alleviating tics in some individuals. A 24-week, double-blind, placebo-controlled double crossover study of 22 children and adolescents found pimozide (mean dose 3.4 mg/day) to be statistically superior to placebo in controlling tics[9]. Outcome in the haloperidol arm of this study (mean dose 3.5 mg/day) was numerically superior to placebo but did not reach statistical significance. Although this study is widely quoted as being positive for pimozide and negative for haloperidol, the absolute difference in response between the two active treatment arms was small. Two children developed severe anxiety and depression during the haloperidol phase that resulted in early termination of treatment. Haloperidol tends to be poorly tolerated by children and adolescents. The high burden of side effects leads to less than a third being willing to continue treatment in the longer term[10,11].

Risperidone has been shown to be more effective than placebo in a small (n = 34), randomised study[12]. Fatigue and increased appetite were problematic in the risperidone arm and a mean weight gain of 2.8 kg over 8 weeks was reported. Although there is a suggestion that risperidone[13] and olanzapine[14] may be more effective than pimozide, weight gain may be more pronounced in children and adolescents than in adults and this may limit the use of atypicals in young people. One small randomised, controlled trial found risperidone and clonidine to be equally effective[15].

Sulpiride has been shown to be effective and relatively well tolerated[15], as has ziprasidone[16]. Open studies support the efficacy of quetiapine[17] and olanzapine[18,19]. Case series suggest aripiprazole is effective and well tolerated[20,21] (also in tics[22]). One very small crossover study (n = 7) found no effect for clozapine[23].

Other drugs

A small (n = 10), double-blind, placebo-controlled, crossover trial of baclofen was suggestive of beneficial effects in overall impairment rather than a specific effect on tics[24]. The numerical benefits shown in this study did not reach statistical significance. Similarly, a double-blind, placebo-controlled trial of nicotine augmentation of haloperidol found beneficial effects in overall impairment rather than a specific effect on tics[25]. These benefits persisted for several weeks after nicotine (in the form of patches) was withdrawn. Nicotine patches were associated with a high prevalence of nausea and vomiting (71% and 40%, respectively). The authors suggest that PRN use may be appropriate. Pergolide (a D_1-D_2-D_3 agonist), given in low doses, significantly reduced tics in a double-blind, placebo-controlled, crossover study in children and adolescents[26]. Side effects included sedation, dizziness, nausea, and irritability. Flutamide, an antiandrogen, has been the subject of a small RCT in adults with TS. Modest, short-lived effects were seen in motor but not phonic tics[27]. A small RCT has shown significant advantages for metoclopramide over placebo[28].

Case reports or case series describing positive effects for ondansetron[29], clomiphene[30] tramadol[31], ketanserin[32], topiramate[33], cyproterone[34], levetiracetam[35], and cannabis[36] have been published. Tetrabenazine may be useful as an add-on treatment[37]. Many other drugs have been reported to be effective in single case reports. Patients in these reports all had co-morbid psychiatric illness, making it difficult to determine the effect of these drugs on Tourette syndrome alone.

Botulinum toxin has been used to reduce the severity of single (especially vocal) tics[1].

There may be a sub-group of children who develop tics and/or obsessive compulsive disorder in association with streptococcal infection. This group has been given the acronym PANDAS (Paediatric Autoimmune Neuropsychiatric Disorder Associated with Streptococcus)[38]. This is thought to be an autoimmune-mediated effect, and there have been trials of immunomodulatory therapy in these children. However, current clinical consensus is that tics or OCD should be treated in the usual way unless a child is part of a research trial. A normal course of antibiotic treatment should be given for any identified active infection (e.g. Strep sore throat in a child who presents acutely with new onset tics and/or OCD).

References

1   Swain JE et al. Tourette syndrome and tic disorders: a decade of progress. J Am Acad Child Adolesc Psychiatry 2007; 46:947–968.
2.   Riddle MA et al. Clinical psychopharmacology for Tourette syndrome and associated disorders. Adv Neurol 2001; 85:343–354.
3.   Piacentini JC et al. Behavioral treatments for tic suppression: habit reversal training. Adv Neurol 2006; 99:227–233.
4.   Goetz CG et al. Clonidine and Gilles de la Tourette syndrome: double-blind study using objective rating methods. Ann Neurol 1987; 21:307–310.
5.   Leckman JF et al. Clonidine treatment of Gilles de la Tourette syndrome. Arch Gen Psychiatry 1991; 48:324–328.
6.   Tourette Syndrome Study Group. Treatment of ADHD in children with tics: a randomized controlled trial. Neurology 2002; 58:527–536.
7.   Du YS et al. Randomized double-blind multicentre placebo-controlled clinical trial of the clonidine adhesive patch for the treatment of tic disorders. Aust N Z J Psychiatry 2008; 42:807–813.
8.   Scahill L et al. A placebo-controlled study of guanfacine in the treatment of children with tic disorders and attention deficit hyperactivity disorder. Am J Psychiatry 2001; 158:1067–1074.
9.   Sallee FR et al. Relative efficacy of haloperidol and pimozide in children and adolescents with Tourette disorder. Am J Psychiatry 1997; 154:1057–1062.
10.   Chappell PB et al. The pharmacologic treatment of tic disorders. Child Adolesc Psychiatr Clin N Am 1995; 4:197–216.
11.   Srour M et al. Psychopharmacology of tic disorders. J Can Acad Child Adolesc Psychiatry 2008; 17:150–159.
12.   Scahill L et al. A placebo-controlled trial of risperidone in Tourette syndrome. Neurology 2003; 60:1130–1135.
13.   Bruggeman R et al. Risperidone versus pimozide in Tourette disorder: a comparative double-blind parallel-group study. J Clin Psychiatry 2001; 62:50–56.
14.   Onofrj M et al. Olanzapine in severe Gilles de la Tourette syndrome: a 52-week double-blind cross-over study vs. low-dose pimozide. J Neurol 2000; 247:443–446.
15.   Robertson MM et al. Management of Gilles de la Tourette syndrome using sulpiride. Clin Neuropharmacol 1990; 13:229–235.
16.   Sallee FR et al. Ziprasidone treatment of children and adolescents with Tourette syndrome: a pilot study. J Am Acad Child Adolesc Psychiatry 2000; 39:292–299.
17.   Mukaddes NM et al. Quetiapine treatment of children and adolescents with Tourette disorder. J Child Adolesc Psychopharmacol 2003; 13:295–299.
18.   Budman CL et al. An open-label study of the treatment efficacy of olanzapine for Tourette disorder. J Clin Psychiatry 2001; 62:290–294.
19.   McCracken JT et al. Effectiveness and tolerability of open label olanzapine in children and adolescents with Tourette syndrome. J Child Adolesc Psychopharmacol 2008; 18:501–508.
20.   Davies L et al. A case series of patients with Tourette syndrome in the United Kingdom treated with aripiprazole. Hum Psychopharmacol 2006; 21:447–453.
21.   Seo WS et al. Aripiprazole treatment of children and adolescents with Tourette disorder or chronic tic disorder. J Child Adolesc Psychopharmacol 2008; 18:197–205.
22.   Yoo HK et al. An open-label study of the efficacy and tolerability of aripiprazole for children and adolescents with tic disorders. J Clin Psychiatry 2007; 68:1088–1093.
23.   Caine ED et al. The trial use of clozapine for abnormal involuntary movement disorders. Am J Psychiatry 1979; 136:317–320.
24.   Gaffney GR et al. Risperidone versus clonidine in the treatment of children and adolescents with Tourette syndrome. J Am Acad Child Adolesc Psychiatry 2002; 41:330–336.
25.   Singer HS et al. Baclofen treatment in Tourette syndrome: a double-blind, placebo-controlled, crossover trial. Neurology 2001; 56:599–604.
26.   Silver AA et al. Transdermal nicotine and haloperidol in Tourette disorder: a double-blind placebo-controlled study. J Clin Psychiatry 2001; 62:707–714.
27.   Gilbert DL et al. Tourette syndrome improvement with pergolide in a randomized, double-blind, crossover trial. Neurology 2000; 54:1310–1315.
28.   Nicolson R et al. A randomized, double-blind, placebo-controlled trial of metoclopramide for the treatment of Tourette disorder. J Am Acad Child Adolesc Psychiatry 2005; 44:640–646.
29.   Toren P et al. Ondansetron treatment in patients with Tourette syndrome. Int Clin Psychopharmacol 1999; 14:373–376.
30.   Sandyk R. Clomiphene citrate in Tourette syndrome. Int J Neurosci 1988; 43:103–106.
31.   Shapira NA et al. Novel use of tramadol hydrochloride in the treatment of Tourette syndrome. J Clin Psychiatry 1997; 58:174–175.
32.   Bonnier C et al. Ketanserin treatment of Tourette syndrome in children. Am J Psychiatry 1999; 156:1122–1123.
33.   Abuzzahab FS et al. Control of Tourette syndrome with topiramate. Am J Psychiatry 2001; 158:968.
34.   Izmir M et al. Cyproterone acetate treatment of Tourette syndrome. Can J Psychiatry 1999; 44:710–711.
35.   Awaad Y et al. Use of levetiracetam to treat tics in children and adolescents with Tourette syndrome. Mov Disord 2005; 20:714–718.
36.   Sandyk R et al. Marijuana and Tourette syndrome. J Clin Psychopharmacol 1988; 8:444–445.
37.   Porta M et al. Tourette syndrome and role of tetrabenazine: review and personal experience. Clin Drug Investig 2008; 28:443–459.
38.   Moretti G et al. What every psychiatrist should know about PANDAS: a review. Clin Pract Epidemol Ment Health 2008; 4:13.

Children

Melatonin in the treatment of insomnia in children and adolescents

Insomnia is a common symptom in childhood. Underlying causes may be behavioural (inappropriate sleep associations or bedtime resistance), physiological (delayed sleep phase syndrome) or related to underlying mood disorders (anxiety, depression, and bipolar disorder). All forms of insomnia are more common in children with learning difficulties, autism, ADHD and sensory impairments (particularly visual). Although behavioural interventions should be the primary intervention and have a robust evidence base, exogenous melatonin is now the 'first-line' medication prescribed for childhood insomnia[1].

Melatonin is a hormone that is produced by the pineal gland in a circadian manner. The evening rise in melatonin, enabled by darkness, precedes the onset of natural sleep by about two hours[2]. Melatonin is involved in the induction of sleep and in synchronisation of the circadian system.

There are a wide variety of unlicensed fast-release, slow-release and liquid preparations of melatonin. Many products rely on food-grade rather than pharmaceutical-grade melatonin, which is a cause of concern. A prolonged release formulation of melatonin (Circadin) was licensed in the UK in April 2008 as a short-term treatment of insomnia in patients over 55 years of age. It has not been evaluated in children and use in this population will be off-label (out of licence). There are a wide number of melatonin analogues already produced or in development[3].

Efficacy

Two meta-analyses on the use of melatonin in sleep disorders have been published[4,5]. Both pooled data from studies in children and adults. The first considered melatonin in primary sleep disorders (not accompanied by any medical or psychiatric disorder likely to account for the sleep problem) and showed improvements in the time take to fall asleep of 11.7 minutes across the group, but nearly 40 minutes if delayed sleep phase syndrome was the underlying cause. The study considering secondary sleep disorders and in this heterogeneous group found no significant effect on sleep latency.

Since these meta-analyses many smaller RCTs comparing melatonin with placebo in children have been published[6–12]. Studies have considered diverse groups including children with sleep phase delay, ADHD, autistic spectrum disorders, intellectual disability, and epilepsy. Results are surprisingly consistent considering the different underlying disorders. Children in these studies fall asleep about 30 minutes quicker (26.9–34 mins) and their total time asleep increases by a similar (19.8–48 mins) amount of time.

Side-effects

Many of the children who have received melatonin in RCTs and published case series had developmental problems and/or sensory deficits. The scope for detecting subtle adverse effects in this population is limited. Screening for side effects was not routine in all studies. Melatonin has been reported to worsen seizures[13] and may also exacerbate asthma[14,15] in the short term. Other reported side effects include headache, depression, restlessness, confusion, nausea, tachycardia, and pruritis[16,17]. Long-term side effects have not been evaluated.

Dose

The cut-off point between physiological and pharmacological doses in children is less than 500 µg. Physiological doses of melatonin may result in very high receptor occupancy. The doses used in

Children

RCTs and published case series vary hugely, between 500 µg and 5 mg being the most common, although much lower and higher doses have been used. The optimal dose is unknown and there is no evidence to support a direct relationship between dose and response[18]. Larger-scale, dose-ranging studies, using objective measures are in progress. In the future the role of objective measures such as actigraphy and salivary melatonin assays to determine which children have delayed sleep phase syndrome may be of value.

References

1. Gringras P. When to use drugs to help sleep. Arch Dis Child 2008; 93:976–981.
2. Macchi MM et al. Human pineal physiology and functional significance of melatonin. Front Neuroendocrinol 2004; 25:177–195.
3. Arendt J et al. Melatonin and its agonists: an update. Br J Psychiatry 2008; 193:267–269.
4. Buscemi N et al. The efficacy and safety of exogenous melatonin for primary sleep disorders. A meta-analysis. J Gen Intern Med 2005; 20:1151–1158.
5. Buscemi N et al. Efficacy and safety of exogenous melatonin for secondary sleep disorders and sleep disorders accompanying sleep restriction: meta-analysis. BMJ 2006; 332:385–393.
6. Van der Heijden KB et al. Effect of melatonin on sleep, behavior, and cognition in ADHD and chronic sleep-onset insomnia. J Am Acad Child Adolesc Psychiatry 2007; 46:233–241.
7. Wasdell MB et al. A randomized, placebo-controlled trial of controlled release melatonin treatment of delayed sleep phase syndrome and impaired sleep maintenance in children with neurodevelopmental disabilities. J Pineal Res 2008; 44:57–64.
8. Braam W et al. Melatonin treatment in individuals with intellectual disability and chronic insomnia: a randomized placebo-controlled trial. J Intellect Disabil Res 2008; 52:256–264.
9. Gupta M et al. Add-on melatonin improves sleep behavior in children with epilepsy: randomized, double-blind, placebo-controlled trial. J Child Neurol 2005; 20:112–115.
10. Coppola G et al. Melatonin in wake–sleep disorders in children, adolescents and young adults with mental retardation with or without epilepsy: a double-blind, cross-over, placebo-controlled trial. Brain Dev 2004; 26:373–376.
11. Weiss MD et al. Sleep hygiene and melatonin treatment for children and adolescents with ADHD and initial insomnia. J Am Acad Child Adolesc Psychiatry 2006; 45:512–519.
12. Garstang J et al. Randomized controlled trial of melatonin for children with autistic spectrum disorders and sleep problems. Child Care Health Dev 2006; 32:585–589.
13. Sheldon SH. Pro-convulsant effects of oral melatonin in neurologically disabled children. Lancet 1998; 351:1254.
14. Maestroni GJ. The immunoneuroendocrine role of melatonin. J Pineal Res 1993; 14:1–10.
15. Sutherland ER et al. Elevated serum melatonin is associated with the nocturnal worsening of asthma. J Allergy Clin Immunol 2003; 112:513–517.
16. Chase JE et al. Melatonin: therapeutic use in sleep disorders. Ann Pharmacother 1997; 31:1218–1226.
17. Jan JE et al. Melatonin treatment of sleep–wake cycle disorders in children and adolescents. Dev Med Child Neurol 1999; 41:491–500.
18. Sack RL et al. Sleep-promoting effects of melatonin: at what dose, in whom, under what conditions, and by what mechanisms? Sleep 1997; 20:908–915.

Children

Rapid tranquillisation (RT) in children and adolescents

As in adults, a comprehensive mental state assessment and appropriately implemented treatment plan along with staff skilled in the use of de-escalation techniques and appropriate placement of the patient are key to minimising the need for enforced parenteral medication.

Oral medication should always be offered before resorting to IM. Monitoring after RT is the same as in adults (see section on rapid tranquillisation, Chapter 7).

Table Recommended drugs for RT in children

Medication	Dose	Onset of action	Comment
Olanzapine[1,2]	2.5–10 mg IM	15–30 min IM	Possibly increased risk of respiratory depression when administered with benzodiazepines. Separate administration by at least one hour
Haloperidol[3]	0.025–0.075 mg/kg/dose (max 2.5 mg) IM Adolescents > 12 years can receive the adult dose (2.5–5 mg)	20–30 min IM	Must have parenteral anticholinergics present in case of laryngeal spasm(young people more vulnerable to severe EPS) **ECG essential**
Lorazepam[3,4]	0.05–0.1 mg/kg/dose IM	20–40 min IM	Slower onset of action than midazolam Flumazenil is the reversing agent
Midazolam[4,5]	0.1–0.15 mg/kg	10–20 min IM (1–3 min IV)	Risk of disinhibition reactions. Quicker onset and shorter duration of action than lorazepam or diazepam Shorter onset and duration of action than haloperidol Can be given as buccal liquid (same dose regimen as shown). Onset of action is 15–30 minutes[6]. Some published data in mental health but only in adults[7] Unlicensed product
Diazepam – IV only (not for IM administration)[8]	0.1 mg/kg/dose by slow IV injection. Max 40 mg total daily dose <12 years and 60 mg >12 years	5–10 min	Flumazenil is the reversing agent. Long half-life that does not correlate with length of sedation. Possibility of accumulation **Never give as IM injection**
Ziprasidone[9–11]	10–20 mg	15–30 min IM	Apparently effective. QT prolongation is of concern in this patient group
Aripiprazole[12]	5.25–15 mg	15–30 min IM	Evidence of effectiveness in adults but no data for children and adolescents

Children

References

1. Breier A et al. A double-blind, placebo-controlled dose-response comparison of intramuscular olanzapine and haloperidol in the treatment of acute agitation in schizophrenia. Arch Gen Psychiatry 2002; 59:441–448.
2. Lindborg SR et al. Effects of intramuscular olanzapine vs. haloperidol and placebo on QTc intervals in acutely agitated patients. Psychiatry Res 2003; 119:113–123.
3. Sorrentino A. Chemical restraints for the agitated, violent, or psychotic pediatric patient in the emergency department: controversies and recommendations. Curr Opin Pediatr 2004; 16:201–205.
4. Nobay F et al. A prospective, double-blind, randomized trial of midazolam versus haloperidol versus lorazepam in the chemical restraint of violent and severely agitated patients. Acad Emerg Med 2004; 11:744–749.
5. Kennedy RM et al. The "ouchless emergency department". Getting closer: advances in decreasing distress during painful procedures in the emergency department. Pediatr Clin North Am 1999; 46:1215–1247.
6. Schwagmeier R et al. Midazolam pharmacokinetics following intravenous and buccal administration. Br J Clin Pharmacol 1998; 46:203–206.
7. Taylor D et al. Buccal midazolam for agitation on psychiatric intensive care wards. Int J Psychiatry Clin Pract 2008; 12:309–311.
8. Nunn K, Dey C. Medication Table. In: Nunn K, Dey C, editors. The Clinician's Guide to Psychotropic Prescribing in Children and Adolescents. 1 ed. Sydney: Glad Publishing; 2003; 383–452.
9. Khan SS et al. A naturalistic evaluation of intramuscular ziprasidone versus intramuscular olanzapine for the management of acute agitation and aggression in children and adolescents. J Child Adolesc Psychopharmacol 2006; 16:671–677.
10. Staller JA. Intramuscular ziprasidone in youth: a retrospective chart review. J Child Adolesc Psychopharmacol 2004; 14:590–592.
11. Hazaray E et al. Intramuscular ziprasidone for acute agitation in adolescents. J Child Adolesc Psychopharmacol 2004; 14:464–470.
12. Sanford M et al. Intramuscular aripiprazole: a review of its use in the management of agitation in schizophrenia and bipolar I disorder. CNS Drugs 2008; 22:335–352.

Children

Doses of commonly used psychotropic drugs in children and adolescents

Suggested approximate oral starting doses (see primary literature for doses in individual indications). Lower dose in suggested range is for children weighing less than 25 kg.

Risperidone	0.25–2 mg	Adjust dose according to response and adverse effects
Olanzapine	2.5–5 mg	Use plasma levels to determine maintenance dose
Clozapine	6.25–12.5 mg	Use plasma levels to determine maintenance dose
Fluoxetine	5–10 mg/day	Adjust dose according to response and adverse effects
Lithium	100–200 mg/day lithium carbonate	Use plasma levels to determine maintenance dose
Valproate	10–20 mg/kg/day in divided doses	Use plasma levels to determine maintenance dose
Carbamazepine	5 mg/kg/day in divided doses	Use plasma levels to determine maintenance dose

Children

chapter 6

Substance misuse

Introduction

Mental and behavioural problems due to psychoactive substance use are common. Many psychoactive substances may be problematic including alcohol, opioids, cannabinoids, sedatives, stimulants, hallucinogens, tobacco, and volatile substances. The World Health Organisation (WHO) in the International Classification of Diseases-10 (ICD-10)[1] identifies acute intoxication, harmful use, dependence syndrome, withdrawal state, withdrawal state with delirium, psychotic disorder, amnesic syndrome, residual and late-onset psychotic disorder, other mental and behavioural disorders and unspecified mental and behavioural disorders as substance-related disorders. Substance misuse is commonly seen in people with severe mental illness (so-called dual diagnosis) and personality disorder. In many units, dual diagnosis is the norm rather than the exception in adult psychiatry.

According to ICD-10[1], dependence syndrome is 'a cluster of physiological, behavioural, and cognitive phenomena in which the use of a substance or a class of substances takes on a much higher priority for a given individual than other behaviours that once had greater value'. A definite diagnosis of dependence should only be made if at least three of the following have been present together in the last year:

- compulsion to take substance
- difficulties controlling substance-taking behaviour
- physiological withdrawal state
- evidence of tolerance
- neglect of alternative interests
- persistent use despite harm.

Substance use disorders should generally be treated with a combination of psychosocial and pharmacological interventions. This chapter will concentrate on pharmacological interventions for alcohol, opioids, and nicotine use. Cocaine, other stimulants, and benzodiazepine use will be discussed briefly. Note that various NICE guidelines and technology appraisals (see relevant sections), Department of Health Substance Misuse Guidelines[2], National Treatment Agency for Substance Misuse guidance[3] also provide a comprehensive overview of treatment approaches, as does a British Association for Psychopharmacology consensus[4].

References

1. World Health Organisation. International Statistical Classification of Diseases and Related Health Problems. 10th revision version for 2007. 2007. http://www.who.int/.
2. Department of Health. Drug misuse and dependence. UK guidelines on clinical management. 2007.
3. Day E. National Treatment Agency for Substance Misuse. Opiate detoxification in an inpatient setting. 2005. http://www.nta.nhs.uk/.
4. Lingford-Hughes AR et al. Evidence-based guidelines for the pharmacological management of substance misuse, addiction and comorbidity: recommendations from the British Association for Psychopharmacology. J Psychopharmacol 2004;18:293–335.

Substance
misuse

Alcohol dependence

Pharmacotherapy for alcohol withdrawal

- Alcohol withdrawal is associated with significant morbidity and mortality when improperly managed.
- All patients need general support; a proportion will need pharmacotherapy to modify the course of reversal of alcohol-induced neuroadaptation.
- Benzodiazepines are recognised as the treatment of choice for alcohol withdrawal. They are cross-tolerant with alcohol and have anticonvulsant properties.
- Parenteral vitamin replacement is an important adjunctive treatment for the prophylaxis and/or treatment of Wernicke–Korsakoff syndrome and other vitamin-related neuropsychiatric conditions.

Management of alcohol withdrawal and detoxification

Most patients undergoing alcohol withdrawal can do so safely at home with regular supervision by their GP and a community team. Some individuals with alcohol dependence will need pharmacological treatment in order to withdraw safely from alcohol. Before any managed episode of alcohol withdrawal there should be consideration of the following. Does the client want to undergo detoxification? What are the goals of treatment? Intended goals usually include symptom suppression, prevention of complications, or subsequent abstinence. Managed withdrawal should be considered within the wider context of the ongoing care/treatment package. Are plans in place for the post-withdrawal period? In addition a risk assessment should be carried out to determine the appropriate setting (see guidelines for in-patient treatment below). Care should be ensured with older patients who might be more safely managed as in-patients.

The majority of patients can be detoxified in the community. However, supervised medically assisted in-patient treatment is indicated where there is:

- severe dependence
- a history of DTs and/or alcohol withdrawal seizures
- a history of concurrent substance misuse (polydrug use)
- a history of failed community detoxification(s)
- poor social support
- cognitive impairment
- psychiatric co-morbidity (anxiety, depression, suicidal intent, psychotic illness)
- poor physical health, e.g. diabetes, liver disease, hypertension, malnutrition, infection.

The alcohol withdrawal syndrome

In alcohol-dependent drinkers, the central nervous system has adjusted to the constant presence of alcohol in the body (neuroadaptation). When the blood alcohol concentration (BAC) is suddenly lowered (as alcohol is metabolised too quickly for the brain to adjust), the brain remains in a hyperactive and hyperexcited state, causing the withdrawal syndrome.

The alcohol withdrawal syndrome is not a uniform entity. It varies significantly in clinical manifestations and severity. Symptoms can range from mild insomnia to delirium tremens (DTs).

The first symptoms and signs occur within hours of the last drink and peak within 24–48 hours. They include restlessness, tremor, sweating, anxiety, nausea, vomiting, loss of appetite, and insomnia. Tachycardia and systolic hypertension are also evident. Generalised seizures occur rarely, usually within 24 hours of cessation. In most alcohol-dependent individuals symptoms of alcohol withdrawal are mild-to-moderate and disappear within 5–7 days after the last drink. In more severe cases (approx. 5% of cases), DTs may develop.

Delirium tremens is a toxic confusional state that occurs when alcohol withdrawal symptoms are severe, and is often associated with medical illness. It is a life-threatening condition with a mortality of approximately 5%. The classic triad of symptoms includes clouding of consciousness and confusion, vivid hallucinations affecting every sensory modality, and marked tremor. Clinical features also include paranoid delusions, agitation, sleeplessness and autonomic hyperactivity (tachycardia, hypertension, sweating, and fever). Symptoms of DTs typically peak between 72–96 hours after the last drink. Prodromal symptoms usually include night-time insomnia, restlessness, fear, and confusion. Treatment of DTs requires early diagnosis and prompt transfer to the general medical setting where intravenous diazepam can be given, medical disorders treated, fluids and electrolytes replaced, and thiamine and other vitamins administered.

Risk factors for DTs and seizures
* severe alcohol dependence
* past experience of DTs
* long history of alcohol dependence with multiple previous episodes of inpatient treatment
* older age
* concomitant acute medical illness
* severe withdrawal symptoms when presenting for treatment.

Alcohol withdrawal assessment
* history (including history of previous episodes of alcohol withdrawal)
* physical examination
* time of most recent drink
* concomitant drug (illicit and prescribed) intake
* severity of withdrawal symptoms
* co-existing medical/psychiatric disorders
* laboratory investigations: FBC, U&E, LFTs, INR, PT, and urinary drug screen
* breathalyser: blood alcohol concentration may be estimated by a breathalyser reading.

Withdrawal scales can be helpful. They can be used as a baseline against which withdrawal severity can be measured over time. Use of these scales can minimise over- and under-dosing with benzodiazepines.

The Clinical Institute Withdrawal Assessment of Alcohol Scale Revised (CIWA-Ar)[1] is a ten-item scale which can be completed in around five minutes (see the following page).

When alcohol withdrawal is severe/complicated it is important to arrange laboratory investigations in order to check for low haemoglobin, macrocytosis, thrombocytopaenia, leucocytosis, and raised liver function tests. Check also for dehydration, hyponatraemia, hypokalaemia, and hypomagnesaemia; also hypoglycaemia or hyperglycaemia.

Clinical Institute Withdrawal Assessment of Alcohol Scale, Revised[1]

Patient:_____ Date:_____

Time:_____ (24 hour clock, midnight = 00:00)

Pulse or heart rate, taken for one minute:_____
Blood pressure:_____

NAUSEA AND VOMITING – Ask 'Do you feel sick to your stomach? Have you vomited?' Observation.
0 no nausea and no vomiting
1 mild nausea with no vomiting
2
3
4 intermittent nausea with dry heaves
5
6
7 constant nausea, frequent dry heaves and vomiting

TREMOR – Arms extended and fingers spread apart. Observation.
0 no tremor
1 not visible, but can be felt fingertip to fingertip
2
3
4 moderate, with patient's arms extended
5
6
7 severe, even with arms not extended

PAROXYSMAL SWEATS – Observation.
0 no sweat visible
1 barely perceptible sweating, palms moist
2
3
4 beads of sweat obvious on forehead
5
6
7 drenching sweats

ANXIETY – Ask 'Do you feel nervous?' Observation.
0 no anxiety, at ease
1 mild anxious
2
3
4 moderately anxious, or guarded, so anxiety is inferred
5
6
7 equivalent to acute panic states as seen in severe delirium or acute schizophrenic reactions

AGITATION – Observation.
0 normal activity
1 somewhat more than normal activity
2
3
4 moderately fidgety and restless
5
6
7 paces back and forth during most of the interview, or constantly thrashes about Scores
Scores
≤10 – mild withdrawal (do not need additional medication)
≤15 – moderate withdrawal
>15 – severe withdrawal

TACTILE DISTURBANCES – Ask 'Have you any itching, pins and needles sensations, any burning, any numbness, or do you feel bugs crawling on or under your skin?' Observation.
0 none
1 very mild itching, pins and needles, burning or numbness
2 mild itching, pins and needles, burning or numbness
3 moderate itching, pins and needles, burning or numbness
4 moderately severe hallucinations
5 severe hallucinations
6 extremely severe hallucinations
7 continuous hallucinations

AUDITORY DISTURBANCES – Ask 'Are you more aware of sounds around you? Are they harsh? Do they frighten you? Are you hearing anything that is disturbing to you? Are you hearing things you know are not there?' Observation.
0 not present
1 very mild harshness or ability to frighten
2 mild harshness or ability to frighten
3 moderate harshness or ability to frighten
4 moderately severe hallucinations
5 severe hallucinations
6 extremely severe hallucinations
7 continuous hallucinations

VISUAL DISTURBANCES – Ask 'Does the light appear to be too bright? Is its colour different? Does it hurt your eyes? Are you seeing anything that is disturbing to you? Are you seeing things you know are not there?' Observation.
0 not present
1 very mild sensitivity
2 mild sensitivity
3 moderate sensitivity
4 moderately severe hallucinations
5 severe hallucinations
6 extremely severe hallucinations
7 continuous hallucinations

HEADACHE, FULLNESS IN HEAD – Ask 'Does your head feel different? Does it feel like there is a band around your head?' Do not rate for dizziness or lightheadedness. Otherwise, rate severity.
0 not present
1 very mild
2 mild
3 moderate
4 moderately severe
5 severe
6 very severe
7 extremely severe

ORIENTATION AND CLOUDING OF SENSORIUM – Ask 'What day is this? Where are you? Who am I?'
0 oriented and can do serial additions
1 cannot do serial additions or is uncertain about date
2 disoriented for date by no more than 2 calendar days
3 disoriented for date by more than 2 calendar days
4 disoriented for place/or person

Total **CIWA-Ar** Score_____
Rater's Initials_____

Maximum Possible Score 67

The CIWA-Ar is not copyrighted and may be reproduced freely.

Withdrawal in the community (community detoxification)

- There should be someone at home who is able to monitor and supervise the withdrawal process. This should ideally be over the full 24-hour period. In situations where the supporter cannot be present full-time, there should be a high level of home supervision.
- Discuss treatment plan with the patient and person who will be supporting them. It is helpful to write this out and keep a copy in the notes. This should include contingency plans. Give a copy to the patient and send a copy to their GP.
- Arrange for medication to be picked up on a daily basis.
- If a patient resumes drinking, stop detoxification.
- Give patient and carer contact details (including a mobile phone number) so they can contact you if there are any problems.

Use of benzodiazepines

- Benzodiazepines are typically given for 7 days[2].
- The choice of benzodiazepine should be contingent upon the circumstances.
- Chlordiazepoxide is the benzodiazepine of choice in uncomplicated withdrawal as it has a low dependence-forming potential[2].
- A shorter-acting benzodiazepine, such as oxazepam, should be used in patients with alcoholic liver disease.
- Longer-acting benzodiazepines may be more effective in preventing seizures and delirium, but there is a risk of accumulation in elderly patients and those with liver failure[2].
- Additional titration using as-required medication may be used to achieve complete symptom suppression in the first 2 days[3].
- Benzodiazepines can be given in a number of ways: (1) in "front-loading" a loading dose is given followed by doses every 90 minutes or so, to achieve light sedation; no further doses are needed; (2) symptom-triggered therapy (in patients without a history of complications)[3] or (3) a tapering dose regimen (described below).

Dose of benzodiazepines

The dose needed will depend on an assessment of:

- Severity of alcohol dependence (clinical history, number of units per drinking day and score on Severity of Alcohol Dependence Questionnaire (SADQ)
- Severity of alcohol withdrawal symptoms. CIWA-Ar (>10–20: moderate and >20: severe) or Short Alcohol Withdrawal Scale (SAWS)[4] >12.

Substance misuse

Table Short Alcohol Withdrawal Scale (SAWS)				
	None (0)	*Mild (1)*	*Moderate (2)*	*Severe (3)*
Anxious				
Sleep disturbance				
Problems with memory				
Nausea				
Restless				
Tremor (shakes)				
Feeling confused				
Sweating				
Miserable				
Heart pounding				

The SAWS is a self-completion questionnaire. Symptoms cover the previous 24-hour period. Total scores above 12 require pharmacotherapy.

Use of chlordiazepoxide[5]

Mild dependence usually requires very small doses of chlordiazepoxide or else may be managed without medication.

Moderate dependence requires a larger dose of chlordiazepoxide. A typical regimen might be 10–20 mg qds, reducing gradually over 5–7 days. Note that 5–7 days' treatment is adequate and *longer treatment is rarely helpful or necessary*. It is advisable to monitor withdrawal and BAC daily prior to providing the day's medication. This may mean that community pharmacologically assisted alcohol withdrawals need to start on Monday to last 5 days. The protocol below may also be used for an inpatient with moderate dependence.

Chlordiazepoxide – moderate dependence
Day 1.. 20 mg qds
Day 2.. 15 mg qds
Day 3.. 10 mg qds
Day 4.. 5 mg qds
Day 5.. 5 mg bd

Severe dependence requires even larger doses of chlordiazepoxide and will often require specialist/in-patient treatment. Intensive daily monitoring is advised for the first 2–3 days, especially for severe dependence (see on the following page). This may require special arrangements over a weekend. Prescribing should not start if the patient is heavily intoxicated, and in such circumstances they should be advised to return when not intoxicated, at an early opportunity.

Inpatient treatment

The approach may be flexible with regard to the number of days prescribing, depending on the individual. Severely dependent patients should get 7 days treatment with the flexibility of "as-required" medication in the first 2 days. If symptoms are controlled within the first 2 days, then it will be easier to implement the reducing regimen. Patients who have a history of DTs, head injury, or cognitive impairment may need lengthier withdrawal regimens, e.g. lasting 10 days.

Chlordiazepoxide should be prescribed according to a flexible regimen over the first 24 (up to 48) hours, with dosage titrated against the rated severity of withdrawal symptoms. This is followed by a fixed 5-day reducing regimen, based upon the dosage requirement estimated during the first 24 (to 48) hours. Occasionally (e.g. in DTs) the flexible regimen may need to be prolonged beyond the first 24 hours. However, rarely (if ever) is it necessary to resort to the use of other drugs, such as antipsychotics (associated with reduced seizure threshold) or intravenous diazepam (associated with risk of overdose).

The intention of the flexible protocol for the first 24 hours is to titrate dosage of chlordiazepoxide against severity of alcohol withdrawal symptoms. It is necessary to avoid either under-treatment (associated with patient discomfort and a higher incidence of complications such as seizures or DTs), or over-treatment (associated with excessive sedation and risk of toxicity/interaction with alcohol consumed prior to admission).

In the inpatient setting it is possible to be more responsive, with constant monitoring of the severity of withdrawal symptoms, linked to the administered dose of chlordiazepoxide.

Prescribing in alcohol withdrawal for severe dependence

First 24 hours (day 1)

On admission, the patient should be assessed by a doctor and prescribed chlordiazepoxide (diazepam is used in some centres). *Observations should be at regular intervals during the first 24 hours.* Three doses of chlordiazepoxide must be specified:

FIRST DOSE (STAT)

This is the first dose of chlordiazepoxide which will be administered by ward staff immediately following admission, as a fixed 'stat' dose. It should be estimated upon:

- clinical signs and symptoms of withdrawal (see below);
- breath alcohol concentration on admission (at least 20 minutes after the last drink to avoid falsely high readings from the mouth) and 1 hour later.

The dose prescribed should usually be within the range of 5–50 mg. However, if withdrawal symptoms on admission are mild, or if the breath alcohol is very high, or rising, the initial dose may be 0 mg (i.e. nothing). It is the relative fall in blood alcohol concentration that determines the need for medication not the absolute figure (hence the need to take two breathalyser readings at an interval soon after admission). Caution is needed if a patient shows a high BAC reading.

INCREMENTAL DOSE (RANGE)

This is the range within which subsequent doses of chlordiazepoxide should be administered during the first 24 hours (see below). A dose of 5–40 mg will cover almost all circumstances.

MAXIMUM DOSE IN 24 HOURS

This is the maximum cumulative dose that may be given during the first 24 hours. It may be estimated according to clinical judgement, but **250 mg should be adequate for most cases.**

Doses above 250 mg a day should not be prescribed without prior discussion with a consultant or specialist registrar.

The cumulative chlordiazepoxide dose administered during the initial 24-hour period assessment is called the *baseline dose*, and this is used to calculate the subsequent reducing regimen.

Days 2–5

After the initial 24-hour assessment period a standardised reducing regimen is used. Chlordiazepoxide is given in divided doses, four times daily. The afternoon and evening doses can be proportionately higher in order to provide night sedation (but note that the effect of chlordiazepoxide and its metabolites is long-lived). The dose should be reduced each day by approximately 20% of the baseline dose, so that no chlordiazepoxide is given on day 6. However, a longer regimen may be required in the case of patients who have DTs or a history of DTs. This should be discussed with a specialist registrar or consultant, and the dose tailored according to clinical need.

> **Note**
> Chlordiazepoxide should not routinely be prescribed on a PRN basis after the initial assessment (first 2 days) is complete. Patients exhibiting significant further symptoms may have psychiatric (or other) complications and should be seen by the ward or duty doctor.

Observations and administration

After chlordiazepoxide has been prescribed as above, the first 'stat' dose is given immediately. Subsequent doses during the first 24 hours are administered with a frequency and dosage that depend upon the observations of alcohol withdrawal status rated by the ward staff.

OBSERVATIONS

Each set of observations consist of:

- alcohol withdrawal scale (e.g. CIWA-Ar) and/or clinical observations
- BP
- heart rate
- breathalyser (first and second observations only).

Observations should be recorded:

- during admission procedure immediately arrival on the ward;
- throughout the first 24-hours approximately every 1–2 hours. The frequency will also depend upon:
  - severity of withdrawal
  - whether or not chlordiazepoxide has been administered
- twice daily observation from days 2–6.

If a patient is asleep (and this is not due to intoxication), they should not be woken up for observations. However, it should be recorded that they were asleep.

During the first 24 hours chlordiazepoxide should be administered when withdrawal symptoms are considered significant (usually a CIWA-Ar score >15). If a patient suffers hallucinations or agitation, an increased dose should be administered, according to clinical judgement.

Table Alcohol withdrawal treatment interventions – summary

Severity	Supportive care	Medical care	Pharmacotherapy for neuroadaptation reversal	Setting
Mild CIWA-Ar ≤10	Moderate-to-high level required	Little required	Little to none required – maybe symptomatic treatment only (e.g. paracetamol)	Home
Moderate CIWA-Ar ≤15	Moderate-to-high level required	Little required	Little to none required – maybe symptomatic treatment only	Home or community
Severe CIWA-Ar >15	High level required	Medical monitoring	Usually required – probably symptomatic and substitution treatment (e.g. chlordiazepoxide)	Community or hospital
Complicated CIWA-Ar >10 Plus medical problems	High level required	Specialist medical care required	Substitution and symptomatic treatments probably required	Hospital

Substance
misuse

An example of a chlordiazepoxide regimen for severe dependence		
		Total (mg)
Day 1 (first 24 hours)	40 mg qds + 40 mg PRN	200
Day 2	40 mg qds	160
Day 3	30 mg tds and 40 mg nocte (or 30 mg qds)	120–130
Day 4	30 mg bd and 20 mg bd (or 25 mg qds)	100
Day 5	20 mg qds	80
Day 6	20 mg bd and 10 mg bd	60
Day 7	10 mg qds	40
Day 8	10 mg tds or 10 mg bd and 5 mg bd	30
Day 9	10 mg bd (or 5 mg qds)	20
Day 10	10 mg nocte	10

Please also see above for first 24 hours dose assessment period.

Medically compromised patients

In patients with liver cirrhosis, give a shorter-acting benzodiazepine, e.g. oxazepam. It is important to check LFTs as soon as possible in order to optimise the dose. Some patients may need, and be able to tolerate, relatively high starting doses, e.g. 40 mg qds, whereas others may only be able to tolerate a lower starting dose e.g. 20 mg qds. Use a withdrawal scale as a marker and be guided by the patient's clinical observations. It is important to note that the risk of alcohol withdrawal seizures may be higher with oxazepam.

Approximate equivalent doses of benzodiazepines are as follows:

- *diazepam 5 mg = chlordiazepoxide 15 mg = oxazepam 15 mg*

Oxazepam is also useful in patients with chronic respiratory disease (N.B. the majority of dependent drinkers are smokers). Always use a withdrawal assessment scale as above.

Vitamin supplementation

"There is insufficient evidence available from randomized controlled clinical trials to guide clinicians in the dose, frequency, route or duration of thiamine treatment for either prophylaxis against or treatment of established WKS (Wernicke Korsakoff Syndrome) due to alcohol misuse. Current recommendations for best practice continue to be guided extrapolations from basic science and case reports"[6].

Prophylactic use of thiamine

It is generally advised that **all patients** undergoing in-patient detoxification should be given **parenteral** thiamine as prophylaxis for Wernicke's encephalopathy (WE). This is probably best given for 5 days and may be followed by oral vitamin B Compound. The only parenteral high-potency

B-complex vitamin therapy licensed in the UK is Pabrinex. Although intravenous Pabrinex remains the treatment of choice in patients in whom a presumptive diagnosis of WE has been made, or for whom the diagnosis is clear, IM Pabrinex is typically given as prophylaxis for in-patients undergoing medically assisted withdrawal.

Clients undergoing community detoxification should also be considered for parenteral prophylaxis with Pabrinex because oral thiamine is not adequately absorbed and there is considerable doubt about the usefulness of oral replacement. However, parenteral administration of thiamine is not always possible in the community setting. In this case, low-risk drinkers without neuropsychiatric complications and with an adequate diet should be offered oral thiamine: a minimum of 300 mg daily during assisted alcohol withdrawal and periods of high alcohol intake[3].

IM thiamine preparations have a lower incidence of anaphylactic reactions than IV preparations, at 1 per 5 million pairs of ampoules of Pabrinex – far lower than many frequently used drugs that carry no special warning in the BNF. However this risk has resulted in fears about using parenteral preparations and the inappropriate use of oral thiamine preparations. Given the nature of Wernicke's encephalopathy, the benefit to risk ratio favours parenteral thiamine[3,6–9]. One pair of IM high-potency Pabrinex ampoules should be administered once daily for 5 days[8]. BNF guidance/CSM advice states that facilities for treating anaphylaxis should be available. This includes the need for staff to be trained in the management of anaphylaxis and administration of adrenaline (epinephrine) IM.

> **Prophylactic treatment** for patients at risk of Wernicke's encephalopathy should be:
> **One pair IM/IV ampoules high potency B-complex vitamins (Pabrinex) daily for 3–5 days**
> (Thiamine 200–300 mg IM daily may be given if pabrinex is unavailable)

Note: All patients should receive this regimen as an absolute minimum.

Wernicke's encephalopathy

The classical triad of ophthalmoplegia, ataxia, and confusion is rarely present in Wernicke's encephalopathy, and the syndrome is much more common than is widely believed[9]. A presumptive diagnosis of Wernicke's encephalopathy should therefore be made in any patient undergoing detoxification who experiences any of the following signs:

* ataxia
* hypothermia and hypotension
* confusion
* ophthalmoplegia/nystagmus
* memory disturbance
* coma/unconsciousness.

Note that alcohol and benzodiazepines can cause ataxia and nystagmus, which may be confused with Wernicke's encephalopathy.

Parenteral B-complex must be administered before glucose is administered in all patients presenting with altered mental status.

Therapeutic treatment for presumed/diagnosed Wernicke's encephalopathy (to be undertaken within the general medical hospital setting) consists of:

> At least two pairs of IV ampoules (i.e. four ampoules) of high-potency B-complex vitamins *three times daily* for 2 days

* If no response, then discontinue treatment.
* If signs/symptoms respond, continue 1 pair IV or IM ampoules daily for 5 days or for as long as improvement continues.

Seizure prophylaxis

A meta-analysis of trials assessing efficacy of drugs preventing alcohol withdrawal seizures has demonstrated that benzodiazepines, particularly long-acting preparations such as diazepam, significantly reduced seizures *de novo*[10]. Most clinicians prefer to use diazepam for medically assisted withdrawal in those with a previous history of seizures. Some units advocate carbamazepine loading in patients with untreated epilepsy; those with a history of more than two seizures during previous withdrawal episodes; or previous seizures despite adequate diazepam loading. Phenytoin does not prevent alcohol-withdrawal seizures and is therefore not indicated. Please note that there is no need to continue an anticonvulsant if it has been used to treat an alcohol withdrawal-related seizure. A recent Cochrane review evaluated anticonvulsants for alcohol withdrawal and found no definitive evidence on the effectiveness in alcohol withdrawal[8]. Please also see BAP guidelines[3].

Those who have a seizure for the first time should be investigated to rule out an organic disease or structural lesion.

Liver disease

For individuals with impaired liver functioning, oxazepam (a short-acting benzodiazepine) may be preferred to chlordiazepoxide, in order to avoid excessive build up of metabolites and over-sedation.

Hallucinations

Mild perceptual disturbances usually respond to chlordiazepoxide. However, hallucinations can be treated with oral haloperidol. Haloperidol may also be given intramuscularly or (very rarely) intravenously if necessary (but BP should be monitored for hypotension and ECG for QT prolongation). Caution is needed because haloperidol can reduce seizure threshold. Have parenteral procyclidine available in case of dystonic reactions.

Symptomatic pharmacotherapy in alcohol withdrawal

Dehydration:	Ensure adequate fluid intake in order to maintain hydration and electrolyte balance. Dehydration can lead to cardiac arrhythmia and death
Pain:	Paracetamol
Nausea and vomiting:	Metoclopramide 10 mg or prochlorperazine 5 mg 4–6 hourly
Diarrhoea:	Diphenoxylate and atropine (Lomotil). Loperamide
Hepatic encephalopathy:	Lactulose (within the general medical hospital)
Skin itching	Antihistamines (occurs commonly and not only in individuals with alcoholic liver disease)

Relapse prevention

There is no place for the continued use of benzodiazepines beyond treatment of the acute alcohol withdrawal syndrome and they should not be prescribed. Acamprosate and supervised disulfiram are licensed for treatment in the UK and can be considered as adjuncts to psychosocial treatment. These should be initiated by a specialist service. After 12 weeks transfer of the prescribing to the GP may be appropriate, although specialist care may continue (shared care).

Acamprosate

Acamprosate is a synthetic taurine analogue, which appears to act centrally on glutamate and gamma-aminobutyric acid (GABA) neurotransmitter systems, although the mechanism has not been fully established. It is licensed to prevent relapse to alcohol use and has been found to have a modest treatment effect[2]. It is best suited to supporting abstinence in individuals who are concerned that craving will lead to a lapse/relapse. Acamprosate should be initiated as soon as possible after abstinence has been achieved and should be maintained if the patient relapses. However continued alcohol use cancels out any benefit. Acamprosate should be prescribed in combination with psychosocial treatment. Contra-indications are severe renal or hepatic impairment and therefore liver and kidney function tests should be performed before commencing acamprosate. It should be avoided in individuals who are pregnant or breastfeeding.

Please see the BNF for current dosages. For adults 18–65 years at 60 kg and over, the starting dose is 666 mg 3 times daily. For adults less than 60 kg, the dose should be reduced to 666 mg (morning), 333 mg (midday) and 333 mg (night).

Naltrexone

Naltrexone is an opioid receptor antagonist and does not have marketing authorisation for the treatment of alcohol dependence in the UK. A systematic review of naltrexone treatment concluded that short-term treatment with naltrexone was effective at reducing craving for alcohol; however there were a number of limitations[9].

Disulfiram (Antabuse)

Some evidence supports the use of supervised disulfiram as part of a comprehensive treatment programme[2,3,9]. Disulfiram inhibits aldehyde dehydrogenase, thus leading to acetaldehyde accumulation after drinking alcohol, which can cause extremely unpleasant physical effects. Continued drinking can lead to arrhythmias, hypotension and collapse. Despite being available for many years, the number of controlled clinical trials is limited.

Because of the known adverse effects of disulfiram, in order to initiate treatment, the clinician must ensure that no alcohol has been consumed for at least 24 hours before commencing treatment. Contra-indications to use include cardiac failure, coronary artery disease, history of cerebrovascular disease, pregnancy and breastfeeding, liver disease, and peripheral neuropathy. Please refer to the BNF for the full range of contra-indications and dosages.

Doses as stated in the BNF are 800 mg for the first dose, reducing to 100–200 mg daily. Patients should ideally have supervised consumption of disulfiram by a relative or pharmacist, with regular review. Halitosis is a common side effect.

Pregnancy and alcohol use

Evidence suggests that alcohol consumption during pregnancy may cause harm to the foetus. The National Institute for Health and Clinical Excellence (NICE) advises that women should not drink any alcohol during pregnancy[10]. If women must drink, NICE advises that they should not do so in the first three months of pregnancy, and should limit their consumption to one or two units once or twice a week for the rest of the pregnancy.

For alcohol-dependent women who have withdrawal symptoms, pharmacological cover for detoxification should be offered, ideally as an inpatient. It is important to carry out a risk–benefit assessment of alcohol withdrawal symptoms versus prescribed benzodiazepines that may carry a risk of foetal abnormalities. This should also be assessed against risk of continued alcohol consumption to the foetus. Chlordiazepoxide has been suggested as being unlikely to pose a substantial risk, however dose-dependent malformations have been observed[11]. The timing of detoxification in relation to the trimester of pregnancy should be risk-assessed against continued alcohol consumption and risks to the foetus[3]. The Regional Drugs and Therapeutics Centre Teratology Service[12] provides national advice for healthcare professionals and like to follow up on pregnancies that require alcohol detoxification. Please refer to the references below. Specialist advice should always be sought. (See also section on pregnancy, Chapter 7).

References

1. Sullivan JT et al. Assessment of alcohol withdrawal: the revised clinical institute withdrawal assessment for alcohol scale (CIWA-Ar). Br J Addict 1989; 84:1353–1357.
2. Mayo-Smith MF. Pharmacological management of alcohol withdrawal. A meta-analysis and evidence-based practice guideline. American Society of Addiction Medicine Working Group on Pharmacological Management of Alcohol Withdrawal. JAMA 1997; 278:144–151.
3. Lingford-Hughes AR et al. Evidence-based guidelines for the pharmacological management of substance misuse, addiction and comorbidity: recommendations from the British Association for Psychopharmacology. J Psychopharmacol 2004; 18:293–335.
4. Gossop M et al. A Short Alcohol Withdrawal Scale (SAWS): development and psychometric properties. Addict Biol 2002; 7:37–43.
5. Duncan D et al. Chlormethiazole or chlordiazepoxide in alcohol detoxification. Psychiatr Bull 1996; 20:599–601.
6. Thomson AD et al. The Royal College of Physicians report on alcohol: guidelines for managing Wernicke's encephalopathy in the accident and Emergency Department. Alcohol Alcohol 2002; 37:513–521.
7. Thomson AD et al. The treatment of patients at risk of developing Wernicke's encephalopathy in the community. Alcohol Alcohol 2006; 41:159–167.
8. Polycarpou A et al. Anticonvulsants for alcohol withdrawal. Cochrane Database Syst Rev 2005;CD005064.
9. Srisurapanont M et al. Opioid antagonists for alcohol dependence. Cochrane Database Syst Rev 2005;CD001867.
10. Royal College of Obstetricians and Gynaecologists. Alcohol consumption and the outcomes of pregnancy. Statement No.5. http://www.rcog.org.uk/. 2006.
11. Flannery W, Wolff K. Substance use disorders in pregnancy. In: O'Keane V, Marsh MS, Senevirante T, editors. Psychiatric Disorders and Pregnancy: Obstetric and Psychiatric Care. London: Taylor and Francis; 2005.
12. Regional Drug & Therapeutics Centre. Teratology. 2009. http://www.nyrdtc.nhs.uk/.

Opioid misuse and dependence

Prescribing for opioid dependence

> **Note:** treatment of opioid dependence usually requires specialist intervention – generalists who do not have specialist experience should always contact substance misuse services before attempting to treat opioid dependence. It is strongly recommended that general adult psychiatrists *do not* initiate opioid substitute treatment unless directly advised by specialist services. It cannot be over-emphasised that the use of methadone is readily fatal; opioid withdrawal is not.

The treatment interventions used for opioid-dependent people in the UK range from low-intensity harm minimisation such as needle exchange through to substitution opioid maintenance therapy and high-intensity structured programmes such as residential abstinence-based psychosocial treatment. Pharmacological treatments can be broadly categorised as maintenance, detoxification or abstinence[1]:

Treatment aims
- to reduce or prevent withdrawal symptoms
- to reduce or eliminate non-prescribed drug use
- to stabilise drug intake and lifestyle
- to reduce drug-related harm (particularly injecting behaviour)
- to engage and provide an opportunity to work with the patient.

Treatment
This will depend upon:

- what pharmacotherapies and/or other interventions are available
- patient's previous history of drug use and treatment
- patient's current drug use and circumstances.

Principles of prescribing[2]
Use licensed medications for heroin dependence treatment (methadone and buprenorphine)

- The prescriber should ensure that the patient is dependent on opioids and that the patient is given a safe initial dose with suitable supervision and review to minimise the risk of toxicity.
- Daily dispensing is advised for at least the first three months of prescribing.
- Supervised consumption in the first three months or until stability achieved.

Evidence of opioid dependence
Before considering prescribing any substitute pharmacotherapy, care should be taken to ensure that the patient does have a diagnosis of opioid dependence as corroborated by:

- a diagnosis of opioid dependence from history and examination of patient
- a positive urine or oral fluid drug screen for opioids
- objective signs of opioid withdrawal (see below)
- recent sites of injection may also be present (depending on route of administration of opioid).

Opioid withdrawal symptoms may include: nausea; stomach cramps; muscular tension; muscle spasms/twitching; aches and pains; insomnia; and the objective signs listed below.

Table Objective opioid withdrawal scales			
Symptoms	*Absent/normal*	*Mild–moderate*	*Severe*
Lacrimation	Absent	Eyes watery	Eyes streaming/wiping eyes
Rhinorrhoea	Absent	Sniffing	Profuse secretion (wiping nose)
Agitation	Absent	Fidgeting	Cannot remain seated
Perspiration	Absent	Clammy skin	Beads of sweat
Piloerection	Absent	Barely palpable hairs standing up	Readily palpable, visible
Pulse rate (BPM)	<80	>80 but <100	>100
Vomiting	Absent	Absent	Present
Shivering	Absent	Absent	Present
Yawning/10 min	<3	3–5	6 or more
Dilated pupils	Normal <4 mm	Dilated 4–6 mm	Widely dilated >6 mm

Untreated heroin withdrawal symptoms typically reach their peak 32–72 hours after the last dose and symptoms will have subsided substantially after 5 days. Untreated methadone withdrawal typically reaches its peak between 4–6 days after the last dose and symptoms do not substantially subside for 10–12 days[3].

Induction and stabilisation of substitute prescribing

It is usually preferable to use a longer-acting opioid agonist or partial agonist (e.g. methadone or buprenorphine respectively) in opioid dependence, as it is generally easier to maintain stability[3]. However, patients with a less severe opioid dependency (e.g. history of using codeine or dihydro-codeine-containing preparations only) may in some cases be better managed by maintaining/detoxifying them using that preparation or equivalent.

Choosing between buprenorphine and methadone for substitute treatment

The 2007 NICE Guidance on the Management of Opioid Dependence recommends oral methadone or buprenorphine as the pharmacotherapeutic options in opioid dependence[1]. The decision of which to use should be based on the client's preference; their past experience of maintenance with either methadone or buprenorphine; their long-terms plans, including a preference for one or other as a detoxification regimen; and in the case of buprenorphine their ability to refrain from heroin use for long enough to avoid precipitated opioid withdrawal symptoms. These considerations are highlighted in the table below; in cases where methadone and buprenorphine appear equally suitable, the NICE Guidance advises prescribing methadone as first choice[1].

Table Considerations when choosing between buprenorphine and methadone for substitute treatment

	Methadone	Buprenorphine
Withdrawal syndrome	Appears to be more marked	Appears to have a milder withdrawal syndrome than methadone and therefore may be preferred for detoxification programs[4,5]
Differences in side-effect profiles may effect patient preference	Methadone may be associated with QTc prolongation and torsade de pointes (see later in this section)	Buprenorphine is often described as less sedating then methadone
Chronic pain	Patients with chronic pain conditions that frequently require additional opioid analgesia may have difficulties being treated with buprenorphine because of the 'blockade' effect	Buprenorphine appears to provide greater 'blockade' effects than doses of methadone <60 mg[6-9]. This may be considered an advantage or disadvantage by patients – see opposite
Effectiveness	Higher-dose methadone maintenance treatment (>60 mg) appears more effective than buprenorphine. However there are no adequate trials of high-dose buprenorphine (16–32 mg) compared with high-dose methadone maintenance treatment[10]	Buprenorphine is less effective than methadone at retaining patients in treatment at the guidance dose ranges[1]
Combining with other medications	Methadone levels may alter with drugs that inhibit/induce CYP3A4 such as erythromycin, several SSRIs, ribovarin, and some anticonvulsants. This may make dose assessment difficult if a person is not consistent in their use of these CYP3A4-inhibiting drugs	Buprenorphine is less affected by such medications, and may be preferable for such patients

Substance misuse

Table Considerations when choosing between buprenorphine and methadone for substitute treatment (Cont.)

	Methadone	Buprenorphine
Pregnancy	Women who are pregnant or planning a pregnancy should consider methadone treatment	There is a risk of buprenorphine-precipitated withdrawal or risk with awaiting spontaneous withdrawal prior to initiation of buprenorphine in pregnant women. However, if a patient already stable on buprenorphine becomes pregnant, a decision may be made to continue with that medication
Diversion	Patients at greater risk of diversion of medication (e.g. past history of this; treatment in a prison setting) may be better served with supervised methadone treatment	Sublingual buprenorphine tablets can be more easily diverted with the risk of injecting tablets. Available in combination with naloxone (Suboxone) – injection then becomes counter-productive
Transfer to buprenorphine		Methadone clients unable to reduce to doses of methadone <60 mg without becoming 'unstable' cannot easily be transferred to buprenorphine Those receiving 100 mg a day methadone will generally go into withdrawal if given buprenorphine[11]

Suboxone

With regards to the risk of diversion and subsequent injecting of buprenorphine, consideration may be given by the prescriber to a buprenorphine/naloxone preparation which theoretically may reduce the risk of diversion: the rationale is that as the presence of naloxone makes injecting the diverted drug less appealing due to the precipitation of opioid withdrawal symptoms. However, at the time of writing it remains the case that "Clinical experience with this new combination product is [currently] extremely limited in the UK, and it is too early to indicate the relative positions of these two versions of buprenorphine"[1]. Extended treatment schedules (12 weeks) tend to be more effective than shorter detoxification regimens[12]. Suboxone is probably more effective in acute detoxification than clonidine[13].

Dosing of this preparation is the same as for buprenorphine.

Methadone

Clinical effectiveness

Methadone, a long-acting opioid agonist, has been shown to be an effective maintenance therapy intervention for the treatment of heroin dependence by retaining patients in treatment and decreasing heroin use more than non-opioid-based replacement therapy[10]. In addition higher doses of methadone (60–100 mg/day) have been shown to be more effective than lower dosages in retaining patients and in reducing illicit heroin and cocaine use during treatment[14]. Methadone is also effective at reducing withdrawal severity when used for detoxification from heroin, however there is a high relapse following termination of treatment[15].

Prescribing information

Methadone is a Controlled Drug with a high dependency potential and a low lethal dose. The initial two weeks of treatment with methadone are associated with a substantially increased risk of overdose mortality[2,16–19]. It is important that appropriate assessment, titration of doses and monitoring is performed during this period.

Prescribing should only commence if:

*   opioid drugs are being taken on a regular basis (typically daily)
*   there is convincing evidence of dependence (see above)
*   consumption of methadone can be supervised initially.

Supervised daily consumption is recommended for new prescriptions, for a minimum of 3 months[2]. If this is not possible, instalment prescriptions for daily dispensing and collection should be used. No more than one week's supply should be dispensed at one time, except in exceptional circumstances[2].

> *Important:* All patients starting a methadone treatment programme must be informed of the risks of toxicity and overdose, and the necessity for safe storage of any take home medication[2,18,19,21]. Safe storage is vital, particularly if there are children in the household, as tragic deaths have occurred when children have ingested methadone.

Substance misuse

METHADONE DOSE

For patients who are *currently prescribed* methadone but who require the medication to be continued by a different doctor (for example if they are admitted to hospital) and if *all* the criteria listed below are met, then it is safe to prescribe the same dose:

> • Dose confirmed in writing by the previous prescriber
> • Last consumption confirmed and supervised (e.g. pharmacy contacted) and is within last 3 days
> • Previous prescriber has stopped prescribing and current prescription is completed or cancelled to date
> • Patient is stable or "comfortable" on dose (no signs of intoxication/withdrawal) and the patient is not presenting as intoxicated with other drugs and/or alcohol
> • No other contra-indications or cautions are present.

Otherwise the following recommendations should be followed.

STARTING DOSE

Consideration must be given to the potential for opioid toxicity, taking into account:

• Tolerance to opioids can be affected by a number of factors and significantly influences an individual's risk of toxicity[22]. Of particular importance in assessing this are the client's reported current quantity, frequency and route of administration; whilst being wary of possible over-reporting. A person's tolerance to methadone can be significantly reduced within three to four days of not using opioids, so caution must be exercised after this time, with careful re-titration from a starting dose.
• Use of other depressant drugs, e.g. alcohol and benzodiazepines.
• Long half-life of methadone, as cumulative toxicity may develop[23,24]. For this reason a patient should be reviewed regularly for signs of intoxication and the dose omitted or reduced if there is any sign of drowsiness or other evidence of opioid toxicity.
• Inappropriate dosing can result in potentially fatal overdose, particularly in the first few days[16-19]. Deaths have occurred following the commencement of a daily dose of 40 mg methadone[2]. It is safer to keep to a low dose that can subsequently be increased at intervals if this dose later proves to be insufficient.

> *Note:* Opioid withdrawal is *not* a life-threatening condition. Opioid toxicity is.

Direct conversion tables for opioids and methadone should be viewed cautiously, as there are a number of factors influencing the values at any given time. It is much safer to titrate the dose against presenting withdrawal symptoms.

The **initial total** daily dose for most cases will be in the range of **10–30 mg** methadone depending on the level of tolerance[1,2]. An initial dose of up to **40 mg** methadone may be prescribed by an experienced competent clinician for patients who are assessed as being heavily dependent and tolerant, but it is unwise to exceed this dose[1,2]. An additional dose of methadone can be given later the same day in cases where there is evidence of ongoing opioid withdrawal, but this should only be undertaken by prescribers with the appropriate competencies[1,2].

Note: onset of action should be evident within half an hour, with peak plasma levels being achieved after approximately two to four hours of dosing.

METHADONE STABILISATION DOSE

- **First week**

  Outpatients should attend daily for the first few days to enable assessment by the prescriber and any dose titration against withdrawal symptoms. Dose increases should not exceed 5–10 mg a day and not usually more than 30 mg in the first week above the initial starting dose[1]. Note that steady-state plasma levels are only achieved approximately five days after the last dose increase. Once the patient has been stabilised on an adequate dose, methadone should be prescribed as a single regular daily dose. It should not be prescribed on a PRN basis or at variable dosage.

- **Subsequent period**

  Subsequent increases of 5–10 mg methadone can continue after the first week, and there should be at least a few days between each successive increase[2]. It may take several weeks to reach the therapeutic daily dose of 60–120 mg[2]. Stabilisation is usually achieved within six weeks but may take longer. However it is important to consider that some patients may require more rapid stabilisation. This would need to be balanced by a high level of supervision and observation thereby allowing the ability to increase doses more rapidly.

METHADONE CAUTIONS

- **Intoxication**

  Methadone should not be given to any patient showing signs of intoxication, especially due to alcohol or other depressant drugs (e.g. benzodiazepines)[22,25]. Risk of fatal overdose is greatly enhanced when methadone is taken concomitantly with alcohol and other respiratory depressant drugs. Concurrent alcohol and illicit drug consumption must be borne in mind when considering subsequent prescribing of methadone due to the increased risk of overdose associated with polysubstance misuse[16,19,25,26].

- **Severe hepatic/renal dysfunction**

  Metabolism and elimination of methadone may be affected, in which case the dose or dosing interval should be adjusted accordingly against clinical presentation. Because of extended plasma half-life, the interval between assessments during initial dosing may need to be extended.

METHADONE OVERDOSE

In the event of methadone overdose, **naloxone** should be administered following the BNF guidelines. Naloxone can be given by intravenous, intramuscular, or subcutatneous route. The emergency services should always be called.

Dose: 0.4–2 mg repeated at intervals of 2–3 minutes to a maximum of 10 mg if respiratory function does not improve. If no response consider alternative causes for overdose.

Although the onset of action will be slower with the intramuscular route, this is the preferred route within the psychiatric setting or addiction service where the intravenous route may be difficult and actually take longer to administer.

In the medical setting a continuous intravenous infusion (2 mg/500 ml) at a rate adjusted according to response may be used.

Naloxone is short-acting and therefore the effect may reverse within 20 minutes to 1 hour, meaning that a patient can revert back into an overdose state. Therefore on-going medical monitoring should be provided after naloxone administration.

| Always Call Emergency Services |

Analgesia for methadone-prescribed patients

Non-opioid analgesics should be used in preference (e.g. paracetamol, NSAIDs) initially where appropriate.

If opioid analgesia (e.g. codeine, dihydrocodeine, morphine), is indicated due to the type and severity of the pain then this should be titrated accordingly for pain relief in line with usual analgesic protocols. The patient's methadone dose should remain constant to prevent withdrawal symptoms from their underlying opioid dependence. Titrating the methadone dose to provide analgesia may be used in certain circumstances but this should only be carried out by experienced specialists.

METHADONE AND RISK OF TORSADES DE POINTES/QT INTERVAL PROLONGATION

It is possible that methadone either alone or combined with other QT prolonging agents may increase the likelihood of QT interval prolongation on the electrocardiogram, which is associated with Torsades de Pointes and can be fatal[27–29].

Recommended ECG monitoring

In 2006, the MHRA recommended that patients with the following risk factors for QT interval prolongation are carefully monitored whilst taking methadone: heart or liver disease, electrolyte abnormalities, concomitant treatment with CYP3A4 inhibitors, or medicines with the potential to cause QT interval prolongation, (e.g. some antipsychotics; erythromycin; amongst others). In addition, any patient requiring more than 100 mg of methadone per day should be closely monitored[30], because of the possible increased risk of QTc prolongation[27]. Thus, in individuals with such risk factors, e.g. those with known heart disease, and those being titrated up to doses of methadone exceeding 100 mg, a baseline ECG and subsequent ECGs should ideally be taken. The timeframe for the latter is not yet subject to a rigorous evidence base; annual checks in the absence of cardiac symptomatology would be a reasonable minimum frequency where there are risk factors as listed. It is also important to check the actions of any medications being prescribed with methadone for CYP3A4 inhibitory activity, to inform the risk–benefit analysis when commencing methadone[31].

Buprenorphine appears to be associated with less QTc prolongation and therefore may be a safer alternative in this respect[32], although there are few studies in this area at present; and there are many other factors to take into account when choosing an appropriate opioid substitute, as described earlier.

Remember that QT should be corrected for heart rate to produce a corrected QT (QTc) in milliseconds (ms). This is normally documented on the ECG recording. The ECG should be read by a professional with experience at reading ECGs. Brief guidelines as to actions to take are documented below. Always seek specialist advice if unsure.

Substance misuse

Table Recommended ECG monitoring for methadone

	Borderline prolonged QTc	Action	Prolonged QTc	Action	Very prolonged QTc	Action
Females	≥470 ms	Repeat ECG Electrolytes Try to modify QT risk factors Regular ECG until normal	≥500 ms	Repeat ECG Electrolytes Try to modify QT risk factors Seek specialist help Consider stopping methadone Regular ECGs until normal	≥550 ms	Urgent specialist referral Repeat ECG Electrolytes Try to modify QT risk factors Stop methadone
Males	≥450 ms					

Buprenorphine

Clinical effectiveness

Buprenorphine (Subutex) is a synthetic partial opioid agonist and with a low intrinsic activity and high affinity at μ opioid receptors. It is an effective treatment for use in maintenance treatment for heroin addiction, although not more effective than methadone at adequate dosages[33]. There is no significant difference between buprenorphine and methadone in terms of completion of detoxification treatment, but withdrawal symptoms may resolve more quickly with buprenorphine[34].

Prescribing information

Buprenorphine is absorbed via the sublingual route which takes approximately 5–10 minutes to complete. It is effective in treating opioid dependence because:

- it alleviates/prevents opioid withdrawal and craving
- it reduces the effects of additional opioid use because of its high receptor affinity[6–8]
- it is long-acting allowing daily (or less frequent) dosing. The duration of action is related to the buprenorphine dose administered: low doses (e.g. 2 mg) exert effects for up to 12 hours; higher doses (e.g. 16–32 mg) exert effects for as long as 48–72 hours.

BUPRENORPHINE STARTING DOSE

The same principles as for methadone apply when starting treatment with buprenorphine. However, of particular interest with buprenorphine is the phenomenon of precipitated withdrawal. Patient education is an important factor in reducing the problems during induction.

INDUCTING HEROIN USERS

The first dose of buprenorphine should be administered when the patient is experiencing opioid withdrawal symptoms to reduce the risk of precipitated withdrawal. The initial dose recommendations are as follows:

Patient in withdrawal and no risk factors	8 mg buprenorphine
Patient not experiencing withdrawal and no risk factors	4 mg buprenorphine
Patient has concomitant risk factors (e.g. medical condition, polydrug misuse, low or uncertain severity of dependence)	2–4 mg buprenorphine

TRANSFERRING FROM METHADONE TO BUPRENORPHINE

Patients transferring from methadone are at risk of experiencing precipitated withdrawal symptoms that may continue at a milder level for 1–2 weeks. Factors affecting precipitated withdrawal are listed in the table below.

Table Factors affecting risk of precipitated withdrawal with buprenorphine

Factor	Discussion	Recommended strategy
Dose of methadone	More likely with doses of methadone above 30 mg. Generally – the higher the dose, the more severe the precipitated withdrawal[35]	Attempt transfer from doses of methadone <40 mg (preferably ≤30 mg). Transfer from >60 mg should not be attempted
Time between last methadone dose and first buprenorphine dose	Interval should be at least 24 hours. Increasing the interval reduces the incidence and severity of withdrawal[36,37]	Cease methadone and delay first dose until patient experiencing withdrawal from methadone
Dose of buprenorphine	Very low doses of buprenorphine (e.g. 2 mg) are generally inadequate to substitute for methadone. High first doses of buprenorphine (e.g. 8 mg) are more likely to precipitate withdrawal	First dose should generally be 4 mg; review patient 2–3 hours later
Patient expectancy	Patients not prepared for precipitated withdrawal are more likely to become distressed and confused by the effect	Inform patients in advance. Have contingency plan for severe symptoms
Use of other medications	Symptomatic medication (e.g. lofexidine) can be useful to relieve symptoms	Prescribe in accordance to management plan

TRANSFERRING FROM METHADONE DOSE <40 MG (IDEALLY ≤30 MG) TO BUPRENORPHINE
Methadone should be ceased abruptly, and the first dose of buprenorphine given at least 24 hours after the last methadone dose. The following conversion rates at the start of treatment are recommended but higher doses may be subsequently needed depending on clinical presentation:

Last methadone dose	Day 1 – initial buprenorphine dose	Day 2 – buprenorphine dose
20–40 mg	4 mg	6–8 mg
10–20 mg	4 mg	4–8 mg
1–10 mg	2 mg	2–4 mg

TRANSFERRING FROM METHADONE DOSE 40–60 MG TO BUPRENORPHINE
- The methadone dose should be reduced as far as possible without the patient becoming unstable or chaotic, and then abruptly stopped.
- The first buprenorphine dose should be delayed until the patient displays clear signs of withdrawal, generally 48–96 hours after the last dose of methadone. Symptomatic medication (lofexidine) may be useful to provide temporary relief.
- An initial dose of 2–4 mg should be given. The patient should then be reviewed 2–3 hours later.

- If withdrawal has been precipitated further symptomatic medication can be prescribed.
- If there has been no precipitation or worsening of withdrawal, an additional 2–4 mg of buprenorphine can be dispensed on the same day.
- The patient should be reviewed the following day at which point the dose should be increased to 8–12 mg.

TRANSFERRING FROM METHADONE DOSES >60 MG TO BUPRENORPHINE

Such transfers should not be attempted in an outpatient setting except in exceptional circumstances by an experienced practitioner. Usually patients would be partially detoxified from methadone and transferred to buprenorphine when the methadone was at or below 30 mg daily. However, if transfer from higher-dose methadone to buprenorphine is required, a referral to an inpatient unit should be considered.

TRANSFERRING FROM OTHER PRESCRIBED OPIOIDS TO BUPRENORPHINE

There is little experience in transferring patients from other prescribed opioids (e.g. codeine, dihydrocodeine, morphine). Basic principles suggest that transferring from opioids with short half-lives should be similar to inducting heroin users; whereas transferring from opioids with longer half-lives will be similar to transferring from methadone.

STABILISATION DOSE OF BUPRENORPHINE

Outpatients should attend regularly for the first few days to enable assessment by the prescriber and any dose titration. Dose increases should be made in increments of 2–4 mg at a time, daily if necessary, up to a maximum daily dose of 32 mg. Effective maintenance doses are usually in the range of 12–24 mg daily[38] and patients should generally be able to achieve maintenance levels within 1–2 weeks of starting buprenorphine.

BUPHRENORPHINE LESS THAN DAILY DOSING

Buprenorphine is licensed in the UK as a medication to be taken daily. International evidence and experience indicates that many clients can be comfortably maintained on one dose every 2–3 days[39–42]. This may be pertinent for patients in buprenorphine treatment who are considered unsuitable for take-away medication because of the risk of diversion. The following conversion rate is recommended:

2-day buprenorphine dose = 2 × daily dose of buprenorphine (to a max. 32 mg)
3-day buprenorphine dose = 3 × daily dose of buprenorphine (to a max. 32 mg)

Note: In the event of patients being unable to stabilise comfortably on buprenorphine (often those transferring from methadone), the option of transferring to methadone should be available. Methadone can be commenced 24 hours after the last buprenorphine dose. Doses should be titrated according to clinical response, being mindful of the residual 'blockade' effect of buprenorphine which may last for several days.

Cautions with buprenorphine

- **Liver function:** There is some evidence suggesting that high-dose buprenorphine can cause changes in liver function in individuals with a history of liver disease[43]. Such patients should have LFTs measured before commencing with follow-up investigations conducted 6–12 weeks after commencing buprenorphine. More frequent testing should be considered in patients of particular concern, e.g. severe liver disease. Elevated liver enzymes in the absence of clinically significant liver disease however does not necessarily contra-indicate treatment with buprenorphine

- **Intoxication:** Buprenorphine should not be given to any patient showing signs of intoxication, especially due to alcohol or other depressant drugs (e.g. benzodiazepines). Buprenorphine in combination with other sedative drugs can result in respiratory depression, sedation, coma, and death. Concurrent alcohol and illicit drug consumption must be borne in mind when considering subsequent prescribing of buprenorphine due to the increased risk of overdose associated with polysubstance misuse.

OVERDOSE WITH BUPRENORPHINE

Buprenorphine as a single drug in overdose is generally regarded as safer than methadone and heroin because it causes less respiratory depression. However, in combination with other respiratory-depressant drugs the effects may be harder to manage. Very high doses of naloxone (e.g. 10–15 mg) may be needed to reverse buprenorphine effects (although lower doses such as 0.8 to 2mg may be sufficient), hence ventilator support is often required in cases where buprenorphine is contributing to respiratory depression (e.g. in polydrug overdose).

Always Call Emergency Services

ANALGESIA FOR BUPRENORPHINE-PRESCRIBED PATIENTS

Non-opioid analgesics should be used in preference (e.g. paracetamol, NSAIDs). Buprenorphine reduces or blocks the effect of full opioid agonists complicating their use as analgesics in patients on buprenorphine. If adequate pain control cannot be achieved then it may be necessary to transfer the patient to a stable methadone dose so that an opioid analgesic can be effectively used for pain control (see note on analgesia for methadone-prescribed patients).

Alternative oral preparations

Oral methadone and buprenorphine should continue to be the mainstay of treatment[2]; other oral options such as slow-release oral morphine (SROM) preparations and dihydrocodeine are not licensed in the UK for the treatment of opiate dependence[2].

However, a specialised clinician may in very exceptional circumstances prescribe oral dihydrocodeine as maintenance therapy, where clients are unable to tolerate methadone or buprenorphine, or in other exceptional circumstances; taking into account the difficulties associated with its short half-life, supervision requirements, and diversion potential[2].

Slow-release oral morphine preparations (SROM) have been shown elsewhere in Europe to be useful as maintenance therapy in those who fail to tolerate methadone; again only for prescribing by specialised clinicians[2].

Injectable opioid maintenance prescribing

With regard to the prescribing of injectable opioids, a small number of patients in the UK continue to receive these under the former 'British system'[2], and a further minority are being treated in trial clinics in the UK[44], modelled on the recent Swiss and Dutch injectable opioid maintenance clinics. The trials in Europe have shown promising results, and the UK results are awaited. Meanwhile, injectable opioid treatment is not currently available in all specialist services in the UK[2]. Notably, a Home Office licence is required to prescribe diamorphine for addictions treatment, and specialist levels of competence are required to prescribe injectable substitute opioids[2].

At present, clients should only be considered for injectable opioid prescribing in combination with psychosocial interventions, as part of a wider package of care, as an option in cases where the individual has not responded adequately to oral opioid substitution treatment, and in an area where it can be supported by locally commissioned and provided mechanisms for supervised consumption[2]. Readers are referred to NTA guidance regarding injectable opioid prescribing for further information[44].

Opioid detoxification and reduction regimens

Opioid maintenance can be continued from the short term to almost indefinitely, depending on clinical need. Some patients are keen to detoxify after short periods of stability and other patients may decide to detoxify after medium- to long-term periods of stability on maintenance prescriptions. All detoxification programmes should be part of a care programme. Given the risk of serious fatal overdose post detoxification, services providing such treatment should educate the patient about these risks and supply and train them with naloxone and overdose training for emergency use[1,45,46].

Regarding the length of detoxification, the NICE guidelines state "dose reduction can take place over anything from a few days to several months, with a higher initial stabilisation dose taking longer to taper", and indicate that "up to 3 months is typical for methadone reduction, while buprenorphine reductions are typically carried out over 14 days to a few weeks"[47]. In practice, a detoxification in the community may extend over a longer period, if this facilitates the client's comfort during the process, compliance with the care-plan, continued abstinence from illicit use during detoxification, and subsequent abstinence following detoxification.

Detoxification in an inpatient setting, the NICE guidelines indicate, may take place over a shorter time than in the community (suggesting 14–21 days for methadone and 7–14 days for buprenorphine) "as the supportive environment helps a service user to tolerate emerging withdrawal symptoms"[48]. As in the community, a stabilisation on the dose of a substitute opioid is first achieved, followed by gradual dose reduction; with additive medications judiciously prescribed for withdrawal symptoms if and as needed.

Community setting

- **Methadone**

  Following a period of stabilisation with methadone or a longer period of maintenance, the patient and prescriber may agree a reduction programme as part of a care plan to reduce the daily methadone dose. The usual reduction would be by 5–10 mg weekly or fortnightly although there can be much variation in the reduction and speed of reduction. In the community setting, patient preference is the most important variable in terms of dose reduction and rate of reduction. The detoxification programme should be reviewed regularly and remain flexible to adjustments and changes, such as relapse to illicit drug use or patient anxieties about speed of reduction. Factors such as an increase in heroin or other drug use or worsening of the patient's physical, psychological or social well-being, may warrant a temporary increase, or stabilisation of the dose or a slowing-down of the reduction rate. Towards the end of the detoxification the dose reduction may be slower than 1–2 mg per week.

- **Buprenorphine**
  The same principles as for methadone apply when planning a buprenorphine detoxification regimen. Dose reduction should be gradual to minimise withdrawal discomfort. Suggested reduction regimen:

Daily buprenorphine dose	Reduction rate
Above 16 mg	4 mg every 1–2 weeks
8–16 mg	2–4 mg every 1–2 weeks
2–8 mg	2 mg per week or fortnight
Below 2 mg	Reduce by 0.4–0.8 mg per week

In-patient setting

- **Methadone**
  Patients should have a starting dose assessment of methadone, over 48 hours by a specialist inpatient team. The dose may then be reduced following a linear regimen over up to four weeks[47].

- **Buprenorphine**
  Buprenorphine can be used effectively for short-term inpatient detoxifications following the same principles as for methadone.

- **Lofexidine**
  Lofexidine, an α_2 adrenergic agonist, can counteract the adrenergic hyperactivity associated with opioid withdrawal[49] (demonstrated by characteristic signs and symptoms, such as tachycardia, sweating, runny nose, hair standing on end, shivering, and goose bumps). Thus, it is licensed for the management of symptoms of opioid withdrawal[47], although additional short-term adjunctive medications may be needed for symptoms not treated by an α_2 adrenergic agonist, such as loperamide for diarrhoea[2]. Detoxification using lofexidine is much faster than with methadone or buprenorphine, typically lasting 5–7 days, and up to a maximum of 10 days. The usual regimen commences at 800 mcg daily, rising to 2.4 mg in split doses, which is then reduced over subsequent days[2]. Side effects may include a dry mouth, drowsiness, and clinically significant hypotension and bradycardia[2]; the latter two in particular must therefore be monitored during lofexidine prescribing.

Although lofexidine is not useful for detoxification of those with substantial opioid dependence[2], there are certain circumstances in which this regimen may have a role: in cases where the client has made an informed and clinically appropriate decision not to use methadone or buprenorphine for detoxification; in cases where they have made a similarly informed and clinically appropriate decision to detoxify within a short time period; and in cases where there is only mild or uncertain opioid dependence (including young people)[47].

Substance misuse

313

Relapse prevention – psychosocial interventions

Psychosocial and behavioural therapies play an important role in the treatment of drug misuse: by helping people develop skills to resist drug misuse and cope with associated problems, they form an important adjunct to pharmacological treatments[2].

These include brief interventions, such as exploring ambivalence about drug use and possible treatment, with the aim of increasing motivation to change behaviour; providing information about self-help groups (e.g. Narcotics Anonymous); behavioural couples therapy; family therapy, community reinforcement approach and other psychosocial therapies[2]. One particular form of therapy is Contingency Management, considered by NICE[48] as having a strong evidence base from a growing body of work in the US. The principle of this therapy is to provide structured external incentives focused on changing specific behaviours. For example, low-monetary-value vouchers may be provided in a structured setting contingent on each presentation of a drug-negative test until stability is achieved. Vouchers of higher monetary value (e.g. £10) should be considered to encourage harm reduction on a one-off basis or over a limited duration for managing physical health problems, such as concordance with or completion of:

- hepatitis B/C and HIV testing
- hepatitis B immunisation
- tuberculosis testing[48].

"The emphasis on reinforcing positive behaviours is consistent with current knowledge about the underlying neuropsychology of many people who misuse drugs and is more likely to be effective than penalising negative behaviours. There is good evidence that contingency management increases the likelihood of positive behaviours and is cost effective"[48]. Further details are beyond the scope of this text, and the interested reader is therefore referred to the 2007 NICE guidelines on psychosocial interventions in drug misuse.

Relapse prevention – naltrexone

Evidence for the effectiveness of naltrexone as a treatment for relapse prevention in opioid misusers has been inconclusive[50]. However, for those who prefer an abstinence programme, are fully informed of the potential adverse effects and benefits of treatment, and are highly motivated to remain on treatment, naltrexone treatment has been found by NICE to be a cost-effective treatment strategy in aiding abstinence from opioid misuse[51].

Close monitoring is particularly important when naltrexone treatment is initiated because of the higher risk of fatal overdose at this time. Discontinuation of naltrexone may also be associated with an increase in inadvertent overdose from illicit opioids. Thus, supervision of naltrexone administration, and careful choice of who is prescribed it (those who are abstinence-focused and motivated) is very important. Moreover, people taking naltrexone often experience adverse effects of unease (dysphoria), depression and insomnia, which can lead to relapse to illicit opioid use while on naltrexone treatment, or failure to continue on treatment. The dysphoria maybe caused by either withdrawal from illicit drugs or by the naltrexone treatment itself, emphasising the importance of prescribing naltrexone as part of a care programme that includes psychosocial therapy and general support[51].

Initiating naltrexone treatment

Naltrexone has the propensity to cause a severe withdrawal reaction in patients who are either currently taking opioid drugs or who were previously taking opioid drugs and there has not been a sufficient "wash-out" period before administering naltrexone.

The minimum recommended interval between stopping the opioid and starting naltrexone depends on the opioid used, duration of use and the amount taken as a last dose. Opioid agonists with long half-lives such as methadone will require a wash-out period of up to 10 days, whereas shorter-acting opioids such as heroin may only require up to 7 days.

Experience with buprenorphine indicates that a wash-out period of up to 7 days is sufficient (final buprenorphine dose >2 mg; duration of use >2 weeks) and in some cases naltrexone may be started within 2–3 days of a patient stopping (final buprenorphine dose <2 mg; duration of use <2 weeks).

A test dose of naloxone (0.2–0.8 mg), which has a much shorter half-life than naltrexone, may be given to the patient as an IM dose prior to starting naltrexone treatment. Any withdrawal symptoms precipitated will be of shorter duration than if precipitated by naltrexone.

Patients *must* be advised of the risk of withdrawal prior to giving the dose. It is worth thoroughly questioning the patient as to whether they have taken any opioid-containing preparation unknowingly (e.g. over-the-counter analgesic).

Important points regarding prescribing naltrexone

Ensure the client is fully informed of the increased risk of fatal opioid overdose:

Following detoxification and any period of abstinence, an individual's tolerance to opioids will decrease markedly. At such a time, using opioids puts the individual at greatly increased risk of overdose.

Discontinuation of naltrexone may also be associated with an increase in inadvertent overdose from illicit opioids, emphasising the need for close monitoring and support of the client at this time.

Dose of naltrexone

An initial dose of 25 mg naltrexone should be administered after a suitable opioid-free interval (and naloxone challenge if appropriate). The patient should be monitored for 4 hours after the first dose, for symptoms of opioid withdrawal. Symptomatic medication for withdrawal (lofexidine) should be available for use, if necessary, on the first day of naltrexone dosing (withdrawal symptoms may last up to 4–8 hours). Once the patient has tolerated this low naltrexone dose, subsequent doses can be increased to 50 mg daily as a maintenance dose.

Pregnancy and opioid use

> Substitute prescribing can occur at any time in pregnancy and carries a lower risk than continuing illicit use[2].

In well-stabilised women, abstinence can be achieved, slowly with a synthetic opioid, and not after the 32nd week (to avoid pre-term delivery)[52]. Some mothers may request detoxification, although during the first trimester it is safest to stabilise them to avoid spontaneous abortion[2]. However, for many other pregnant opioid users, this will not be the aim: enforcing it is likely to deter some clients from seeking help, and the majority will then return to opioid use at some point during their pregnancy[52]; fluctuating opioid concentrations in the maternal blood from intermittent use of illicit opioids may then lead to foetal withdrawal or overdose[53,54]. Given the value of a comprehensive care package, pregnant women attending treatment usually have better general health than those using drugs who are not in treatment, even if the former continue to also use illicit drugs[2]. The emphasis must therefore be on early engagement in treatment[2], and, methadone maintenance treatment during pregnancy, in the context of a multidisciplinary team (including obstetricians, neonatologists and addictions specialists) and detailed holisitic package of care, (including comprehensive psychosocial input)[52]; this is currently regarded as the gold standard[53,54].

The majority of neonates born to methadone-maintained mothers will, however, require treatment for neonatal abstinence syndrome (NAS)[52]: NAS is characterised by a variety of signs and symptoms relating to the autonomic nervous system, gastrointestinal tract, and respiratory system[53]; with methadone usually commenced after 48 hours[55]. In the case of any mother using drugs or in opioid substitution treatment, it is important to have access to skilled neonatal paediatric care, to monitor the neonate and treat as required.

Specialist advice should be obtained before initiating opioid substitution treatment or detoxification, particularly with regards to management and treatment plan during pregnancy. Maternal metabolism of methadone may increase towards the third trimester of pregnancy. At this time an increased methadone dose may be required or occasionally split dosing on the medication to prevent withdrawal.

Limited controlled data are available on the treatment of opioid dependence in pregnancy[52,54,56], and particularly the use of buprenorphine in pregnancy[52,57]. However, the buprenorphine cases recorded to date suggest that buprenorphine, compared with methadone, may lead to a less severe abstinence syndrome in the neonate[52].

It is useful to anticipate potential problems for women prescribed opioids during pregnancy with regard to opioid pain relief: such women should be managed in specialist antenatal clinics due to the increased associated risks. Antenatal assessment by anaesthetists may be recommended with regard to anticipating any anaesthetic risks, any analgesic requirements, and problems with venous access.

Pregnancy and breastfeeding – methadone

Although the newborn may experience a withdrawal syndrome, as described, there is no evidence of an increase in congenital defects with methadone.

Methadone is considered compatible with breastfeeding, although other risk factors such as HIV, hepatitis C, use of benzodiazepines, cocaine and other drugs need to be considered and may mean that breastfeeding is contra-indicated. The Clinical Guidelines[2] recommend that breast feeding should still be encouraged, but that with regards to methadone and breast feeding "the dose is kept as low as possible while maintaining stability, and the infant monitored to avoid sedation".

Pregnancy and breastfeeding – buprenorphine

Currently there is insufficient evidence regarding the use of buprenorphine as an opioid substitute treatment during pregnancy or breastfeeding to be able to define its safety profile. More evidence is available on the safety of methadone, which, for that reason, makes it the preferred choice. However, women well maintained on buprenorphine prior to pregnancy may remain on buprenorphine following full informed consent and advice that safety of buprenorphine in pregnancy has not been demonstrated[2]. Please note buprenorphine is not licensed for use in pregnancy and should not be initiated in this circumstance by a non-specialist[2].

Opioid overdose and use of naloxone

All addictions services and psychiatric units should have naloxone available.

1. Call 999
2. Check airways and breathing
3. Administer IM naloxone; Repeat dose if needed
4. Stay with the client and await the ambulance

Opioid overdose with heroin or other opioids can be recognised by;

* Pin-point pupils
* Respiratory depression (<8 breaths per minute)
* Cold to touch/blue lips
* Unconsciousness.

Actions to be taken on discovering an opioid overdose

* Check area safe, then try to rouse overdose victim
* If unrousable – call for help/ambulance
* Check airway and breathing
  – If not breathing, give 2 rescue breaths (optional)
  – If breathing – place in recovery position
* Administer 0.4 mg naloxone IM
* Repeat this dose if there is no response after 2–3 minutes
* Consider use of high-flow oxygen (where available)
* Await emergency team/ambulance
* Patient to have medical monitoring for several hours after naloxone as the effects of naloxone are short acting (between 30 minutes to one hour) and the effects of an opioid overdose may re-emerge. Patients may need additional doses of naloxone.

'Take home' naloxone

Research trials have assessed the impact of providing take home naloxone and overdose management training to opioid-using patients. Although no randomised controlled trials are available, the available evidence is promising for reducing heroin-related overdose deaths[45,46]. Some services are providing one dose of take home naloxone (400 mcg) in combination with opioid overdose management training (as above) to opioid-using clients in treatment.

References

1. National Institute for Clinical Excellence. Methadone and buprenorphine for the management of opioid dependence. Technology Appraisal 114. http://www.nice.org.uk. 2007.
2. Department of Health. Drug misuse and dependence. UK guidelines on clinical management. 2007.
3. Department of Health. Drug misuse and dependence: guidelines on clinical management. Norwich: Department of Health; 1999.
4. Seifert J et al. Detoxification of opiate addicts with multiple drug abuse: a comparison of buprenorphine vs. methadone. Pharmacopsychiatry 2002; 35:159–164.

Substance misuse

5. Jasinski DR et al. Human pharmacology and abuse potential of the analgesic buprenorphine: a potential agent for treating narcotic addiction. Arch Gen Psychiatry 1978; 35:501–516.
6. Bickel WK et al. Buprenorphine: dose-related blockade of opioid challenge effects in opioid dependent humans. J Pharmacol Exp Ther 1988; 247:47–53.
7. Walsh SL et al. Acute administration of buprenorphine in humans: partial agonist and blockade effects. J Pharmacol Exp Ther 1995; 274:361–372.
8. Comer SD et al. Buprenorphine sublingual tablets: effects on IV heroin self-administration by humans. Psychopharmacology 2001; 154:28–37.
9. Donny EC et al. High-dose methadone produces superior opioid blockade and comparable withdrawal suppression to lower doses in opioid-dependent humans. Psychopharmacology 2002; 161:202–212.
10. Mattick RP et al. Buprenorphine maintenance versus placebo or methadone maintenance for opioid dependence. Cochrane Database Syst Rev 2003;CD002207.
11. Rosado J et al. Sublingual buprenorphine/naloxone precipitated withdrawal in subjects maintained on 100mg of daily methadone. Drug Alcohol Depend 2007; 90:261–269.
12. Woody GE et al. Extended vs short-term buprenorphine-naloxone for treatment of opioid-addicted youth: a randomized trial. JAMA 2008; 300: 2003–2011.
13. Ziedonis DM et al. Predictors of outcome for short-term medically supervised opioid withdrawal during a randomized, multicenter trial of buprenorphine-naloxone and clonidine in the NIDA clinical trials network drug and alcohol dependence. Drug Alcohol Depend 2009; 99:28–36.
14. Faggiano F et al. Methadone maintenance at different dosages for opioid dependence. Cochrane Database Syst Rev 2003; CD002208.
15. Amato L et al. Methadone at tapered doses for the management of opioid withdrawal. Cochrane Database Syst Rev 2005; CD003409.
16. Harding-Pink D. Methadone: one person's maintenance dose is another's poison. Lancet 1993; 341:665–666.
17. Drummer OH et al. Methadone toxicity causing death in ten subjects starting on a methadone maintenance program. Am J Forensic Med Pathol 1992; 13:346–350.
18. Caplehorn JR. Deaths in the first two weeks of maintenance treatment in NSW in 1994: identifying cases of iatrogenic methadone toxicity. Drug Alcohol Rev 1998; 17:9–17.
19. Zador D et al. Deaths in methadone maintenance treatment in New South Wales, Australia 1990–1995. Addiction 2000; 95:77–84.
20. Department of Health TFtRSfDM. Report of an independent review of drug treatment services in England. 1996. http://www.dh.gov.uk/.
21. Hall W. Reducing the toll of opioid overdose deaths in Australia. Drug Alcohol Rev 1999; 18:213–220.
22. White JM et al. Mechanisms of fatal opioid overdose. Addiction 1999; 94:961–972.
23. Wolff K et al. The pharmacokinetics of methadone in healthy subjects and opiate users. Br J Clin Pharmacol 1997; 44:325–334.
24. Rostami-Hodjegan A et al. Population pharmacokinetics of methadone in opiate users: characterization of time-dependent changes. Br J Clin Pharmacol 1999; 48:43–52.
25. Farrell M et al. Suicide and overdose among opiate addicts. Addiction 1996; 91:321–323.
26. Neale J. Methadone, methadone treatment and non-fatal overdose. Drug Alcohol Depend 2000; 58:117–124.
27. Krantz MJ et al. Torsade de pointes associated with very-high-dose methadone. Ann Intern Med 2002; 137:501–504.
28. Kornick CA et al. QTc interval prolongation associated with intravenous methadone. Pain 2003; 105:499–506.
29. Martell BA et al. The impact of methadone induction on cardiac conduction in opiate users. Ann Intern Med 2003; 139:154–155.
30. Medicines and Healthcare Products Regulatory Agency. Risk of QT interval prolongation with methadone. Current Problems in Pharmacovigilance 2006; 31:6.
31. Cruciani RA. Methadone: to ECG or not to ECG...That is still the question. J Pain Symptom Manage 2008; 36:545–552.
32. Wedam EF et al. QT-interval effects of methadone, levomethadyl, and buprenorphine in a randomized trial. Arch Intern Med 2007; 167:2469–2475.
33. Mattick RP et al. Buprenorphine maintenance versus placebo or methadone maintenance for opioid dependence. Cochrane Database Syst Rev 2008;CD002207.
34. Gowing L et al. Buprenorphine for the management of opioid withdrawal. Cochrane Database Syst Rev 2009;CD002025.
35. Walsh SL et al. Effects of buprenorphine and methadone in methadone-maintained subjects. Psychopharmacology 1995; 119:268–276.
36. Strain EC et al. Acute effects of buprenorphine, hydromorphone and naloxone in methadone-maintained volunteers. J Pharmacol Exp Ther 1992; 261:985–993.
37. Strain EC et al. Buprenorphine effects in methadone-maintained volunteers: effects at two hours after methadone. J Pharmacol Exp Ther 1995; 272: 628–638.
38. Ling W et al. Buprenorphine maintenance treatment of opiate dependence: a multicenter, randomized clinical trial. Addiction 1998; 93:475–486.
39. Amass L et al. Alternate-day buprenorphine dosing is preferred to daily dosing by opioid-dependent humans. Psychopharmacology 1998; 136: 217–225.
40. Amass L et al. Alternate-day dosing during buprenorphine treatment of opioid dependence. Life Sci 1994; 54:1215–1228.
41. Johnson RE et al. Buprenorphine treatment of opioid dependence: clinical trial of daily versus alternate-day dosing. Drug Alcohol Depend 1995; 40:27–35.
42. Eissenberg T et al. Controlled opioid withdrawal evaluation during 72 h dose omission in buprenorphine-maintained patients. Drug Alcohol Depend 1997; 45:81–91.
43. Berson A et al. Hepatitis after intravenous buprenorphine misuse in heroin addicts. J Hepatol 2001; 34:346–350.
44. National Treatment Agency for Substance Misuse. Injectable heroin (and injectable methadone). Potential roles in drug treatment. Full Guidance Report. http://www.nta.nhs.uk/. 2003.
45. Baca CT et al. Take-home naloxone to reduce heroin death. Addiction 2005; 100:1823–1831.
46. Strang J et al. Emergency naloxone for heroin overdose. BMJ 2006; 333:614–615.
47. National Institute for Clinical Excellence. Drug misuse: opioid detoxification. Clinical Guidance 52. 2007.
48. National Institute for Clinical Excellence. Drug misuse: psychosocial interventions. Clinical Guidance 51. 2007. http://www.nice.org.uk/.
49. Yu E et al. A Phase 3 placebo-controlled, double-blind, multi-site trial of the alpha-2-adrenergic agonist, lofexidine, for opioid withdrawal. Drug Alcohol Depend 2008; 97:158–168.
50. Kirchmayer U et al. Naltrexone maintenance treatment for opioid dependence. Cochrane Database Syst Rev 2003;CD001333.
51. National Institute for Clinical Excellence. Naltrexone for the management of opioid dependence. Technology Appraisal 115. http://www.nice.org.uk. 2007.
52. Winklbaur B et al. Treating pregnant women dependent on opioids is not the same as treating pregnancy and opioid dependence: a knowledge synthesis for better treatment for women and neonates. Addiction 2008; 103:1429–1440.
53. Finnegan LP. Neonatal Abstinence Syndrome. In: Hoekelman RA, Friedman SB, Nelson N, Seidel HM, editors. Primary Pediatric Care. St Louis: Mosby; 1992; 1367–1378.
54. Winklbaur B et al. Opioid dependence and pregnancy. Curr Opin Psychiatry 2008; 21:255–259.
55. Fischer G et al. Methadone versus buprenorphine in pregnant addicts: a double-blind, double-dummy comparison study. Addiction 2006; 101: 275–281.
56. Minozzi S et al. Maintenance agonist treatments for opiate dependent pregnant women. Cochrane Database Syst Rev 2008;CD006318.
57. Kayemba-Kay's S et al. Buprenorphine withdrawal syndrome in newborns: a report of 13 cases. Addiction 2003; 98:1599–1604.

Drug misuse: opioid detoxification

NICE Clinical Guideline 52
July 2007[47]

- Detoxification should be an available option for those who have expressed an informed choice to become abstinent.
- Give detailed information about detoxification and the associated risks, including the loss of opioid tolerance following detoxification, the ensuing increased risk of overdose and death from illicit drug use; and the importance of continued support to maintain abstinence and reduce the risk of adverse outcomes.
- Methadone or buprenorphine should be offered as the first-line treatment in opioid detoxification.
- Ultra-rapid detoxification under general anaesthesia or heavy sedation (where the airway needs to be supported) must not be offered. This is because of the risk of serious adverse events, including death.
- Offer a community-based programme to all service users considering opioid detoxification. Exceptions to this may include service users who:
  - have not benefited from previous formal community-based detoxification
  - need care because of significant comorbid physical or mental health problems
  - require complex polydrug detoxification, e.g. concurrent detoxification from alcohol or benzodiazepines are experiencing significant social problems that will limit the benefit of community-based detoxification.

Drug misuse: psychological interventions

NICE Clinical Guidance 51
July 2007[48]

Brief interventions

- Opportunistic brief interventions focused on motivation should be offered to people in limited contact with drug services (e.g., those attending a needle and syringe exchange).
- These interventions should aim to increase motivation to change behaviour, and provide non-judgemental feedback.

Self help

- Provide people who misuse drugs with information about self-help groups, e.g. Narcotics Anonymous and Cocaine Anonymous.

Contingency management

- Introduce contingency management to reduce illicit drug use and/or promote engagement with services for people receiving methadone maintenance treatment.

Methadone and buprenorphine for the management of opioid dependence

NICE Technology Appraisal Guidance 114
January 2007[1]

- Methadone and buprenorphine (oral formulations), using flexible dosing regimens, are recommended as options for maintenance therapy in the management of opioid dependence.
- The decision about which drug to use should be made on a case-by-case basis, taking into account a number of factors, including the person's history of opioid dependence, their commitment to a particular long-term management strategy, and an estimate of the risks and benefits of each treatment made by the responsible clinician in consultation with the person. If both drugs are equally suitable, methadone should be prescribed as the first choice.
- Methadone and buprenorphine should be administered daily, under supervision, for at least the first 3 months. Supervision should be relaxed only when the patient's compliance is assured. Both drugs should be given as part of a programme of supportive care.

Naltrexone for the management of opioid dependence

NICE Technology Appraisal Guidance 115
January 2007[51]

- Naltrexone is recommended as a treatment option in detoxified formerly opioid-dependent people who are highly motivated to remain in an abstinence programme.
- Naltrexone should only be administered under adequate supervision to people who have been fully informed of the potential adverse effects of treatment. It should be given as part of a programme of supportive care.
- The effectiveness of naltrexone in preventing opioid misuse in people being treated should be reviewed regularly. Discontinuation of naltrexone treatment should be considered if there is evidence of such misuse.

Nicotine and smoking cessation

NICE guidance on smoking cessation

Harmful effects from nicotine dependence are generally related to the harm caused by smoking cigarettes and therefore the primary goal of treatment is complete cessation of smoking. The three main treatments licensed in the UK for smoking cessation are nicotine replacement (all formulations are available over the counter), the antidepressant bupropion prolonged-release and varenicline tartrate. Nicotine replacement therapy (NRT) and bupropion have been investigated in a large number of well-conducted RCTs, and varenicline in four similar trials. NICE has developed treatment guidance for nicotine dependence and smoking cessation.

NICE has also made recommendations on brief interventions and referral to NHS smoking cessation services' some of which are outlined below[1].

- Everyone who smokes should be advised to stop.
- All smokers should be asked how interested they are in quitting.
- Healthcare workers (including GPs and hospital doctors) should offer referral to smoking cessation services and if the person does not want to attend these services, can initiate pharmacotherpy as per NICE guidelines[2] if sufficiently experienced.

The original NICE guidance assessed bupropion and nicotine replacement therapy (NRT) and the new guidance includes varenicline. NICE has made several recommendations for treatment.

- NRT and bupropion are recommended for those who want to stop smoking.
- NRT and bupropion should only be prescribed as part of an "abstinent-contingent treatment" model in which smokers make a commitment to stop smoking on a particular date and medication is only continued if the user remains abstinent from smoking at follow-ups. To increase cost-efficacy, the total treatment course is dispensed in divided prescriptions. NRT should initially be prescribed to last for 2 weeks after the quit date and bupropion for 3–4 weeks after the quit date. Subsequent prescriptions should be given if the smoker is making good progress at their quit attempt.
- Bupropion should not be used in the under 18s, pregnant or breastfeeding women.
- NHS-funded smoking cessation treatments should not usually be offered within 6 months of an unsuccessful attempt at smoking cessation with either NRT or bupropion, unless there are external circumstances which led to relapse.
- The evidence is insufficient to recommend NRT combined with bupropion.
- Factors to consider when deciding which treatment to initiate include:
  - motivation to stop
  - availability of counselling
  - previous experience with smoking cessation aids
  - contra-indications to use (particularly for bupropion)
  - personal preference of smoker.

Nicotine replacement therapy (NRT)
Clinical effectiveness

A Cochrane review of 23 randomised controlled trials of NRT against placebo or non-NRT for smoking cessation with at least 6 month follow-up[3] concluded that all six commercially available forms of NRT are effective. NRT increases the odds of quitting by approximately 1.5 to 2 fold regardless of clinical setting. NRT significantly reduces the severity of nicotine withdrawal symptoms and urge to smoke and should be given as per recommended doses in the BNF and outlined below. The dosages may vary according to the degree of nicotine dependence as indicated by markers such as daily cigarette consumption, latency to first cigarette in the morning and severity of withdrawal symptoms on previous quit attempts.

Notes: The MHRA recently issued new advice on the use of NRT to widen access in at-risk patient groups. NRT may now be used by:

- Adolescents aged 12–18, but as there are limited data on the safety and efficacy, duration should be restricted to 12 weeks. Treatment should only be continued longer than 12 weeks on the advice of a healthcare professional.
- Pregnant women – ideally they should stop smoking without using NRT but, if this is not possible, NRT may be recommended to assist a quit attempt as it is considered that the risk to the foetus of continued smoking by the mother outweighs any potential adverse effects of NRT. The decision to use NRT should be made following a risk–benefit assessment as early in pregnancy as possible. The aim should be to discontinue NRT use after 2–3 months. Intermittent (oral) forms of NRT are preferable during pregnancy although a patch may be appropriate if nausea and/or vomiting are a problem. If patches are used, they should be removed before going to bed at night. Generally clinicians are advised to use only 16-hour patches with pregnant women as then the onus is not on the woman to remember to remove the patch. If she forgets to take the 16-hour one off there is no further nicotine delivery.
- Breastfeeding – NRT can be used by women who are breastfeeding. The amount of nicotine the infant is exposed to from breast milk is relatively small and less hazardous than the second-hand smoke they would otherwise be exposed to if the mother continued to smoke. If possible, patches should be avoided. NRT products taken intermittently (oral forms) are preferred as their use can be adjusted to allow the maximum time between their administration and feeding of the baby, to minimise the amount of nicotine in the milk.
- Cardiovascular disease - dependent smokers with a myocardial infarction (MI), severe dysrhythmia or recent cerebrovascular accident (CVA) who are in hospital, should be encouraged to stop smoking with non-pharmacological interventions. If this fails NRT may be considered but as data on safety in these patient groups are limited, initiation of NRT should only be done under medical supervision. For patients with stable cardiovascular disease, NRT is a lesser risk than continuing to smoke.
- Diabetes – nicotine releases catecholamines, which can affect carbohydrate metabolism. Diabetic patients should be advised to monitor their blood sugar levels more closely than usual when starting NRT.
- Renal or hepatic impairment – NRT should be used with caution in patients with moderate to severe hepatic impairment and/or severe renal impairment, as the clearance of nicotine or its metabolites may be decreased, with the potential for increased adverse effects.
- Drug interactions with NRT – drug interactions may occur as a *result of quitting smoking* rather from NRT per se. The only interaction that is possibly directly attributable to NRT is with adenosine (adverse haemodynamic effects).

Preparations and dose
All NRTs should be used for about 8–12 weeks but may be continued beyond this time if needed to prevent relapse. They can also be used in combination if required, usually the patch plus a faster-acting oral NRT for relief of situational urges to smoke. Cochrane report an odds ratio of 1.42 for combination NRT versus patch alone for long-term abstinence[3].

- Sublingual tablet (2 mg): recommended dose of one tablet per hour or, for heavy smokers (smoking more than 20 cigarettes per day), two tablets per hour (maximum 40 x 2 mg daily).
- Gum (2 mg or 4 mg chewed slowly when urge to smoke occurs) up to maximum of 15 pieces daily. Gum needs to be rested against the gums or buccal mucosa for absorption to occur.

- Patch: two different types are available (24 hour or 16 hour). There is no difference in efficacy. Both types come in 3 strengths to allow gradual weaning. Recently a 25 mg 16 hour patch was introduced.
  - 16 hour patches deliver nicotine over a 16-hour period and are removed at bedtime (dose 25 mg, 15 mg, 10 mg, 5 mg)
  - 24 hour patches are worn throughout the night and taken off and replaced in the morning (21 mg, 14 mg, 7 mg).
- Nasal spray (each metered spray delivers 0.5 mg nicotine. A dose = 1 spray to each nostril, up to maximum of 2 doses per hour or 32 doses per day). Most suitable for highly dependent smokers.
- Inhalator (10 mg/cartridge) used with a plastic mouthpiece. Dose initially up to 12 cartridges per day – puffed for 20 min every hour.
- Lozenge (1 mg, 2 mg and 4 mg) up to maximum of 15 per day. Lozenges need to be rested against the gums or buccal mucosa to allow absorption of nicotine.

Side effects
Mainly mild local irritant effects such as skin irritation, stinging in the mouth/throat/nose depending on formulation. These usually disappear with continued use as tolerance develops rapidly.

Bupropion (amfebutamone)
Clinical effectiveness
Bupropion (Zyban) is an atypical antidepressant, with dopaminergic and noradrenergic actions, and has been advocated by NICE for smoking cessation. A systematic review of 19 randomised controlled trials of bupropion revealed a doubling of smoking cessation as compared to the placebo control. Trials show it significantly reduces the severity of nicotine withdrawal symptoms and urges to smoke and in some patients will make smoking less pleasurable and rewarding.

There is a risk of about 1 in 1000 of seizures associated with bupropion use and therefore this must be considered before initiation of treatment.

Bupropion is contra-indicated in patients with a history of seizures, eating disorders, a CNS tumour, bipolar disorder, pregnancy, breast feeding or those experiencing acute benzodiazepine or alcohol withdrawal. As many drugs reduce seizure threshold, including other antidepressants, a risk–benefit assessment must be made in such cases and if bupropion is prescribed it should be at half dose.

Side effects
Insomnia, dry mouth, headache (common ~30%). Seizure, hypersensitivity reaction or rash (rare ~0.1%).

Start 1–2 weeks before the planned 'quit date' at 150 mg daily for 6 days, then 150 mg twice daily for a maximum of 7–9 weeks. The dose will need to be reduced in the elderly or in those experiencing side effects. Not recommended for those < 18 years old.

Varenicline (Champix)
Varenicline tartrate was launched in the UK in December 2006. It has been recommended by NICE for use as part of a programme of behavioural support[4]. It is a partial agonist binding with high affinity to the $\alpha_4\beta_2$ nicotinic acetylcholine receptor. Two large-scale randomised placebo-controlled trials comparing it directly with bupropion suggest it is nearly 80% more effective[5,6]. It is also more effective than 24-hour NRT[7]. Like NRT and bupropion, varenicline significantly reduces nicotine

withdrawal symptoms, and there is also evidence it makes smoking less rewarding so may help prevent 'slips' develop into full relapse.

Dose
Days 1–3: 0.5 mg once daily, Days 4–7: 0.5 mg twice daily and Day 8–end of week 12, 1 mg twice daily. Smokers should set a 'quit date' between Days 8–14. For patients who have successfully stopped smoking at the end of 12 weeks, an additional course of 12 weeks treatment at 1 mg twice daily may be considered. The only contra-indication is hypersensitivity to the drug or excipients. There are no known drug interactions.

Warnings and precautions
Smoking cessation, with or without pharmacotherapy, has been associated with exacerbation of underlying psychiatric illness (e.g. depression). There is no clinical experience with varenicline in patients with epilepsy or psychiatric illness. It should not be used in the under 18s, pregnant or breastfeeding women, or in those with end-stage renal disease. Those with severe renal impairment may require a dosage reduction.

Side effects
The main side effect is nausea (30%). Depression and suicidality have also been reported[8] and care should be taken to monitor patients for any signs of agitation, mood changes, or suicidal thoughts[9].

Note: Stopping smoking may alter the pharmacokinetics or pharmacodynamics of other drugs, including several used in psychiatry, for which dosage adjustment may be necessary (examples include alprazolam, theophylline, chlorpromazine, diazepam, warfarin, insulin, clomipramine, clozapine, desipramine, doxepin, fluphenazine, haloperidol, imipramine and oxazepam). Stopping smoking is not thought to alter blood levels of chlordiazepoxide, ethanol, lorazepam, midazolam, or trizolam. It is unclear whether quitting affects blood levels of amitriptyline and nortriptyline[4]. Smoking cessation usually results in an increase in plasma levels of CYP1A2 substrates (smoking induces CYP1A2). See section on smoking (chapter 8).

Pregnancy and nicotine use
As stated earlier ideally women should stop smoking without using NRT but, if this is not possible, NRT may be recommended to assist a quit attempt. Please see above.

References
1. National Institute for Clinical Excellence. Brief interventions and referral for smoking cessation in primary care and other settings. Public Health Intervention Guidance No.1. http://www.nice.org.uk/. 2006.
2. National Institute for Clinical Excellence. The clinical effectiveness and cost effectiveness of bupropion (Zyban) and Nicotine Replacement Therapy for smoking cessation. Technical Appraisal 39. http://www.nice.org.uk. 2002.
3. Stead LF et al. Nicotine replacement therapy for smoking cessation. Cochrane Database Syst Rev 2008;CD000146.
4. Desai HD et al. Smoking in patients receiving psychotropic medications: a pharmacokinetic perspective. CNS Drugs 2001; 15:469–494.
5. Gonzales D et al. Varenicline, an alpha4beta2 nicotinic acetylcholine receptor partial agonist, vs sustained-release bupropion and placebo for smoking cessation: a randomized controlled trial. JAMA 2006; 296:47–55.
6. Jorenby DE et al. Efficacy of varenicline, an alpha4beta2 nicotinic acetylcholine receptor partial agonist, vs placebo or sustained-release bupropion for smoking cessation: a randomized controlled trial. JAMA 2006; 296:56–63.
7. Aubin HJ et al. Varenicline versus transdermal nicotine patch for smoking cessation: results from a randomised open-label trial. Thorax 2008; 63:717–724.
8. McIntyre RS. Varenicline and suicidality: a new era in medication safety surveillance. Expert Opin Drug Saf 2008; 7:511–514.
9. Medicines and Healthcare Products Regulatory Agency. Varenicline: adverse psychiatric reactions including depression. Drug Safety Update 2008; 2:2–3.

Pharmacological treatment of dependence on stimulant drugs

The most common drugs abused in this class are cocaine (exists as hydrochloride which is usually snorted, and as free base or 'crack' which is usually smoked) and amphetamines. There is no effective pharmacotherapy for the treatment of stimulant dependence. A wide variety of pharmacological agents have been assessed and found lacking[1]; although research is ongoing[2].

The recommended treatment for dependence on stimulants is psychosocial; in particular contingency management[3], although benefit has also been shown for cognitive behavioural and relapse prevention approaches[4].

Cocaine

Detoxification

There are no evidence-based pharmacological treatments for the management of cocaine withdrawal. Symptoms of withdrawal include depressed mood, agitation and insomnia[6]. These are usually self-limiting. It should be noted that given cocaine's short half-life and the binge nature of cocaine use, many patients detoxify themselves regularly, with no pharmacological therapy. Symptomatic relief such as the short-term use of hypnotics may be helpful in some but note that these agents may be diverted for illicit use or become agents of dependence themselves[5].

Substitution treatment

There is no evidence for substitution therapy for the treatment of cocaine misuse. This should not be prescribed[5].

Amphetamines

A wide variety of amphetamines are misused including "street" amphetamine and dexamphetamine. Any drug in this class is likely to have abuse potential. As with cocaine there is no evidence base for pharmacological treatment of withdrawal[5,7,8], although the number of agents that have been investigated is limited[7,8].

Detoxification

Treatment should focus on symptomatic relief, although many symptoms of amphetamine withdrawal (low mood, listlessness, fatigue, etc.) are short-lived and may not be amenable to pharmacological treatment. Insomnia can be treated with short courses of hypnotics.

Maintenance

Dexamphetamine maintenance should not be initiated. There is no good evidence for this practice[5]. There are, however, patients that have been prescribed dexamphetamine as a maintenance treatment for drug dependence for many years. Ideally it should be gradually detoxified over several months. For some the consequences of enforced detoxification may be worse than continuing to be prescribed dexamphetamine. A decision to continue prescribing dexamphetamine should only be made by an addiction specialist[5].

Polysubstance abuse

In those that are dependent on opiates and cocaine, the provision of effective substitution therapy with either methadone or buprenorphine can lead to a reduction in cocaine use[5].

References

1. de Lima MS et al. Pharmacological treatment of cocaine dependence: a systematic review. Addiction 2002; 97:931–949.
2. Sofuoglu M et al. Novel approaches to the treatment of cocaine addiction. CNS Drugs 2005; 19:13–25.
3. National Institute for Clinical Excellence. Drug misuse: psychosocial interventions. Clinical Guidance 51. 2007. http://www.nice.org.uk/.
4. Dutra L et al. A meta-analytic review of psychosocial interventions for substance use disorders. Am J Psychiatry 2008; 165:179–187.
5. Department of Health. Drug misuse and dependence. UK guidelines on clinical management. 2007.
6. Rounsaville BJ. Treatment of cocaine dependence and depression. Biol Psychiatry 2004; 56:803–809.
7. Shoptaw SJ et al. Treatment for amphetamine withdrawal. Cochrane Database Syst Rev 2009;CD003021.
8. Srisurapanont M et al. Treatment for amphetamine dependence and abuse. Cochrane Database Syst Rev 2001;CD003022.

Benzodiazepine use (see section in Chapter 4)

Benzodiazepine prescribing has increased since the 1970s, mainly because of the discontinuation of barbiturates and the perceived improved safety profile of benzodiazepines. However, benzodiazepines have a high potential for causing dependence. Prescriptions originally started for other disorders may have been continued long term and allowed to develop into dependence. A Cochrane review evaluated the evidence for pharmacological interventions for benzodiazepine mono-dependence. This concluded that a gradual reduction of benzodiazepines was preferable to an abrupt discontinuation[1] (see section on benzodiazepines in Chapter 4 for suggested regimens). A more recent review suggested that withdrawal over a period of less than 6 months is appropriate for most patients[2].

A large number of patients presenting to addictions services may be using illicit benzodiazepines on top of their primary substance of abuse. Although some services provide prescriptions of benzodiazepines, there is no evidence that substitute prescribing of benzodiazepines reduces benzodiazepine use. In exceptional circumstances, if benzodiazepines are prescribed, this should be for a short-term, time-limited (2–3 weeks) prescription.

If patients have been prescribed benzodiazepines for a substantial period of time, it may be preferable to convert to equivalents of diazepam as this is longer acting. Benzodiazepine dependence as part of polysubstance dependence should also be treated by a gradual withdrawal of the medication. Benzodiazepines prescribed at greater than 30 mg diazepam equivalent per day may cause harm[3] and so this should be avoided. Psychosocial interventions including contingency management have had some success at reducing benzodiazepine use.

Pregnancy and benzodiazepine use

There is a risk of teratogenicity with benzodiazepine use, so ideally benzodiazepine prescriptions should be gradually discontinued before a planned pregnancy. If a woman is prescribed benzodiazepines and found to be pregnant, the prescription should be gradually withdrawn over as short a time as possible. A risk–benefit analysis should be undertaken and specialist advice sought at the time but generally speaking, benzodiazepines should be avoided in pregnancy (see pregnancy section in Chapter 7).

References

1. Denis C et al. Pharmacological interventions for benzodiazepine mono-dependence management in outpatient settings. Cochrane Database Syst Rev 2006;CD005194.
2. Lader M et al. Withdrawing benzodiazepines in primary care. CNS Drugs 2009; 23:19–34.
3. Department of Health. Drug misuse and dependence: guidelines on clinical management. Norwich: Department of Health; 1999.

Substance misuse

Drugs of misuse – a summary

One in ten adults uses illicit drugs in any one year[1], and at least a third of those with mental illness can be classified as having a 'dual diagnosis'[2,3]. There is now compelling evidence that cannabis use increases the risk of psychosis or depression[4]. It is therefore important to be aware of the main mental state changes associated with drugs of abuse. Note also that substance misuse in fully compliant individuals increases relapse rate to the levels seen in non-compliant individuals with schizophrenia[5]. Urine-testing for illicit drugs is routine on many psychiatric wards. It is important to be aware of the duration of detection of drugs in urine and of other commonly used substances and drugs that can give a false-positive result. Some false positives are unexpected and so not readily predictable, for example quetiapine has given a false positive for methadone[6] and amisulpride for buprenorphine[7].

Table Drugs of misuse – a summary

Drug	Physical signs/symptoms of intoxication	Most common mental state changes[8]
Amfetamine[12]	Tachycardia; increased BP; anorexia; tremor; restlessness	Visual/tactile/olfactory auditory hallucinations; paranoia; decreased concentration; elation
Benzodiazepines	Sedation (possible); dizziness; respiratory depression	Relaxation; visual hallucinations; disorientation; sleep disturbance
Barbiturates	Headache; hypotension; respiratory depression	Restlessness/ataxia; confusion/excitement; drowsiness
Cannabis[13,9]	Tachycardia; lack of co-ordination; red eyes; postural hypotension	Elation; psychosis; perceptual distortions; disturbance of memory/judgement, twofold increase in risk of developing schizophrenia[14]
Cocaine	Tachycardia/tachypnoea; increased BP/headache; respiratory depression; chest pain	Euphoria; paranoid psychosis; panic attacks/anxiety; insomnia/excitement
Heroin	Pinpoint pupils; clammy skin; respiratory depression	Drowsiness; euphoria; hallucinations
Methadone	Respiratory depression; pulmonary oedema	As above

Withdrawal symptoms	Duration of withdrawal	Duration of detection in the urine[9,10,11]	Other substances which give a positive result[11]
Extreme fatigue; hunger depression	Peaks 7–34 hours; lasts maximum of 5 days	Up to 72 hours	Cough and decongestant preparations, selegiline, large quantities of tryramine, tranylcypromine, chloroquine, ranitidine
Seizures; psychosis; paraesthesia	Usually short-lived but may last weeks to months	Up to 28 days: depending on half-life of drug taken	Zopiclone Nefopam
Similar to alcohol: tremor, vomiting, seizures, delirium tremens	Depends on half-life – likely to be at least several days	Up to 21 days, depending on half-life	None known
Restlessness; irritability; insomnia; anxiety[10]	Uncertain Probably less than 1 month[9] (longer in heavy users[10])	Single use: 3 days; chronic heavy use: up to 21 days	Passive 'smoking' of cannabis Efavirenz
Profound lethargy; decreased consciousness	12–18 hours	Up to 96 hours	Food/tea containing coco leaves Codeine Ephedrine Pseudoephedrine
Nausea pains/gooseflesh; general aches and runny nose/eyes; diarrhoea	Peaks after 36–72 hours	Up to 72 hours	Food/tea containing poppy seed Procaine Any opiate analgesic Diphenoxylate, Naltrexone
As above but milder and longer lasting	Peaks after 4–6 days; can last 3 weeks	Up to 7 days with chronic use	Imipramine Pethidine Chlorpheniramine (high doses) Diphenydramine Cetirizine Doxylamine

References

1. Hoare J, Flately J. Drug Misuse Declared: Findings from the 2007/08 British Crime Survey. England and Wales. http://www.homeoffice.gov.uk/. 2008.
2. Menezes PR et al. Drug and alcohol problems among individuals with severe mental illness in south London. Br J Psychiatry 1996; 168:612–619.
3. Phillips P. et al. Drug and alcohol misuse among in-patients with psychotic illnesses in three inner-London psychiatric units. Psychiatr Bull 2003; 27:217–220.
4. Moore TH et al. Cannabis use and risk of psychotic or affective mental health outcomes: a systematic review. Lancet 2007; 370:319–328.
5. Hunt GE et al. Medication compliance and comorbid substance abuse in schizophrenia: impact on community survival 4 years after a relapse. Schizophr Res 2002; 54:253–264.
6. Widschwendter CG et al. Quetiapine cross reactivity with urine methadone immunoassays. Am J Psychiatry 2007; 164:172.
7. Couchman L et al. Amisulpride and sulpiride interfere in the CEDIA DAU buprenorphine test. Ann Clin Psychiatry 2008; 45 Suppl 1.
8. Micromedex® Healthcare Series. CD-ROM, version 5.1. http://www.micromedex.com. 2004
9. Johns A. Psychiatric effects of cannabis. Br J Psychiatry 2001; 178:116–122.
10. Budney AJ et al. Review of the validity and significance of cannabis withdrawal syndrome. Am J Psychiatry 2004; 161:1967–1977.
11. Euromed. Technical Bulletin – January 2006. www.euromedltd.com. 2006
12. Shoptaw SJ et al. Treatment for amphetamine psychosis. Cochrane Database Syst Rev 2009;CD003026.
13. Hall W et al. Long-term cannabis use and mental health. Br J Psychiatry 1997; 171:107–108.
14. Arseneault L et al. Causal association between cannabis and psychosis: examination of the evidence. Br J Psychiatry 2004; 184:110–117.

Substance
misuse

Interactions between 'street drugs' and prescribed psychotropic drugs

There are some significant interactions between 'street drugs' and drugs that are prescribed for the treatment of mental illness. Information comes from case reports or theoretical assumptions, rarely from systematic investigation. A summary can be found in the table below, but remember that the knowledge base is poor. Always be cautious.

In all patients who misuse street drugs:

- Infection with hepatitis B and C is common. This may lead to a reduced ability to metabolise other drugs and increased sensitivity to side effects.
- Infection with HIV is common[1,2]. Antiretroviral drugs are involved in pharmacokinetic interactions with a number of prescribed drugs; see HIV section for a summary. Interactions with street drugs are likely.
- Prescribed drugs may be used in the same way as illicit drugs (i.e. erratically and not as intended). Large quantities of prescribed drugs should not be given to outpatients.
- Additive or synergistic effects of respiratory depressants may play a contributory role in deaths from overdose with methadone or other opioid agonists[3]. Caution is needed in prescribing sedative medicines.

Acute behavioural disturbance

Acute intoxication with street drugs may result in behavioural disturbance. Non-drug management is preferable. If at all possible, a urine drug screen should be done to determine the drugs that have been taken, before prescribing any psychotropic. A physical examination should be done if possible (BP, TPR and ECG).

If intervention with a psychotropic is unavoidable, haloperidol 5 mg *or* olanzapine 10 mg po/IM is probably the safest option. Temperature, pulse, respiration and blood pressure *must* be monitored afterwards. Benzodiazepines are commonly misused with other street drugs and so standard doses may be ineffective in tolerant users. Interactions are also possible (see following table). Try to avoid.

References

1. Vocci FJ et al. Medication development for addictive disorders: the state of the science. Am J Psychiatry 2005; 162:1432–1440.
2. Tsuang J et al. Pharmacological treatment of patients with schizophrenia and substance abuse disorders. Addict Disord Treat 2005; 4:127–137.
3. National Institute for Clinical Excellence. Drug misuse: opioid detoxification. Clinical Guidance 52. 2007. Ref Type: Pamphlet.
4. Department of Health. Drug misuse and dependence. UK guidelines on clinical management. 2007.
5. Johns A. Psychiatric effects of cannabis. Br J Psychiatry 2001;178:116–122.
6. Ashton CH. Pharmacology and effects of cannabis: a brief review. Br J Psychiatry 2001; 178:101–106.
7. Miller BL, Mena I, Giombetti R, Villanueva-Meyer J, Djenderedjian AH. Neuropsychiatric Effects of Cocaine: SPECT Measurements. In: Paredes A, Gorelick DA, editors. Cocaine: Physiological and Physiopathological Effects. 1 ed. New York: Haworth Press; 1993. 47–58.
8. Gowing LR et al. The health effects of ecstasy: a literature review. Drug Alcohol Rev 2002; 21:53–63.
9. Zullino DF et al. Tobacco and cannabis smoking cessation can lead to intoxication with clozapine or olanzapine. Int Clin Psychopharmacol 2002; 17:141–143.
10. Green AI et al. Alcohol and cannabis use in schizophrenia: effects of clozapine vs. risperidone. Schizophr Res 2003; 60:81–85.
11. Wines JD, Jr. et al. Opioid withdrawal during risperidone treatment. J Clin Psychopharmacol 1999; 19:265–267.
12. Uehlinger C et al. Increased (R)-methadone plasma concentrations by quetiapine in cytochrome P450s and ABCB1 genotyped patients. J Clin Psychopharmacol 2007; 27:273–278.
13. Poling J et al. Risperidone for substance dependent psychotic patients. Addict Disord Treat 2005; 4:1–3.
14. Albanese MJ et al. Risperidone in cocaine-dependent patients with comorbid psychiatric disorders. J Psychiatry Pract 2006; 12:306–311.
15. Sattar SP et al. Potential benefits of quetiapine in the treatment of substance dependence disorders. J Psychiatry Neurosci 2004; 29:452–457.
16. Grabowski J et al. Risperidone for the treatment of cocaine dependence: randomized, double-blind trial. J Clin Psychopharmacol 2000; 20:305–310.
17. Kampman KM et al. A pilot trial of olanzapine for the treatment of cocaine dependence. Drug Alcohol Depend 2003; 70:265–273.
18. Farren CK et al. Significant interaction between clozapine and cocaine in cocaine addicts. Drug Alcohol Depend 2000; 59:153–163.
19. Benowitz NL et al. Effects of delta-9-tetrahydrocannabinol on drug distribution and metabolism. Antipyrine, pentobarbital, and ethanol. Clin Pharmacol Ther 1977; 22:259–268.
20. Hemeryck A et al. Selective serotonin reuptake inhibitors and cytochrome P-450 mediated drug–drug interactions: an update. Curr Drug Metab 2002; 3:13–37.
21. Bush E et al. A case of serotonin syndrome and mutism associated with methadone. J Palliat Med 2006; 9:1257–1259.
22. Lima MS et al. Antidepressants for cocaine dependence. Cochrane Database Syst Rev 2003;CD002950.
23. Fletcher PJ et al. Fluoxetine, but not sertraline or citalopram, potentiates the locomotor stimulant effect of cocaine: possible pharmacokinetic effects. Psychopharmacology (Berl) 2004; 174:406–413.
24. Silins E et al. Qualitative review of serotonin syndrome, ecstasy (MDMA) and the use of other serotonergic substances: hierarchy of risk. Aust N Z J Psychiatry 2007; 41:649–655.
25. Roldan, C.J. and Habal, R. Toxicity, cocaine. http://www.emedicine.com. 2004

Further reading

Cleary M et al. Psychosocial interventions for people with both severe mental illness and substance misuse. Cochrane Database Syst Rev 2008;CD001088.
Howard LA et al. The role of pharmacogenetically-variable cytochrome P450 enzyme in drug abuse and dependence. Pharmacogenomics 2002; 3:185–199.
Williams R et al. Substance use and misuse in psychiatric wards. Psychiatr Bull 2000; 24:43–46.

Substance misuse

Table Interactions between 'street drugs' and psychotropics (for references, see previous page)

	Cannabis	Heroin/methadone[4]	Cocaine, Amfetamines, Ecstasy	Alcohol
General considerations	• Usually smoked in cigarettes (induces CYP1A2) • Can be sedative[5] • Dose-related tachycardia[6]	• Can produce sedation/respiratory depression • QTc prolongation also reported with methadone (see section on methadone)	• Stimulants (cocaine can be sedative in higher doses) • Arrhythmia possible • Cerebral/cardiac ischaemia with cocaine[7] – may be fatal • Hyperthermia/dehydration with ecstasy[8]	• Sedative • Liver damage possible
Older antipsychotics	• Antipsychotics reduce the psychotropic effects of almost all drugs of abuse by blocking dopamine receptors (dopamine is the neurotransmitter responsible for 'reward') • Patients prescribed antipsychotics may increase their consumption of illicit substances to compensate • Patients who have taken ecstasy may be more prone to EPS • Cardiotoxic or very sedative antipsychotics are best avoided, at least initially. Sulpiride is a reasonably safe first choice			
Atypicals	• Risk of additive sedation • Cannabis can reduce serum levels of olanzapine and clozapine via induction of CYP1A2[9] • Clozapine might reduce cannabis and alcohol consumption[10]	• Risk of additive sedation • Case report of methadone withdrawal being precipitated by risperidone[11] • Isolated report of quetiapine increasing methadone levels, especially in those with slowed CYP2D6 hepatic metabolism[12]	• Antipsychotics may reduce craving and cocaine-induced euphoira[13–16] • Olanzapine may worsen cocaine dependency[17] • Clozapine may increase cocaine levels but diminish subjective response[18]	• Increased risk of hypotension with olanzapine (and possibly other α-blockers)

Table Interactions between 'street drugs' and psychotropics (for references, see previous page) (Cont.)

	Cannabis	Heroin/methadone[4]	Cocaine, Amfetamines, Ecstasy	Alcohol
Antidepressants	• Tachycardia has been reported (monitor pulse and take care with TCAs[19])	• Avoid very sedative antidepressants • Some SSRIs can increase methadone plasma levels[20] (citalopram is SSRI of choice) • Case report of serotonin syndrome occurring when sertraline prescribed with methadone for a palliative care patient[21]	• Avoid TCAs (arrhythmia) • MAOIs contra-indicated (hypertension) • SSRI antidepressants are generally ineffective at attenuating withdrawal effects from cocaine[22] • Risk of SSRIs increasing cocaine levels, especially fluoxetine[23] • Concomitant use of SSRIs, cocaine or other stimulants could precipitate a serotonin syndrome[24]	• Avoid very sedative antidepressants • Avoid antidepressants that are toxic in OD • Impaired psycho-motor skills (*not* SSRIs)
Anticholinergics	• Misuse is likely. Try to avoid if at all possible (by using an atypical if an antipsychotic is required) • Can cause hallucinations, elation and cognitive impairment			
Lithium	• Very toxic if taken erratically • Always consider the effects of dehydration (particularly problematic with alcohol or ecstasy)			
Carbamazepine/ valproate		• Carbamazepine (CBZ) decreases methadone levels[7] (danger if CBZ stopped suddenly) • Valproate seems less likely to interact	• Carbamazepine induces CYP3A4, which leads to increased formation of norcocaine (hepatotoxic and more cardiotoxic than cocaine)[25]	• Monitor LFTs
Benzodiazepines (Always remember that benzodiazepines are liable to misuse)	• Monitor level of sedation	• Oversedation (and respiratory depression possible • Concomitant use can lead to accidental overdose • Possible pharmacokinetic interaction (increased methadone levels)	• Oversedation (if high doses of cocaine have been taken) • Widely used after cocaine intoxication • Future misuse possible detoxification	• Oversedation (and respiratory depression) possible • Widely used in alcohol

chapter 7

Use of psychotropics in special patient groups

Depression and psychosis in epilepsy

The prevalence of clinical depression in people with epilepsy is reported to range from 9% to 22%[1,2] and depressive symptoms may occur in up to 60% of people with intractable epilepsy[3]. This association may be explained in part by serotonin; depletion increases the risk of both depression and epilepsy[4]. Suicide rates in epilepsy have been estimated to be 4–5 times that of the general population[1,2]. The prevalence of psychotic illness in people with epilepsy is at least 4%[4]. A diagnosis of temporal lobe epilepsy does not seem to confer additional risk[5].

Peri-ictal depression or psychosis (that is, symptoms temporally related to seizure activity) should initially be treated by optimising anticonvulsant therapy[6]. Interictal depression or psychosis (symptoms occurring independently of seizures) are likely to require treatment with antidepressants or antipsychotics[2,6].

Use of antidepressants and antipsychotics in epilepsy

The prevalence of active epilepsy in adults under the age of 65 is 0.6% and the annual incidence 0.03%[7]. It is notable that the incidence of unprovoked seizures in the placebo arms of randomised controlled trials of antidepressants and antipsychotics is approximately 15-fold higher, suggesting that both depression and psychosis are risk factors for seizures[8]. Reports of seizures associated with drug treatment should be interpreted within the context of this background risk and single case reports treated with caution. Note also that almost all antidepressants and antipsychotics have been associated with hyponatraemia (see section on hyponatraemia) and seizures may occur if this is severe[9]. The majority of antipsychotics and antidepressants can reduce the seizure threshold[1,2,10,11] and the risk is dose-related.

There are few systematic studies of antipsychotics or antidepressants in people with epilepsy. Data are mainly derived from animal studies, clinical trials, case reports, and spontaneous reporting to regulatory bodies. The table at the end of this section gives some general guidance. Treatment should be commenced at the lowest dose and this should be gradually increased until a therapeutic dose is achieved[2,11,12]. As a general rule, the more sedating a drug is, the more likely it is to induce seizures[11].

Electroconvulsive therapy (ECT) has anticonvulsive properties and is worth considering in the treatment of depression in patients with unstable epilepsy[1,2].

Depression and psychosis associated with anticonvulsant drugs

Anticonvulsant drugs have been associated with new-onset depression and psychosis[1]. If anticonvulsants have recently been changed, this should always be considered as a potential cause of a new/worsening depressive or psychotic illness. Lowering of folate levels by some anticonvulsants may also influence the expression of depression[1]. Folate levels should be checked and remedied where necessary.

Psychosis[13]

Summaries of Product Characteristics and/or case reports associate the following anticonvulsants with the onset of psychotic symptoms: carbamazepine, ethosuximide, gabapentin, lamotrigine[14], levetiracetam[15], piracetam, pregabalin[16], primidone, tiagabine, topiramate[17], valproate, vigabatrin, and zonisamide[18]. Some of these reports may relate to the process of 'forced normalisation' in which a diminished frequency of seizures allows psychotic symptoms to emerge.

Depression[13,19]

Summaries of Product Characteristics and case reports associate the following anticonvulsants with the onset of depressive symptoms: acetazolamide, barbiturates, carbamazepine, ethosuximide, gabapentin, phenytoin, piracetam, tiagabine, topiramate, and vigabatrin.

Interactions

Pharmacokinetic interactions between anticonvulsants and antidepressants/antipsychotics are common. These interactions are primarily mediated through cytochrome P450 enzymes[1,2]. Fluoxetine and paroxetine are potent inhibitors of several hepatic CYP enzyme systems (CYP2D6, CYP3A4). Sertraline is a less potent inhibitor, but this effect is dose-related and higher doses of sertraline are commonly used. Citalopram is a weak inhibitor. Carbamazepine and phenytoin have a narrow therapeutic index and plasma levels can be increased by enzyme inhibitors. This is particularly dangerous with phenytoin. Plasma levels should be monitored and dosage adjustment may be required.

Carbamazepine is an enzyme inducer (mainly CYP3A4) and can lower plasma levels of some antipsychotic drugs[20]. Many other medicines can cause problems in people with epilepsy by raising or reducing the seizure threshold or interacting with anticonvulsant drugs. Check Appendix 1 of the BNF or contact pharmacy for advice (see also table on anticonvulsant interactions).

Epilepsy and driving

People with epilepsy may not drive a car if they have had a seizure while awake in the previous year or, if seizures occur only during sleep, this has been an established nocturnal pattern for at least 3 years. The consequences of inducing seizures with antidepressants or antipsychotics can therefore be significant. For further information see www.dvla.gov.uk.

Table Psychotropics in epilepsy*

Antidepressant	Safety in epilepsy	Special considerations
Moclobemide[21]	Good choice	Not known to be pro-convulsive
SSRIs[22]	Good choice	May be anticonvulsant at therapeutic doses[8]; no clear difference between drugs[7]
Mirtazapine[23]/ reboxetine/venlafaxine[24,25]	Care required	Less data and clinical experience than with SSRIs. Venlafaxine pro-convulsive in OD. Use with care
Duloxetine[9,13]	Care required	Very limited data and clinical experience. Seizures have been reported rarely
Amitriptyline Dosulepin (dothiepin)[26] Clomipramine[27] Bupropion[8]	Avoid	Most TCAs are epileptogenic. Ideally, should be avoided completely
Lithium[2]	Care required	Low pro-convulsive effect at therapeutic doses. Marked pro-convulsive activity in overdose
Antipsychotic		
Trifluoperazine/ haloperidol[2,11,28,29]	Good choice	Low pro-convulsive effect. Carbamazepine increases the metabolism of some antipsychotics and larger doses of an antipsychotic may be required
Sulpiride[30]	Good choice	Low pro-convulsive effect (less clinical experience). No known interactions with anticonvulsants
Risperidone[8] Olanzapine[8] Quetiapine[8] Amisulpride[31,32]	Care required	Relatively limited clinical experience but probably safe. Olanzapine may affect EEG[33] and myoclonic seizures have been reported[34]. Seizures rarely reported with quetiapine[35] but also shown to have anticonvulsant activity in ECT[30]
Aripiprazole	Care required	Very limited data and clinical experience. Seizures have been reported rarely[36]
Clozapine[6,10,37]	Avoid if possible	Very epileptogenic. Approximately 5% who receive more than 600 mg/day develop seizures. Sodium valproate is the anticonvulsant of choice as it has a lower incidence of leucopoenia than carbamazepine
Chlorpromazine[6] Loxapine	Avoid	Most epileptogenic of the older drugs. Ideally best avoided completely
Zotepine	Avoid	Has established dose-related pro-convulsive effect. Best avoided completely
Depot antipsychotics	Avoid	None of the depot preparations currently available are thought to be epileptogenic, however: • the kinetics of depots are complex (seizures may be delayed) • if seizures do occur, the offending drug may not be easily withdrawn. Depots should be used with extreme care

*This table contains information about the pro-convulsive effects of antidepressants and antipsychotics when used in therapeutic doses. See section on psychotropics in overdose for information about supra-therapeutic doses.

Special groups

References

1. Harden CL et al. Mood disorders in patients with epilepsy: epidemiology and management. CNS Drugs 2002; 16:291–302.
2. Curran S et al. Selecting an antidepressant for use in a patient with epilepsy. Safety considerations. Drug Saf 1998; 18:125–133.
3. Lambert MV et al. Depression in epilepsy: etiology, phenomenology, and treatment. Epilepsia 1999; 40 Suppl 10:S21–S47.
4. Bagdy G et al. Serotonin and epilepsy. J Neurochem 2007; 100:857–873.
5. Adams SJ et al. Neuropsychiatric morbidity in focal epilepsy. Br J Psychiatry 2008; 192:464–469.
6. Blumer D et al. Treatment of the interictal psychoses. J Clin Psychiatry 2000; 61:110–122.
7. Montgomery SA. Antidepressants and seizures: emphasis on newer agents and clinical implications. Int J Clin Pract 2005; 59:1435–1440.
8. Alper K et al. Seizure incidence in psychopharmacological clinical trials: an analysis of Food and Drug Administration (FDA) summary basis of approval reports. Biol Psychiatry 2007; 62:345–354.
9. Maramattom BV. Duloxetine-induced syndrome of inappropriate antidiuretic hormone secretion and seizures. Neurology 2006; 66:773–774.
10. Pisani F et al. Effects of psychotropic drugs on seizure threshold. Drug Saf 2002; 25:91–110.
11. Marks RC et al. Antipsychotic medications and seizures. Psychiatr Med 1991; 9:37–52.
12. Rosenstein DL et al. Seizures associated with antidepressants: a review. J Clin Psychiatry 1993; 54:289–299.
13. Datapharm Communications Ltd. Electronic Medicines Compendium. http://medguidesmedicines org uk/; 2006
14. Brandt C et al. Development of psychosis in patients with epilepsy treated with lamotrigine: report of six cases and review of the literature. Epilepsy Behav 2007; 11:133–139.
15. Youroukos S et al. Acute psychosis associated with levetiracetam. Epileptic Disord 2003; 5:117–119.
16. Olaizola I et al. Pregabalin-associated acute psychosis and epileptiform EEG-changes. Seizure 2006; 15:208–210.
17. Karslioaylu EH et al. Topiramate-induced psychotic exacerbation: case report and review of literature. Int J Psychiatry Clin Pract 2007; 11:285–290.
18. Michael CT et al. Psychosis following initiation of zonisamide. Am J Psychiatry 2007; 164:682.
19. Besag FM. Behavioural effects of the newer antiepileptic drugs: an update. Expert Opin Drug Saf 2004; 3:1–8.
20. Tiihonen J et al. Carbamazepine-induced changes in plasma levels of neuroleptics. Pharmacopsychiatry 1995; 28:26–28.
21. Schiwy W et al. Therapeutic and side-effect profile of a selective and reversible MAO-A inhibitor, brofaromine. Results of dose-finding trials in depressed patients. J Neural Transm Suppl 1989; 28:33–44.
22. Wedin GP et al. Relative toxicity of cyclic antidepressants. Ann Emerg Med 1986; 15:797–804.
23. Zia Ul HM et al. Mirtazapine precipitated seizures: a case report. Prog Neuropsychopharmacol Biol Psychiatry 2008; 32:1076–1078.
24. Juckel G et al. Epileptiform EEG patterns induced by mirtazapine in both psychiatric patients and healthy volunteers. J Clin Psychopharmacol 2003; 23:421–422.
25. Alldredge BK. Seizure risk associated with psychotropic drugs: clinical and pharmacokinetic considerations. Neurology 1999; 53:S68–S75.
26. Buckley NA et al. Greater toxicity in overdose of dothiepin than of other tricyclic antidepressants. Lancet 1994; 343:159–162.
27. Stimmel GL et al. Psychotrophic drug-induced reductions in seizure threshold: incidence and consequences. CNS Drugs 1996; 5:3750.
28. Markowitz JC et al. Seizures with neuroleptics and antidepressants. Gen Hosp Psychiatry 1987; 9:135–141.
29. Darby JK et al. Haloperidol dose and blood level variability: toxicity and interindividual and intraindividual variability in the nonresponder patient in the clinical practice setting. J Clin Psychopharmacol 1995; 15:334–340.
30. Gazdag G et al. The impact of neuroleptic medication on seizure threshold and duration in electroconvulsive therapy. Ideggyogy Sz 2004; 57:385–390.
31. Patat A et al. Effects of 50mg amisulpride on EEG, psychomotor and cognitive functions in healthy sleep-deprived subjects. Fundam Clin Pharmacol 1999; 13:582–594.
32. Tracqui A et al. Amisulpride poisoning: a report on two cases. Hum Exp Toxicol 1995; 14:294–298.
33. Amann BL et al. EEG abnormalities associated with antipsychotics: a comparison of quetiapine, olanzapine, haloperidol and healthy subjects. Hum Psychopharmacol 2003; 18:641–646.
34. Camacho A et al. Olanzapine-induced myoclonic status. Clin Neuropharmacol 2005; 28:145–147.
35. Dogu O et al. Seizures associated with quetiapine treatment. Ann Pharmacother 2003; 37:1224–1227.
36. Tsai JF. Aripiprazole-associated seizure. J Clin Psychiatry 2006; 67:995–996.
37. Toth P et al. Clozapine and seizures: a review. Can J Psychiatry 1994; 39:236–238.

Further reading

Centorrino F et al. EEG abnormalities during treatment with typical and atypical antipsychotics. Am J Psychiatry 2002; 159:109–115.

Farooq S. Interventions for psychotic symptoms concomitant with epilepsy. Cochrane Database Syst Rev 2008;CD006118.

Schmitz B. Antidepressant drugs: indications and guidelines for use in epilepsy. Epilepsia 2002; 43(Suppl. 2):14–18.

Van der Feltz-Cornelis CM. Treatment of interictal psychiatric disorder in epilepsy. I. Affective and anxiety disorders. Acta Neuropsychiatr 2002; 14:39–43.

Van der Feltz-Cornelis CM. Treatment of interictal psychiatric disorder in epilepsy. II. Chronic psychosis. Acta Neuropsychiatr 2002; 14:44–48.

Van der Feltz-Cornelis CM. Treatment of interictal psychiatric disorder in epilepsy. III. Personality disorder, aggression and mental retardation. Acta Neuropsychiatr 2002; 14:49–54.

Special groups

Pharmacokinetic drug interactions between antiepileptic drugs and other psychotropic drugs[1-4]

Antiepileptic drug	Increases level of	Decreases level of	Level increased by	Level decreased by
Carbamazepine	Phenytoin	Clobazam Clonazepam Ethosuximide Lamotrigine Midazolam Phenytoin Primidone Tiagabine Topiramate Valproic acid Zonisamide Aripiprazole Chlorpromazine Clozapine Fluphenazine Haloperidol Olanzapine Quetiapine Risperidone Sertindole Zotepine Citalopram Mianserin Mirtazepine Paroxetine ?Sertraline TCAs Trazodone Benzodiazepines Bupropion Donepezil Methadone Methylphenidate Modafinil Thyroxine	Valproic acid and primidone increase levels of 10, 11-epoxide (metabolite of carbamazepine) Clobazam Lamotrigine Oxcarbazepine Fluoxetine Fluvoxamine Sertraline Trazodone	Oxcarbazepine Phenobarbitone Phenytoin Primidone St John's Wort Valproate

Table Pharmacokinetic drug interactions between antiepileptic drugs and other psychotropic drugs (Cont.)

Antiepileptic drug	Increases level of	Decreases level of	Level increased by	Level decreased by
Phenytoin	Carbamazepine Phenobarbital Valproate	Carbamazepine Ethosuximide Lamotrigine Phenobarbitone Primidone Tiagabine Topiramate Valproate Zonisamide Clonazepam Oxazepam Aripiprazole Clozapine Haloperidol Quetiapine Phenothiazines Risperidone Sertindole Mianserin Mirtazapine Paroxetine TCAs Benzodiazepines Bupropion Donepezil Methadone Thyroxine	Carbamazepine Ethosuximide Oxcarbazepine Phenobarbitone Primidone Topiramate Valproate Phenothiazines ?Zotepine Fluoxetine Fluvoxamine Paroxetine Sertraline TCAs Trazodone Clobazam Clonazepam Chlordiazepoxide Diazepam Disulfiram Modafanil Thyroxine	Carbamazepine Clonazepam Diazepam Phenobarbitone Primidone Valproate Vigabatrin Alcohol (chronic) Phenothiazines St John's Wort
Lamotrigine	Oxcarbazepine Risperidone	None known	Sertraline Valproate	Carbamazepine Oxcarbazepine Phenobarbitone Phenytoin Primidone
Valproate	Clozapine Ethosuximide Free phenytoin Lamotrigine Oxcarbazepine Phenobarbitone Primidone Benzodiazepines Bupropion TCAs	Topiramate 10-monohydroxy metabolite of oxcarbazepine Total phenytoin	Risperidone	Carbamazepine Phenobarbitone Phenytoin Primidone Topiramate ?Fluoxetine
Gabapentin	None known	None known	None known	None known
Levetiracetam	None known	None known	None known	None known

Table Pharmacokinetic drug interactions between antiepileptic drugs and other psychotropic drugs (Cont.)

Antiepileptic drug	Increases level of	Decreases level of	Level increased by	Level decreased by
Vigabatrin	Carbamazepine	?Phenobarbitone Phenytoin Primidone	None known	None known
Oxcarbazepine	10,11-epoxide, metabolite of carbamazepine Phenobarbitone Phenytoin	Carbamazepine Lamotrigine	None known	Carbamazepine Phenobarbitone Phenytoin Valproate
Phenobarbital	Phenytoin	Carbamazepine Clonazepam Ethosuximide Lamotrigine Oxcarbazepine Phenytoin Tiagabine Topiramate Valproate Zotepine Aripiprazole ?Chlorpromazine Clozapine Haloperidol Promethazine Quetiapine Mianserin TCAs Paroxetine Bupropion Modafinil Thyroxine Zonisamide	Carbamazepine Oxcarbazepine Phenytoin Valproate Alcohol (acute) Methylphenidate	Vigabatrin Alcohol (chronic) St John's Wort
Tiagabine	None known	Valproate	None known	Carbamazepine Phenobarbitone Phenytoin Primidone
Topiramate	Phenytoin	?Valproate	None known	Carbamazepine Phenobarbitone Phenytoin Valproate
Ethosuximide	?Phenytoin	None known	Valproate	Carbamazepine Phenobarbitone Phenytoin Primidone

References

1. British Medical Association and Royal Pharmaceutical Society of Great Britain. British National Formulary (57th edition). London: BMJ Group and RPS Publishing; 2009.
2. Stockley's Drug Interactions. London: The Pharmaceutical Press; 2008.
3. Patsalos PN et al. The importance of drug interactions in epilepsy therapy. Epilepsia 2002; 43:365–385.
4. Schmitz B. Antidepressant drugs: indications and guidelines for use in epilepsy. Epilepsia 2002; 43 Suppl 2:14–18.

Special groups

Withdrawing anticonvulsant drugs

Patients with epilepsy

Optimal treatment with anticonvulsant drugs will render seizure-free two-thirds of people with epilepsy[1,2]. Many patients ask about drug withdrawal. It should be noted that this is a specialist area of practice and it is strongly recommended that patients are referred for a neurological opinion.

The withdrawal of anticonvulsants in people with epilepsy has been associated with relapse rates of between 12 and 63%[2]. This wide variation probably reflects the heterogeneous nature of the patients studied. It should be noted that patients who remain on anticonvulsant drugs also relapse[3].

The following factors are associated with unsuccessful withdrawal[2,4,5].

Onset of epilepsy during or after adolescence

Family history of epilepsy

Epilepsy of proven or suspected organic origin

Mental retardation

Abnormal neurological examination

Poor initial response to treatment

Ongoing seizures during treatment

Prescription of two or more anticonvulsant drugs

Ongoing abnormal EEG

Abnormal EEG developing during withdrawal period

The dose of anticonvulsant drugs should be gradually tapered over a period of 6 months. If the patient is taking more than one anticonvulsant (note that such a patient is at increased risk of relapse), each drug should be withdrawn sequentially. The risk of seizure recurrence is greatest during the period of anticonvulsant withdrawal and steadily decreases over the first year; 70–80% of relapses occur within a year[3]. For those patients who discontinue their anticonvulsant medication because they are seizure free and whose seizures later return, approximately 1 in 4 may continue to have seizures after anticonvulsants are reinstated[6].

Recommendation

Patients with epilepsy should be referred to a neurologist for advice about withdrawing anticonvulsant drugs.

Patients with affective disorders

There is little research that addresses the risk of relapse in patients who take anticonvulsant drugs for their mood-stabilising properties. There are three possibilities:

1. **The natural course of the illness is improved by a period of treatment with mood-stabilising drugs.** There is no evidence to suggest that this is true. Patients with bipolar illness tend to have more episodes and shorter periods of stability as they get older.

2. **The illness resumes its natural course.** It then follows that the more effective the mood-stabilising medication has been, the greater the chance of relapse when it is stopped.

3. **Prognosis may be worsened in some way that is poorly understood.** This has been demonstrated for lithium (see section on lithium). Treatment with lithium for at least 3 years followed by gradual taper over at least 1 month minimises this risk. One naturalistic retrospective study suggested that the relapse rate in the first 3 months after anticonvulsants have been discontinued may be as high as 80%[7]; an important caveat is that it is not known whether relapse was a cause or consequence of medication discontinuation. There is some evidence to suggest that the risk of completed suicide is high in the month after (presumably abrupt) discontinuation of either lithium or valproate[8].

Recommendation

When used as mood-stabilisers, it would be prudent to withdraw anticonvulsant drugs slowly. The optimum duration of taper is unknown. A period of at least 1 month is suggested.

References

1. Cockerell OC et al. Remission of epilepsy: results from the National General Practice Study of Epilepsy. Lancet 1995; 346:140–144.
2. Cockerell OC et al. Prognosis of epilepsy: a review and further analysis of the first nine years of the British National General Practice Study of Epilepsy, a prospective population-based study. Epilepsia 1997; 38:31–46.
3. Britton JW. Antiepileptic drug withdrawal: literature review. Mayo Clin Proc 2002; 77:1378–1388.
4. Medical Research Council Antiepileptic Drug Withdrawal Study Group. Randomised study of antiepileptic drug withdrawal in patients in remission. Lancet 1991; 337:1175–1180.
5. Schmidt D et al. A practical guide to when (and how) to withdraw antiepileptic drugs in seizure-free patients. Drugs 1996; 52:870–874.
6. Sillanpaa M et al. Prognosis of seizure recurrence after stopping antiepileptic drugs in seizure-free patients: A long-term population-based study of childhood-onset epilepsy. Epilepsy Behav 2006; 8:713–719.
7. Franks MA et al. Bouncing back: is the bipolar rebound phenomenon peculiar to lithium? A retrospective naturalistic study. J Psychopharmacol 2008; 22:452–456.
8. Goodwin FK et al. Suicide risk in bipolar disorder during treatment with lithium and divalproex. JAMA 2003; 290:1467–1473.

Special groups

Drug choice in pregnancy

A 'normal' outcome to pregnancy can never be guaranteed. The spontaneous abortion rate in confirmed early pregnancy is 10–20% and the risk of spontaneous major malformation is 2–3% (approximately 1 in 40 pregnancies)[1].

Lifestyle factors have an important influence on pregnancy outcome. It is well established that smoking cigarettes, eating a poor diet and drinking alcohol during pregnancy can have adverse consequences for the foetus. More recent data suggest that moderate maternal caffeine consumption is associated with low birth weight[2], and that pre-pregnancy obesity increases the risk of neural tube defects (obese women seem to require higher doses of folate supplementation than women who have a BMI in the healthy range[3]).

In addition, psychiatric illness during pregnancy is an independent risk factor for congenital malformations and perinatal mortality[4]. Affective illness increases the risk of pre-term delivery[5].

Drugs account for a very small proportion of abnormalities (approximately 5% of the total). Potential risks of drugs include major malformation (first-trimester exposure), neonatal toxicity (third-trimester exposure), and long-term neurobehavioural effects.

The safety of psychotropics in pregnancy cannot be clearly established because robust, prospective trials are obviously unethical. Individual decisions on psychotropic use in pregnancy are therefore based, at best on database studies that have many limitations including failure to control for the effects of illness and other medication, prospective data from teratology information centres and published case reports which are known to be biased towards adverse outcomes. At worst there may be no human data at all, only animal data from early preclinical studies. With new drugs early reports of adverse outcomes may or may not be replicated and a 'best guess' assessment must be made of the risks and benefits associated with withdrawal or continuation of drug treatment. Pregnancy does not protect against mental illness and may even elevate overall risk. The patient's view of risks and benefits will have paramount importance. This section provides a brief summary of the relevant issues and evidence to date.

General principles of prescribing in pregnancy

In all women of child bearing potential
- Always discuss the possibility of pregnancy – many pregnancies are unplanned
- Try to avoid using drugs that are contra-indicated during pregnancy in women of reproductive age (especially valproate and carbamazepine). If these drugs are prescribed, women should be made fully aware of their teratogenic properties even if not planning pregnancy. Consider prescribing folate

If mental illness is newly diagnosed in a pregnant woman
- Try to avoid all drugs in the first trimester (when major organs are being formed) unless benefits outweigh risks
- If non-drug treatments are not effective/appropriate, use an established drug at the lowest effective dose

If a woman taking psychotropic drugs is planning a pregnancy
- Consideration should be given to discontinuing treatment if the woman is well and at low risk of relapse
- Discontinuation of treatment for women with SMI and at high risk of relapse is unwise, but consideration should be given to switching to a low-risk drug. Be aware that switching drugs may increase the risk of relapse

If a woman taking psychotropic medication discovers that she is pregnant
- Abrupt discontinuation of treatment post-conception for women with SMI and at a high risk of relapse is unwise; relapse may ultimately be more harmful to the mother and child than continued, effective drug therapy
- Consider remaining with current (effective) medication rather than switching, to minimise the number of drugs to which the foetus is exposed

If the patient smokes (smoking is more common in pregnant women with psychiatric illness)[6]
- Always encourage switching to nicotine replacement therapy – smoking has numerous adverse outcomes, NRT does not[7]

In all pregnant women
- Ensure that the prospective parents are as involved as possible in all decisions
- Use the lowest effective dose
- Use the drug with the lowest risk to mother and foetus
- Prescribe as few drugs as possible both simultaneously and in sequence
- Be prepared to adjust doses as pregnancy progresses and drug handling is altered. Dose increases are frequently required in the third trimester[8] when blood volume expands by around 30%. Plasma level monitoring is helpful, where available. Note that hepatic enzyme activity changes markedly during pregnancy; CYP2D6 activity is increased by almost 50% by the end of pregnancy while the activity of CYP1A2 is reduced by up to 70%[9]
- Consider referral to specialist perinatal services
- Ensure adequate foetal screening
- Be aware of potential problems with individual drugs around the time of delivery
- Inform the obstetric team of psychotropic use and possible complications
- Monitor the neonate for withdrawal effects after birth
- Document all decisions

What to include in discussions with pregnant women[10]

Discussions should include:

- the risk of relapse or deterioration in symptoms and the woman's ability to cope with untreated or sub-threshold symptoms
- severity of previous episodes, response to treatment, and the woman's preference
- the possibility that stopping a drug with known teratogenic risk after pregnancy is confirmed may not remove the risk of malformations
- the risks from stopping medication abruptly
- the need for prompt treatment because of the potential impact of an untreated mental disorder on the foetus or infant
- the increased risk of harm associated with drug treatments during pregnancy and the postnatal period, including the risk in overdose (and acknowledge uncertainty surrounding risks)
- the background risk of foetal malformations for pregnant women without a mental disorder.

Where possible, written material should be provided to explain the risks (preferably individualised). Absolute and relative risks should be discussed. Risks should be described using natural frequencies rather than percentages (for example, 1 in 10 rather than 10%) and common denominators (for example, 1 in 100 and 25 in 100, rather than 1 in 100 and 1 in 4).

Psychosis during pregnancy and postpartum

- Pregnancy does not protect against relapse.
- Psychiatric illness during pregnancy predicts post-partum psychosis[11].
- The risk of perinatal psychosis is 0.1–0.25% in the general population, but is about 50% in women with a history of bipolar disorder.
- During the month after childbirth there is a 20-fold increase (to 30–50%) in the relative risk of psychosis.
- The risk of recurrent post-partum psychosis is 50–90%.
- The mental health of the mother in the perinatal period influences foetal well-being, obstetric outcome and child development.

The risks of not treating psychosis include:

- harm to the mother through poor self-care or judgement, lack of obstetric care or impulsive acts
- harm to the foetus or neonate (ranging from neglect to infanticide)[12].

It has long been established that people with schizophrenia are more likely to have minor physical anomalies than the general population[13]. Some of these anomalies may be apparent at birth[4], while others are more subtle and may not be obvious until later in life. This background risk complicates assessment of the effects of antipsychotic drugs[14]. (Psychiatric illness itself during pregnancy is an independent risk factor for congenital malformations and perinatal mortality[4].)

Treatment with antipsychotics

Older, **first-generation antipsychotics** are generally considered to have minimal risk of teratogenicity[15,16], although data are less than convincing, as might be expected.

- Most data originate from studies that included primarily women with hyperemesis gravidarum (a condition associated with an increased risk of congenital malformations) treated with low doses of phenothiazines[14]. The modest increase in risk identified in some of these studies, along with no clear clustering of congenital abnormalities suggest that the condition being treated may be responsible rather than drug treatment[17].

- There may be an association between haloperidol and limb defects, but if real, the risk is likely to be extremely low[14,16].
- Neonatal dyskinesia has been reported with FGAs[18].
- Neonatal jaundice has been reported with phenothiazines[14].

It remains uncertain whether FGAs are entirely without risk to the foetus or to later development[19]. However, this continued uncertainty and the wide use of these drugs over several decades suggest that any risk is small – an assumption borne out by most studies[15].

Data relating to **second-generation antipsychotics** are growing.

- The extent of placental passage is highest for olanzapine followed by risperidone followed by quetiapine[20].
- There are most data for olanzapine which has been associated with both lower birth weight and increased risk of intensive care admission[17], and with macrosomia[21]; the last of these is consistent with the reported increase in the risk of gestational diabetes[14,22,23]. Although olanzapine seems to be relatively safe with respect to congenital malformations, it has been associated with a range of problems including hip dysplasia[24], meningocele, ankyloblepharon[25], and neural tube defects[14] (an effect that could be related to pre-pregnancy obesity rather than drug exposure[2]). Importantly there is no clustering of congenital malformations.
- Limited data suggest that neither risperidone[14,23,26–28], nor quetiapine[23] are major teratogens in humans. There are virtually no published data relating to other SGAs[14].
- The use of clozapine appears to present no increased risk of malformation, although gestational diabetes and neonatal seizures may be more likely to occur[22]. There is a single case report of maternal overdose resulting in foetal death[14] and there are theoretical concerns about the risk of agranulocytosis in the foetus/neonate[14]. NICE recommends that pregnant women should be switched from clozapine to another antipsychotic[10]. However, for almost all women on clozapine, a switch to a different antipsychotic will result in relapse. On the balance of the available evidence, clozapine should usually be continued.

Overall, these data do not allow an assessment of relative risks associated with different agents and certainly do not confirm absolutely the safety of any particular drug. At least one study has suggested a small increased risk of malformation and caesarean section in people receiving antipsychotics[17]. Older drugs may still be preferred in pregnancy, but, considering data available on some newer drugs, it may not now be appropriate always to switch to these first-generation drugs, should continued treatment be necessary. As with other drugs, decisions must be based on the latest available information and an individualised assessment of probable risks and benefits. If possible, specialist advice should be sought, and primary reference sources consulted.

Recommendations – psychosis in pregnancy
• Patients with a history of psychosis who are maintained on antipsychotic medication should be advised to discuss a planned pregnancy as early as possible • Be aware that drug-induced hyperprolactinaemia may prevent pregnancy. Consider switching to alternative drug • Such patients, particularly if they have suffered repeated relapses, are best maintained on antipsychotics during and after pregnancy. This may minimise foetal exposure by avoiding the need for higher doses, and/or multiple drugs should relapse occur • There is most experience with **chlorpromazine** (constipation and sedation can be a problem), **trifluoperazine, haloperidol, olanzapine** and **clozapine** (gestational diabetes may be a problem with both SGAs). If the patient is established on another antipsychotic, the most up-to-date advice should always be obtained. Experience with other drugs is growing and a change in treatment may not be necessary or wise • NICE recommends avoiding depot preparations and anticholinergic drugs in pregnancy • A few authorities recommend discontinuation of antipsychotics 5–10 days before anticipated delivery to minimise the chances of neonatal effects. This may, however, put mother and infant at risk and needs to be considered carefully. Antipsychotic discontinuation symptoms can occur in the neonate (e.g. crying, agitation, increased suckling). Some centres used mixed (breast/bottle) feeding to minimise withdrawal. With SGAs, discontinuation may not be necessary or desirable.

Depression during pregnancy and postpartum[29,30]

- Approximately 10% of pregnant women develop a depressive illness and a further 16% a self-limiting depressive reaction. Much post-partum depression begins before birth.
- There is a significant increase in new psychiatric episodes in the first 3 months after delivery. At least 80% are mood disorders, primarily depression.
- Women who have had a previous episode of depressive illness (postpartum or not) are at higher risk of further episodes during pregnancy and post-partum. The risk is highest in women with bipolar illness.
- Affective illness may increase the risk of pre-term delivery[5] (some evidence to the contrary[31]).
- The mental health of the mother influences foetal well-being, obstetric outcome, and child development.

The risks of not treating depression include:

- harm to the mother through poor self-care, lack of obstetric care or self-harm
- harm to the foetus or neonate (ranging from neglect to infanticide).

Treatment with antidepressants

The use of antidepressants during pregnancy is common; in the Netherlands, up to 2% of women are prescribed antidepressants during the first trimester[32], and in the US up to 8% of women are prescribed antidepressants at some point during their pregnancy[33]. The majority of prescriptions are for SSRIs. **Relapse rates are high** in those with a history of depression who discontinue medication. One study found that 68% of women who were well on antidepressant treatment and stopped during pregnancy relapsed, compared with 26% who continued antide-pressants[30]. There are conflicting data on the issue of the influence of duration of antidepressant use[34,35].

Tricyclic antidepressants

- Foetal exposure to tricyclics (via umbilicus and amniotic fluid) is high[36,37].
- TCAs have been widely used throughout pregnancy without apparent detriment to the foetus[38,39] and have for many years been agents of choice in pregnancy.
- Limited data suggests in utero exposure to tricyclics has no effects on later development[40,41].
- Some authorities recommend the use of nortriptyline and desipramine (not available in the UK) because these drugs are less anticholinergic and hypotensive than amitriptyline and imipramine (respectively, their tertiary amine parent molecules).
- TCA use during pregnancy increases the risk of pre-term delivery[38,39,42].
- Use of TCAs in the third trimester is well known to produce neonatal withdrawal effects; agitation, irritability, seizures, respiratory distress and endocrine and metabolic disturbances[38]. These are usually mild and self-limiting.
- Little is known of the developmental effects of prenatal exposure to tricyclics, although one small study detected no adverse consequences[40].

SSRIs

- Sertraline appears to result in the least placental exposure[43].
- SSRIs appear not to be major teratogens[35,38], with most data supporting the safety of fluoxetine[40,44–47]. Note however that one study revealed a slight overall increase in rate of malformation with SSRIs[48]. Database and case-control studies have reported an association between SSRIs and anencephaly, craniosynostosis, omphalocele, and persistent pulmonary hypertension of the newborn[49,50]. These associations have not been replicated.
- Paroxetine has been specifically associated with cardiac malformations[51] particularly after high-dose (>25 mg/day), first trimester exposure[52]. However some studies have failed to replicate this finding for paroxetine[38,53], and have implicated other SSRIs[54,55]. Other studies have found no association between any SSRI and an increased risk of cardiac septal defects[50].
- SSRIs have also been associated with decreased gestational age (mean 1 week), spontaneous abortion[56] and decreased birth weight (mean 175 g)[44,45,57]. The longer the duration of in-utero exposure, the greater the chance of low birth weight and respiratory distress[34]; SSRIs may therefore compound the effects of depression with regard to pre-term birth[58].
- Three groups of symptoms are seen in neonates exposed to antidepressants in late pregnancy; those associated with serotonergic toxicity, those associated with antidepressant discontinuation symptoms and those related to early birth[59]. Third-trimester exposure to sertraline has been associated with reduced early APGAR scores[44]. Third-trimester use of paroxetine may give rise to neonatal complications, presumably related to abrupt withdrawal[60,61]. Other SSRIs have similar, possibly less severe effects[61,62].
- Data relating to neurodevelopmental outcome of foetal exposure to SSRIs suggest that these drugs are safe, although data are less than conclusive[40,41,63,64]. Depression itself may have more obvious adverse effects on development[40].
- Although associated with an increased risk of bleeding overall, SSRIs do not seem to confer a disproportionate risk of postpartum haemorrhage[65].

Other antidepressants

- Rather more scarce data suggest the absence of teratogenic potential with **mocobemide**[66], **reboxetine**[67], and **venlafaxine** (although neonatal withdrawal may occur)[45,68,69], but none of these drugs can be specifically recommended. Similarly, **trazodone**, **bupropion** (amfebutamone), and **mirtazapine** cannot be recommended because there are few data supporting their safety[45,70,71]. Recent data suggest that both bupropion and mirtazapine are not associated with malformations but, like SSRIs, may be linked to an increased rate of spontaneous abortion[72,73].

Special groups

- **MAOIs** should be avoided in pregnancy because of a suspected increased risk of congenital malformation and because of the risk of hypertensive crisis[74].
- There is no evidence to suggest that **ECT** causes harm to either the mother or foetus during pregnancy[75] although general anaesthesia is, of course, not without risks. In resistant depression, NICE recommend that ECT is used before/instead of drug combinations.
- **Omega-3 fatty acids** may also be a treatment option[76] although efficacy and safety data are scant.

Recommendations – depression in pregnancy

- Patients who are already receiving antidepressants and are at high risk of relapse are best maintained on antidepressants during and after pregnancy
- Those who develop a moderate or severe depressive illness during pregnancy should be treated with antidepressant drugs
- There is most experience with **amitriptyline, imipramine** (constipation and sedation can be a problem with both; withdrawal symptoms may occur), and **fluoxetine** (increased chance of earlier delivery and reduced birth weight). If the patient is established on another anti-depressant, always obtain the most up-to-date advice. Experience with other drugs is growing and a change in treatment may not be necessary or wise. **Paroxetine may be less safe than other SSRIs**
- The neonate may experience discontinuation symptoms such as agitation and irritability, or even convulsions (with SSRIs). The risk is assumed to be particularly high with short half-life drugs such as paroxetine and venlafaxine. Continuing to breast feed and then 'weaning' by switching to mixed (breast/bottle) feeding may help reduce the severity of reactions
- When taken in late pregnancy, **SSRIs** may increase the risk of persistent pulmonary hypertension of the newborn.

Bipolar illness during pregnancy and postpartum

- The risk of relapse during pregnancy if mood-stabilising medication is discontinued is high; one study found that bipolar women who were euthymic at conception and discontinued mood-stabilisers were twice as likely to relapse and spent 5 times as long ill than women who continued mood-stabilisers[77].
- The risk of relapse after delivery is hugely increased: up to eight-fold in the first month post-partum.
- The mental health of the mother influences foetal well-being, obstetric outcome, and child development.

The risks of not stabilising mood include:

- harm to the mother through poor self-care, lack of obstetric care, or self-harm
- harm to the foetus or neonate (ranging from neglect to infanticide).

Treatment with mood-stabilisers

- **Lithium** completely equilibrates across the placenta[78].
- Although the overall risk of major malformations in infants exposed in utero has probably been overestimated, lithium should be avoided in pregnancy if possible. Slow discontinuation before conception is the preferred course of action[22,79] because abrupt discontinuation is suspected of worsening the risk of relapse. The relapse rate post-partum may be as high as 70% in women

who discontinued lithium before conception[80]. If discontinuation is unsuccessful during pregnancy – restart and continue.

- Lithium use during pregnancy has a well-known association with the cardiac malformation Ebstein's anomaly (relative risk is 10–20 times more than control, but the absolute risk is low at 1:1000)[81]. The period of maximum risk to the foetus is 2–6 weeks after conception[82], before many women know that they are pregnant. The risk of atrial and ventricular septal defects may also be increased[17].
- If lithium is continued during pregnancy, high-resolution ultrasound and echocardiography should be performed at 6 and 18 weeks of gestation.
- In the third trimester, the use of lithium may be problematic because of changing pharmacokinetics: an increasing dose of lithium is required to maintain the lithium level during pregnancy as total body water increases, but the requirements return abruptly to pre-pregnancy levels immediately after delivery[83]. Lithium plasma levels should be monitored every month during pregnancy and immediately after birth. Women taking lithium should deliver in hospital where fluid balance can be monitored and maintained.
- Neonatal goitre, hypotonia, lethargy, and cardiac arrhythmia can occur.

Most data relating to **carbamazepine** and **valproate** come from studies in epilepsy, a condition associated with increased neonatal malformation. These data may not be precisely relevant to use in mental illness.

- Both carbamazepine and valproate have a clear causal link with increased risk of a variety of foetal abnormalities, particularly spina bifida[84]. Both drugs should be avoided, if possible, and an antipsychotic prescribed instead. Valproate confers a higher risk than carbamazepine[85,86]. Although 1 in 20 women of child-bearing age who are in long-term contact with mental health services are prescribed mood-stabilising drugs, awareness of the teratogenic potential of these drugs amongst psychiatrists is low[84].
- Where continued use of valproate or carbamazepine is deemed essential, low-dose monotherapy is strongly recommended, as the teratogenic effect is probably dose-related[87,88]. NICE recommends that the dose of valproate should be limited to 1000 mg a day.
- Vulnerability to valproate-induced neural tube defects may be genetically determined via genes that code for folate metabolism/handling[89].
- Ideally, all patients should take folic acid (5 mg daily) for at least a month before conception (this may reduce the risk of neonatal neural tube defects). Note, however, that some authorities recommend a lower dose[90], presumably because of a risk of twin births[91].
- Use of carbamazepine in the third trimester may necessitate maternal vitamin K.
- Data for **lamotrigine** suggest a low risk of foetal malformations when used as monotherapy[90,92,93], although a substantially increased risk of cleft palate has been reported[94]. Clearance of lamotrigine seems to increase radically during pregnancy[95]. NICE suggests that lamotrigine should not be routinely prescribed in pregnancy.

Special groups

Recommendations – bipolar disorder in pregnancy

- For women who have had a long period without relapse, the possibility of switching to a safer drug (antipsychotic) or withdrawing treatment completely before conception and for at least the first trimester should be considered
- The risk of relapse both pre- and post-partum is very high if medication is discontinued abruptly
- Women with severe illness or who are known to relapse quickly after discontinuation of a mood-stabiliser should be advised to continue their medication following discussion of the risks
- No mood-stabiliser is clearly safe. Women prescribed lithium should undergo level 2 ultrasound of the foetus at 6 and 18 weeks' gestation to screen for Ebstein's anomaly. Those prescribed valproate or carbamazepine (both teratogenic) should receive prophylactic folic acid to reduce the incidence of neural tube defects, and receive appropriate antenatal screening tests
- If carbamazepine is used, prophylactic vitamin K should be administered to the mother and neonate after delivery
- Valproate (the most teratogenic) and combinations of mood-stabilisers should be avoided
- Lamotrigine may be associated with cleft palate
- NICE recommends the use of mood-stabilising antipsychotics as a preferable alternative to continuation with a mood-stabiliser
- In acute mania in pregnancy use an antipsychotic and if ineffective consider ECT
- In bipolar depression during pregnancy use CBT for moderate depression and an SSRI for more severe depression.

Epilepsy during pregnancy and post-partum

- In pregnant women with epilepsy, there is an increased risk of maternal complications such as severe morning sickness, eclampsia, vaginal bleeding, and premature labour. Women should get as much sleep and rest as possible and comply with medication (if prescribed) in order to minimise the risk of seizures.
- The risk of having a child with minor malformations may be increased regardless of treatment with antiepileptic drugs (AEDs).

The risks of not treating epilepsy are as follows:

- If seizures are inadequately controlled, there is an increased risk of accidents resulting in foetal injury. Post-partum the mother may be less able to look after herself and her child.
- The risk of seizures during delivery is 1–2%, potentially worsening maternal and neonatal mortality.

Treatment with anticonvulsant drugs

It is established that treatment with anticonvulsant drugs increases the risk of having a child with major congenital malformation to two- to three-fold that seen in the general population. Congenital heart defects (1.8%) and facial clefts (1.7%) are the most common congenital malformations. Both carbamazepine and valproate are associated with a hugely increased incidence of spina bifida at 0.5–1% and 1–2%, respectively. The risk of other neural tube defects is also increased. In women with epilepsy, the risk of foetal malformations with carbamazepine is 2.3%; with lamotrigine, 3%; and with valproate, 7.2%[96], possibly even higher[86,88]. Higher doses (particularly doses of valproate exceeding 1000 mg/day) and anticonvulsant polypharmacy are particularly problematic[88,97]. Cognitive deficits have been reported in older children who have been exposed to valproate in utero. Those exposed to carbamazepine may not be similarly disadvantaged[98]. Early data with lamotrigine[92,99] and oxcarbazepine[100] suggest a relatively lower risk of malformation, but confirmation is required (and note risk of cleft palate with lamotrigine[94]).

Pharmacokinetics change during pregnancy, and there is marked inter-individual variation[101]. Dosage adjustment may be required to keep the patient seizure-free[102]. Serum levels usually return to pre-pregnancy levels within a month of delivery often much more rapidly. Doses may need to be reduced at this point.

Best practice guidelines recommend that a woman should receive the lowest possible dose of a single anticonvulsant.

Recommendations – epilepsy in pregnancy

- For women who have been seizure free for a long period, the possibility of withdrawing treatment before conception and for at least the first trimester should be considered
- No anticonvulsant is clearly safer. Women prescribed valproate or carbamazepine should receive prophylactic folic acid to reduce the risk of neural tube defects. Prophylactic vitamin K should be administered to the mother and neonate after delivery
- Valproate and combinations of anticonvulsants should be avoided if possible
- All women with epilepsy should have a full discussion with their neurologist to quantify the risks and benefits of continuing anticonvulsant drugs during pregnancy.

Sedatives
Anxiety disorders and insomnia are commonly seen in pregnancy[103]. Preferred treatments are CBT and sleep-hygiene measures respectively.

- First-trimester exposure to **benzodiazepines** has been associated with an increased risk of oral clefts in new-borns[104], although a recent study has failed to confirm this association[105].
- Benzodiazepines have been associated with pylorostenosis and alimentary tract atresia[105]; replication of these findings is required.
- There is an association between benzodiazepine use in pregnancy and low birth weight[105].
- Third-trimester use is commonly associated with neonatal difficulties (floppy baby syndrome)[106].
- **Promethazine** has been used in hyperemesis gravidarum and appears not to be teratogenic, although data are limited.
- NICE recommends the use of low-dose chlorpromazine or amitriptyline.

Rapid tranquillisation
There is almost no published information on the use of rapid tranquillisation in pregnant women. The acute use of short-acting benzodiazepines such as lorazepam and of the sedative antihistamine promethazine is unlikely to be harmful. Presumably, the use of either drug will be problematic immediately before birth. NICE also recommends the use of an antipsychotic but does not specify a particular drug[10]. Intramuscular olanzapine is probably preferable to intramuscular haloperidol because of the lower risk of EPS.

Special groups

353

Recommendations – psychotropics in pregnancy

Psychotropic group	Recommendations
Antidepressants	Nortriptyline Amitriptyline Imipramine Fluoxetine
Antipsychotics	**Conventional drugs** have been widely used, although safety is not fully established. Most experience with **chlorpromazine, haloperidol**, and **trifluoperazine**. No clear evidence that any antipsychotic is a major teratogen, although data for SGAs other than olanzapine and clozapine are scarce
Mood-stabilisers	Consider using an **antipsychotic** as a mood-stabiliser rather than an anticonvulsant drug Avoid **anticonvulsants** unless risks and consequences of relapse outweigh the known risk of teratogenesis. Women of childbearing potential taking carbamazepine or valproate should receive prophylactic **folic acid**. Avoid valproate and combinations where possible
Sedatives	**Non-drug measures are preferred** **Benzodiazepines** are probably not teratogenic but are best avoided in late pregnancy. **Promethazine** is widely used but supporting safety data are scarce

References

1. McElhatton PR. Pregnancy: (2) General principles of drug use in pregnancy. Pharm J 2003; 270:232–234.
2. CARE Study Group. Maternal caffeine intake during pregnancy and risk of fetal growth restriction: a large prospective observational study. BMJ 2008; 337:a2332.
3. Rasmussen SA et al. Maternal obesity and risk of neural tube defects: a metaanalysis. Am J Obstet Gynecol 2008; 198:611–619.
4. Schneid-Kofman N et al. Psychiatric illness and adverse pregnancy outcome. Int J Gynaecol Obstet 2008; 101:53–56.
5. MacCabe JH et al. Adverse pregnancy outcomes in mothers with affective psychosis. Bipolar Disord 2007; 9:305–309.
6. Goodwin RD et al. Mental disorders and nicotine dependence among pregnant women in the United States. Obstet Gynecol 2007; 109:875–883.
7. Tobacco Advisory group of the Royal College of Physicians. Harm reduction in nicotine addiction. Helping people who can't quit. 2007. http://www.rcplondon.ac.uk/.
8. Sit DK et al. Changes in antidepressant metabolism and dosing across pregnancy and early postpartum. J Clin Psychiatry 2008; 69:652–658.
9. Ter Horst PG et al. Pharmacological aspects of neonatal antidepressant withdrawal. Obstet Gynecol Surv 2008; 63:267–279.
10. National Institute for Clinical Excellence. Antenatal and postnatal mental health. Clinical management and service guidance (reissued April 2007). 2007. http://www.nice.org.uk/.
11. Harlow BL et al. Incidence of hospitalization for postpartum psychotic and bipolar episodes in women with and without prior prepregnancy or prenatal psychiatric hospitalizations. Arch Gen Psychiatry 2007; 64:42–48.
12. Spinelli MG. A systematic investigation of 16 cases of neonaticide. Am J Psychiatry 2001; 158:811–813.
13. Ismail B et al. Minor physical anomalies in schizophrenic patients and their siblings. Am J Psychiatry 1998; 155:1695–1702.
14. Gentile S. Antipsychotic therapy during early and late pregnancy. A systematic review. Schizophr Bull 2008;Epub ahead of print.
15. Trixler M et al. Use of antipsychotics in the management of schizophrenia during pregnancy. Drugs 2005; 65:1193–1206.
16. Diav-Citrin O et al. Safety of haloperidol and penfluridol in pregnancy: a multicenter, prospective, controlled study. J Clin Psychiatry 2005; 66:317–322.
17. Reis M et al. Maternal use of antipsychotics in early pregnancy and delivery outcome. J Clin Psychopharmacol 2008; 28:279–288.
18. Collins KO et al. Maternal haloperidol therapy associated with dyskinesia in a newborn. Am J Health Syst Pharm 2003; 60:2253–2255.
19. Webb RT et al. Antipsychotic drugs for non-affective psychosis during pregnancy and postpartum. Cochrane Database Syst Rev 2004;CD004411.
20. Newport DJ et al. Atypical antipsychotic administration during late pregnancy: placental passage and obstetrical outcomes. Am J Psychiatry 2007; 164:1214–1220.
21. Newham JJ et al. Birth weight of infants after maternal exposure to typical and atypical antipsychotics: prospective comparison study. Br J Psychiatry 2008; 192:333–337.
22. Ernst CL et al. The reproductive safety profile of mood stabilizers, atypical antipsychotics, and broad-spectrum psychotropics. J Clin Psychiatry 2002; 63 Suppl 4:42–55.
23. McKenna K et al. Pregnancy outcome of women using atypical antipsychotic drugs: a prospective comparative study. J Clin Psychiatry 2005; 66:444–449.
24. Spyropoulou AC et al. Hip dysplasia following a case of olanzapine exposed pregnancy: a questionable association. Arch Womens Ment Health 2006; 9:219–222.
25. Arora M et al. Meningocele and ankyloblepharon following in utero exposure to olanzapine. Eur Psychiatry 2006; 21:345–346.
26. Ratnayake T et al. No complications with risperidone treatment before and throughout pregnancy and during the nursing period. J Clin Psychiatry 2002; 63:76–77.
27. Dabbert D et al. Follow-up of a pregnancy with risperidone microspheres. Pharmacopsychiatry 2006; 39:235.
28. Kim SW et al. Use of long-acting injectable risperidone before and throughout pregnancy in schizophrenia. Prog Neuropsychopharmacol Biol Psychiatry 2007; 31:543–545.
29. Llewellyn AM et al. Depression during pregnancy and the puerperium. J Clin Psychiatry 1997; 58 Suppl 15:26–32.

30. Cohen LS et al. Relapse of major depression during pregnancy in women who maintain or discontinue antidepressant treatment. JAMA 2006; 295:499–507.
31. Larsson C et al. Health, sociodemographic data, and pregnancy outcome in women with antepartum depressive symptoms. Obstet Gynecol 2004; 104:459–466.
32. Ververs T et al. Prevalence and patterns of antidepressant drug use during pregnancy. Eur J Clin Pharmacol 2006; 62:863–870.
33. Andrade SE et al. Use of antidepressant medications during pregnancy: a multisite study. Am J Obstet Gynecol 2008; 198:194–195.
34. Oberlander TF et al. Effects of timing and duration of gestational exposure to serotonin reuptake inhibitor antidepressants: population-based study. Br J Psychiatry 2008; 192:338–343.
35. Ramos E et al. Duration of antidepressant use during pregnancy and risk of major congenital malformations. Br J Psychiatry 2008; 192:344–350.
36. Loughhead AM et al. Placental passage of tricyclic antidepressants. Biol Psychiatry 2006; 59:287–290.
37. Loughhead AM et al. Antidepressants in amniotic fluid: another route of fetal exposure. Am J Psychiatry 2006; 163:145–147.
38. Davis RL et al. Risks of congenital malformations and perinatal events among infants exposed to antidepressant medications during pregnancy. Pharmacoepidemiol Drug Saf 2007; 16:1086–1094.
39. Kallen B. Neonate characteristics after maternal use of antidepressants in late pregnancy. Arch Pediatr Adolesc Med 2004; 158:312–316.
40. Nulman I et al. Child development following exposure to tricyclic antidepressants or fluoxetine throughout fetal life: a prospective, controlled study. Am J Psychiatry 2002; 159:1889–1895.
41. Nulman I et al. Neurodevelopment of children exposed in utero to antidepressant drugs. N Engl J Med 1997; 336:258–262.
42. Maschi S et al. Neonatal outcome following pregnancy exposure to antidepressants: a prospective controlled cohort study. BJOG 2008; 115:283–289.
43. Hendrick V et al. Placental passage of antidepressant medications. Am J Psychiatry 2003; 160:993–996.
44. Hallberg P et al. The use of selective serotonin reuptake inhibitors during pregnancy and breast-feeding: a review and clinical aspects. J Clin Psychopharmacol 2005; 25:59–73.
45. Gentile S. The safety of newer antidepressants in pregnancy and breastfeeding. Drug Saf 2005; 28:137–152.
46. Kallen BA et al. Maternal use of selective serotonin re-uptake inhibitors in early pregnancy and infant congenital malformations. Birth Defects Res A Clin Mol Teratol 2007; 79:301–308.
47. Einarson TR et al. Newer antidepressants in pregnancy and rates of major malformations: a meta-analysis of prospective comparative studies. Pharmacoepidemiol Drug Saf 2005; 14:823–827.
48. Wogelius P et al. Maternal use of selective serotonin reuptake inhibitors and risk of congenital malformations. Epidemiology 2006; 17:701–704.
49. Chambers CD et al. Selective serotonin-reuptake inhibitors and risk of persistent pulmonary hypertension of the newborn. N Engl J Med 2006; 354:579–587.
50. Alwan S et al. Use of selective serotonin-reuptake inhibitors in pregnancy and the risk of birth defects. N Engl J Med 2007; 356:2684–2692.
51. Thormahlen GM. Paroxetine use during pregnancy: is it safe? Ann Pharmacother 2006; 40:1834–1837.
52. Berard A et al. First trimester exposure to paroxetine and risk of cardiac malformations in infants: the importance of dosage. Birth Defects Res B Dev Reprod Toxicol 2006; 80:18–27.
53. Einarson A et al. Evaluation of the risk of congenital cardiovascular defects associated with use of paroxetine during pregnancy. Am J Psychiatry 2008; 165:749–752.
54. Diav-Citrin O et al. Paroxetine and fluoxetine in pregnancy: a prospective, multicentre, controlled, observational study. Br J Clin Pharmacol 2008; 66:695–705.
55. Louik C et al. First-trimester use of selective serotonin-reuptake inhibitors and the risk of birth defects. N Engl J Med 2007; 356:2675–2683.
56. Hemels ME et al. Antidepressant use during pregnancy and the rates of spontaneous abortions: a meta-analysis. Ann Pharmacother 2005; 39:803–809.
57. Oberlander TF et al. Neonatal outcomes after prenatal exposure to selective serotonin reuptake inhibitor antidepressants and maternal depression using population-based linked health data. Arch Gen Psychiatry 2006; 63:898–906.
58. Suri R et al. Effects of antenatal depression and antidepressant treatment on gestational age at birth and risk of preterm birth. Am J Psychiatry 2007; 164:1206–1213.
59. Boucher N et al. A new look at the neonate's clinical presentation after in utero exposure to antidepressants in late pregnancy. J Clin Psychopharmacol 2008; 28:334–339.
60. Haddad PM et al. Neonatal symptoms following maternal paroxetine treatment: serotonin toxicity or paroxetine discontinuation syndrome? J Psychopharmacol 2005; 19:554–557.
61. Sanz EJ et al. Selective serotonin reuptake inhibitors in pregnant women and neonatal withdrawal syndrome: a database analysis. Lancet 2005; 365:482–487.
62. Koren G. Discontinuation syndrome following late pregnancy exposure to antidepressants. Arch Pediatr Adolesc Med 2004; 158:307–308.
63. Gentile S. SSRIs in pregnancy and lactation: emphasis on neurodevelopmental outcome. CNS Drugs 2005; 19:623–633.
64. Casper RC et al. Follow-up of children of depressed mothers exposed or not exposed to antidepressant drugs during pregnancy. J Pediatr 2003; 142:402–408.
65. Salkeld E et al. The risk of postpartum hemorrhage with selective serotonin reuptake inhibitors and other antidepressants. J Clin Psychopharmacol 2008; 28:230–234.
66. Rybakowski JK. Moclobemide in pregnancy. Pharmacopsychiatry 2001; 34:82–83.
67. Pharmacia Ltd. Erdronax: Use on pregnancy, renally and hepatically impaired patients. Personal Communication. 2003.
68. Einarson A et al. Pregnancy outcome following gestational exposure to venlafaxine: a multicenter prospective controlled study. Am J Psychiatry 2001; 158:1728–1730.
69. Ferreira E et al. Effects of selective serotonin reuptake inhibitors and venlafaxine during pregnancy in term and preterm neonates. Pediatrics 2007; 119:52–59.
70. Einarson A et al. A multicentre prospective controlled study to determine the safety of trazodone and nefazodone use during pregnancy. Can J Psychiatry 2003; 48:106–110.
71. Rohde A et al. Mirtazapine (Remergil) for treatment resistant hyperemesis gravidarum: rescue of a twin pregnancy. Arch Gynecol Obstet 2003; 268:219–221.
72. Djulus J et al. Exposure to mirtazapine during pregnancy: a prospective, comparative study of birth outcomes. J Clin Psychiatry 2006; 67:1280–1284.
73. Cole JA et al. Bupropion in pregnancy and the prevalence of congenital malformations. Pharmacoepidemiol Drug Saf 2007; 16:474–484.
74. Hendrick V et al. Management of major depression during pregnancy. Am J Psychiatry 2002; 159:1667–1673.
75. Miller LJ. Use of electroconvulsive therapy during pregnancy. Hosp Community Psychiatry 1994; 45:444–450.
76. Freeman MP et al. An open trial of Omega-3 fatty acids for depression in pregnancy. Acta Neuropsychiatr 2006; 18:21–24.
77. Viguera AC et al. Risk of recurrence in women with bipolar disorder during pregnancy: prospective study of mood stabilizer discontinuation. Am J Psychiatry 2007; 164:1817–1824.
78. Newport DJ et al. Lithium placental passage and obstetrical outcome: implications for clinical management during late pregnancy. Am J Psychiatry 2005; 162:2162–2170.
79. Dodd S et al. The pharmacology of bipolar disorder during pregnancy and breastfeeding. Expert Opin Drug Saf 2004; 3:221–229.
80. Viguera AC et al. Risk of recurrence of bipolar disorder in pregnant and nonpregnant women after discontinuing lithium maintenance. Am J Psychiatry 2000; 157:179–184.
81. Cohen LS et al. A reevaluation of risk of in utero exposure to lithium. JAMA 1994; 271:146–150.
82. Yonkers KA et al. Lithium during pregnancy: drug effects and therapeutic implications. CNS Drugs 1998; 4:269.
83. Blake LD et al. Lithium toxicity and the parturient: case report and literature review. Int J Obstet Anesth 2008; 17:164–169.

Special groups

355

84. James L et al. Informing patients of the teratogenic potential of mood stabilising drugs; a case notes review of the practice of psychiatrists. J Psychopharmacol 2007; 21:815–819.
85. Wide K et al. Major malformations in infants exposed to antiepileptic drugs in utero, with emphasis on carbamazepine and valproic acid: a nation-wide, population-based register study. Acta Paediatr 2004; 93:174–176.
86. Wyszynski DF et al. Increased rate of major malformations in offspring exposed to valproate during pregnancy. Neurology 2005; 64:961–965.
87. Vajda FJ et al. Critical relationship between sodium valproate dose and human teratogenicity: results of the Australian register of anti-epileptic drugs in pregnancy. J Clin Neurosci 2004; 11:854–858.
88. Vajda FJ et al. Maternal valproate dosage and foetal malformations. Acta Neurol Scand 2005; 112:137–143.
89. Duncan S. Teratogenesis of sodium valproate. Curr Opin Neurol 2007; 20:175–180.
90. Yonkers KA et al. Management of bipolar disorder during pregnancy and the postpartum period. Am J Psychiatry 2004; 161:608–620.
91. Czeizel AE. Folic acid and the prevention of neural-tube defects. N Engl J Med 2004; 350:2209–2211.
92. Sabers A et al. Epilepsy and pregnancy: lamotrigine as main drug used. Acta Neurol Scand 2004; 109:9–13.
93. Cunnington M et al. Lamotrigine and the risk of malformations in pregnancy. Neurology 2005; 64:955–960.
94. Holmes LB et al. Increased risk for non-syndromic cleft palate among infants exposed to lamotrigine during pregnancy. Birth Defects Research 2006; 76:318.
95. de Haan GJ et al. Gestation-induced changes in lamotrigine pharmacokinetics: a monotherapy study. Neurology 2004; 63:571–573.
96. National Institute of Clinical Excellence. The clinical effectiveness and cost effectiveness of newer drugs for epilepsy in adults. Technology Appraisal 76. http://www.nice.org.uk. 2004
97. Vajda FJ et al. The Australian Register of Antiepileptic Drugs in Pregnancy: the first 1002 pregnancies. Aust N Z J Obstet Gynaecol 2007; 47:468–474.
98. Gaily E et al. Normal intelligence in children with prenatal exposure to carbamazepine. Neurology 2004; 62:28–32.
99. Vajda FJ et al. The Australian registry of anti-epileptic drugs in pregnancy: experience after 30 months. J Clin Neurosci 2003; 10:543–549.
100. Meischenguiser R et al. Oxcarbazepine in pregnancy: clinical experience in Argentina. Epilepsy Behav 2004; 5:163–167.
101. Brodtkorb E et al. Seizure control and pharmacokinetics of antiepileptic drugs in pregnant women with epilepsy. Seizure 2008; 17:160–165.
102. Adab N. Therapeutic monitoring of antiepileptic drugs during pregnancy and in the postpartum period: is it useful? CNS Drugs 2006; 20:791–800.
103. Ross LE et al. Anxiety disorders during pregnancy and the postpartum period: A systematic review. J Clin Psychiatry 2006; 67:1285–1298.
104. Dolovich LR et al. Benzodiazepine use in pregnancy and major malformations or oral cleft: meta-analysis of cohort and case-control studies. BMJ 1998; 317:839–843.
105. Wikner BN et al. Use of benzodiazepines and benzodiazepine receptor agonists during pregnancy: neonatal outcome and congenital malformations. Pharmacoepidemiol Drug Saf 2007; 16:1203–1210.
106. McElhatton PR. The effects of benzodiazepine use during pregnancy and lactation. Reprod Toxicol 1994; 8:461–475.

Further reading

Donnelly A et al. Safety of selective serotonin reuptake inhibitors in pregnancy. Psychiatr Bull 2007; 31:183–1.
Einarson A et al. Abrupt discontinuation of psychotropic drugs during pregnancy: fear of teratogenic risk and impact of counselling. J Psychiatry Neurosci 2001; 26:44–48.
Gentile S. Clinical utilization of atypical antipsychotics in pregnancy and lactation. Ann Pharmacother 2004; 38:1265–1271.
Gentile S. Prophylactic treatment of bipolar disorder during pregnancy and breastfeeding: focus on emerging mood stabilizers. Bipolar Disord 2006; 8:207–220.
Hallberg P et al. The use of selective serotonin reuptake inhibitors during pregnancy and breast-feeding: a review and clinical aspects. J Clin Psychopharmacol 2005;25:59–73.
National Institute for Clinical Excellence . Antenatal and postnatal mental health. Clinical management and service guidance (reissued April 2007) http://guidance.nice.org.uk/
Paton C. Prescribing in pregnancy. Br J Psychiatry 2008; 192:321–322.
Ruchkin V et al. SSRIs and the developing brain. Lancet 2005; 365:451–453.
Sanz EJ et al. Selective serotonin reuptake inhibitors in pregnant women and neonatal withdrawal syndrome: a database analysis. Lancet 2005; 365:482–487.`
Wisner KL et al. Major depression and antidepressant treatment: impact on pregnancy and neonatal outcome. Am J Psychiatry 2009; 166: 557–566.

Other sources of information

National Teratology Information Service. http://www.hpa.org.uk/

Special groups

Psychotropics in breast-feeding

Breast-feeding guidelines

Data on the safety of psychotropic medication in breast-feeding are largely derived from small studies or case reports and case series. With the majority of data, only acute adverse effects (or their absence) are reported. Long-term safety cannot therefore be guaranteed for the psychotropics mentioned. The information presented must be interpreted with caution with respect to the limited data from which it is derived and the need for such information to be regularly updated.

General principles of prescribing psychotropics in breast-feeding

- In each case, the benefits of breast-feeding to the mother and infant must be weighed against the risk of drug exposure in the infant.
- Premature infants and infants with renal, hepatic, cardiac, or neurological impairment are at a greater risk from exposure to drugs.
- The infants should be monitored for any specific adverse effects of the drugs as well as for feeding patterns and growth and development.
- It is usually inappropriate to withhold treatment to allow breast-feeding where there is a high risk of relapse. Treatment of maternal illness is the highest priority.
- Where a mother has taken a particular psychotropic drug during pregnancy and until delivery, continuation with the drug while breast-feeding may be appropriate as this may minimise withdrawal symptoms in the infant.
- Women receiving sedating medication should be strongly advised not to sleep with the baby in bed with them.

Wherever possible:

- use the lowest effective dose
- avoid polypharmacy
- time the feeds to avoid peak drug levels in the milk or express milk to give later (this may be impractical in small infants feeding every 1–3 hours).

Summary of recommendations (see full review below for details)

Drug group	Recommended drugs
Antidepressants	**Paroxetine** or **sertraline** (others may be used – see table)
Antipsychotics	**Sulpiride; olanzapine** (others may be used – see table)
Mood-stabilisers	Often best to switch to **mood-stabilising antipsychotic** (see table). **Valproate** can be used but only where there is adequate protection against pregnancy (breast-feeding itself is not adequate protection). Beware risk of hepatotoxicity in breast-fed infants
Sedatives	**Lorazepam** for anxiety; **zolpidem** for sleep (others may be used – see table)

Special groups

Antidepressants in breast-feeding

Drug	Comment
Tricyclic antidepressants (TCAs)[1-8]	All TCAs are excreted in human breast milk. Infant serum levels range from undetectable to low. Adverse effects have not been reported in infants exposed to amitriptyline, nortriptyline, clomipramine, imipramine, dothiepin (dosulepin), and desipramine. There are two case reports of doxepin exposure during breast-feeding leading to adverse effects in the infant. In one, an 8-week-old infant experienced respiratory depression, which resolved 24 hours after stopping nursing. In the other, poor suckling, muscle hypotonia, and drowsiness were observed in a newborn, again resolving 24 hours after removing doxepin exposure
	A study of 15 children did not show a negative outcome on cognitive development in children 3–5 years post-partum, following breast milk exposure to dothiepin
	NICE states that imipramine and nortriptyline are present in breast milk 'at relatively low levels'[9]. Thus these drugs are at least tacitly recommended by NICE
	Data on TCAs not mentioned in this section were not available and their use can therefore not be recommended unless used during pregnancy
Citalopram[10,11-17]	Citalopram is excreted in breast milk. Infant serum levels appear to be low or undetectable, although higher than reported with fluvoxamine, sertraline, and paroxetine. Breast milk peak levels have been observed 3–9 hours after maternal dose
	There is one case report of uneasy sleep in an infant exposed to citalopram while breast-feeding. This resolved on halving the mother's dose. Irregular breathing, sleep disorder, hypo- and hypertonia were observed up to 3 weeks after delivery in another breast-feeding infant exposed to citalopram in utero. The symptoms were attributed to withdrawal syndrome from citalopram despite the mother continuing citalopram post partum
	In a study of 31 infants exposed to citalopram via breast milk, one case each of colic, decreased feeding, and irritability/restlessness was reported
	The manufacturers of citalopram advise against its use in breast-feeding
Escitalopram[18-20]	Escitalopram is excreted in breast milk but adverse effects were not seen in two separate case reports. In a study of 8 women, breast milk peak levels of escitalopram were observed 2–11 hours post maternal dose. No adverse effects were noted in the infants. Serum levels were found to be low or undetectable in all 5 of the infants from whom blood could to be taken
	The manufacturers of escitalopram advise against its use in breast-feeding
Fluvoxamine[21,22-27]	Fluvoxamine is excreted in breast milk. The levels detected in infants exposed to fluvoxamine while breast-feeding vary from undetectable to up to half the maternal serum level. No adverse effects were noted in these infants. Peak drug levels in breast milk have been observed 4 hours after maternal dose
	The manufacturers of fluvoxamine advise against its use in breast-feeding

Table	Antidepressants in breast feeding (Cont.)
Drug	**Comment**
Fluoxetine[28,29–35]	Of the SSRIs, most data relate to fluoxetine. Fluoxetine is excreted into breast milk. Infant serum levels appear to be low, although higher than reported with paroxetine, fluvoxamine, and sertraline, and close to those reported for citalopram. Adverse effects have not been reported for the majority of fluoxetine-exposed infants. However, in two infants, reported adverse effects included excessive crying, decreased sleep, diarrhoea, and vomiting in one and somnolence, decreased feeding, hypotonia, moaning, grunting, and fever in the other. In another, seizure activity at 3 weeks, 4 months and then 5 months was reported. The mother was taking a combination of fluoxetine and carbamazepine. A retrospective study found the growth curves of breast-fed infants of mothers taking fluoxetine to be significantly below those of infants receiving breast milk free of fluoxetine. However, in another study of 11 infants exposed to fluoxetine during pregnancy and lactation, neurological developments and weight gain were found to be normal. No developmental abnormalities were noted in another four infants exposed to fluoxetine during breast-feeding. In a study of 11 infants exposed to fluoxetine whilst breastfeeding, a drop in platelet serotonin was noted in one of the infants. The manufacturers of fluoxetine advise against its use in breast-feeding if possible. They further recommend prescribing the lowest possible dose in women who are breast-feeding
Paroxetine[36,37,38,39–45]	Paroxetine is excreted in breast milk. Infant serum levels vary from low to undetectable There is a single case of adverse consequences arising from maternal paroxetine consumption. Vomiting and irritability were reported in a breast-feeding baby of 18 months. The symptoms were attributed to severe hyponatraemia in the infant. The maternal paroxetine dose was 40 mg. Paroxetine levels were not determined in the breast milk or infant serum Adverse effects were not noted in the other cases cited Breast-fed infants of 27 women taking paroxetine reached the usual developmental milestones at 3, 6 and 12 months, similar to a control group The manufacturers of paroxetine advise that its use in breastfeeding can be considered
Sertraline[46,47,48]	Sertraline is excreted in breast milk. Infant serum levels appear to be low. Peak drug levels in breast milk have been observed 7–10 hours after the maternal dose. No adverse effects were noted in these infants Withdrawal symptoms (agitation, restlessness, insomnia, and an enhanced startle reaction) developed in a breast-fed neonate, after abrupt withdrawal of maternal sertraline. The neonate was exposed to sertraline in utero The manufacturers of sertraline advise against its use in breast-feeding, but NICE states that breast milk levels of sertraline are relatively lower (than what, it is not clear) and so tacitly recommends the use of sertraline[9]

Drug	Comment
Reboxetine[49]	Reboxetine is excreted in breast milk. Infant serum levels ranged from low to undetectable and no adverse effects were noted in 4 infants. In addition, normal developmental milestones were reached by 3 of the infants. The fourth had developmental problems thought not to be related to maternal reboxetine therapy. Breast milk peak levels were observed 1–9 hours after maternal dose The manufacturers of reboxetine advise that its use in breast-feeding can be considered if the benefits outweigh the risk to the child
Venlafaxine[50,51–53]	Venlafaxine is excreted in breast milk. Infant serum levels were found to be low. Although not directly compared, these levels appear to be higher than those seen with fluvoxamine, sertraline, and paroxetine. No adverse effects have been observed Symptoms of lethargy, jitteriness, rapid breathing, poor suckling, and dehydration seen 2 days after delivery of an infant exposed to venlafaxine in utero, subsided over a week on exposure to venlafaxine via breastmilk. It was suggested in this case that breast-feeding may have helped manage the withdrawal symptoms experienced post partum The manufacturers of venlafaxine advise against its use in breast-feeding
MAOIs	No published data could be found
Moclobemide[54,55]	Moclobemide is excreted in breast milk. Infant serum levels appear to be low. No adverse effects were detected in these infants. Peak drug levels in breast milk were seen at 3 hours The manufacturers of moclobemide advise that its use in breastfeeding can be considered if the benefits outweigh the risk to the child
Mianserin[56]	Mianserin is excreted in breast milk. Adverse effects were not seen in 2 infants studied
Mirtazapine[57–59]	Mirtazapine is excreted in breast milk. Infant serum levels range from undetectable to low. No adverse effects have been noted in exposed infants. Psychomotor development was tested in one infant after 6 weeks of exposure and found to be normal No adverse effects were noted in any of the 8 infants in a study of exposure to mirtazapine in breast milk. In addition, developmental milestones were being achieved by all infants at the time of the study. However, the weights for 3 of the infants were observed to be between the 10th to 25th percentiles. All 3 were noted to also have a low birth weight The manufacturers of mirtazapine advise against its use in breast-feeding
Trazodone[60]	Trazodone is excreted into breast milk in small quantities based on assessments after a single maternal dose The manufacturers of trazodone advise that the possibility of excretion of trazodone into breast milk should be considered

Special groups

Antipsychotics in breast-feeding

Drug	Comment
Butyrophenones[2,61–64]	Haloperidol is excreted in breast milk. The extent appears variable. Normal development was noted in one infant. However, delayed development was noted in three infants exposed to a combination of haloperidol and chlorpromazine in breast milk
	Data on butyrophenones not mentioned in this section were not available
Phenothiazines[2,63,65,66]	Most of the data relate to chlorpromazine. Chlorpromazine is excreted in breast milk. There is a wide variation in the breast milk concentrations quoted. Similarly, infant serum levels vary greatly. Lethargy was reported in one infant whose mother was taking chlorpromazine while breast-feeding. In another case, however, an infant exposed to much higher levels showed no signs of lethargy. There is a report of delayed development in three infants exposed to a combination of chlorpromazine and haloperidol while breast-feeding
	In the one case of perphenazine exposure and two cases of trifluoperazine exposure, no adverse effects were noted in the infants
	Data on phenothiazines not mentioned in this section were not available
Thioxanthenes[67–70]	There are two cases of infant exposure to flupentixol and seven to zuclopentixol. Both drugs are excreted in breast milk. No adverse effects or developmental abnormalities have been noted were in exposed infant exposed to flupentixol. The clinical status of the other infant was not reported
Sulpiride[71–75]	There are a number of small studies in which sulpiride has been shown to improve lactation in nursing mothers. The amounts excreted in breast milk were low. No adverse effects were noted in the nursing infants
	The manufacturers of sulpiride advise against its use in breast-feeding
Amisulpride	To our knowledge there are no published data available. Breast-feeding is contra-indicated by the manufacturers of amisulpride
Aripiprazole[76]	Aripiprazole is excreted in breast milk. To our knowledge no infant data are available as yet. There is one case of a woman's failure to lactate after being treated with aripiprazole during pregnancy
	The manufacturers of aripiprazole advise against its use in breast-feeding
Clozapine[2,77–80]	Clozapine is excreted in breast milk. In a study of four infants exposed to clozapine in breast milk, sedation was noted in one and another developed agranulocytosis, which resolved on stopping clozapine. No adverse effects were noted in the other two. Decreased sucking reflex, irritability, seizures, and cardiovascular instability have also been reported in nursing infants exposed to clozapine
	There is one case report of delayed speech acquisition in an infant who was exposed to clozapine during breast-feeding. The infant was also exposed to clozapine in utero
	Because of the risk of neutropenia and seizures, it is advisable to avoid breast-feeding while on clozapine until more data become available
	The manufacturers of clozapine advise against its use in breast-feeding

Special groups

Table Antipsychotics in breast-feeding (Cont.)

Drug	Comment
Olanzapine[81–88]	Olanzapine is excreted in breast milk. Estimates of infant serum levels range from undetectable to low. There is one case of an infant developing jaundice and sedation on exposure to olanzapine during breast-feeding. This continued on cessation of breast-feeding. This infant was exposed to olanzapine in utero and had cardiomegaly. In another, no adverse effects were noted
	No adverse effects were reported in four of seven breast-fed infants of mothers taking olanzapine. Of the rest, one was not assessed, one had a lower developmental age than chronological age (but the mother had also been taking additional psychotropic medication), and drowsiness was noted in another, which resolved on halving the maternal dose. The median maximum concentration in the milk was found at around 5 hours after maternal ingestion
	The manufacturers of olanzapine advise against its use in breast-feeding
Quetiapine[89–95]	Quetiapine is excreted in breast milk
	Adverse effects were not noted in infants in three separate case reports. One of these infants was exposed to a combination of quetiapine and paroxetine
	In addition, no adverse effects were noted in an infant exposed to a combination of quetiapine and fluvoxamine whilst breastfeeding. The baby reached developmental milestones
	In a separate small study of quetiapine augmentation of maternal antidepressant therapy, two out of six babies showed mild developmental delays not thought to be related to quetiapine treatment. The doses in this study ranged from 25–400 mg/day
	There is one reported case of an infant 'sleeping more than expected' whilst exposed to quetiapine, mirtazapine, and a benzodiazepine in breast milk. The drowsiness is thought to be a result of exposure to the benzodiazepine
	The manufacturers of quetiapine advise against its use in breast-feeding
Risperidone[96–99]	Risperidone is excreted in breast milk. In five cases reported in the literature, no adverse effects were noted. In two cases where development was assessed, no abnormalities were observed
	The manufacturers of risperidone advise against its use in breast-feeding
Sertindole	No published data could be found
Ziprasidone	No published data could be found

Mood-stabilisers in breast-feeding

Drug	Comment
Carbamazepine[100–103]	Carbamazepine is excreted in breast milk. Infant serum levels range from 6% to 65% of maternal serum levels. Adverse effects have been reported in a number of infants exposed to carbamazepine during breast-feeding. These include one case of cholestatic hepatitis, and one of transient hepatic dysfunction with hyperbilirubinaemia and elevated GGT. The adverse effects in the first case resolved after discontinuation of breast-feeding and the second resolved despite continued feeding. Other adverse effects reported include seizure-like activity, drowsiness, irritability, and high-pitched crying in one infant whose mother was on multiple agents, hyperexcitability in two infants and poor feeding in another three. In contrast, in a number of infants, no adverse effects were noted The manufacturers of carbamazepine advise that breastfeeding can be considered if the benefits outweigh the risk to the child. The infant must be observed for possible adverse reactions
Lamotrigine[104–110]	Lamotrigine is excreted in breast milk. Infant serum levels range between 18% and 50% of maternal serum levels No adverse effects were noted in 30 nursing infants exposed to lamotrigine. In particular none of the infants developed a rash. In addition, no change in the hepatic and electrolyte profiles was noted in ten of the infants for whom clinical laboratory data were available. However, thrombocytosis was noted in seven infants Because of the theoretical risk of life-threatening rashes, it is advisable to avoid lamotrigine while breast-feeding until more data on its effects become available The manufacturers of lamotrigine advise that the benefits be weighed against the risk to the child
Lithium[103,111–113]	Lithium is excreted in breast milk. Infant serum levels range from 5% to 200% of maternal serum concentrations. Adverse effects have been reported in infants exposed to lithium while breast-feeding. One infant developed cyanosis, lethargy, hypothermia, hypotonia, and a heart murmur, all of which resolved within 3 days of stopping breast-feeding. The infant was exposed to lithium in utero. Non-specific signs of toxicity have been reported in others. There are also reports of no adverse effects in some infants exposed to lithium while breast-feeding Opinions on the use of lithium while breast-feeding vary from absolute contra-indication to mother's informed choice. Conditions which may alter the infant's electrolyte balance and state of hydration must be borne in mind. If it is used, the infant must be carefully monitored for signs of toxicity Breast-feeding is contra-indicated by the manufacturers of lithium
Valproate[103,114–118]	Valproate is excreted into breast milk. Infant serum levels vary from undetectable to 40% of maternal serum levels. Thrombocytopenia and anaemia were reported in a 3-month-old infant exposed to valproate in utero and while breast-feeding. This reversed on stopping breast-feeding The manufacturers of valproate state that there appears to be no contra-indication to its use in breastfeeding. However, hepatotoxicity due to valproate is much more likely in the young so there is a theoretical and important risk in breast-fed infants

Sedatives in breast-feeding

Drug	Comment
Benzodiazepines[119–126]	Diazepam is excreted in breast milk. Infant serum levels vary from undetectable to around 14% of the maternal serum levels. In some infants, no adverse effects were noted. In others, reported adverse effects included sedation, lethargy, and weight loss. Lorazepam, temazepam, and clonazepam are excreted in breast milk in small amounts. Apart from one case report of persistent apnoea in one infant exposed to clonazepam in utero and during breast-feeding, no adverse effects were reported
	Benzodiazepines with a long half-life, such as diazepam, should be avoided in breast-feeding. Any infant exposed to benzodiazepines in breast milk should be monitored for CNS depression and apnoea
Promethazine	No published data could be found. The manufacturers of promethazine issue no specific advice on its use in breastfeeding
Zopiclone, zolpidem and zaleplon[127–129]	All three are excreted into breast milk in small amounts. No adverse effects were noted in exposed infants
	Peak concentrations of zolpidem in breast milk were found 4 hours after ingestion of a single 20-mg dose. Zaleplon peak breast milk levels were found 1 hour after the dose and breast milk concentrations were approximately 50% of plasma concentrations
	The manufacturers of zopiclone, zolpidem, and zaleplon advise against their use in breast-feeding

References

1. Burt VK et al. The use of psychotropic medications during breast-feeding. Am J Psychiatry 2001; 158:1001–1009.
2. Yoshida K et al. Psychotropic drugs in mothers' milk: a comprehensive review of assay methods, pharmacokinetics and of safety of breast-feeding. J Psychopharmacol 1999; 13:64–80.
3. Misri S et al. Benefits and risks to mother and infant of drug treatment for postnatal depression. Drug Saf 2002; 25:903–911.
4. Yoshida K et al. Investigation of pharmacokinetics and of possible adverse effects in infants exposed to tricyclic antidepressants in breast-milk. J Affect Disord 1997; 43:225–237.
5. Frey OR et al. Adverse effects in a newborn infant breast-fed by a mother treated with doxepin. Ann Pharmacother 1999; 33:690–693.
6. Ilett KF et al. The excretion of dothiepin and its primary metabolites in breast milk. Br J Clin Pharmacol 1992; 33:635–639.
7. Kemp J et al. Excretion of doxepin and N-desmethyldoxepin in human milk. Br J Clin Pharmacol 1985; 20:497–499.
8. Buist A et al. Effect of exposure to dothiepin and northiaden in breast milk on child development. Br J Psychiatry 1995; 167:370–373.
9. National Institute for Clinical Excellence. Antenatal and postnatal mental health. Clinical management and service guidance (reissued April 2007). 2007. http://www.nice.org.uk/.
10. Burt VK et al. The use of psychotropic medications during breast-feeding. Am J Psychiatry 2001; 158:1001–1009.
11. Lee A et al. Frequency of infant adverse events that are associated with citalopram use during breast-feeding. Am J Obstet Gynecol 2004; 190:218–221.
12. Heikkinen T et al. Citalopram in pregnancy and lactation. Clin Pharmacol Ther 2002; 72:184–191.
13. Jensen PN et al. Citalopram and desmethylcitalopram concentrations in breast milk and in serum of mother and infant. Ther Drug Monit 1997; 19:236–239.
14. Spigset O et al. Excretion of citalopram in breast milk. Br J Clin Pharmacol 1997; 44:295–298.
15. Rampono J et al. Citalopram and demethylcitalopram in human milk; distribution, excretion and effects in breast fed infants. Br J Clin Pharmacol 2000; 50:263–268.
16. Schmidt K et al. Citalopram and breast-feeding: serum concentration and side effects in the infant. Biol Psychiatry 2000; 47:164–165.
17. Franssen EJ et al. Citalopram serum and milk levels in mother and infant during lactation. Ther Drug Monit 2006; 28:2–4.
18. Gentile S. Escitalopram late in pregnancy and while breast-feeding (Letter). Ann Pharmacother 2006; 40:1696–1697.
19. Castberg I et al. Excretion of escitalopram in breast milk. J Clin Psychopharmacol 2006; 26:536–538.
20. Rampono J et al. Transfer of escitalopram and its metabolite demethylescitalopram into breastmilk. Br J Clin Pharmacol 2006; 62:316–322.
21. Burt VK et al. The use of psychotropic medications during breast-feeding. Am J Psychiatry 2001; 158:1001–1009.
22. Hendrick V et al. Use of sertraline, paroxetine and fluvoxamine by nursing women. Br J Psychiatry 2001; 179:163–166.
23. Piontek CM et al. Serum fluvoxamine levels in breastfed infants. J Clin Psychiatry 2001; 62:111–113.
24. Yoshida K et al. Fluvoxamine in breast-milk and infant development. Br J Clin Pharmacol 1997; 44:210–211.
25. Hagg S et al. Excretion of fluvoxamine into breast milk. Br J Clin Pharmacol 2000; 49:286–288.
26. Arnold LM et al. Fluvoxamine concentrations in breast milk and in maternal and infant sera. J Clin Psychopharmacol 2000; 20:491–492.
27. Kristensen JH et al. The amount of fluvoxamine in milk is unlikely to be a cause of adverse effects in breastfed infants. J Hum Lact 2002; 18:139–143.
28. Burt VK et al. The use of psychotropic medications during breast-feeding. Am J Psychiatry 2001; 158:1001–1009.
29. Yoshida K et al. Fluoxetine in breast-milk and developmental outcome of breast-fed infants. Br J Psychiatry 1998; 172:175–178.
30. Lester BM et al. Possible association between fluoxetine hydrochloride and colic in an infant. J Am Acad Child Adolesc Psychiatry 1993; 32:1253–1255.
31. Hendrick V et al. Fluoxetine and norfluoxetine concentrations in nursing infants and breast milk. Biol Psychiatry 2001; 50:775–782.

32. Hale TW et al. Fluoxetine toxicity in a breastfed infant. Clin Pediatr 2001; 40:681–684.
33. Malone K et al. Antidepressants, antipsychotics, benzodiazepines, and the breastfeeding dyad. Perspect Psychiatr Care 2004; 40:73–85.
34. Heikkinen T et al. Pharmacokinetics of fluoxetine and norfluoxetine in pregnancy and lactation. Clin Pharmacol Ther 2003; 73:330–337.
35. Epperson CN et al. Maternal fluoxetine treatment in the postpartum period: effects on platelet serotonin and plasma drug levels in breastfeeding mother–infant pairs. Pediatrics 2003; 112:e425.
36. Burt VK et al. The use of psychotropic medications during breast-feeding. Am J Psychiatry 2001; 158:1001–1009.
37. Hendrick V et al. Use of sertraline, paroxetine and fluvoxamine by nursing women. Br J Psychiatry 2001; 179:163–166.
38. Malone K et al. Antidepressants, antipsychotics, benzodiazepines, and the breastfeeding dyad. Perspect Psychiatr Care 2004; 40:73–85.
39. Begg EJ et al. Paroxetine in human milk. Br J Clin Pharmacol 1999; 48:142–147.
40. Stowe ZN et al. Paroxetine in human breast milk and nursing infants. Am J Psychiatry 2000; 157:185–189.
41. Misri S et al. Paroxetine levels in postpartum depressed women, breast milk, and infant serum. J Clin Psychiatry 2000; 61:828–832.
42. Ohman R et al. Excretion of paroxetine into breast milk. J Clin Psychiatry 1999; 60:519–523.
43. Berle JO et al. Breastfeeding during maternal antidepressant treatment with serotonin reuptake inhibitors: infant exposure, clinical symptoms, and cytochrome p450 genotypes. J Clin Psychiatry 2004; 65:1228–1234.
44. Merlob P et al. Paroxetine during breast-feeding: infant weight gain and maternal adherence to counsel. Eur J Pediatr 2004; 163:135–139.
45. Abdul Aziz A et al. Severe paroxetine induced hyponatremia in a breast fed infant. J Bahrain Med Soc 2004; 16:195–198.
46. Malone K et al. Antidepressants, antipsychotics, benzodiazepines, and the breastfeeding dyad. Perspect Psychiatr Care 2004; 40:73–85.
47. Berle JO et al. Breastfeeding during maternal antidepressant treatment with serotonin reuptake inhibitors: infant exposure, clinical symptoms, and cytochrome p450 genotypes. J Clin Psychiatry 2004; 65:1228–1234.
48. Llewellyn A et al. Psychotropic medications in lactation. J Clin Psychiatry 1998; 59 Suppl 2:41–52.
49. Hackett LP et al. Transfer of reboxetine into breastmilk, its plasma concentrations and lack of adverse effects in the breastfed infant. Eur J Clin Pharmacol 2006; 62:633–638.
50. Malone K et al. Antidepressants, antipsychotics, benzodiazepines, and the breastfeeding dyad. Perspect Psychiatr Care 2004; 40:73–85.
51. Berle JO et al. Breastfeeding during maternal antidepressant treatment with serotonin reuptake inhibitors: infant exposure, clinical symptoms, and cytochrome p450 genotypes. J Clin Psychiatry 2004; 65:1228–1234.
52. Koren G et al. Can venlafaxine in breast milk attenuate the norepinephrine and serotonin reuptake neonatal withdrawal syndrome. J Obstet Gynaecol Can 2006; 28:299–302.
53. Ilett KF et al. Distribution of venlafaxine and its O-desmethyl metabolite in human milk and their effects in breastfed infants. Br J Clin Pharmacol 2002; 53:17–22.
54. Pons G et al. Moclobemide excretion in human breast milk. Br J Clin Pharmacol 1990; 29:27–31.
55. Buist A et al. Plasma and human milk concentrations of moclobemide in nursing mothers. Hum Psychopharmacol 1998; 13:579–582.
56. Buist A et al. Mianserin in breast milk (Letter). Br J Clin Pharmacol 1993; 36:133–134.
57. Aichhorn W et al. Mirtazapine and breast-feeding. Am J Psychiatry 2004; 161:2325.
58. Klier CM et al. Mirtazapine and breastfeeding: maternal and infant plasma levels. Am J Psychiatry 2007; 164:348–349.
59. Kristensen JH et al. Transfer of the antidepressant mirtazapine into breast milk. Br J Clin Pharmacol 2007; 63:322–327.
60. Verbeeck RK et al. Excretion of trazodone in breast milk. Br J Clin Pharmacol 1986; 22:367–370.
61. Burt VK et al. The use of psychotropic medications during breast-feeding. Am J Psychiatry 2001; 158:1001–1009.
62. Malone K et al. Antidepressants, antipsychotics, benzodiazepines, and the breastfeeding dyad. Perspect Psychiatr Care 2004; 40:73–85.
63. Yoshida K et al. Breast-feeding and psychotropic drugs. Int Rev Psychiatry 1996; 8:117–124.
64. Patton SW et al. Antipsychotic medication during pregnancy and lactation in women with schizophrenia: evaluating the risk. Can J Psychiatry 2002; 47:959–965.
65. Burt VK et al. The use of psychotropic medications during breast-feeding. Am J Psychiatry 2001; 158:1001–1009.
66. Patton SW et al. Antipsychotic medication during pregnancy and lactation in women with schizophrenia: evaluating the risk. Can J Psychiatry 2002; 47:959–965.
67. Burt VK et al. The use of psychotropic medications during breast-feeding. Am J Psychiatry 2001; 158:1001–1009.
68. Matheson I et al. Milk concentrations of flupenthixol, nortriptyline and zuclopenthixol and between-breast differences in two patients. Eur J Clin Pharmacol 1988; 35:217–220.
69. Kirk L et al. Concentrations of Cis(Z)-flupentixol in maternal serum, amniotic fluid, umbilical cord serum, and milk. Psychopharmacology 1980; 72:107–108.
70. aes-Jorgensen T et al. Zuclopenthixol levels in serum and breast milk. Psychopharmacology (Berl) 1986; 90:417–418.
71. Ylikorkala O et al. Treatment of inadequate lactation with oral sulpiride and buccal oxytocin. Obstet Gynecol 1984; 63:57–60.
72. Aono T et al. Augmentation of puerperal lactation by oral administration of sulpiride. J Clin Endocrinol Metab 1970; 48:478–482.
73. Ylikorkala O et al. Sulpiride improves inadequate lactation. Br Med J 1982; 285:249–251.
74. Aono T et al. Effect of sulpiride on poor puerperal lactation. Am J Obstet Gynecol 1982; 143:927–932.
75. Polatti F. Sulpiride isomers and milk secretion in puerperium. Clin Exp Obstet Gynecol 1982; 9:144–147.
76. Schlotterbeck P et al. Aripiprazole in human milk. Int J Neuropsychopharmacol 2007; 10:433.
77. Burt VK et al. The use of psychotropic medications during breast-feeding. Am J Psychiatry 2001; 158:1001–1009.
78. Malone K et al. Antidepressants, antipsychotics, benzodiazepines, and the breastfeeding dyad. Perspect Psychiatric Care 2004; 40:73–85.
79. Patton SW et al. Antipsychotic medication during pregnancy and lactation in women with schizophrenia: evaluating the risk. Can J Psychiatry 2002; 47:959–965.
80. Mendhekar DN. Possible delayed speech acquisition with clozapine therapy during pregnancy and lactation. J Neuropsychiatry Clin Neurosci 2007; 19:196–197.
81. Burt VK et al. The use of psychotropic medications during breast-feeding. Am J Psychiatry 2001; 158:1001–1009.
82. Malone K et al. Antidepressants, antipsychotics, benzodiazepines, and the breastfeeding dyad. Perspect Psychiatr Care 2004; 40:73–85.
83. Goldstein DJ et al. Olanzapine-exposed pregnancies and lactation: early experience. J Clin Psychopharmacol 2000; 20:399–403.
84. Croke S et al. Olanzapine excretion in human breast milk: estimation of infant exposure. Int J Neuropsychopharmacol 2002; 5:243–247.
85. Gardiner SJ et al. Transfer of olanzapine into breast milk, calculation of infant drug dose, and effect on breast-fed infants. Am J Psychiatry 2003; 160:1428–1431.
86. Ambresin G et al. Olanzapine excretion into breast milk: a case report. J Clin Psychopharmacol 2004; 24:93–95.
87. Whitworth A et al. Olanzapine and breast-feeding: changes of plasma concentrations of olanzapine in a breast-fed infant over a period of 5 months. J Psychopharmacol 2008; Epub ahead of print.
88. Lutz UC et al. Olanzapine treatment during breast-feeding: a case report. Ther Drug Monit 2008; 30:399–401.
89. Lee A et al. Excretion of quetiapine in breast milk. Am J Psychiatry 2004; 161:1715–1716.
90. Gentile S. Quetiapine-fluvoxamine combination during pregnancy and while breastfeeding (Letter). Arch Womens Ment Health 2006; 9:158–159.
91. Misri S et al. Quetiapine augmentation in lactation: a series of case reports. J Clin Psychopharmacol 2006; 26:508–511.
92. Ritz S. Quetiapine monotherapy in post-partum onset bipolar disorder with a mixed affective state. Eur Neuropsychopharmacol 2005; 15 Suppl 3:S407.
93. Rampono J et al. Quetiapine and breast-feeding. Ann Pharmacother 2007; 41:711–714.
94. Seppala J. Quetiapine (Seroquel) is effective and well tolerated in the treatment of psychotic depression during breast-feeding. Eur Neuropsychopharmacol 2004;S245.

365

95. Kruninger U et al. Pregnancy and lactation under treatment with quetiapine. Psychiatr Prax 2007; 34 Suppl 1:S75–S76.
96. Ratnayake T et al. No complications with risperidone treatment before and throughout pregnancy and during the nursing period. J Clin Psychiatry 2002; 63:76–77.
97. Hill RC et al. Risperidone distribution and excretion into human milk: case report and estimated infant exposure during breast-feeding. J Clin Psychopharmacol 2000; 20:285–286.
98. Aichhorn W et al. Risperidone and breast-feeding. J Psychopharmacol 2005; 19:211–213.
99. Ilett KF et al. Transfer of risperidone and 9-hydroxyrisperidone into human milk. Ann Pharmacother 2004; 38:273–276.
100. Burt VK et al. The use of psychotropic medications during breast-feeding. Am J Psychiatry 2001; 158:1001–1009.
101. Chaudron LH et al. Mood stabilizers during breastfeeding: a review. J Clin Psychiatry 2000; 61:79–90.
102. Wisner KL et al. Serum levels of valproate and carbamazepine in breastfeeding mother-infant pairs. J Clin Psychopharmacol 1998; 18:167–169.
103. Ernst CL et al. The reproductive safety profile of mood stabilizers, atypical antipsychotics, and broad-spectrum psychotropics. J Clin Psychiatry 2002; 63 Suppl 4:42–55.
104. Ohman I et al. Lamotrigine in pregnancy: pharmacokinetics during delivery, in the neonate, and during lactation. Epilepsia 2000; 41:709–713.
105. Liporace J et al. Concerns regarding lamotrigine and breast-feeding. Epilepsy Behav 2004; 5:102–105.
106. Gentile S. Lamotrigine in pregnancy and lactation (Letter). Arch Womens Ment Health 2005; 8:57–58.
107. Page-Sharp M et al. Transfer of lamotrigine into breast milk (Letter). Ann Pharmacother 2006; 40:1470–1471.
108. Rambeck B et al. Concentrations of lamotrigine in a mother on lamotrigine treatment and her newborn child. Eur J Clin Pharmacol 1997; 51:481–484.
109. Tomson T et al. Lamotrigine in pregnancy and lactation: a case report. Epilepsia 1997; 38:1039–1041.
110. Newport DJ et al. Lamotrigine in breast milk and nursing infants: determination of exposure. Pediatrics 2008; 122:e223–e231.
111. Chaudron LH et al. Mood stabilizers during breastfeeding: a review. J Clin Psychiatry 2000; 61:79–90.
112. Moretti ME et al. Monitoring lithium in breast milk: an individualized approach for breast-feeding mothers. Ther Drug Monit 2003; 25:364–366.
113. Viguera AC et al. Lithium in breast milk and nursing infants: clinical implications. Am J Psychiatry 2007; 164:342–345.
114. Burt VK et al. The use of psychotropic medications during breast-feeding. Am J Psychiatry 2001; 158:1001–1009.
115. Chaudron LH et al. Mood stabilizers during breastfeeding: a review. J Clin Psychiatry 2000; 61:79–90.
116. Wisner KL et al. Serum levels of valproate and carbamazepine in breastfeeding mother-infant pairs. J Clin Psychopharmacol 1998; 18:167–169.
117. Piontek CM et al. Serum valproate levels in 6 breastfeeding mother-infant pairs. J Clin Psychiatry 2000; 61:170–172.
118. Bjornsson E. Hepatotoxicity associated with antiepileptic drugs. Acta Neurol Scand 2008; 118:281–290.
119. Burt VK et al. The use of psychotropic medications during breast-feeding. Am J Psychiatry 2001; 158:1001–1009.
120. Malone K et al. Antidepressants, antipsychotics, benzodiazepines, and the breastfeeding dyad. Perspect Psychiatr Care 2004; 40:73–85.
121. Spigset O et al. Excretion of psychotropic drugs into breast milk: Pharmacokinetic overview and therapeutic implications. CNS Drugs 1998; 9:111–134.
122. Hagg S et al. Anticonvulsant use during lactation. Drug Saf 2000; 22:425–440.
123. Iqbal MM et al. Effects of commonly used benzodiazepines on the fetus, the neonate, and the nursing infant. Psychiatr Serv 2002; 53:39–49.
124. Buist A et al. Breastfeeding and the use of psychotropic medication: a review. J Affect Disord 1990; 19:197–206.
125. Fisher JB et al. Neonatal apnea associated with maternal clonazepam therapy: a case report. Obstet Gynecol 1985; 66:34S–35S.
126. Davanzo R et al. Benzodiazepine e allattamento materno. Medico e Bambino 2008; 27:109–114.
127. Darwish M et al. Rapid disappearance of zaleplon from breast milk after oral administration to lactating women. J Clin Pharmacol 1999; 39:670–674.
128. Pons G et al. Excretion of psychoactive drugs into breast milk. Pharmacokinetic principles and recommendations. Clin Pharmacokinet 1994; 27:270–289.
129. Matheson I et al. The excretion of zopiclone into breast milk. Br J Clin Pharmacol 1990; 30:267–271.

Further reading

Field T. Breastfeeding and antidepressants. Infant Behav Dev 2008; 31:481–487.
Gentile S et al. SSRIs during breastfeeding: spotlight on milk-to-plasma ratio. Arch Womens Ment Health 2007; 10:39–51.
Gentile S. Infant safety with antipsychotic therapy in breast-feeding: a systematic review. J Clin Psychiatry 2008; 69:666–673.

Special groups

Renal impairment

- Using drugs in patients with renal impairment needs careful consideration. This is because some drugs are nephrotoxic and also because pharmacokinetics (absorption, distribution, metabolism, excretion) of drugs are altered in renal impairment.
- Essentially, **patients with renal impairment have a reduced capacity to excrete drugs** and their metabolites.

Prescribing in renal impairment – general principles

1. **Estimate the excretory capacity of the kidney** by calculating the glomerular filtration rate (GFR). GFR can be directly measured by collection of urine over 24 hours, isotope determination or estimated in *adults* in one of two ways[1]; that is creatinine clearance (CrCl) using the Cockroft and Gault equation or estimated GFR (eGFR) using the MDRD below.

(a) Cockroft and Gault equation*

$$\text{CrCl (ml/min)} = \frac{F\,(140 - \text{age (in years)} \times \text{ideal body weight (kg)})}{\text{Serum creatinine } (\mu\text{mol/l})}$$

F = 1.23 (men) and 1.04 (women)

Ideal body weight should be used for patients at extremes of body weight or else the calculation is inaccurate

For men, ideal body weight (kg) = 50 kg + 2.3 kg per inch over 5 feet

For women, ideal body weight (kg) = 45.5 kg + 2.3 kg per inch over 5 feet

*This equation is not accurate if plasma creatinine is unstable, in pregnant women, children or in diseases causing production of abnormal amounts of creatinine and has only been validated in Caucasian patients. Creatinine clearance is less representative of GFR in severe renal failure.

When calculating drug doses use estimated CrCl from the Cockroft and Gault equation.
Do not use MDRD formula (on the following page) for dose calculation because most current dose recommendations are based on the creatinine clearance estimations from Cockroft and Gault.

(b) Modification of Diet in Renal Disease (MDRD) formula

- This gives an estimated GFR (eGFR) for a $1.73\,m^2$ body surface area. If the body surface area is more or less than $1.73\,m^2$ then calculated eGFR becomes less accurate (use correction below).
- Body surface area (BSA) can be calculated as follows

$$m^2 = \sqrt{\frac{\text{height (cm)} \times \text{weight (kg)}}{3600}}$$

- The equation below is what pathology departments use to report eGFR.

  eGFR $(ml/min/1.73\,m^2) = 175 \times [(\text{serum creatinine } (\mu mol/l)/84.4)^{-1.154}] \times$ age $(\text{years})^{-0.203}$
  $\times\ 0.742$ if female
  $\times\ 1.21$ if African American or African Caribbean
  An online calculator is available at www.renal.org/eGFRcalc/GFR.pl

- Actual GFR can be calculated as follows
     Actual GFRw = (eGFR x BSA/1.73)
- **Use Cockroft and Gault for drug dose calculation**

2. **Classify the stage of kidney disease:**

Stage	Description
1	GFR >90 ml/min/1.73 m^2 with other evidence of chronic kidney damage*
2	Mild impairment; GFR 60–89 ml/min/1.73 m^2 with other evidence of kidney damage*
3	Moderate impairment, GFR 30–59 ml/min/1.73 m^2
4	Severe impairment, GFR 15–29 ml/min/1.73 m^2
5	Established renal failure, GFR <15 ml/min/1.73 m^2 **or** on dialysis

*Other evidence of chronic kidney damage is one or more of the following; persistent microalbuminuria; persistent proteinuria; persistent haematuria; structural kidney abnormalities; biopsy proven chronic glomerulonephritis.

3. **Elderly patients (>65 years) are assumed to have mild renal impairment.** Their creatinine may not be raised because they have a smaller muscle mass.
4. **Avoid drugs that are nephrotoxic** (e.g. lithium) in moderate or severe renal failure.
5. **Choose a drug that is safer to use in renal impairment** (see tables below).
6. **Be cautious when using drugs that are extensively renally cleared** (e.g. sulpiride, amisulpride, lithium).
7. **Start at a low dose and increase slowly** because, in renal impairment, the half-life of a drug and the time for it to reach steady state are often prolonged. Plasma level monitoring may be useful for some drugs.
8. **Avoid long-acting drugs** (e.g. depot preparations). Their dose and frequency cannot be easily adjusted should renal function change.
9. **Prescribe as few drugs as possible.** Patients with renal failure take many medications requiring regular review. Interactions and side effects can be avoided if fewer drugs are used.
10. **Monitor patient for adverse effects.** Patients with renal impairment are more likely to experience side effects and they may take longer to develop than in healthy patients. Adverse effects such as sedation, confusion, and postural hypotension can be more common.

11. **Be cautious when using drugs with anticholinergic effects,** since they may cause urinary retention.
12. There are **few clinical studies** of the use of psychotropic drugs in people with renal impairment. Advice about drug use in renal impairment is often based on knowledge of the drug's pharmacokinetics in healthy patients.
13. **The effect of renal replacement therapies on drugs is difficult to predict.** Dosing advice is available from tables and data on each drug's volume of distribution and protein-binding affinity. Seek specialist advice.
14. **Avoid drugs known to prolong QTc interval.** In established renal failure electrolyte changes are common so probably best to avoid antipsychotics with the greatest risk of QTc prolongation (see section on QT prolongation).
15. **Monitor weight carefully.** Weight gain predisposes to diabetes which can cause rhabdomyolysis[2] and renal failure. Psychotropic medications commonly cause weight gain.
16. **Be vigilant for dystonias and neuroleptic malignant syndrome (NMS),** as the resulting rhabdomyolysis can cause or worsen renal failure and there are case reports of rhabdomyolysis occurring with antipsychotics without other symptoms of NMS[3–5].

Table Antipsychotics in renal impairment	
Drug	*Comments*
Amisulpride[6–9]	Primarily renally excreted. 50% excreted unchanged in urine. Limited experience in renal disease. Manufacturer states no data with doses of >50 mg but recommends following dosing: 50% of dose if GFR 30–60 ml/min; 33% of dose if GFR is 10–30 ml/min; no recommendations for GFR <10 ml/min so best avoided in established renal failure
Aripiprazole[6,7,9–11]	Less than 1% of unchanged aripiprazole renally excreted. Manufacturer states no dose adjustment required in renal failure as pharmacokinetics are similar in healthy and severely renally diseased patients
Chlorpromazine[6,7,9,12,13]	Less than 1% excreted unchanged in urine. Manufacturer advises avoiding in renal dysfunction. Dosing: GFR 10–50 ml/min, dose as in normal renal function; GFR <10 ml/min, start with a small dose because of an increased risk of anticholinergic, sedative and hypotensive side effects. Monitor carefully
Clozapine[7,9,14–17]	Only trace amounts of unchanged clozapine excreted in urine; however there are rare case reports of interstitial nephritis and acute renal failure. Nocturnal enuresis and urinary retention are common side effects. Contra-indicated by manufacturer in severe renal disease. Anticholinergic, sedative and hypotensive side effects occur more frequently in patients with renal disease. Dosing: GFR 10–50 ml/min as in normal renal function but with caution; GFR <10 ml/min start with a low dose and titrate slowly (based on renal specialist opinion). Levels are useful to guide dosing. May cause and aggravate diabetes, a common cause of renal disease
Flupentixol[6,7,9]	Negligible renal excretion of unchanged flupentixol. Dosing: GFR 10–50 ml/min dose as in normal renal function; GFR <10 ml/min start with ¼ to ½ of normal dose and titrate slowly. May cause hypotension and sedation in renal impairment and can accumulate. Manufacturer recommends caution in renal failure. Avoid depot preparations in renal impairment

Table	Antipsychotics in renal impairment (Cont.)
Drug	**Comments**
Fluphenazine[7,9]	Little information available; manufacturer contra-indicates in renal insufficiency and renal failure. Dosing: GFR 10–50 ml/min dose as in normal renal function; GFR <10 ml/min start with a low dose and titrate slowly. Avoid depot preparations in renal impairment
Haloperidol[4,6,7,9,13,18,19]	Less than 1% excreted unchanged in the urine. Manufacturer advises caution in renal failure. Dosing: GFR 10–50 ml/min, dose as in normal renal function; GFR <10 ml/min start with a lower dose as can accumulate with repeated dosing. A case report of haloperidol use in renal failure suggests starting at a low dose and increasing slowly. Avoid depot preparations in renal impairment
Olanzapine[3,6,7,9,19]	57% of olanzapine is excreted mainly as metabolites (7% excreted unchanged) in urine. Dosing: GFR <10–50 ml/min initially, 5 mg daily and titrate as necessary. Avoid depot preparation in renal impairment unless the oral dose is well tolerated and effective. Manufacturer recommends a lower depot starting dose of 150 mg 4 weekly in patients with renal impairment. May cause and aggravate diabetes, a common cause of renal disease
Paliperidone[6,7,9]	Paliperidone is a metabolite of risperidone. 59% excreted unchanged in urine. Dosing: GFR 30–80 ml/min, 3 mg daily and increase according to response to max of 6 mg daily; GFR 10–30 ml/min, 3 mg alternate days increasing to 3 mg daily according to response. Use with caution as clearance is markedly reduced in end-stage disease. Manufacturer contraindicates use if GFR <10 ml/min due to lack of experience. Avoid depot preparation
Pimozide[6,7,9]	Less than 1% of pimozide is excreted unchanged in the urine; dose reductions not usually needed in renal impairment. Dosing: GFR 10–50 ml/min, dose as in normal renal function; GFR <10 ml/min start at a low dose and increase according to response. Manufacturer cautions in renal failure
Pipotiazine[7]	Little information available; contra-indicated in renal failure by manufacturer. Avoid depot preparations in renal impairment
Quetiapine[6,7,9,20,21]	Less than 5% of quetiapine excreted unchanged in the urine. Plasma clearance reduced by an average of 25% in patients with a GFR <30 ml/min. In patients with GFR of <10–50 ml/min start at 25 mg/day and increase in daily increments of 25–50 mg to an effective dose. Two separate case reports, one of thrombotic thrombocytopenic purpura and another of non-NMS rhabdoymolysis both resulting in acute renal failure with quetiapine have been described
Risperidone[6,7,9,19,22,23]	Clearance of risperidone and the active metabolite of risperidone is reduced by 60% in patients with moderate to severe renal disease. Dosing : GFR <50 ml/min 0.5 mg twice daily for at least 1 week then increasing by 0.5 mg twice daily to 1–2 mg bd. The manufacturer advises caution when using risperidone in renal impairment. The long-acting injection should only be used after titration with oral risperidone as described above. If 2 mg orally is tolerated, 25 mg intramuscularly every 2 weeks can be administered. A case report of the successful use of risperidone use in a child with steroid-induced psychosis and nephrotic syndrome has been described

Table	Antipsychotics in renal impairment (Cont.)
Drug	**Comments**
Sertindole[6,7,24]	Less than 1% of sertindole is excreted into urine. A single-dose study of sertindole found no dose adjustment needed in mild, moderate or severe renal impairment. The manufacturers state no dose adjustment needed in renal impairment. Dosing: GFR 10–50 ml/min dose as in normal renal function; GFR <10 ml/min dose as normal renal function but start at a low dose and increase according to response
Sulpiride[2,6,7,9,25]	Almost totally renally excreted, with 95% excreted in urine and faeces as unchanged sulpiride. Dosing regimen: GFR 30–60 ml/min, give 70% of normal dose; GFR 10–30 ml/min give 50% of normal dose; GFR <10 ml/min give 34% of normal dose. There is a case report of renal failure with sulpiride due to diabetic coma and rhabdomyolysis. Manufacturer contra-indicates in severe renal disease. Probably best avoided in renal impairment
Trifluoperazine[9]	Less than 1% excreted unchanged in the urine. Dose GFR <10–50 ml/min as for normal renal function – start with a low dose
Ziprasidone[6,19,26,27]	<1% is renally excreted unchanged. No dose adjustment needed for GFR >10 ml/min but care needed with using the injection as it contains a renally eliminated excipient (cyclodextrin sodium)
Zotepine[6,9,28]	<0.1% is excreted as unchanged zotepine in urine. Patients with renal dysfunction have higher plasma levels than healthy patients, so start low, gradually titrate and reduce the maximum daily dose. The manufacturer suggests a starting dose of 25 mg twice daily, gradually titrating to a maximum of 75 mg twice daily in patients with established renal impairment. Can increase creatinine levels, avoid in nephrolithiasis
Zuclopentixol[6,7,9]	10–20% of unchanged drug and metabolites excreted unchanged in urine. Manufacturer cautions use in renal disease as can accumulate. Dosing: 10–50 ml/min dose as in normal renal function; GFR <10 ml/min start with 50% of the dose and titrate slowly. Avoid depot preparation in renal impairment

Table Antidepressants in renal impairment

Drug	Comments
Amitriptyline[6,7,9,13,19,29-31]	<2% excreted unchanged in urine; no dose adjustment needed in renal failure. Dose as in normal renal function but start at a low dose and increase slowly. Monitor patient for urinary retention, confusion, sedation, and postural hypotension. Has been used to treat pain in those with renal disease. Plasma level monitoring may be useful
Bupropion[6,7,9,13,19,32,33] (amfebutamone)	0.5% excreted unchanged in the urine. Dosing: GFR <50 ml/min, 150 mg once daily. A single-dose study in haemodialysis patients (stage 5 disease) recommended a dose of 150 mg every 3 days. Metabolites may accumulate in renal impairment and clearance is reduced. Elevated levels increase risk of seizures
Citalopram[6,7,9,19,34-37]	<13% of citalopram is excreted unchanged in the urine. Single-dose studies in mild and moderate renal impairment show no change in the pharmacokinetics of citalopram. Dosing is as for normal renal function; however, use with caution if GFR <10 ml/min due to reduced clearance. The manufacturer does not advise use if GFR <20 ml/min. Renal failure has been reported with citalopram overdose. Has been shown to treat depression in chronic renal failure and improve quality of life
Clomipramine[6,7,9,13,38]	2% of unchanged clomipramine is excreted in the urine. Dosing: GFR 20-50 ml/min, dose as for normal renal function; GFR <20 ml/min, effects unknown, start at a low dose and monitor patient for urinary retention, confusion, sedation, and postural hypotension as accumulation can occur. There is a case report of clomipramine-induced interstitial nephritis and reversible acute renal failure
Dosulepin[6,9,39] (dothiepin)	56% of mainly active metabolites renally excreted. They have a long half-life and may accumulate, resulting in excessive sedation. Dosing: GFR 20-50 ml/min, dose as for normal renal function; GFR <20 ml/min, start with a small dose and titrate to response. Monitor patient for urinary retention, confusion, sedation, and postural hypotension
Doxepin[6,7,9,13]	<1% excreted unchanged in urine. Dose as in normal renal function but monitor patient for urinary retention, confusion, sedation and postural hypotension. Manufacturer advises using with caution. Haemolytic anaemia with renal failure has been reported with doxepin
Duloxetine[6,9]	Manufacturer states no dose adjustment is necessary for GFR >30 ml/min; however, starting at a low dose and increasing slowly is advised. Duloxetine is contra-indicated in patients with a GFR <30 ml/min as it can accumulate in chronic kidney disease. Licensed to treat diabetic neuropathic pain. Diabetes is a common cause of renal impairment
Escitalopram[6,9,40,41]	8% excreted unchanged in urine. The manufacturer states dosage adjustment is not necessary in patients with mild or moderate renal impairment but caution is advised if GFR <30 ml/min so start with a low dose and increase slowly. A case study of reversible renal tubular defects and another of renal failure have been reported with escitalopram
Fluvoxamine[6,9,13,19]	Little information on its use in renal impairment. Manufacturer cautions in renal impairment. Dosing: GFR 10-50 ml/min dose as for normal renal function; GFR <10 ml/min dose as for normal renal function but start on a low dose and titrate slowly

Table Antidepressants in renal impairment (Cont.)

Drug	Comments
Fluoxetine[6,7,9,13,19,42–44]	2.5–5% of fluoxetine and 10% of the active metabolite norfluoxetine are excreted in the urine. Dosing: GFR 20–50 ml/min dose as normal renal function; GFR <20 ml/min use a low dose or on alternate days and increase according to response. Plasma levels after 2 months treatment (in patients on dialysis with GFR <10 ml/min) are similar to those with normal renal function. One small placebo-controlled study of fluoxetine in patients on chronic dialysis found no significant differences in depression scores between the two groups
Imipramine[6,7,9,13,29]	<5% excreted unchanged in the urine. No specific dose adjustment necessary in renal impairment (GFR <10–50 ml/min). Monitor patient for urinary retention, confusion, sedation, and postural hypotension. Renal impairment with imipramine has been reported and manufacturer advises caution in severe renal impairment. Renal damage reported rarely
Lofepramine[6,7,9,45]	There is little information about the use of lofepramine in renal impairment. Less than 5% is excreted unchanged in the urine. Dosing: GFR 10–50 ml/min dose as in normal renal function; GFR <10 ml/min start with a small dose and titrate slowly. Manufacturer contra-indicates in severe renal impairment
Mirtazapine[6,7,9,46]	75% excreted unchanged in the urine. Clearance is reduced by 30% in patients with a GFR of 11–39 ml/min and by 50% in patients with a GFR <10 ml/min. Dosing advice: GFR 10–50 ml/min dose as for normal renal function; GFR <10 ml/min start at a low dose and monitor closely. Mirtazapine has been used to treat pruritis caused by renal failure but is associated with kidney calculus formation
Moclobemide[6,7,9,47,48]	<1% of parent drug excreted unchanged in the urine. However, an active metabolite was found to be raised in patients with renal impairment but was not thought to affect dosing. The manufacturer advises that dose adjustments are not required in renal impairment. Dosing: GFR <10–50 ml/min dose as in normal renal function
Nortriptyline[6,9,13,19,29,49]	If GFR 10–50 ml/min, dose as in normal renal function; if GFR <10 ml/min start at a low dose. Plasma level monitoring recommended at doses of >100 mg/day, as plasma concentrations of active metabolites are raised in renal impairment. Worsening of GFR in elderly patients has also been reported. Plasma level monitoring can be useful
Paroxetine[6,7,9,13,50–53]	Less than 2% of oral dose is excreted unchanged in the urine. Single-dose studies show increased plasma concentrations of paroxetine when GFR <30 ml/min. Dosing advice differs: GFR 30–50 ml/min dose as normal renal function; GFR <10–30 ml/min start at 10 mg/day (other source says start at 20 mg) and increase dose according to response. Paroxetine 10 mg daily and psychotherapy have been used successfully to treat depression in patients on chronic haemodialysis. Rarely associated with Fanconi syndrome and acute renal failure
Phenelzine[6,9]	Approximately 1% excreted unchanged in the urine. No dose adjustment required in renal failure

Table Antidepressants in renal impairment (Cont.)

Drug	Comments
Reboxetine[6,7,9,54,55]	Approximately 10% of unchanged drug is excreted unchanged in the urine. Dosing: GFR <20 ml/min, 2 mg twice daily, adjusting dose according to response. Half-life is prolonged as renal function decreases
Sertraline[6,7,9,13,56]	<0.2% of unchanged sertraline excreted in urine. Pharmacokinetics in renal impairment are unchanged in single-dose studies but no published data on multiple dosing. Dosing is as for normal renal function. Sertraline has been used to treat dialysis-associated hypotension; however acute renal failure has been reported so it should be used with caution
Trazodone[6,7,9,57]	<5% excreted unchanged in urine but care needed as approximately 70% of active metabolite also excreted. Dosing: GFR 20–50 ml/min, dose as normal renal function; GFR 10–20 ml/min, dose as normal renal function but start with small dose and increase gradually; GFR <10 ml/min, start with small doses and increase gradually
Trimipramine[6,9,13,29,58,59]	No dose reduction required in renal impairment; however, elevated urea, acute renal failure, and interstitial nephritis have been reported. As with all tricyclic antidepressants, monitor patient for urinary retention, confusion, sedation, and postural hypotension as patients with renal impairment are at increased risk of having these side effects
Venlafaxine[6,7,13,60–62]	1–10% is excreted unchanged in the urine (30% as the active metabolite). Clearance is decreased and half-life prolonged in renal impairment. Dosing advice differs: GFR 30–50 ml/min, dose as in normal renal function or reduce by 50%; GFR 10–30 ml/min reduce dose by 50% and give tablets once daily; GFR <10 ml/min, reduce dose by 50% and give once daily, however manufacturer advises avoiding use in these patients. Avoid using the XL preparation if GFR <30 ml/min. Rhabdomyolysis and renal failure have been reported rarely with venlafaxine. Has been used to treat peripheral diabetic neuropathy in haemodialysis patients

Table Mood-stabilisers in renal impairment

Drug	Comments
Carbamazepine[6,7,9,63–69]	2–3% of the dose is excreted unchanged in urine. Dose reduction not necessary in renal disease, although cases of renal failure, tubular necrosis, and tubulointerstitial nephritis have been reported rarely and metabolites may accumulate
Lamotrigine[6,7,9,70–73]	<10% of lamotrigine is excreted unchanged in the urine. Single-dose studies in renal failure show pharmacokinetics are little affected: however, inactive metabolites can accumulate (effects unknown) and half-life can be prolonged. Renal failure and interstitial nephritis have also been reported. Dosing: GFR <10–50 ml/min, use cautiously, start with a low dose, increase slowly and monitor closely. One source suggests in GFR <10 ml/min use 100 mg every other day
Lithium[6,7,9,13,74,75]	Lithium is nephrotoxic and contraindicated in severe renal impairment; 95% is excreted unchanged in the urine. Long-term treatment may result in impaired renal function ('creeping creatinine'), permanent changes in kidney histology and both reversible and irreversible kidney damage. If lithium is used in renal impairment, toxicity is more likely. The manufacturer contra-indicates lithium in renal impairment. Dosing: GFR 10–50 ml/min, avoid or reduce dose (50–75% of normal dose) and monitor levels; GFR <10 ml/min, avoid if possible, however if used it is essential to reduce dose (25–50% of normal dose). Renal damage is more likely with chronic toxicity than with acute
Valproate[6,7,9,76–82]	Approximately 2% excreted unchanged. Dose adjustment usually not required in renal impairment; however, free valproate levels may be increased. Renal impairment, interstitial nephritis, Fanconi's syndrome, renal tubular acidosis, and renal failure have been reported. Dose as in normal renal function, however in severe impairment (GFR <10 ml/min) it may be necessary to alter doses according to free (unbound) valproate levels

Table	Anxiolytics and hypnotics in renal impairment
Drug	**Comments**
Buspirone[6,7,9,13]	Less than 1% is excreted unchanged; however, active metabolite is renally excreted. Dosing advice contradictory, suggest: GFR 10–50 ml/min dose as normal; GFR <10 ml/min avoid if possible due to accumulation of active metabolites; if essential, reduce dose by 25–50% if patient is anuric. Manufacturer contra-indicates in severe renal impairment
Clomethiazole[6,7,9,83] (chlormethiazole)	0.1–5% of unchanged drug excreted unchanged in urine. Dose as in normal renal function but monitor for excessive sedation. Manufacturer recommends caution in renal disease
Chlordiazepoxide[7,9,13]	1–2% excreted unchanged but chlordiazepoxide has a long-acting active metabolite that can accumulate. Dosing: GFR 10–50 ml/min, dose as normal renal function; GFR <10 ml/min, reduce dose by 50%. Monitor for excessive sedation
Clonazepam[6,7,9]	<0.5% of clonazepam excreted unchanged in urine. Dose adjustment not required in impaired renal function; however with long-term administration, active metabolites may accumulate so start at a low dose and increase according to response. Monitor for excessive sedation
Diazepam[6,9,13,84]	Less than 0.5% is excreted unchanged. Dosing: GFR 20–50 ml/min, dose as in normal renal function; GFR <20 ml/min, use small doses and titrate to response. Long-acting, active metabolites accumulate in renal impairment; monitor patients for excessive sedation and encephalopathy. One case of interstitial nephritis with diazepam has been reported in a patient with chronic renal failure
Lorazepam[6,7,9,13,85–89]	<1% excreted unchanged in urine, dose as in normal renal function but carefully according to response as some may need lower doses. Monitor for excessive sedation. Impaired elimination reported in two patients with severe renal impairment and also reports of propylene glycol in lorazepam injection causing renal impairment and acute tubular necrosis
Nitrazepam[7,9]	Less than 5% excreted unchanged in the urine. Dosing GFR 10–50 ml/min as per normal renal function; GFR <10 ml/min start with small dose and increase slowly. Manufacturer advises reducing dose in renal impairment. Monitor patient for sedation
Oxazepam[6,9,13,90]	Less than 1% excreted unchanged in the urine. Dose adjustment needed in severe renal impairment. Oxazepam may take longer to reach steady state in patients with renal impairment. Dosing: GFR 10–50 ml/min, dose as in normal renal function; GFR <10 ml/min, start at a low dose and increase according to response. Monitor for excessive sedation
Promethazine[6,7,9,13]	Dose reduction usually not necessary; however, promethazine has a long half-life so monitor for excessive sedative effects in patients with renal impairment. Manufacturer advises caution in renal impairment
Temazepam[6,7,9,13]	<2% excreted unchanged in urine. In renal impairment the inactive metabolite can accumulate. Monitor for excessive sedative effects. Dosing: GFR 20–50 ml/min, dose as normal renal function; GFR <10–20 ml/min, dose as in normal renal function but start with small doses

Table	Anxiolytics and hypnotics in renal impairment (Cont.)
Drug	**Comments**
Zaleplon[6,7,91,92]	In renal impairment inactive metabolites accumulate. No dose adjustment appears to be necessary in patients with a GFR >20 ml/min. Zaleplon is not recommended if GFR <20 ml/min, however it has been used in patients on haemodialysis
Zolpidem[6,7,9,91]	Clearance moderately reduced in renal impairment. No dose adjustment required in renal impairment; however there are no published studies of zolpidem in severe renal impairment
Zopiclone[6,7,9,93,94]	Less than 5% excreted unchanged in urine. Manufacturer states no accumulation of zopiclone in renal impairment but suggests starting at 3.75 mg. Dosing: GFR <10 ml/min, start with lower dose. Can cause interstitial nephritis rarely

Summary – psychotropics in renal impairment

Drug group	Recommended drugs
Antipsychotics	No agent clearly preferred to another, however: • avoid sulpiride and amisulpride • avoid highly anticholinergic agents because they may cause urinary retention • first-generation antipsychotic – suggest **haloperidol** 2–6 mg a day • second-generation antipsychotic – suggest **olanzapine** 5 mg a day
Antidepressants	No agent clearly preferred to another, however: • **citalopram** and **sertraline** are suggested as reasonable choices
Mood-stabilisers	No agent clearly preferred to another, however: • avoid lithium • suggest start one of the following at a low dose and increase slowly, monitor for adverse effects: **valproate, carbamazepine,** and **lamotrigine**
Anxiolytics and hypnotics	No agent clearly preferred to another, however: • excessive sedation is more likely to occur in patients with renal impairment, so monitor all patients carefully • **lorazepam** and **zopiclone** are suggested as reasonable choices

References

1. Devaney A et al. Chronic kidney disease — new approaches to classification. Hospital Pharmacist 2006; 13:410.
2. Toprak O et al. New-onset type II diabetes mellitus, hyperosmolar non-ketotic coma, rhabdomyolysis and acute renal failure in a patient treated with sulpiride. Nephrol Dial Transplant 2005; 20:662–663.
3. Baumgart U et al. Olanzapine-induced acute rhabdomyolysis-a case report. Pharmacopsychiatry 2005; 38:36–37.
4. Marsh SJ et al. Rhabdomyolysis and acute renal failure during high-dose haloperidol therapy. Ren Fail 1995; 17:475–478.
5. Smith RP et al. Quetiapine overdose and severe rhabdomyolysis. J Clin Psychopharmacol 2004; 24:343.
6. Micromedex® Healthcare Series. DRUGDEX® System. 2009. Englewood, Colorado, first quarter.
7. Datapharm Communications Ltd. Electronic Medicines Compendium. 2009. http://emc.medicines.org.uk/
8. Noble S et al. Amisulpride: a review of its clinical potential in dysthymia. CNS Drugs 1999; 12:471–483.
9. Ashley C, Currie A. The Renal Drug Handbook, 3rd Edn. Oxford: Radcliffe Publishing Ltd; 2009.
10. Aragona M. Tolerability and efficacy of aripiprazole in a case of psychotic anorexia nervosa comorbid with epilepsy and chronic renal failure. Eat Weight Disord 2007; 12:e54–e57.
11. Mallikaarjun S et al. Effects of hepatic or renal impairment on the pharmacokinetics of aripiprazole. Clin Pharmacokinet 2008; 47:533–542.
12. Fabre J et al. Influence of renal insufficiency on the excretion of chloroquine, phenobarbital, phenothiazines and methacycline. Helv Med Acta 1967; 33:307–316.
13. Aronoff GR, Berns JS, Brier ME, Golper TA, Morrison G, Singer I. Drug Prescribing in Renal Failure: Dosing Guidelines for Adults and Children. 5th edn. Philadelphia: American College of Physicians; 2007.
14. Fraser D et al. An unexpected and serious complication of treatment with the atypical antipsychotic drug clozapine. Clin Nephrol 2000; 54:78–80.
15. Au AF et al. Clozapine-induced acute interstitial nephritis. Am J Psychiatry 2004; 161:1501.
16. Elias TJ et al. Clozapine-induced acute interstitial nephritis. Lancet 1999; 354:1180–1181.
17. Siddiqui BK et al. Simultaneous allergic interstitial nephritis and cardiomyopathy in a patient on clozapine. NDT Plus 2008; 1:55–56.
18. Lobeck F et al. Haloperidol concentrations in an elderly patient with moderate chronic renal failure. J Geriatr Drug Ther 1986; 1:91–97.

Special groups

19. Cohen LM et al. Update on psychotropic medication use in renal disease. Psychosomatics 2004; 45:34–48.
20. Thyrum PT et al. Single-dose pharmacokinetics of quetiapine in subjects with renal or hepatic impairment. Prog Neuropsychopharmacol Biol Psychiatry 2000; 24:521–533.
21. Huynh M et al. Thrombotic thrombocytopenic purpura associated with quetiapine. Ann Pharmacother 2005; 39:1346–1348.
22. Snoeck E et al. Influence of age, renal and liver impairment on the pharmacokinetics of risperidone in man. Psychopharmacology 1995; 122:223–229.
23. Herguner S et al. Steroid-induced psychosis in an adolescent: treatment and prophylaxis with risperidone. Turk J Pediatr 2006; 48:244–247.
24. Wong SL et al. Pharmacokinetics of sertindole and dehydrosertindole in volunteers with normal or impaired renal function. Eur J Clin Pharmacol 1997; 52:223–227.
25. Bressolle F et al. Pharmacokinetics of sulpiride after intravenous administration in patients with impaired renal function. Clin Pharmacokinet 1989; 17:367–373.
26. Aweeka F et al. The pharmacokinetics of ziprasidone in subjects with normal and impaired renal function. Br J Clin Pharmacol 2000; 49:27S–33S.
27. Pfizer. Geodon (ziprasidone) prescribing information. 2009. http://www.pfizer.com/
28. Moviano. Combined Summary of Product Characteristics. Zoleptil. 2006.
29. Lieberman JA et al. Tricyclic antidepressant and metabolite levels in chronic renal failure. Clin Pharmacol Ther 1985; 37:301–307.
30. Murphy EJ. Acute pain management pharmacology for the patient with concurrent renal or hepatic disease. Anaesth Intensive Care 2005; 33:311–322.
31. Mitas JA et al. Diabetic neuropathic pain: control by amitriptyline and fluphenazine in renal insufficiency. South Med J 1983; 76:462–463, 467.
32. Worrall SP et al. Pharmacokinetics of bupropion and its metabolites in haemodialysis patients who smoke. A single dose study. Nephron Clin Pract 2004; 97:c83–c89.
33. Turpeinen M et al. Effect of renal impairment on the pharmacokinetics of bupropion and its metabolites. Br J Clin Pharmacol 2007; 64:165–173.
34. Spigset O et al. Citalopram pharmacokinetics in patients with chronic renal failure and the effect of haemodialysis. Eur J Clin Pharmacol 2000; 56:699–703.
35. Joffe P et al. Single-dose pharmacokinetics of citalopram in patients with moderate renal insufficiency or hepatic cirrhosis compared with healthy subjects. Eur J Clin Pharmacol 1998; 54:237–242.
36. Kelly CA et al. Adult respiratory distress syndrome and renal failure associated with citalopram overdose. Hum Exp Toxicol 2003; 22:103–105.
37. Kalender B et al. Antidepressant treatment increases quality of life in patients with chronic renal failure. Ren Fail 2007; 29:817–822.
38. Onishi A et al. Reversible acute renal failure associated with clomipramine-induced interstitial nephritis. Clin Exp Nephrol 2007; 11:241–243.
39. Rees JA. Clinical interpretation of pharmacokinetic data on dothiepin hydrochloride (Dosulepin, Prothiaden). J Int Med Res 1981; 9:98–102.
40. Adiga GU et al. Renal tubular defects from antidepressant use in an older adult: An uncommon but reversible adverse drug effect. Clin Drug Invest 2006; 26:607–610.
41. Miriyala K et al. Renal failure in a depressed adolescent on escitalopram. J Child Adolesc Psychopharmacol 2008; 18:405–408.
42. Blumenfield M et al. Fluoxetine in depressed patients on dialysis. Int J Psychiatry Med 1997; 27:71–80.
43. Bergstrom RF et al. The effects of renal and hepatic disease on the pharmacokinetics, renal tolerance, and risk-benefit profile of fluoxetine. Int Clin Psychopharmacol 1993; 8:261–266.
44. Rabindranath KS et al. Physical measures for treating depression in dialysis patients. Cochrane Database Syst Rev 2005;CD004541.
45. Lancaster SG et al. Lofepramine. A review of its pharmacodynamic and pharmacokinetic properties, and therapeutic efficacy in depressive illness. Drugs 1989; 37:123–140.
46. Davis MP et al. Mirtazapine for pruritus. J Pain Symptom Manage 2003; 25:288–291.
47. Schoerlin MP et al. Disposition kinetics of moclobemide, a new MAO-A inhibitor, in subjects with impaired renal function. J Clin Pharmacol 1990; 30:272–284.
48. Stoeckel K et al. Absorption and disposition of moclobemide in patients with advanced age or reduced liver or kidney function. Acta Psychiatr Scand Suppl 1990; 360:94–97.
49. Pollock BG et al. Metabolic and physiologic consequences of nortriptyline treatment in the elderly. Psychopharmacol Bull 1994; 30:145–150.
50. Doyle GD et al. The pharmacokinetics of paroxetine in renal impairment. Acta Psychiatr Scand Suppl 1989; 350:89–90.
51. Kaye CM et al. A review of the metabolism and pharmacokinetics of paroxetine in man. Acta Psychiatr Scand Suppl 1989; 350:60–75.
52. Koo JR et al. Treatment of depression and effect of antidepression treatment on nutritional status in chronic hemodialysis patients. Am J Med Sci 2005; 329:1–5.
53. Ishii T et al. A rare case of combined syndrome of inappropriate antidiuretic hormone secretion and Fanconi syndrome in an elderly woman. Am J Kidney Dis 2006; 48:155–158.
54. Coulomb F et al. Pharmacokinetics of single-dose reboxetine in volunteers with renal insufficiency. J Clin Pharmacol 2000; 40:482–487.
55. Dostert P et al. Review of the pharmacokinetics and metabolism of reboxetine, a selective noradrenaline reuptake inhibitor. Eur Neuropsychopharmacol 1997; 7 Suppl 1:S23–S35.
56. Brewster UC et al. Addition of sertraline to other therapies to reduce dialysis-associated hypotension. Nephrology (Carlton) 2003; 8:296–301.
57. Catanese B et al. A comparative study of trazodone serum concentrations in patients with normal or impaired renal function. Boll Chim Farm 1978; 117:424–427.
58. Simpson GM et al. A preliminary study of trimipramine in chronic schizophrenia. Curr Ther Res Clin Exp 1966; 99:248.
59. Leighton JD et al. Trimipramine-induced acute renal failure (Letter). N Z Med J 1986; 99:248.
60. Troy SM et al. The effect of renal disease on the disposition of venlafaxine. Clin Pharmacol Ther 1994; 56:14–21.
61. Pascale P et al. Severe rhabdomyolysis following venlafaxine overdose. Ther Drug Monit 2005; 27:562–564.
62. Guldiken S et al. Complete relief of pain in acute painful diabetic neuropathy of rapid glycaemic control (insulin neuritis) with venlafaxine HCL. Diabetes Nutr Metab 2004; 17:247–249.
63. Verrotti A et al. Renal tubular function in patients receiving anticonvulsant therapy: a long-term study. Epilepsia 2000; 41:1432–1435.
64. Hogg RJ et al. Carbamazepine-induced acute tubulointerstitial nephritis. J Pediatr 1981; 98:830–832.
65. Hegarty J et al. Carbamazepine-induced acute granulomatous interstitial nephritis. Clin Nephrol 2002; 57:310–313.
66. Nicholls DP et al. Acute renal failure from carbamazepine (Letter). Br Med J 1972; 4:490.
67. Jubert P et al. Carbamazepine-induced acute renal failure. Nephron 1994; 66:121.
68. Imai H et al. Carbamazepine-induced granulomatous necrotizing angiitis with acute renal failure. Nephron 1989; 51:405–408.
69. Tutor-Crespo MJ et al. Relative proportions of serum carbamazepine and its pharmacologically active 10,11-epoxy derivative: effect of polytherapy and renal insufficiency. Ups J Med Sci 2008; 113:171–180.
70. Fillastre JP et al. Pharmacokinetics of lamotrigine in patients with renal impairment: influence of haemodialysis. Drugs Exp Clin Res 1993; 19:25–32.
71. Wootton R et al. Comparison of the pharmacokinetics of lamotrigine in patients with chronic renal failure and healthy volunteers. Br J Clin Pharmacol 1997; 43:23–27.
72. Schaub JE et al. Multisystem adverse reaction to lamotrigine. Lancet 1994; 344:481.
73. Fervenza FC et al. Acute granulomatous interstitial nephritis and colitis in anticonvulsant hypersensitivity syndrome associated with lamotrigine treatment. Am J Kidney Dis 2000; 36:1034–1040.
74. Gitlin M. Lithium and the kidney: an updated review. Drug Saf 1999; 20:231–243.
75. Lepkifker E et al. Renal insufficiency in long-term lithium treatment. J Clin Psychiatry 2004; 65:850–856.
76. Smith GC et al. Anticonvulsants as a cause of Fanconi syndrome. Nephrol Dial Transplant 1995; 10:543–545.
77. Fukuda Y et al. Immunologically mediated chronic tubulo-interstitial nephritis caused by valproate therapy. Nephron 1996; 72:328–329.
78. Zaki EL et al. Renal injury from valproic acid: case report and literature review. Pediatr Neurol 2002; 27:318–319.

Special groups

79. Tanaka H et al. Distal type of renal tubular acidosis after anti-epileptic therapy in a girl with infantile spasms. Clin Exp Nephrol 1999; 3:311–313.
80. Knorr M et al. Fanconi syndrome caused by antiepileptic therapy with valproic acid. Epilepsia 2004; 45:868–871.
81. Watanabe T et al. Secondary renal Fanconi syndrome caused by valproate therapy. Pediatr Nephrol 2005; 20:814–817.
82. Rahman MH et al. Acute hemolysis with acute renal failure in a patient with valproic acid poisoning treated with charcoal hemoperfusion. Hemodial Int 2006; 10:256–259.
83. Pentikainen PJ et al. Pharmacokinetics of chlormethiazole in healthy volunteers and patients with cirrhosis of the liver. Eur J Clin Pharmacol 1980; 17:275–284.
84. Sadjadi SA et al. Allergic interstitial nephritis due to diazepam. Arch Intern Med 1987; 147:579.
85. Verbeeck RK et al. Impaired elimination of lorazepam following subchronic administration in two patients with renal failure. Br J Clin Pharmacol 1981; 12:749–751.
86. Reynolds HN et al. Hyperlactatemia, increased osmolar gap, and renal dysfunction during continuous lorazepam infusion. Crit Care Med 2000; 28:1631–1634.
87. Yaucher NE et al. Propylene glycol-associated renal toxicity from lorazepam infusion. Pharmacotherapy 2003; 23:1094–1099.
88. Hayman M et al. Acute tubular necrosis associated with propylene glycol from concomitant administration of intravenous lorazepam and trimethoprim-sulfamethoxazole. Pharmacotherapy 2003; 23:1190–1194.
89. Zar T et al. Acute kidney injury, hyperosmolality and metabolic acidosis associated with lorazepam. Nat Clin Pract Nephrol 2007; 3:515–520.
90. Murray TG et al. Renal disease, age, and oxazepam kinetics. Clin Pharmacol Ther 1981; 30:805–809.
91. Drover DR. Comparative pharmacokinetics and pharmacodynamics of short-acting hypnosedatives: zaleplon, zolpidem and zopiclone. Clin Pharmacokinet 2004; 43:227–238.
92. Sabbatini M et al. Zaleplon improves sleep quality in maintenance hemodialysis patients. Nephron Clin Pract 2003; 94:c99–103.
93. Goa KL et al. Zopiclone. A review of its pharmacodynamic and pharmacokinetic properties and therapeutic efficacy as an hypnotic. Drugs 1986; 32:48–65.
94. Hussain N et al. Zopiclone-induced acute interstitial nephritis. Am J Kidney Dis 2003; 41:E17.

Hepatic impairment

Patients with hepatic impairment may have:

- **reduced capacity to metabolise** biological waste products, dietary proteins, and foreign substances such as drugs. Clinical consequences include hepatic encephalopathy and increased dose-related side-effects from drugs
- **reduced ability to synthesise** plasma proteins and vitamin K-dependent clotting factors. Clinical consequences include hypoalbuminaemia, leading in extreme cases to ascites. Increased toxicity from highly protein-bound drugs should be anticipated. There is also an increased risk of bleeding from GI-irritant drugs and perhaps with SSRIs
- **reduced hepatic blood flow**. Clinical consequences include oesophageal varices and elevated plasma levels of drugs subject to first pass metabolism.

General principles

Liver function tests (LFTs) are a poor marker of hepatic metabolising capacity, as the hepatic reserve is large. Note that many patients with chronic liver disease are asymptomatic or have fluctuating clinical symptoms. Always consider the clinical presentation rather than adhere to rigid rules involving LFTs.

There are few clinical studies relating to the use of psychotropic drugs in people with hepatic disease. The following principles should be adhered to:

1. Prescribe as **few drugs** as possible.
2. Use **lower starting doses**, particularly of drugs that are highly protein bound. TCAs, SSRIs (except citalopram), trazodone, and antipsychotics may have increased free plasma levels, at least initially. This will not be reflected in measured (total) plasma levels. Use lower doses of drugs known to be subject to extensive first-pass metabolism. Examples include TCAs and haloperidol.
3. Be **cautious with drugs that are extensively hepatically metabolised** (most psychotropic drugs). Lower doses may be required. Exceptions are sulpiride, amisulpride, lithium, and gabapentin, which all undergo no or minimal hepatic metabolism.
4. **Leave longer intervals between dosage increases**. Remember that the half-life of most drugs is prolonged in hepatic impairment, so it will take longer for plasma levels to reach steady state.
5. Always **monitor carefully for side effects**, which may be delayed.
6. **Avoid drugs that are very sedative** because of the risk of precipitating hepatic encephalopathy.
7. **Avoid drugs that are very constipating** because of the risk of precipitating hepatic encephalopathy.
8. **Avoid drugs that are known to be hepatotoxic** in their own right (e.g. MAOIs, chlorpromazine).
9. **Choose a low-risk drug** (see tables on the following pages) and **monitor LFTs** weekly, at least initially. If LFTs deteriorate after a new drug is introduced, consider switching to another drug.

These rules should always be observed in severe liver disease (low albumin, increased clotting time, ascites, jaundice, encephalopathy, etc.). The information above, and on the following pages, should be interpreted in the context of the patient's clinical presentation.

Table Antipsychotics in hepatic impairment

Drug	Comments
Amisulpride[1,2]	Predominantly renally excreted, so dosage reduction should not be necessary as long as renal function is normal *but* there are no clinical studies in people with hepatic impairment and little clinical experience. Caution required
Aripiprazole[1]	Extensively hepatically metabolised. Limited data that hepatic impairment has minimal effect on pharmacokinetics. SPC states no dosage reduction required in mild–moderate hepatic impairment, but caution required in severe impairment. Limited clinical experience. Caution required. Small number of reports of hepatotoxicity; ↑LFTs, hepatitis and jaundice
Clozapine[1-3]	Very sedative and constipating. Contra-indicated in active liver disease associated with nausea, anorexia or jaundice, progressive liver disease or hepatic failure. In less severe disease, start with 12.5 mg and increase slowly, using plasma levels to gauge metabolising capacity and guide dosage adjustment. Transient elevations in AST, ALT, and GGT to over twice the normal range occur in over 10% of physically healthy people. Clozapine-induced hepatitis, jaundice, cholestasis, and liver failure have been reported. If jaundice develops, clozapine should be discontinued
Flupentixol/ zuclopenthixol[1,2,4,5]	Both are extensively hepatically metabolised. Small, transient elevations in transaminases have been reported in some patients treated with zuclopenthixol. No other literature reports of use or harm. Both drugs have been in use for many years. Depot preparations are best avoided, as altered pharmacokinetics will make dosage adjustment difficult and side effects from dosage accumulation more likely
Haloperidol[1,6]	Drug of choice in clinical practice and no problems reported although UK SPC states 'caution in liver disease'. Isolated reports of cholestatic hepatitis
Olanzapine[1-3]	Although extensively hepatically metabolised, the pharmacokinetics of olanzapine seem to change little in severe hepatic impairment. It is sedative and anticholinergic (can cause constipation) so caution is advised. Start with 5 mg/day and consider using plasma levels to guide dosage (aim for 20–40 µg/L). Dose-related, transient, asymptomatic elevations in ALT and AST reported in physically healthy adults. People with liver disease may be at increased risk. Rare cases of hepatitis in the literature
Paliperidone[7]	Mainly excreted unchanged by the kidneys so no dosage adjustment required. However, no data are available with respect to severe hepatic impairment and clinical experience is limited. Caution required
Phenothiazines[1,2,8-10]	All cause sedation and constipation. Associated with cholestasis and some reports of fulminant hepatic cirrhosis. Best avoided completely in hepatic impairment. Chlorpromazine is particularly hepatotoxic
Quetiapine[1,2,11-14]	Extensively hepatically metabolised but short half-life. Clearance reduced by a mean of 30% in hepatic impairment so small dosage adjustments may be required. Can cause sedation and constipation. Little clinical experience in hepatic impairment so caution recommended. One case of fatal hepatic failure reported in the literature

Special groups

Table	Antipsychotics in hepatic impairment (Cont.)
Drug	**Comments**
Risperidone[1–3]	Extensively hepatically metabolised and highly protein bound. Manufacturers recommend a reduced starting dose, slower dose titration and a maximum dose of 4 mg in hepatic impairment. Transient, asymptomatic elevations in LFTs, cholestatic hepatitis, and rare cases of hepatic failure have been reported. Steatohepatitis may arise as a result of weight gain. Clinical experience limited in hepatic impairment so caution recommended
Sulpiride[1,2,15,16]	Almost completely renally excreted with a low potential to cause sedation or constipation. Dosage reduction should not be required. Some clinical experience in hepatic impairment with few problems. Fairly old established drug. Isolated case reports of cholestatic jaundice and primary biliary cirrhosis. SPC states contra-indicated in severe hepatic disease

Table	Antidepressants in hepatic impairment
Drug	**Comments**
Fluoxetine[1,2,17–21]	Extensively hepatically metabolised with a long half-life. Kinetic studies demonstrate accumulation in compensated cirrhosis. Although dosage reduction (of at least 50%) or alternate-day dosing could be used, it would take many weeks to reach steady-state serum levels, making fluoxetine complex to use. Asymptomatic increases in LFTs found in 0.5% of healthy adults. Rare cases of hepatitis reported. Avoid in liver disease where PT is prolonged.
Other SSRIs[1,2,21–31]	All are hepatically metabolised and accumulate on chronic dosing. Dosage reduction may be required. Sertraline has been found to be both safe and effective in a placebo-controlled RCT of the management of cholestatic pruritis[32]. Raised LFTs and rare cases of hepatitis, including chronic active hepatitis, have been reported with paroxetine. Sertraline and fluvoxamine have also been associated with hepatitis. Citalopram and escitalopram have minimal effects on hepatic enzymes and may be the SSRI of choice although clinical experience is limited and occasional hepatotoxicity has been reported. Paroxetine is used by some specialised liver units with few apparent problems. Avoid in liver disease where PT is prolonged.
Tricyclics[1,2,33]	All are hepatically metabolised, highly protein bound and will accumulate. They vary in their propensity to cause sedation and constipation. All are associated with raised LFTs and rare cases of hepatitis. There is most clinical experience with imipramine. Sedative TCAs such as trimipramine, dothiepin (dosulepin), and amitriptyline are best avoided. Lofepramine is possibly the most hepatotoxic and should be avoided completely
Venlafaxine[1,2,34,35]	Dosage reduction of 50% advised in moderate hepatic impairment. Little clinical experience. Rare cases of hepatitis reported. Caution advised
MAOIs[1,2,36,37]	People with hepatic impairment reported to be more sensitive to the side effects of MAOIs. MAOIs are also more hepatotoxic than other antidepressants, so best avoided completely
Moclobemide[1,2,38,39]	Clinical experience limited but probably safer than the irreversible MAOIs. 50% reduction in dose advised by manufacturers. Rare cases of hepatotoxicity reported. Caution advised

Table Antidepressants in hepatic impairment (Cont.)

Drug	Comments
Reboxetine[1,2,40]	50% reduction in starting dose recommended. Clinical experience limited. Does not seem to be associated with hepatotoxicity. Caution advised
Mirtazapine[1,2]	Hepatically metabolised and sedative. 50% dose reduction recommended based on kinetic data, but clinical experience limited. Mild, asymptomatic increases in LFTs seen in healthy adults. Caution advised
Duloxetine[1,2,41]	Hepatically metabolised. Clearance markedly reduced even in mild impairment. Reports of hepatocellular injury and, less commonly, jaundice. Isolated case report of fulminant hepatic failure. Limited experience. Best avoided
Agomelatine[42]	Limited data suggest increased plasma levels in hepatic impairment. Dose adjustment may not be required. Agomelatine has a slightly increased rate of LFT change compared with placebo. LFT monitoring required

Table Mood-stabilisers in hepatic impairment[1,2,43]

Drug	Comments
Carbamazepine	Extensively hepatically metabolised and potent inducer of CYP450 enzymes. Contraindicated in acute liver disease. In chronic stable disease, caution advised. Reduce starting dose by 50%, and titrate up slowly, using plasma levels to guide dosage. Stop if LFTs deteriorate. Associated with hepatitis, cholangitis, cholestatic and hepatocellular jaundice, and hepatic failure (rare). Adverse hepatic effects are most common in the first month of treatment. Hepatocellular damage is often associated with a poor outcome[43]. Vulnerability to carbamazepine-induced hepatic damage may be genetically determined[43]
Lamotrigine	Manufacturers recommend 50% reduction in initial dose, dose escalation and maintenance dose in moderate hepatic impairment and 75% in severe hepatic impairment. Discontinue if lamotrigine-induced rash (which can be serious). Extreme caution advised, particularly if co-prescribed with valproate. Elevated LFTs and hepatitis reported
Lithium[44,45]	Not metabolised so dosage reduction not required as long as renal function is normal. Use serum levels to guide dosage and monitor more frequently if ascites status changes (volume of distribution will change). One case of ascites and one of hyperbilirubinaemia reported over many decades of lithium use worldwide
Valproate[46]	Highly protein bound and hepatically metabolised. Dosage reduction with close monitoring of LFTs in moderate hepatic impairment. Use plasma levels (free levels if possible) to guide dosage. Caution advised. Contra-indicated in severe and/or active hepatic impairment; impairment of usual metabolic pathway can lead to generation of hepatotoxic metabolites via alternative pathway. Associated with elevated LFTs and serious hepatotoxicity including fulminant hepatic failure. Mitochondrial disease, learning disability, polypharmacy, metabolic disorders, and underlying hepatic disease may be risk factors. Particularly hepatotoxic in very young children. The greatest risk is in the first 3 months of treatment

Table	Summary – psychotropics in hepatic impairment
Drug group	**Recommended drugs**
Antipsychotics	**Haloperidol**: low dose *or* **Sulpiride/amisulpride**: no dosage reduction required if renal function is normal
Antidepressants	**Imipramine**: start with 25 mg/day and titrate slowly (weekly at most) if required *or* **Paroxetine** or **citalopram**: start at 10 mg if severe hepatic impairment. Titrate slowly (if required) as above (but note increased risk of bleeding)
Mood-stabilisers	**Lithium**: use plasma levels to guide dosage. Care needed if ascites status changes
Sedatives	**Lorazepam, oxazepam, temazepam**: as short half-life with no active metabolites. Use low doses with caution, as sedative drugs can precipitate hepatic encephalopathy **Zopiclone**: 3.75 mg with care in moderate hepatic impairment

Drug-induced hepatic damage

Hy's rule, defined as ALT >3 times the upper limit of normal combined with serum bilirubin >2 times the upper limit of normal is recommended by the FDA to assess the hepatotoxicity of new drugs[43].

Drug-induced hepatic damage can be due to:

- Direct dose-related hepatotoxicity (Type 1 ADR). A small number of drugs fall into this category, e.g. paracetamol; alcohol
- Hypersensitivity reactions (Type 2 ADR). These can present with rash, fever, and eosinophilia. Almost all drugs have been associated with cases of hepatotoxicity; frequency varies.

Almost any type of liver damage can occur, ranging from mild transient asymptomatic increases in LFTs to fulminant hepatic failure. See tables above for details of the hepatotoxic potential of individual drugs.

Risk factors for drug-induced hepatotoxicity include[47]:

- Increasing age
- Female gender
- Alcohol consumption
- Co-prescription of enzyme-inducing drugs
- Genetic predisposition
- Obesity
- Pre-existing liver disease (small effect).

When interpreting LFTs, remember that[47]:

- 12% of the healthy adult population have one LFT outside (above or below) the normal reference range.
- Up to 10% of patients with clinically significant hepatic disease have normal LFTs.
- Individual LFTs lack specificity for the liver, but >1 abnormal test greatly increases the likelihood of liver pathology.
- The absolute values of LFTs are a poor indicator of disease severity.

When monitoring LFTs:

- Ideally LFTs should be measured before treatment starts so that 'baseline' values are available.
- LFT elevations of <2 times the upper limit of the normal reference range are rarely clinically significant.
- Most drug-related LFT elevations occur early in treatment (first month) and are transient. They may indicate adaptation of the liver to the drug rather than damage per se. Transient LFT elevations may also occur during periods of weight gain[48].
- If LFTs are persistently elevated >3 fold, continuing to rise or accompanied by clinical symptoms, the suspected drugs should be withdrawn.
- When tracking change, >20% change in liver enzymes is required to exclude biological or analytical variation

References

1. Datapharm Communications Ltd. Electronic Medicines Compendium. 2009. http://emc.medicines.org.uk/.
2. Micromedex® Healthcare Series . Volume 138 http://www.micromedex com/
3. Atasoy N et al. A review of liver function tests during treatment with atypical antipsychotic drugs: a chart review study. Prog Neuropsychopharmacol Biol Psychiatry 2007; 31:1255–1260.
4. Amdisen A et al. Zuclopenthixol acetate in viscoleo - a new drug formulation. An open Nordic multicentre study of zuclopenthixol acetate in Viscoleo in patients with acute psychoses including mania and exacerbation of chronic psychoses. Acta Psychiatr Scand 1987; 75:99–107.
5. Wistedt B et al. Zuclopenthixol decanoate and haloperidol decanoate in chronic schizophrenia: a double-blind multicentre study. Acta Psychiatr Scand 1991; 84:14–21.
6. Ozcanli T et al. Severe liver enzyme elevations after three years of olanzapine treatment: a case report and review of olanzapine associated hepatotoxicity. Prog Neuropsychopharmacol Biol Psychiatry 2006; 30:1163–1166.
7. Vermeir M et al. Absorption, metabolism, and excretion of paliperidone, a new monoaminergic antagonist, in humans. Drug Metab Dispos 2008; 36:769–779.
8. Regal RE et al. Phenothiazine-induced cholestatic jaundice. Clin Pharm 1987; 6:787–794.
9. Zimmerman HJ et al. Drug-induced cholestasis. Med Toxicol 1987; 2:112–160.
10. de Abajo FJ et al. Acute and clinically relevant drug-induced liver injury: a population based case-control study. Br J Clin Pharmacol 2004; 58:71–80.
11. Thyrum PT et al. Single-dose pharmacokinetics of quetiapine in subjects with renal or hepatic impairment. Prog Neuropsychopharmacol Biol Psychiatry 2000; 24:521–533.
12. Nemeroff CB et al. Quetiapine: preclinical studies, pharmacokinetics, drug interactions, and dosing. J Clin Psychiatry 2002; 63 Suppl 13:5–11.
13. Green B. Focus on quetiapine. Curr Med Res Opin 1999; 15:145–151.
14. El H, I et al. Subfulminant liver failure associated with quetiapine. Eur J Gastroenterol Hepatol 2004; 16:1415–1418.
15. Melzer E et al. Severe cholestatic jaundice due to sulpiride. Isr J Med Sci 1987; 23:1259–1260.
16. Ohmoto K et al. Symptomatic primary biliary cirrhosis triggered by administration of sulpiride. Am J Gastroenterol 1999; 94:3660–3661.
17. Schenker S et al. Fluoxetine disposition and elimination in cirrhosis. Clin Pharmacol Ther 1988; 44:353–359.
18. Cai Q et al. Acute hepatitis due to fluoxetine therapy. Mayo Clin Proc 1999; 74:692–694.
19. Friedenberg FK et al. Hepatitis secondary to fluoxetine treatment. Am J Psychiatry 1996; 153:580.
20. Johnston DE et al. Chronic hepatitis related to use of fluoxetine. Am J Gastroenterol 1997; 92:1225–1226.
21. Hale AS. New antidepressants: use in high-risk patients. J Clin Psychiatry 1993; 54 Suppl:61–70.
22. Benbow SJ et al. Paroxetine and hepatotoxicity. BMJ 1997; 314:1387.
23. Odeh M et al. Severe hepatotoxicity with jaundice associated with paroxetine. Am J Gastroenterol 2001; 96:2494–2496.
24. Dunbar GC. An interim overview of the safety and tolerability of paroxetine. Acta Psychiatr Scand Suppl 1989; 350:135–137.
25. Kuhs H et al. A double-blind study of the comparative antidepressant effect of paroxetine and amitriptyline. Acta Psychiatr Scand Suppl 1989; 350:145–146.
26. De Bree H et al. Fluvoxamine maleate: disposition in men. Eur J Drug Metab Pharmacokinet 1983; 8:175–179.
27. Green BH. Fluvoxamine and hepatic function. Br J Psychiatry 1988; 153:130–131.
28. Milne RJ et al. Citalopram. A review of its pharmacodynamic and pharmacokinetic properties, and therapeutic potential in depressive illness. Drugs 1991; 41:450–477.
29. Lopez-Torres E et al. Hepatotoxicity related to citalopram (Letter). Am J Psychiatry 2004; 161:923–924.
30. Colakoglu O et al. Toxic hepatitis associated with paroxetine. Int J Clin Pract 2005; 59:861–862.
31. Rao N. The clinical pharmacokinetics of escitalopram. Clin Pharmacokinet 2007; 46:281–290.
32. Mayo MJ et al. Sertraline as a first-line treatment for cholestatic pruritus. Hepatology 2007; 45:666–674.
33. Committee on Safety in Medicines. Lofepramine (Gamanil) and abnormal blood tests of liver function. Current Problems 1988; 23:2.
34. Cardona X et al. Venlafaxine-associated hepatitis. Ann Intern Med 2000; 132:417.
35. Phillips BB et al. Hepatitis associated with low-dose venlafaxine for postmenopausal vasomotor symptoms. Ann Pharmacother 2006; 40:323–327.
36. Gomez-Gil E et al. Phenelzine-induced fulminant hepatic failure. Ann Intern Med 1996; 124:692–693.
37. Bonkovsky HL et al. Severe liver injury due to phenelzine with unique hepatic deposition of extracellular material. Am J Med 1986; 80:689–692.
38. Stoeckel K et al. Absorption and disposition of moclobemide in patients with advanced age or reduced liver or kidney function. Acta Psychiatr Scand Suppl 1990; 360:94–97.
39. Timmings P et al. Intrahepatic cholestasis associated with moclobemide leading to death. Lancet 1996; 347:762–763.
40. Tran A et al. Pharmacokinetics of reboxetine in volunteers with hepatic impairment. Clin Drug Invest 2000; 19:473–477.
41. Hanje AJ et al. Case report: fulminant hepatic failure involving duloxetine hydrochloride. Clin Gastroenterol Hepatol 2006; 4:912–917.
42. Dolder CR et al. Agomelatine treatment of major depressive disorder. The Annals of Pharmacotherapy 2008; 42:1822–1831.
43. Bjornsson E. Hepatotoxicity associated with antiepileptic drugs. Acta Neurol Scand 2008; 118:281–290.
44. Cohen LS et al. Lithium-induced hyperbilirubinemia in an adolescent. J Clin Psychopharmacol 1991; 11:274–275.
45. Hazelwood RE. Ascites: a side effect of lithium? Am J Psychiatry 1981; 138:257.
46. Krahenbuhl S et al. Mitochondrial diseases represent a risk factor for valproate-induced fulminant liver failure. Liver 2000; 20:346–348.
47. Rosalki SB et al. Liver function profiles and their interpretation. Br J Hosp Med 1994; 51:181–186.
48. Rettenbacher MA et al. Association between antipsychotic-induced elevation of liver enzymes and weight gain: a prospective study. J Clin Psychopharmacol 2006; 26:500–503.

Special groups

Prescribing in the elderly

General principles

The pharmacokinetics and pharmacodynamics of most drugs are altered to an important extent in the elderly. These changes in drug handling and action must be taken into account if treatment is to be effective and adverse effects minimised. The elderly often have a number of concurrent illnesses and may require treatment with several drugs. This leads to a greater chance of problems arising because of drug interactions and to a higher rate of drug-induced problems in general[1]. It is reasonable to assume that all drugs are more likely to cause adverse effects in the elderly than in younger patients.

How drugs affect the ageing body (altered pharmacodynamics)

As we age, control over reflex actions such as blood pressure and temperature regulation is reduced. Receptors may become more sensitive. This results in an increased incidence and severity of side effects. For example, drugs that decrease gut motility are more likely to cause constipation (e.g. anti-cholinergics and opioids) and drugs that affect blood pressure are more likely to cause falls (e.g. TCAs and diuretics). The elderly are more sensitive to the effects of benzodiazepines than younger adults. Therapeutic response can also be delayed; the elderly may take longer to respond to antidepressants than younger adults[2].

The elderly may be more prone to develop serious side effects from some drugs such as agranulo-cytosis with clozapine[3], stroke with antipsychotic drugs[4], and bleeding with SSRIs.

How ageing affects drug therapy (altered pharmacokinetics)[5]

ABSORPTION

Gut motility decreases with age, as does secretion of gastric acid. This leads to drugs being absorbed more slowly, resulting in a slower onset of action. The same *amount* of drug is absorbed as in a younger adult, but the rate of absorption is slower.

DISTRIBUTION

The elderly have more body fat, less body water, and less albumin than younger adults. This leads to an increased volume of distribution and a longer duration of action for some fat-soluble drugs (e.g. diazepam), higher concentrations of some drugs at the site of action (e.g. digoxin) and a reduction in the amount of drug bound to albumin (increased amounts of active 'free drug'; e.g. warfarin, phenytoin).

METABOLISM

The majority of drugs are hepatically metabolised. Liver size is reduced in the elderly, but in the absence of hepatic disease or significantly reduced hepatic blood flow, there is no significant reduction in metabolic capacity. The magnitude of pharmacokinetic interactions is unlikely to be altered but the pharmacodynamic consequences of these interactions may be amplified.

EXCRETION

Renal function declines with age: 35% of function is lost by the age of 65 years and 50% by the age of 80.

More function is lost if there are concurrent medical problems such as heart disease, diabetes, or hypertension. Measurement of serum creatinine or urea can be misleading in the elderly because muscle mass is reduced, so less creatinine is produced. It is particularly important that e-GFR[6] is used as a measure of renal function in this age group. It is best to assume that all elderly patients have at most two-thirds of normal renal function.

Special groups

Most drugs are eventually (after metabolism) excreted by the kidney. A few do not undergo biotransformation first. Lithium and sulpiride are important examples. Drugs primarily excreted via the kidney will accumulate in the elderly, leading to toxicity and side effects. Dosage reduction is likely to be required (see section on renal effects of psychotropics).

Drug interactions

Some drugs have a narrow therapeutic index (a small increase in dose can cause toxicity and a small reduction in dose can cause a loss of therapeutic action). The most commonly prescribed ones are: digoxin, warfarin, theophylline, phenytoin, and lithium. Changes in the way these drugs are handled in the elderly and the greater chance of interaction with other drugs mean that toxicity and therapeutic failure are more likely. These drugs can be used safely but extra care must be taken and blood levels should be measured where possible.

Some drugs inhibit or induce hepatic metabolising enzymes. Important examples include the SSRIs, erythromycin, and carbamazepine. This may lead to the metabolism of another drug being altered. Many drug interactions occur through this mechanism. Details of individual interactions and their consequences can be found in Appendix 1 of the *BNF*. Most can be predicted by a sound knowledge of pharmacology.

Reducing drug-related risk

Adherence to the following principles will reduce drug-related morbidity and mortality:

- Use drugs only when absolutely necessary.
- Avoid, if possible, drugs that block α_1 adrenoceptors, have anticholinergic side effects, are very sedative, have a long half-life or are potent inhibitors of hepatic metabolising enzymes.
- Start with a low dose and increase slowly but do not undertreat. Some drugs still require the full adult dose.
- Try not to treat the side effects of one drug with another drug. Find a better-tolerated alternative.
- Keep therapy simple; that is, once-daily administration whenever possible.

Administering medicines in foodstuffs[7,8]

Sometimes patients may refuse treatment with medicines, even when such treatment is thought to be in their best interests. Where the patient has a mental illness or has capacity, the Mental Health Act should be used, but if the patient lacks capacity, this option may not be desirable. Medicines should never be administered covertly to elderly patients with dementia without a full discussion with the MDT and the patient's relatives. The outcome of this discussion should be clearly documented in the patient's clinical notes. Medicine should be administered covertly only if the clear and express purpose is to reduce suffering for the patient. (See section on covert administration, this chapter).

References

1. Royal College of Physicians. Medication for older people. Summary and recommendations of a report of a working party of The Royal College of Physicians. J R Coll Physicians Lond 1997; 31:254–257.
2. Paykel ES et al. Residual symptoms after partial remission: an important outcome in depression. Psychol Med 1995; 25:1171–1180.
3. Munro J et al. Active monitoring of 12,760 clozapine recipients in the UK and Ireland. Beyond pharmacovigilance. Br J Psychiatry 1999; 175:576–580.
4. Douglas IJ et al. Exposure to antipsychotics and risk of stroke: self controlled case series study. BMJ 2008; 337:a1227.
5. Mayersohn M. Special pharmacokinetic considerations in the elderly. In: Evans WE, Schentag JJ, Jusko WJ, editors. Applied Pharmacokinetics Principles of Therapeutic Drug Monitoring. Spokane, WA: Applied Therapeutics Inc; 1986; 229–293.
6. Morriss R et al. Lithium and eGFR: a new routinely available tool for the prevention of chronic kidney disease. Br J Psychiatry 2008; 193:93–95.
7. Treloar A et al. Concealing medication in patients' food. Lancet 2001; 357:62–64.
8. Treloar A et al. Administering medicines to patients with dementia and other organic cognitive syndromes. Adv Psychiatr Treat 2001; 7:444–450.

Special groups

Further reading

National Service Framework for Older People. London: Department of Health, 2001.

Dementia

Dementia is a progressive degenerative neurological syndrome affecting about 6% of those aged over 65 years. This age-related disorder is characterised by cognitive decline, impaired memory and thinking, and a gradual loss of skills needed to carry out activities of daily living. Often, other mental functions may also be affected, including changes in mood, personality, and social behaviour[1].

The various types of dementia are classified according to the different disease processes affecting the brain. The most common cause of dementia is Alzheimer's disease, accounting for almost 60% of all cases. Vascular dementia and dementia with Lewy bodies (DLB) are responsible for most other cases. Alzheimer's disease and vascular dementia may co-exist and are often difficult to separate clinically. Dementia is also encountered in about 30–70% of patients with Parkinson's disease[2] (see separate section on Parkinson's disease).

Alzheimer's disease

Mechanism of action of cognitive enhancers used in Alzheimer's disease

ACETYLCHOLINESTERASE (AChE) INHIBITORS

The cholinergic hypothesis of Alzheimer's disease is based on the observation that the cognitive deterioration associated with the disease results from progressive loss of cholinergic neurons and decreasing levels of acetylcholine (ACh) in the brain[3]. Both acetylcholinesterase (AChE) and butyrylcholinesterase (BuChE) have been found to play an important role in the degradation of ACh[4].

Three inhibitors of AChE are currently licensed in the UK for the treatment of mild to moderate dementia in Alzheimer's disease: donepezil, rivastigmine, and galantamine. In addition, rivastigmine is licensed in the treatment of mild to moderate dementia associated with Parkinson's disease. Cholinesterase inhibitors differ in pharmacological action: donepezil selectively inhibits AChE, rivastigmine affects both AChE and BuChE, and galantamine selectively inhibits AChE and also affects nicotinic receptors[5]. To date, these differences have not been shown to result in differences in efficacy or tolerability. (See table below for comparison of AChE inhibitors).

MEMANTINE

Memantine is licensed in the UK for the treatment of moderately severe to severe Alzheimer's disease. It acts as an antagonist at *N*-methyl-D-aspartate (NMDA) receptors, an action which, in theory, may be neuroprotective and thus disease modifying[6]. (See table on next page.)

Table Characteristics of cognitive enhancers[7-11]

Characteristic	Donepezil (Aricept®-Pfizer, Eisai)	Rivastigmine (Exelon®-Novartis)	Galantamine (Reminyl®-Shire/Janssen-Cilag)	Memantine (Exiba®-Lundbeck)
Primary mechanism	AChE-I (selective and reversible)	AChE-I (pseudo-irreversible)	AChE-I (selective and reversible)	NMDA receptor antagonist
Other mechanism	None	BuChE-I	Nicotine modulator	5-HT3 receptor antagonist
Starting dose	5 mg daily	1.5 mg bd	4 mg bd (or 8 mg XL daily)	5 mg daily
Usual treatment dose (max dose)	10 mg daily	6 mg bd or 9.5 mg/24hrs patch	12 mg bd (or 24 mg XL daily)	10 mg bd
Recommended minimum interval between dose increases	4 weeks (increase by 5 mg/day)	2 weeks (increase by 1.5 mg bd)	4 weeks (increase by 4 mg bd)	1 week (increase by 5 mg/day)
Adverse effects[8-11] very common*: ≥1/10 and common: ≥1/100	Nausea*, headache*, diarrhoea*, vomiting, insomnia, muscle cramps, fatigue, syncope dizziness, abdominal disturbance, rash, urinary incontinence	Nausea*, vomiting*, diarrhoea*, dizziness*, anorexia*, agitation, confusion, headache, somnolence, tremor, abdominal pain and dyspepsia, sweating, fatigue, malaise, weight loss	Nausea*, vomiting*, diarrhoea, abdominal pain and dyspepsia, anorexia, fatigue, dizziness, headache, somnolence, weight loss, syncope, depression, insomnia, confusion hypertension	Headache, dizziness, constipation, somnolence, hypertension
Half life (h)	~70	~1	7-8	60-100
Metabolism	CYP 2D6 CYP 3A4	Non-hepatic	CYP 2D6 CYP 3A4	Primarily non-hepatic
Drug–drug interactions	Yes (see separate table)	Interactions unlikely	Yes (see separate table)	Yes (see separate table)
Effect of food on absorption	None	Delays rate and extent of absorption	Delays rate but not extent of absorption	None
Cost of preparations[7] (for 1-month treatment at usual dose)	Tablets: £89.06 Orodispersible tablets: £89.06	Capsules: £66.51 Oral solution (2 mg/ml): £163.30 Patches: £77.97	Tablets: £79.80 Capsules m/r: £84 Oral solution (4mg/mL): £201.60	Tablets: £69.01 Oral drops: £69.01 Note: 5 mg = 10 drops

Special groups

389

Efficacy of drugs used in dementia

All three AChE-Is seem to have broadly similar clinical effects, as measured with the Mini Mental State Examination (MMSE), a 30-point basic evaluation of cognitive function and the Alzheimer's Disease Assessment Scale – cognitive subscale (ADAS-cog), a 70-point evaluation largely of cognitive dysfunction. Pivotal trials of donepezil[12–14] suggest an advantage over placebo of 2.5–3.1 points on the ADAS-cog scale. For rivastigmine[15,16], the advantage is 2.6–4.9 points and for galantamine[17–19] 2.9–3.9. Estimates of the number needed to treat (NNT) (improvement of >4 points ADAS-cog) range from 4 to 12. The table on the following page summarises the efficacy of the four cognitive enhancers used in Alzheimer's disease.

Cochrane reviews for all three AChE-Is have been carried out, both collectively as a group and individually for each drug separately. In the review for all AChE-Is, which included 10 RCTs, results demonstrated that treatment over 6 months produced improvements in cognitive function, of on average –2.7 points (95% CI –3.0 to –2.3, p < 0.00001) on the ADAS-cog scale. Benefits were also noted on measures of Activities of Daily Living (ADL) and behaviour, although none of these treatment effects were large[20].

Direct comparisons of anticholinesterases have given equivocal results – a Pfizer-sponsored study suggested the superiority of donepezil to galantamine[21], a Janssen-sponsored study suggested the converse[22] and a Novartis-sponsored study showed that patients not responding adequately to or declining while taking donepezil may improve or stabilise after switching immediately to rivastigmine, with good tolerability[23]. A double-blind RCT included in the Cochrane review of AChE-Is, which compared donepezil with rivastigmine, however, found no evidence of a difference between the two agents for cognitive function, ADL, or behavioural disturbances at 2 years[20].

Results from the donepezil Cochrane review showed statistically significant improvements for both 5 and 10 mg/day at 24 weeks compared with placebo on the ADAS-cog scale with a 2.01 point and a 2.80 point reduction, respectively[24]. For rivastigmine, high dose (6–12 mg daily) was associated with a 2.1 point improvement in cognitive function on the ADAS-cog score compared with placebo and a 2.2 point improvement in ADL at 26 weeks. At lower doses (4 mg daily or lower) differences were in the same direction but were only statistically significant for cognitive function[25]. The galantamine review showed that treatment with the drug led to significantly greater proportion of subjects with improved or unchanged global rating scale rating at all doses except for 8 mg/day. Point estimate of effect was lower for 8 mg/day but similar for 16–36 mg/day. Treatment effect for 24 mg/day over 6 months was 3.1 point reduction in ADAS-cog[26].

Rivastigmine transdermal patch has been shown to be as effective as the highest doses of capsules but with a superior tolerability profile in a 6-month double-blind, placebo-controlled RCT[27].

Trials of memantine in severe dementia[28] suggest an advantage over placebo of around 2 points on the ADAS-cog scale and NNTs (improvement) of 3–8[29]. Improvement was also seen in other domains of functioning. Early data suggest memantine is effective in mild to moderate Alzheimer's disease with an advantage over placebo of 1.9 points on ADAS-cog[30]. A Cochrane review of memantine concluded that it had a small beneficial effect at 6 months in moderate to severe Alzheimer's disease. Statistically significant effects were detected on cognition, ADL, and behaviour[31].

Table Summary – effect sizes for outcomes of benefit (in at least two studies)[32]

Outcome measures	Donepezil (Aricept®)	Rivastigmine (Exelon®)	Galantamine (Reminyl®)	Memantine (Exiba®)
	Magnitude of effect (95% CI)	Magnitude of effect (95% CI)	Magnitude of effect (95% CI)	Magnitude of effect (95% CI)
ADAS-cog[33] (–ve is better)	–2.83 (–3.29 to –2.37) p < 0.001	–3.91 (–5.48 to –2.34) p < 0.001	–2.46 (–3.47 to –1.44) p < 0.001	
MMSE[34] (+ve is better)	1.14 (0.76 to 1.53) p < 0.001	–0.04 (–1.28 to 1.20) p = 0.95		
CIBIC-plus[32,35] (–ve is better)	–0.45 (–0.54 to –0.36) p < 0.0001	–0.36 (–0.45 to –0.27) p < 0.001	1.22 (1.12 to 1.33)	–0.27 (–0.43 to –0.10) p = 0.002
NPI[36] (–ve is better)	–3.99 (–6.85 to –1.12) p = 0.006		–1.72 (–3.12 to –0.33) p = 0.015	–3.19 (–5.09 to –1.29) p = 0.001

ADAS-cog[33] = Alzheimer's Disease Assessment Scale – cognitive subscale, MMSE[34] = Mini Mental State Examination, CIBIC-plus[32,35] = clinician-based impression of change scale, with caregiver input, NPI[36] = Neuropsychiatric Inventory.

All the above results need to be interpreted with caution, because of the different populations studied but especially as so few head-to-head studies have been published. Alzheimer's disease is usually characterised by inexorable cognitive decline, which is generally well quantified by tests such as ADAS-cog and MMSE. The average rate of decline is 4–6 points on the ADAS-cog over one year, but the range is large. It is therefore difficult to accurately assess treatment effect in individual patients. The effect of anticholinesterases is, on average, to improve modestly cognitive function for several months (scores return to baseline after about 9–12 months)[14,18].

This average incorporates and to some extent conceals three groups of patients: 'non-responders', who continue to decline at the anticipated rate; 'non-decliners', who neither improve significantly nor decline; and 'improvers', who improve to a clinically relevant extent. This last group is usually defined as those who show a >4 point improvement on ADAS-cog. In trials of around 6 months, approximately 25–35% of those on anticholinesterases will be classified as 'improvers' compared with around 15–25% on placebo. Around 55–70% of patients treated with anticholinesterases will show no cognitive decline during a 5–6 month trial[16,18] – about 20% more patients in absolute terms than those on placebo. Note that, for the most part, results of trials so far conducted relate only to patients with mild-to-moderate Alzheimer's disease (those giving a score of 10–26 on MMSE), although data on those with more severe illness are encouraging[37], particularly with galantamine which has been shown to be effective (albeit marginally so) in subjects with MMSE scores of 5–12 points[38].

Taking into account trial differences and all assessments made, available anticholinesterases can be said to have broadly similar efficacy against cognitive symptoms in clinical trials. Any minor differences observed may be accounted for by differences in trial design or patient characteristics. In the absence of sufficient 'head-to-head' studies, the available drugs should be assumed to have equal efficacy. Overall, in a cohort of patients given anticholinesterases at optimal doses under clinical trial conditions, approximately one-third would be expected to improve over 6 months

Special groups

and around another third would be expected not to deteriorate. These observations appear to be broadly reflected in practice.

The benefits of treatment with AChE-Is are rapidly lost when drug administration is interrupted[39] and may not be fully regained when drug treatment is reinitiated[40]. Failure to benefit from one ACEh-I does not necessarily mean that a patient will not respond to another and similarly, poor tolerability with one agent does not rule out good tolerability with another[41].

Other effects
AChE inhibitors may also affect non-cognitive aspects of Alzheimer's disease and other dementia. Several studies have investigated their safety and efficacy in managing the Behavioural and Psychological Symptoms of Dementia (BPSD). For more information about the management of these symptoms, see the following section.

Dosing
Different titration schedules do, to some extent, differentiate anticholinesterases (see table for dosing information). Donepezil has been perhaps the easiest to use as it is given once daily whereas both rivastigmine and galantamine (until recently) needed to be given twice daily and have prolonged titration schedules. These factors may be important to prescribers, patients, and carers. This was demonstrated in a retrospective analysis of the patterns of use of AChE-I, where it was demonstrated that donepezil was significantly more likely to be prescribed at an effective dose than either rivastigmine or galantamine[42]. Galantamine is now usually given once daily as the controlled-release formulation and rivastigmine is now available as a patch. Memantine once-daily dosing has been found to be similar in safety and tolerability as twice-daily dosing and may be more practical[43].

Tolerability
Drug tolerability may differ between anticholinesterases, but, again, in the absence of sufficient direct comparisons, it is difficult to draw definitive conclusions. Overall tolerability can be broadly evaluated by reference to the numbers withdrawing from clinical trials. Withdrawal rates in trials of donepezil[12,13] ranged from 4% to 16% (placebo 1–7%). With rivastigmine[15,16], rates ranged from 7% to 29% (placebo 7%) and with galantamine[17–19] from 7% to 23% (placebo 7–9%). (These figures relate to withdrawals specifically associated with adverse effects.)

Tolerability seems to be affected by speed of titration and, perhaps less clearly, by dose. Most adverse effects occurred in trials during titration, and slower titration schedules are recommended in clinical use. This may mean that these drugs are equally well tolerated in practice. Rivastigmine patch may offer convenience and a superior tolerability profile to capsules[27]. Memantine appears to be well tolerated[44,45].

Adverse effects
When adverse effects occur, they are largely predictable: excess cholinergic stimulation can lead to nausea, vomiting, dizziness, insomnia, and diarrhoea[46]. Urinary incontinence has also been reported[47]. There appear to be no important differences between drugs in respect to type or frequency of adverse events, although clinical trials do suggest a relatively lower frequency of adverse events for donepezil. This may simply be a reflection of the aggressive titration schedules used in trials of other drugs.

In view of their pharmacological action, AChE-inhibitors may have vagotonic effects on heart rate (i.e. bradycardia). The potential for this action may be of particular importance in patients with 'sick sinus syndrome' or other supraventricular cardiac conduction disturbances, such as sinoatrial or atrioventricular block[8–10].

Concerns over the potential cardiac adverse effects associated with AChE-Is were raised following findings from controlled trials of galantamine in Mild Cognitive Impairment (MCI) in which increased mortality was associated with galantamine compared with placebo (1.5% versus 0.5% respectively)[48]. Although no specific cause of death was predominant, half the deaths reported were due to cardiovascular disorders. As a result, the FDA issued a warning restricting galantamine in patients with MCI. The relevance in Alzheimer's disease remains unclear[49]. A Cochrane review of pooled data from RCTs of the AChIs revealed that there was a significantly higher incidence of syncope amongst the AChE-I groups compared with the placebo groups (3.43 v. 1.87%, p = 0.02). The manufacturers of all three agents therefore advise that the drugs should be used with caution in patients with cardiovascular disease or taking concurrent medicines that reduce heart rate, e.g. digoxin or beta blockers. Although a pre- treatment mandatory ECG has been suggested[49], a recent review of published evidence showed that the incidence of cardiovascular side effects is low and that serious adverse effects are rare. In addition, the value of pre-treatment screening and routine ECGs is questionable and is not currently recommended by NICE[50]. Rivastigmine may be the safest choice in patients with cardiovascular disease in view of its lack of interaction potential with other drugs. It is also therefore the most suitable in patients receiving multiple medicines.

Interactions

Potential for interaction may also differentiate currently available cholinesterase inhibitors. Donepezil[51] and galantamine[52] are metabolised by cytochromes 2D6 and 3A4 and so drug levels may be altered by other drugs affecting the function of these enzymes. Anticholinesterases themselves may also interfere with the metabolism of other drugs, although this is perhaps a theoretical consideration. Rivastigmine has almost no potential for interaction since it is metabolised at the site of action and does not affect hepatic cytochromes. Overall, rivastigmine appears to be least likely to cause problematic drug interactions, a factor that may be important in an elderly population subject to polypharmacy (see drugs interactions table).

A recent analysis of the French pharmacovigilance database found that the majority of reported drug interactions concerning AChE-I were found to be pharmacodynamic in nature and most frequently involved the combination of AChE-I and bradycardic drugs (beta blockers, digoxin, amiodarone, calcium channel antagonists). Almost a third of these interactions resulted in cardiovascular adverse drug reactions (ADRs) such as bradycardia, atrioventricular block, and arterial hypotension. The second most frequent drug interaction reported was the combination of AChE-I with anticholinergic drugs leading to pharmacological antagonism[53].

Table Drug–drug interactions[8–11]

Drug	Metabolism	Plasma levels increased by	Plasma levels decreased by	Pharmacodynamic interactions
Donepezil (Aricept®)	Substrate at 3A4 and 2D6	**Ketoconazole** **Itraconazole** **Erythromycin** **Quinidine** **Fluoxetine**	**Rifampicin** **Phenytoin** **Carbamazepine** **Alcohol** **Phenobarbital** **Dexamethasone**	Interaction with **anticholinergic drugs**. Potential for synergistic activity with concomitant **cholinomimetics** such as **neuro-muscular blocking agents** (e.g. **succinylcholine**), **cholinergic agonists**, or **beta blockers** which have effects on cardiac conduction
Rivastigmine (Exelon®)	Non-hepatic metabolism	Metabolic interactions appear unlikely Rivastigmine may inhibit the butyryl-cholinesterase mediated metabolism of other substances, e.g. **cocaine**		Avoid use with **anticholinergic** and **cholinomimetic** drugs. Rivastigmine may exaggerate effects of **succinylcholine-type muscle relaxants** or **cholinergic agonists** e.g. **bethanecol**
Galantamine (Reminyl®)	Substrate at 3A4 and 2D6	**Ketoconazole** **Erythromycin** **Ritonavir** **Quinidine** **Paroxetine** **Fluoxetine** **Fluvoxamine** **Amitriptyline**	None known	Avoid use with **anticholinergic** and **cholinomimetics**. Possible interaction with agents that significantly reduce heart rate, e.g. **digoxin**, **beta blockers**, certain **calcium-channel blockers**, and **amiodarone**. Caution with agents that can cause torsades de pointes (manufacturers recommend ECG in such cases)
Memantine (Exiba®)	Primarily non-hepatic metabolism Renally eliminated	**Cimetidine** **Ranitidine** **Procainamide** **Quinidine** **Quinine** **Nicotine** *(all these use the same renal cation transport system as memantine– potential increase in levels of both drugs)* Alkaline urine–(PH ~8)– may be caused by **carbonic anhydrase inhibitors, sodium bicarbonate**	None known	Action of **L-dopa, dopaminergic agonists**, and **anticholinergics** may be enhanced by memantine Effects of **barbiturates, neuroleptics**, and **hydrochlorothiazide** may be reduced Avoid concomitant use with **amantadine, ketamine**, and **dextromethorphan** (other NMDA antagonists - risk of pharmacotoxic psychosis) Dosage adjustment required for **antispasmotic agents, dantrolene**, and **baclofen** when given with memantine

NICE recommendations

Using a protocol like that originally suggested by NICE[54] may mean that, of a cohort of patients referred for treatment, only three-quarters may be considered suitable for treatment, and only one-third of these may continue treatment for a year or more[55]. In contrast, in the artificial environment of a clinical trial, nearly half of patients continued for 2 years or more[56]. (Note that long-term, double-blind trials may underestimate real-life benefits of treatment because non-responders or poor responders are continued on drug treatment[57]). While NICE guidance has now changed (below) a similar (or lower) rate of take-up and persistence with treatment should be anticipated.

Summary of NICE guidance on anticholinesterases[58]

- The three acetylcholinesterase inhibitors donepezil, galantamine, and rivastigmine are recommended as options in the management of people with Alzheimer's disease of moderate severity (MMSE score of between 10 and 20)
- The initiation of medication is a clinical decision and should not be mechanistically determined by MMSE score, factors such as (but not restricted to) co-existing learning disability, physical impairment (e.g. of sight or hearing), education, language skills, cultural background, individual impact of the dementia and even high pre-morbid function need to be considered so that practice is not discriminatory as articulated in the High Court judgments against NICE guidance
- Only specialists in the care of people with dementia should initiate treatment
- Carers' view on the patient's condition at baseline and follow-up should be sought
- Patients who continue on the drug should be reviewed every 6 months by MMSE score and global, functional and behavioural assessment. The drug should only be continued if the MMSE remains at or above 10 and the drug effect is considered to be worthwhile. (Note, however, that abrupt discontinuation of AChE inhibitors in patients whose MMSE score drops below this level is not advised – a careful trial of graduated discontinuation is preferred)
- Therapy with AChE inhibitor should be initiated with a drug with the lowest acquisition cost. An alternative may be considered on the basis of adverse effects profile, concordance, medical co-morbidity, and possibility of drug interactions
- People with mild Alzheimer's disease currently receiving AChE inhibitors may be continued on therapy until they, their carers, and/or specialist consider it appropriate to stop

---

Combination treatment

A wide range of drug combinations have been evaluated but few have involved more modern treatments such as anticholinesterases and memantine[59], perhaps the most obvious combination to use. Nonetheless, a combination of memantine and donepezil has been shown to be more effective than donepezil in patients with moderate to severe Alzheimer's disease[60]. The combination appears to be well tolerated[60,61]. Similarly, the combination of rivastigmine and memantine has also been investigated in a prospective open-label study in patients who failed to respond to donepezil or galantamine. The combination was found to be beneficial without increased side effects[62]. Studies have confirmed that there are no pharmacokinetic or pharmacodynamic interactions between donepezil and memantine[63] or galantamine and memantine[64].

Other treatments

Ginkgo biloba has been widely used as a cognitive enhancer and there have previously been some experimental data to suggest that it has neuroprotective effects[65]. There are also well-controlled human trial data which suggest that *G. biloba* is effective in mild to moderate Alzheimer's disease with an advantage over placebo of around 1.4 points on ADAS-cog[66]. However, recent community-based double-blind, placebo-controlled clinical trials, found that *Ginkgo biloba* 120 mg daily did not confer benefit in mild–moderate dementia over 6 months[67] and 120 mg twice daily was not effective in reducing either overall incidence rate of dementia or Alzheimer's disease incidence in elderly individuals with normal cognition or those with mild cognitive impairment[68]. A Cochrane review concluded that although *Ginkgo biloba* appears to be safe with no excess side effects compared with placebo, many of the trials were too small and used unsatisfactory methods. There was also evidence of publication bias. Therefore, its clinical benefit in dementia or cognitive impairment is somewhat inconsistent and unconvincing[69]. Several reports have noted that gingko may increase the risk of bleeding[70]. The drug is widely used in Germany but less so elsewhere.

A Cochrane review of **vitamin E** for Alzheimer's disease (AD) and mild cognitive impairment (MCI) examined two studies meeting the inclusion criteria. The authors' conclusions were that there is no evidence of efficacy of vitamin E in prevention or treatment of people with AD or MCI and that further research is required in order to identify its role in this area[71].

A placebo-controlled pilot RCT of 1 mg **folic acid** supplementation of AChE-Is over 6 months in 57 patients with Alzheimer's disease showed significant benefit in combined Instrumental Activities of Daily Living and Social Behaviour scores (folate + 1.50 (SD 5.32) vs placebo −2.29 (SD 6.16) (p = 0.03)) but no change in MMSE scores[72].

Another RCT examining the efficacy of **multivitamins and folic acid** as an adjunctive to AChE-Is over 26 weeks in 89 patients with Alzheimer's disease found no statistically significant benefits between the two groups on cognition or ADL function[73].

Omega-3 supplementation in mild to moderate Alzheimer's disease has been evaluated in 174 patients in a placebo-controlled RCT but there were no significant overall effects on neuropsychiatric symptoms, on activities of daily living or on caregiver's burden, although some possible positive effects were seen on depressive symptoms (assessed by MADRS) and agitation symptoms (assessed by NPI)[74].

A prospective open-label study of **ginseng** in AD measured cognitive performance in 97 patients randomly assigned ginseng or placebo for 12 weeks and then 12 weeks after the ginseng had been discontinued. After ginseng treatment, the cognitive subscales of ADAS and MMSE score began to show improvement continued up to 12 weeks (p = 0.029 and p = 0.009 vs baseline respectively) but scores declined to levels of the control group following discontinuation of ginseng[75].

Dimebon, a non-selective antihistamine previously approved in Russia but later discontinued for commercial reasons has been assessed for safety, tolerability, and efficacy in the treatment of patients with mild to moderate Alzheimer's disease. It acts as a weak inhibitor of butyrylcholinesterase and acetylcholinesterase, weakly blocks the NMDA-receptor signalling pathway and inhibits the mitochondrial permeability transition pore opening. The company-sponsored study included 183 patients and found that dimebon resulted in significant benefits in all five outcome measures (ADAS-cog, MMSE, ADCS-ADL, NPI, and CIBIC-plus) compared with placebo (ITT-LOCF). Dimebon was well tolerated and there was no difference in the percentage of adverse effects between the two groups. The most commonly reported adverse effects for dimebon were dry mouth and depressed mood[76]. Further controlled trials are underway.

Vascular dementia

Vascular dementia has been reported to comprise 10–50% of dementia cases. It is caused by ischaemic damage to the brain and is associated with cognitive impairment and behavioural disturbances. The management options are currently very limited and focus on controlling the underlying risk factors for cerebrovascular disease[77]. Mixed dementia is the most common form of dementia after Alzheimer's disease.

None of the currently available drugs is formally licensed in the UK for vascular dementia. The management of vascular dementia has been summarised in two recent papers[78,79]. There is growing evidence for donepezil[80,81], rivastigmine[82,83], galantamine[84–86], and memantine[87,88]. However, Cochrane reviews for galantamine[89] and rivastigmine[90] concluded that galantamine's efficacy in vascular dementia was not consistent[91] and that there is currently no evidence for the benefit of rivastigmine in vascular dementia in view of the absence of large RCTs. Furthermore a meta-analysis of RCTs found that cholinesterase inhibitors and memantine produce small benefits in cognition of uncertain clinical significance and concluded that data were insufficient to support widespread use of these agents in vascular dementia[77].

Note that it is impossible to diagnose with certainty vascular or Alzheimer's dementia and much dementia has mixed causation.

Dementia with Lewy bodies
It has been suggested that dementia with Lewy bodies (DLB) may account for up to 15–25% of cases of dementia. Characteristic symptoms are dementia marked with fluctuation of cognitive ability, early and persistent visual hallucinations, and spontaneous motor features of parkinsonism. Falls, syncope, transient disturbances of consciousness, neuroleptic sensitivity, and hallucinations are also common[92].

A Cochrane review found no convincing evidence for the efficacy of AChE-Is for dementia with Lewy bodies. This review however, included just one RCT of rivastigmine; the only study that met their inclusion criteria[92]. A comparative analysis of cholinesterase inhibitors in DLB, which included open label trials as well as the placebo-controlled randomised trial of rivastigmine, found that there is so far no compelling evidence that one AChE-I is better that the other in DLB[93].

References

1. Saddichha S et al. Alzheimer's and non-alzheimer's dementia: a critical review of pharmacological and nonpharmacological strategies. Am J Alzheimers Dis Other Demen 2008; 23:150–161.
2. National Institute for Clinical Excellence. Dementia: Supporting people with dementia and their carers in health and social care. Clinical Guidance 42. http://www.nice.org.uk. 2006.
3. Francis PT et al. The cholinergic hypothesis of Alzheimer's disease: a review of progress. J Neurol Neurosurg Psychiatry 1999; 66:137–147.
4. Mesulam M et al. Widely spread butyrylcholinesterase can hydrolyze acetylcholine in the normal and Alzheimer brain. Neurobiol Dis 2002; 9:88–93.
5. Weinstock M. Selectivity of cholinesterase inhibition: clinical implications for the treatment of Alzheimer's disease. CNS Drugs 1999; 12:307–323.
6. Danysz W et al. Neuroprotective and symptomatological action of memantine relevant for Alzheimer's disease – a unified glutamatergic hypothesis on the mechanism of action. Neurotox Res 2000; 2:8–97.
7. British Medical Association and Royal Pharmaceutical Society of Great Britain. British National Formulary. 57th edition. London: BMJ Group and RPS Publishing; 2009.
8. Eisai. Summary of Product Characteristics. Aricept. 2009. http://emc.medicines.org.uk/.
9. Novartis Pharmaceuticals UK Ltd. Summary of Product Characteristics. Exelon. 2009. http://emc.medicines.org.uk/.
10. Shire Pharmaceuticals Limited. Summary of Product Characteristics. Reminyl Tablets. http://emc.medicines.org.uk/. 2008.
11. Lundbeck Limited. Summary of Product Characteristics. Ebixa 10mg/g oral drops, 20mg and 10mg tablets and Treatment Initiation Pack. http://emc. medicines.org.uk/ . 2009.
12. Rogers SL et al. Donepezil improves cognition and global function in Alzheimer disease: a 15-week, double-blind, placebo-controlled study. Donepezil Study Group. Arch Intern Med 1998; 158:1021–1031.
13. Rogers SL et al. A 24-week, double-blind, placebo-controlled trial of donepezil in patients with Alzheimer's disease. Donepezil Study Group. Neurology 1998; 50:136–145.
14. Rogers SL et al. Long-term efficacy and safety of donepezil in the treatment of Alzheimer's disease: final analysis of a US multicentre open-label study. Eur Neuropsychopharmacol 2000; 10:195–203.
15. Corey-Bloom J et al. A randomized trial evaluating the efficacy and safety of ENA 713 (rivastigmine tartrate), a new acetylcholinesterase inhibitor, in patients with mild to moderately severe Alzheimer's disease. Int J Geriatr Psychopharmacol 1998; 1:55–64.
16. Rosler M et al. Efficacy and safety of rivastigmine in patients with Alzheimer's disease: international randomised controlled trial. BMJ 1999; 318:633–638.
17. Tariot PN et al. A 5-month, randomized, placebo-controlled trial of galantamine in AD. The Galantamine USA-10 Study Group. Neurology 2000; 54:2269–2276.
18. Raskind MA et al. Galantamine in AD: A 6-month, placebo-controlled trial with a 6-month extension. The Galantamine USA-1 Study Group. Neurology 2000; 54:2261–2268.
19. Wilcock GK et al. Efficacy and safety of galantamine in patients with mild to moderate Alzheimer's disease: multicentre randomised controlled trial. Galantamine International-1 Study Group. BMJ 2000; 321:1445–1449.
20. Birks J. Cholinesterase inhibitors for Alzheimer's disease. Cochrane Database Syst Rev 2006; CD005593.
21. Jones RW et al. A multinational, randomised, 12-week study comparing the effects of donepezil and galantamine in patients with mild to moderate Alzheimer's disease. Int J Geriatr Psychiatry 2004; 19:58–67.
22. Wilcock G et al. A long-term comparison of galantamine and donepezil in the treatment of Alzheimer's disease. Drugs Aging 2003; 20:777–789.
23. Figiel GS et al. Safety and efficacy of rivastigmine in patients with Alzheimer's disease not responding adequately to donepezil: an open-label study. Prim Care Companion J Clin Psychiatry 2008; 10:291–298.

Special groups

24. Birks J et al. Donepezil for dementia due to Alzheimer's disease. Cochrane Database Syst Rev 2006;CD001190.
25. Birks J et al. Rivastigmine for Alzheimer's disease. Cochrane Database Syst Rev 2009;CD001191.
26. Loy C et al. Galantamine for Alzheimer's disease. Cochrane Database Syst Rev 2004;CD001747.
27. Winblad B et al. A six-month double-blind, randomized, placebo-controlled study of a transdermal patch in Alzheimer's disease – rivastigmine patch versus capsule. Int J Geriatr Psychiatry 2007; 22:456–467.
28. Winblad B et al. Memantine in severe dementia: results of the 9M-Best Study (Benefit and efficacy in severely demented patients during treatment with memantine). Int J Geriatr Psychiatry 1999; 14:135–146.
29. Livingston G et al. The place of memantine in the treatment of Alzheimer's disease: a number needed to treat analysis. Int J Geriatr Psychiatry 2004; 19:919–925.
30. Peskind ER et al. Memantine treatment in mild to moderate Alzheimer disease: a 24-week randomized, controlled trial. Am J Geriatr Psychiatry 2006; 14:704–715.
31. McShane R et al. Memantine for dementia. Cochrane Database Syst Rev 2006;CD003154.
32. Raina P et al. Effectiveness of cholinesterase inhibitors and memantine for treating dementia: evidence review for a clinical practice guideline. Ann Intern Med 2008; 148:379–397.
33. Rosen WG et al. A new rating scale for Alzheimer's disease. Am J Psychiatry 1984; 141:1356–1364.
34. Folstein MF et al. "Mini-mental state". A practical method for grading the cognitive state of patients for the clinician. J Psychiatr Res 1975; 12:189–198.
35. Schneider LS et al. Validity and reliability of the Alzheimer's Disease Cooperative Study-Clinical Global Impression of Change. The Alzheimer's Disease Cooperative Study. Alzheimer Dis Assoc Disord 1997; 11 Suppl 2:S22–S32.
36. Cummings JL. The Neuropsychiatric Inventory: assessing psychopathology in dementia patients. Neurology 1997; 48:S10–S16.
37. Birks J et al. Donepezil for dementia due to Alzheimer's disease. Cochrane Database Syst Rev 2006;CD001190.
38. Burns A et al. Safety and efficacy of galantamine (Reminyl) in severe Alzheimer's disease (the SERAD study): a randomised, placebo-controlled, double-blind trial. The Lancet Neurology 2009; 8:39–47.
39. Burns A et al. Efficacy and safety of donepezil over 3 years: an open-label, multicentre study in patients with Alzheimer's disease. Int J Geriatr Psychiatry 2007; 22:806–812.
40. Doody RS et al. Open-label, multicenter, phase 3 extension study of the safety and efficacy of donepezil in patients with Alzheimer disease. Arch Neurol 2001; 58:427–433.
41. Farlow MR et al. Effective pharmacologic management of Alzheimer's disease. Am J Med 2007; 120:388–397.
42. Dybicz SB et al. Patterns of cholinesterase-inhibitor use in the nursing home setting: a retrospective analysis. Am J Geriatr Pharmacother 2006; 4:154–160.
43. Jones RW et al. Safety and tolerability of once-daily versus twice-daily memantine: a randomised, double-blind study in moderate to severe Alzheimer's disease. Int J Geriatr Psychiatry 2007; 22:258–262.
44. Parsons CG et al. Memantine is a clinically well tolerated N-methyl-D-aspartate (NMDA) receptor antagonist—a review of preclinical data. Neuropharmacology 1999; 38:735–767.
45. Reisberg B et al. Memantine in moderate-to-severe Alzheimer's disease. N Engl J Med 2003; 348:1333–1341.
46. Dunn NR et al. Adverse effects associated with the use of donepezil in general practice in England. J Psychopharmacol 2000; 14:406–408.
47. Hashimoto M et al. Urinary incontinence: an unrecognised adverse effect with donepezil. Lancet 2000; 356:568.
48. FDA Alert for Healthcare Professionals. Galantamine hydrobromide (marketed as Razadyne, formerly Reminyl). http://www.fda.gov/. 2005.
49. Malone DM et al. Cholinesterase inhibitors and cardiovascular disease: a survey of old age psychiatrists' practice. Age Ageing 2007; 36:331–333.
50. Rowland JP et al. Cardiovascular monitoring with acetylcholinesterase inhibitors: a clinical protocol. Adv Psychiatr Treat 2007; 13:178–184.
51. Dooley M et al. Donepezil: a review of its use in Alzheimer's disease. Drugs Aging 2000; 16:199–226.
52. Scott LJ et al. Galantamine: a review of its use in Alzheimer's disease. Drugs 2000; 60:1095–1122.
53. Tavassoli N et al. Drug interactions with cholinesterase inhibitors: an analysis of the French pharmacovigilance database and a comparison of two national drug formularies (Vidal, British National Formulary). Drug Saf 2007; 30:1063–1071.
54. National Institute of Clinical Excellence. Guidance on the use of donepezil, rivastigmine and galantamine for the treatment of Azheimer's disease. Technology Appraisal 19. http://www.nice.org.uk. 2001.
55. Matthews HP et al. Donepezil in Alzheimer's disease: eighteen month results from Southampton Memory Clinic. Int J Geriatr Psychiatry 2000; 15:713–720.
56. Ieni JR et al. Safety of donepezil in extended treatment of Alzheimer's disease. Eur Neuropsycho pharmacol 1999; 9 (Suppl. 5):328–329.
57. AD2000 Collaborative Group. Long-term donepezil treatment in 565 patients with Alzheimer's disease (AD2000): randomised double-blind trial. Lancet 2004; 363:2105–2115.
58. National Institute for Clinical Excellence. Donepezil, galantamine, rivastigmine (review) and memantine for the treatment of Alzheimer's disease. Technology Appraisal No. 111. http://www.nice.org.uk. 2006.
59. Schmitt B et al. Combination therapy in Alzheimer's disease: a review of current evidence. CNS Drugs 2004; 18:827–844.
60. Tariot PN et al. Memantine treatment in patients with moderate to severe Alzheimer disease already receiving donepezil: a randomized controlled trial. JAMA 2004; 291:317–324.
61. Hartmann S et al. Tolerability of memantine in combination with cholinesterase inhibitors in dementia therapy. Int Clin Psychopharmacol 2003; 18:81–85.
62. Dantoine T et al. Rivastigmine monotherapy and combination therapy with memantine in patients with moderately severe Alzheimer's disease who failed to benefit from previous cholinesterase inhibitor treatment. Int J Clin Pract 2006; 60:110–118.
63. Periclou AP et al. Lack of pharmacokinetic or pharmacodynamic interaction between memantine and donepezil. Ann Pharmacother 2004; 38:1389–1394.
64. Grossberg GT et al. Rationale for combination therapy with galantamine and memantine in Alzheimer's disease. J Clin Pharmacol 2006; 46:17S–26S.
65. Ahlemeyer B et al. Pharmacological studies supporting the therapeutic use of Ginkgo biloba extract for Alzheimer's disease. Pharmacopsychiatry 2003; 36 Suppl 1:S8–14.
66. Kanowski S et al. Ginkgo biloba extract EGb 761 in dementia: intent-to-treat analyses of a 24-week, multi-center, double-blind, placebo-controlled, randomized trial. Pharmacopsychiatry 2003; 36:297–303.
67. McCarney R et al. Ginkgo biloba for mild to moderate dementia in a community setting: a pragmatic, randomised, parallel-group, double-blind, placebo-controlled trial. Int J Geriatr Psychiatry 2008; 23:1222–1230.
68. DeKosky ST et al. Ginkgo biloba for prevention of dementia: a randomized controlled trial. JAMA 2008; 300:2253–2262.
69. Birks J et al. Ginkgo biloba for cognitive impairment and dementia. Cochrane Database Syst Rev 2009;CD003120.
70. Bent S et al. Spontaneous bleeding associated with ginkgo biloba: a case report and systematic review of the literature: a case report and systematic review of the literature. J Gen Intern Med 2005; 20:657–661.
71. Issac MG et al. Vitamin E for Alzheimer's disease and mild cognitive impairment. Cochrane Database Syst Rev 2008;CD002854.
72. Connelly PJ et al. A randomised double-blind placebo-controlled trial of folic acid supplementation of cholinesterase inhibitors in Alzheimer's disease. Int J Geriatr Psychiatry 2008; 23:155–160.
73. Sun Y et al. Efficacy of multivitamin supplementation containing vitamins B6 and B12 and folic acid as adjunctive treatment with a cholinesterase inhibitor in Alzheimer's disease: a 26-week, randomized, double-blind, placebo-controlled study in Taiwanese patients. Clin Ther 2007; 29:2204–2214.
74. Freund-Levi Y et al. Omega-3 supplementation in mild to moderate Alzheimer's disease: effects on neuropsychiatric symptoms. Int J Geriatr Psychiatry 2008; 23:161–169.
75. Lee ST et al. Panax ginseng enhances cognitive performance in Alzheimer disease. Alzheimer Dis Assoc Disord 2008; 22:222–226.
76. Doody RS et al. Effect of dimebon on cognition, activities of daily living, behaviour, and global function in patients with mild-to-moderate Alzheimer's disease: a randomised, double-blind, placebo-controlled study. Lancet 2008; 372:207–215.

77. Kavirajan H et al. Efficacy and adverse effects of cholinesterase inhibitors and memantine in vascular dementia: a meta-analysis of randomised controlled trials. Lancet Neurol 2007; 6:782–792.
78. Bocti C et al. Management of dementia with a cerebrovascular component. Alzheimer's and Dementia 2007; 3:398–403.
79. Demaerschalk BM et al. Treatment of vascular dementia and vascular cognitive impairment. Neurologist 2007; 13:37–41.
80. Roman GC et al. Donepezil in vascular dementia: combined analysis of two large-scale clinical trials. Dement Geriatr Cogn Disord 2005; 20:338–344.
81. Malouf R et al. Donepezil for vascular cognitive impairment. Cochrane Database Syst Rev 2004;CD004395.
82. Moretti R et al. Rivastigmine superior to aspirin plus nimodipine in subcortical vascular dementia: an open, 16-month, comparative study. Int J Clin Pract 2004; 58:346–353.
83. Moretti R et al. Rivastigmine in subcortical vascular dementia: a randomized, controlled, open 12-month study in 208 patients. Am J Alzheimers Dis Other Demen 2003; 18:265–272.
84. Small G et al. Galantamine in the treatment of cognitive decline in patients with vascular dementia or Alzheimer's disease with cerebrovascular disease. CNS Drugs 2003; 17:905–914.
85. Kurz AF et al. Long-term safety and cognitive effects of galantamine in the treatment of probable vascular dementia or Alzheimer's disease with cerebrovascular disease. Eur J Neurol 2003; 10:633–640.
86. Erkinjuntti T et al. Efficacy of galantamine in probable vascular dementia and Alzheimer's disease combined with cerebrovascular disease: a randomised trial. Lancet 2002; 359:1283–1290.
87. Wilcock G et al. A double-blind, placebo-controlled multicentre study of memantine in mild to moderate vascular dementia (MMM500). Int Clin Psychopharmacol 2002; 17:297–305.
88. Orgogozo JM et al. Efficacy and safety of memantine in patients with mild to moderate vascular dementia: a randomized, placebo-controlled trial (MMM 300). Stroke 2002; 33:1834–1839.
89. Craig D et al. Galantamine for vascular cognitive impairment. Cochrane Database Syst Rev 2006;CD004746.
90. Craig D et al. Rivastigmine for vascular cognitive impairment. Cochrane Database Syst Rev 2005;CD004744.
91. Auchus AP et al. Galantamine treatment of vascular dementia: a randomized trial. Neurology 2007; 69:448–458.
92. Wild R et al. Cholinesterase inhibitors for dementia with Lewy bodies. Cochrane Database Syst Rev 2003;CD003672.
93. Bhasin M et al. Cholinesterase inhibitors in dementia with Lewy bodies: a comparative analysis. Int J Geriatr Psychiatry 2007; 22:890–895.

Further reading

Loy C et al. Galantamine for Alzheimer's disease and mild cognitive impairment. Cochrane Database Syst Rev 2006;CD001747.
Burns A et al. Clinical practice with anti-dementia drugs: a consensus statement from British Association for Psychopharmacology. J Psychopharmacol 2006; 20:732–755.

Special groups

Behavioural and psychological symptoms of dementia

Behavioural and psychological symptoms of dementia (BPSD) is the collective term used to describe the group of non-cognitive symptoms experienced in dementia. These can include: psychosis, agitation, and mood disorder[1] and affects 50–80% of patients to varying degrees[2]. The management of these symptoms is the subject of a longstanding debate because, for a variety of reasons, treatment is not well informed by properly conducted studies[3] and many available agents have been linked to serious adverse effects.

Antipsychotics
First-generation antipsychotics (FGAs) have been widely used for decades in behavioural disturbance associated with dementia. They are probably effective[4] but, because of extrapyramidal and other adverse effects, are less well tolerated[5,6] than second-generation antipsychotics (SGAs). SGAs have been shown to be comparable in efficacy to FGAs for behavioural symptoms of dementia[7–9], with one study finding the atypical risperidone to be superior to the typical (FGA) haloperidol[10].

Risperidone is the only drug licensed in the UK for BPSD. It is indicated for the short-term treatment (up to 6 weeks) of persistent aggression in patients with moderate to severe Alzheimer's dementia unresponsive to non-pharmacological approaches and when there is a risk of harm to self or others[11].

SGAs were once widely recommended in dementia-related behaviour disturbance[12] but their use is now highly controversial[13,14]. There are three reasons for this: effect size is small[15–18], tolerability is poor[18–20], and there is a tentative association with increased mortality[21].

Efficacy of SGAs
Various reviews and trials support the efficacy of olanzapine[7,22], risperidone[23–27], quetiapine[9,28–30], aripiprazole[31–33] and amisulpride[34,35]. Studies comparing olanzapine with risperidone[17] and quetiapine with risperidone[36] in BPSD found no significant differences between treatment groups. One study found clozapine to be beneficial in treatment-resistant agitation associated with dementia[37].

The first CATIE-AD study[38] showed very minor effectiveness advantages for olanzapine and risperidone (but not for quetiapine) over placebo in terms of time to discontinuation, but all drugs were poorly tolerated because of sedation, confusion, and EPS (the last of these was not a problem with quetiapine). Similarly, in the second CATIE-AD study[39] greater improvement was noted with olanzapine or risperidone on certain neuropsychiatric rating scales compared with placebo (but not with quetiapine). A Cochrane review[40] of atypical antipsychotics for aggression and psychosis in Alzheimer's disease found that evidence suggests that risperidone and olanzapine are useful in reducing aggression and risperidone reduces psychosis. However the authors concluded that because of modest efficacy and significant increase in adverse effects, neither risperidone nor olanzapine should be routinely used to treat dementia patients unless there is severe distress or a serious risk of physical harm to those living or working with the patient.

Increased mortality with antipsychotics in dementia
Following analysis of published and unpublished data in 2004, initial warnings were issued in the UK and USA regarding increased mortality in patients with dementia with certain atypical antipsychotics (mainly risperidone and olanzapine)[41–43]. These warnings have been extended to include all atypical antipsychotics as well as conventional antipsychotics[44,45] in view of more recent data. The inclusion of a warning about a possible risk of cerebrovascular events has now been added to SPCs for all typical and atypical antipsychotics.

Several published analyses support the warnings[21,46], suggesting an association between some SGAs and stroke[47,48]. Other studies have detected no clear adverse outcome[49–52]. Increased mortality with FGAs, or typical antipsychotics, has been shown to be similar[53–55] to that with SGAs and possibly even greater[56–60]. One study suggested that the risk of cerebrovascular adverse events (CVAEs) in elderly users of antipsychotics may not be cumulative[61]. The risk was found to be elevated especially during the first weeks of treatment but then decreases over time, returning to base level after 3 months. In contrast, a long-term study (24–54 months) found that mortality was progressively increased over time for antipsychotic-treated (risperidone and FGAs) patients compared with those receiving placebo[62]. At 12 months survival was 70% (antipsychotics) vs 77% (placebo); 46% vs 71% at 24 months and 30% vs 59% at 36 months. This study clearly suggests that antipsychotics should be avoided, if at all possible.

A recent assessment report by the European Medicines Agency (EMEA)[44] concluded that despite study limitations, the available evidence suggests that conventional antipsychotics are also associated with increased mortality in elderly people with dementia. Although the results of some studies suggest an excess mortality observed with conventional antipsychotics compared with atypical antipsychotics, the report concluded that this could not be confirmed because of the methodological limitations of the studies. In addition, there was not enough evidence to determine whether the risk differs from one medicine to another, so the risk is assumed to apply to all medicines in the class.

Several mechanisms have been postulated for the underlying causes of CVAEs with antipsychotics[63]. Orthostatic hypotension may aggravate the deficit in cerebral perfusion in an individual with cerebrovascular insufficiency or atherosclerosis, thus causing a CVA. Tachycardia may similarly decrease cerebral perfusion or dislodge a thrombus in a patient with atrial fibrillation (see section on psychotropics in AF). Following an episode of orthostatic hypotension, there could be a rebound excess of catecholamines with vasoconstriction thus aggravating cerebral insufficiency. In addition, hyperprolactinaemia could in theory accelerate atherosclerosis and sedation might cause dehydration and haemoconcentration, each of which is a possible mechanism for increased risk of cerebrovascular events[63].

In the UK, concerns about a link to stroke and increased mortality have led to a reduction in the use of those antipsychotics identified as potential causative agents and which were implicated in the studies linking them with stroke. Some centres use amisulpride but its use is only minimally supported[34,35] and its safety in this group of patients unknown.

Both typical[64] and atypical antipsychotics[65] may also hasten cognitive decline in dementia, although there is recent evidence to refute this[36,66,67].

Others pharmacological agents

Donepezil[68,69], rivastigmine[70–73], and galantamine[74] may afford some benefit in reducing behavioural disturbance in dementia. Their effect seems apparent only after several weeks of treatment[75]. However, the evidence is somewhat inconsistent and a recent study of donepezil in agitation associated with dementia found no apparent benefit compared with placebo[76]. Rivastigmine has shown positive results for neuropsychiatric symptoms associated with vascular[70] and Lewy body dementia[70,77], although NICE guidance has not considered AChEIs for dementias other than Alzheimer's disease[78]. Growing evidence for memantine also suggests benefits for neuropsychiatric symptoms associated with dementia[79–81]. Despite apparently positive findings in (often manufacturer-sponsored) studies the use of cognitive-enhancing agents for behavioural disturbance remains controversial.

Special groups

Benzodiazepines[82,83] and trazodone[84,85] are widely used but poorly supported. Benzodiazepines have been associated with cognitive decline[82] and may contribute to increase frequency of falls and hip fractures[83,86] in the elderly population. SSRIs are of doubtful efficacy[87,88]. Mood-stabilisers have also been used[89,90]. One RCT of valproate that included an open-label extension found valproate to be partly effective in controlling symptoms[91].

Non-drug measures

A variety of non-pharmacological methods[92] have been developed and some are reasonably well supported by cogent research[93–95]. Behavioural management techniques and caregiver psychoeducation centred on individual patient's behaviour are generally successful and the effects can last for months[94]. Music therapy, Snoezelen[96] (specially designed rooms with soothing and stimulating environment), and some types of sensory stimulation are useful during the sessions but have no longer-term effects[94]. A number of different complementary therapies[97] have been used in dementia including massage, reflexology, administration of herbal medicines, and aromatherapy. Aromatherapy[98] is the fastest growing of these therapies, with extracts from lavender and Melissa balm most commonly used[92]. Some positive results from controlled trials have shown significant reduction in agitation[99] although the evidence base is still sparse and the side-effect profile unexplored[100]. Given concerns over almost all drug therapies, non-pharmacological measures should always be considered first.

Summary

The evidence base available to guide treatment in this area is insufficient to allow specific recommendations on appropriate management and drug choice. Whichever drug is chosen, the following approach should be followed:

- Exclude physical illness potentially precipitating BPSD e.g. constipation, infection, pain
- Target the symptoms requiring treatment
- Consider non-pharmacological methods
- Carry out a risk/benefit analysis tailored to individual patient needs when selecting a drug
- Discuss treatment options and explain the risks to patient (if they have capacity) and family/carers
- Titrate drug from a low starting dose and maintain the lowest dose possible for the shortest period necessary
- Review appropriateness of treatment regularly so that ineffective drug is not continued unnecessarily
- Monitor for adverse effects
- Document clearly treatment choices and discussions with patient, family, or carers

---

References

1. Aalten P et al. Behavioral problems in dementia: a factor analysis of the neuropsychiatric inventory. Dement Geriatr Cogn Disord 2003; 15:99–105.
2. Lyketsos CG et al. Prevalence of neuropsychiatric symptoms in dementia and mild cognitive impairment: results from the cardiovascular health study. JAMA 2002; 288:1475–1483.
3. Salzman C et al. Elderly patients with dementia-related symptoms of severe agitation and aggression: consensus statement on treatment options, clinical trials methodology, and policy. J Clin Psychiatry 2008; 69:889–898.
4. Devanand DP et al. A randomized, placebo-controlled dose-comparison trial of haloperidol for psychosis and disruptive behaviors in Alzheimer's disease. Am J Psychiatry 1998; 155:1512–1520.
5. Chan WC et al. A double-blind randomised comparison of risperidone and haloperidol in the treatment of behavioural and psychological symptoms in Chinese dementia patients. Int J Geriatr Psychiatry 2001; 16:1156–1162.
6. Tariot PN et al. Quetiapine treatment of psychosis associated with dementia: a double-blind, randomized, placebo-controlled clinical trial. Am J Geriatr Psychiatry 2006; 14:767–776.
7. Verhey FR et al. Olanzapine versus haloperidol in the treatment of agitation in elderly patients with dementia: results of a randomized controlled double-blind trial. Dement Geriatr Cogn Disord 2006; 21:1–8.

Special groups

8. De Deyn PP et al. A randomized trial of risperidone, placebo, and haloperidol for behavioral symptoms of dementia. Neurology 1999; 53:946–955.
9. Savaskan E et al. Treatment of behavioural, cognitive and circadian rest-activity cycle disturbances in Alzheimer's disease: haloperidol vs. quetiapine. Int J Neuropsychopharmacol 2006; 9:507–516.
10. Suh GH et al. Comparative efficacy of risperidone versus haloperidol on behavioural and psychological symptoms of dementia. Int J Geriatr Psychiatry 2006; 21:654–660.
11. Janssen-Cilag Ltd. Summary of Product Characteristics. Risperdal tablets, liquid and quicklet. 2009. http://emc.medicines.org.uk/.
12. Lee PE et al. Atypical antipsychotic drugs in the treatment of behavioural and psychological symptoms of dementia: systematic review. BMJ 2004; 329:75.
13. Jeste DV et al. Atypical antipsychotics in elderly patients with dementia or schizophrenia: review of recent literature. Harv Rev Psychiatry 2005; 13:340–351.
14. Jeste DV et al. ACNP White Paper: update on use of antipsychotic drugs in elderly persons with dementia. Neuropsychopharmacology 2008; 33:957–970.
15. Aupperle P. Management of aggression, agitation, and psychosis in dementia: focus on atypical antipsychotics. Am J Alzheimers Dis Other Demen 2006; 21:101–108.
16. Yury CA et al. Meta-analysis of the effectiveness of atypical antipsychotics for the treatment of behavioural problems in persons with dementia. Psychother Psychosom 2007; 76:213–218.
17. Deberdt WG et al. Comparison of olanzapine and risperidone in the treatment of psychosis and associated behavioral disturbances in patients with dementia. Am J Geriatr Psychiatry 2005; 13:722–730.
18. Schneider LS et al. Efficacy and adverse effects of atypical antipsychotics for dementia: meta-analysis of randomized, placebo-controlled trials. Am J Geriatr Psychiatry 2006; 14:191–210.
19. Anon. How safe are antipsychotics in dementia? Drug Ther Bull 2007; 45:81–86.
20. Rosack J. Side-effect risk often tempers antipsychotic use for dementia. Psychiatr News 2006; 41:1.
21. Schneider LS et al. Risk of death with atypical antipsychotic drug treatment for dementia: meta-analysis of randomized placebo-controlled trials. JAMA 2005; 294:1934–1943.
22. Street JS et al. Olanzapine treatment of psychotic and behavioral symptoms in patients with Alzheimer disease in nursing care facilities: a double-blind, randomized, placebo-controlled trial. The HGEU Study Group. Arch Gen Psychiatry 2000; 57:968–976.
23. Bhana N et al. Risperidone: a review of its use in the management of the behavioural and psychological symptoms of dementia. Drugs Aging 2000; 16:451–471.
24. Katz I et al. The efficacy and safety of risperidone in the treatment of psychosis of Alzheimer's disease and mixed dementia: a meta-analysis of 4 placebo-controlled clinical trials. Int J Geriatr Psychiatry 2007; 22:475–484.
25. Onor ML et al. Clinical experience with risperidone in the treatment of behavioral and psychological symptoms of dementia. Prog Neuropsychopharmacol Biol Psychiatry 2007; 31:205–209.
26. Rabinowitz J et al. Treating behavioral and psychological symptoms in patients with psychosis of Alzheimer's disease using risperidone. Int Psychogeriatr 2007; 19:227–240.
27. Kurz A et al. Effects of risperidone on behavioral and psychological symptoms associated with dementia in clinical practice. Int Psychogeriatr 2005; 17:605–616.
28. McManus DQ et al. Quetiapine, a novel antipsychotic: experience in elderly patients with psychotic disorders. Seroquel Trial 48 Study Group. J Clin Psychiatry 1999; 60:292–298.
29. Onor ML et al. Efficacy and tolerability of quetiapine in the treatment of behavioral and psychological symptoms of dementia. Am J Alzheimers Dis Other Demen 2006; 21:448–453.
30. Zhong KX et al. Quetiapine to treat agitation in dementia: a randomized, double-blind, placebo-controlled study. Curr Alzheimer Res 2007; 4:81–93.
31. Laks J et al. Use of aripiprazole for psychosis and agitation in dementia. Int Psychogeriatr 2006; 18:335–340.
32. De Deyn P et al. Aripiprazole for the treatment of psychosis in patients with Alzheimer's disease: a randomized, placebo-controlled study. J Clin Psychopharmacol 2005; 25:463–467.
33. Mintzer JE et al. Aripiprazole for the treatment of psychoses in institutionalized patients with Alzheimer dementia: a multicenter, randomized, double-blind, placebo-controlled assessment of three fixed doses. Am J Geriatr Psychiatry 2007; 15:918–931.
34. Mauri M et al. Amisulpride in the treatment of behavioural disturbances among patients with moderate to severe Alzheimer's disease. Acta Neurol Scand 2006; 114:97–101.
35. Lim HK et al. Amisulpride versus risperidone treatment for behavioral and psychological symptoms in patients with dementia of the Alzheimer type: a randomized, open, prospective study. Neuropsychobiology 2006; 54:247–251.
36. Rainer M et al. Quetiapine versus risperidone in elderly patients with behavioural and psychological symptoms of dementia: efficacy, safety and cognitive function. Eur Psychiatry 2007; 22:395–403.
37. Lee HB et al. Clozapine for treatment-resistant agitation in dementia. J Geriatr Psychiatry Neurol 2007; 20:178–182.
38. Schneider LS et al. Effectiveness of atypical antipsychotic drugs in patients with Alzheimer's disease. N Engl J Med 2006; 355:1525–1538.
39. Sultzer DL et al. Clinical symptom responses to atypical antipsychotic medications in Alzheimer's disease: phase 1 outcomes from the CATIE-AD effectiveness trial. Am J Psychiatry 2008; 165:844–854.
40. Ballard C et al. The effectiveness of atypical antipsychotics for the treatment of aggression and psychosis in Alzheimer's disease. Cochrane Database Syst Rev 2006;CD003476.
41. Duff G. Atypical antipsychotic drugs and stroke. http://www.mhra.gov.uk. 2004
42. FDA. Deaths with antipsychotics in elderly patients with behavioral disturbances. http://www.fda.gov/. 2005.
43. Pharmacovigilance Working Party. Antipsychotics and cerebrovascular accident. SPC wording for antipsychotics . http://www.mhra.gov.uk. 2005.
44. European Medicines Agency. CHMP Assessment Report on conventional antipsychotics. 2008. http://www.emea.europa.eu
45. FDA Alert for Healthcare Professionals. Antipsychotics. 2008. http://www.fda.gov
46. Kryzhanovskaya LA et al. A review of treatment-emergent adverse events during olanzapine clinical trials in elderly patients with dementia. J Clin Psychiatry 2006; 67:933–945.
47. Herrmann N et al. Do atypical antipsychotics cause stroke? CNS Drugs 2005; 19:91–103.
48. Douglas IJ et al. Exposure to antipsychotics and risk of stroke: self controlled case series study. BMJ 2008; 337:a1227.
49. Gill SS et al. Atypical antipsychotic drugs and risk of ischaemic stroke: population based retrospective cohort study. BMJ 2005; 330:445.
50. Finkel S et al. Risperidone treatment in elderly patients with dementia: relative risk of cerebrovascular events versus other antipsychotics. Int Psychogeriatr 2005; 17:617–629.
51. Raivio MM et al. Neither atypical nor conventional antipsychotics increase mortality or hospital admissions among elderly patients with dementia: a two-year prospective study. Am J Geriatr Psychiatry 2007; 15:416–424.
52. Barnett MJ et al. Comparison of risk of cerebrovascular events in an elderly VA population with dementia between antipsychotic and nonantipsychotic users. J Clin Psychopharmacol 2007; 27:595–601.
53. Kales HC et al. Mortality risk in patients with dementia treated with antipsychotics versus other psychiatric medications. Am J Psychiatry 2007; 164:1568–1576.
54. Herrmann N et al. Atypical antipsychotics and risk of cerebrovascular accidents. Am J Psychiatry 2004; 161:1113–1115.
55. Trifiro G et al. All-cause mortality associated with atypical and typical antipsychotics in demented outpatients. Pharmacoepidemiol Drug Saf 2007; 16:538–544.
56. Nasrallah HA et al. Lower mortality in geriatric patients receiving risperidone and olanzapine versus haloperidol: preliminary analysis of retrospective data. Am J Geriatr Psychiatry 2004; 12:437–439.

57. Gill SS et al. Antipsychotic drug use and mortality in older adults with dementia. Ann Intern Med 2007; 146:775–786.
58. Sacchetti E et al. Risk of stroke with typical and atypical anti-psychotics: a retrospective cohort study including unexposed subjects. J Psychopharmacol 2008; 22:39–46.
59. Wang PS et al. Risk of death in elderly users of conventional vs. atypical antipsychotic medications. N Engl J Med 2005; 353:2335–2341.
60. Hollis J et al. Antipsychotic medication dispensing and risk of death in veterans and war widows 65 years and older. Am J Geriatr Psychiatry 2007; 15:932–941.
61. Kleijer BC et al. Risk of cerebrovascular events in elderly users of antipsychotics. J Psychopharmacol 2008; Epub ahead of print.
62. Ballard C et al. The dementia antipsychotic withdrawal trial (DART-AD): long-term follow-up of a randomised placebo-controlled trial. Lancet Neurol 2008; 8:151–157.
63. Smith DA et al. Association between risperidone treatment and cerebrovascular adverse events: examining the evidence and postulating hypotheses for an underlying mechanism. J Am Med Dir Assoc 2004; 5:129–132.
64. McShane R et al. Do neuroleptic drugs hasten cognitive decline in dementia? Prospective study with necropsy follow up. BMJ 1997; 314:266–270.
65. Ballard C et al. Quetiapine and rivastigmine and cognitive decline in Alzheimer's disease: randomised double blind placebo controlled trial. BMJ 2005; 330:874.
66. Livingston G et al. Antipsychotics and cognitive decline in Alzheimer's disease: the LASER-Alzheimer's disease longitudinal study. J Neurol Neurosurg Psychiatry 2007; 78:25–29.
67. Paleacu D et al. Quetiapine treatment for behavioural and psychological symptoms of dementia in Alzheimer's disease patients: a 6-week, double-blind, placebo-controlled study. Int J Geriatr Psychiatry 2008; 23:393–400.
68. Terao T et al. Can donepezil be considered a mild antipsychotic in dementia treatment? A report of donepezil use in 6 patients. J Clin Psychiatry 2003; 64:1392–1393.
69. Weiner MF et al. Effects of donepezil on emotional/behavioral symptoms in Alzheimer's disease patients. J Clin Psychiatry 2000; 61:487–492.
70. Figiel G et al. A systematic review of the effectiveness of rivastigmine for the treatment of behavioral disturbances in dementia and other neurological disorders. Curr Med Res Opin 2008; 24:157–166.
71. Finkel SI. Effects of rivastigmine on behavioral and psychological symptoms of dementia in Alzheimer's disease. Clin Ther 2004; 26:980–990.
72. Rosler M et al. Effects of two-year treatment with the cholinesterase inhibitor rivastigmine on behavioural symptoms in Alzheimer's disease. Behav Neurol 1998; 11:211–216.
73. Cummings JL et al. Effects of rivastigmine treatment on the neuropsychiatric and behavioral disturbances of nursing home residents with moderate to severe probable Alzheimer's disease: a 26-week, multicenter, open-label study. Am J Geriatr Pharmacother 2005; 3:137–148.
74. Cummings JL et al. Reduction of behavioral disturbances and caregiver distress by galantamine in patients with Alzheimer's disease. Am J Psychiatry 2004; 161:532–538.
75. Barak Y et al. Donepezil for the treatment of behavioral disturbances in Alzheimer's disease: a 6-month open trial. Arch Gerontol Geriatr 2001; 33:237–241.
76. Howard RJ et al. Donepezil for the treatment of agitation in Alzheimer's disease. N Engl J Med 2007; 357:1382–1392.
77. McKeith I et al. Efficacy of rivastigmine in dementia with Lewy bodies: a randomised, double-blind, placebo-controlled international study. Lancet 2000; 356:2031–2036.
78. National Institute for Clinical Excellence. Dementia: Supporting people with dementia and their carers in health and social care. Clinical Guidance 42. http://www.nice.org.uk . 2006.
79. Cummings JL et al. Behavioral effects of memantine in Alzheimer disease patients receiving donepezil treatment. Neurology 2006; 67:57–63.
80. Wilcock GK et al. Memantine for agitation/aggression and psychosis in moderately severe to severe Alzheimer's disease: a pooled analysis of 3 studies. J Clin Psychiatry 2008; 69:341–348.
81. Gauthier S et al. Improvement in behavioural symptoms in patients with moderate to severe Alzheimer's disease by memantine: a pooled data analysis. Int J Geriatr Psychiatry 2007; 23:537–545.
82. Verdoux H et al. Is benzodiazepine use a risk factor for cognitive decline and dementia? A literature review of epidemiological studies. Psychol Med 2005; 35:307–315.
83. Lagnaoui R et al. Benzodiazepine utilization patterns in Alzheimer's disease patients. Pharmacoepidemiol Drug Saf 2003; 12:511–515.
84. Martinon-Torres G et al. Trazodone for agitation in dementia. Cochrane Database Syst Rev 2004; CD004990.
85. Lopez-Pousa S et al. Trazodone for Alzheimer's disease: a naturalistic follow-up study. Arch Gerontol Geriatr 2008; 47:207–215.
86. Chang CM et al. Benzodiazepine and risk of hip fractures in older people: a nested case-control study in Taiwan. Am J Geriatr Psychiatry 2008; 16:686–692.
87. Deakin JB et al. Paroxetine does not improve symptoms and impairs cognition in frontotemporal dementia: a double-blind randomized controlled trial. Psychopharmacology 2004; 172:400–408.
88. Finkel SI et al. A randomized, placebo-controlled study of the efficacy and safety of sertraline in the treatment of the behavioral manifestations of Alzheimer's disease in outpatients treated with donepezil. Int J Geriatr Psychiatry 2004; 19:9–18.
89. Lonergan ET et al. Valproic acid for agitation in dementia. Cochrane Database Syst Rev 2004;CD003945.
90. Tariot PN et al. Efficacy and tolerability of carbamazepine for agitation and aggression in dementia. Am J Psychiatry 1998; 155:54–61.
91. Sival RC et al. Sodium valproate in aggressive behaviour in dementia: a twelve-week open label follow-up study. Int J Geriatr Psychiatry 2004; 19:305–312.
92. Douglas S et al. Non-pharmacological interventions in dementia. Adv Psychiatr Treat 2004; 10:171–177.
93. Ayalon L et al. Effectiveness of nonpharmacological interventions for the management of neuropsychiatric symptoms in patients with dementia: a systematic review. Arch Intern Med 2006; 166:2182–2188.
94. Livingston G et al. Systematic review of psychological approaches to the management of neuropsychiatric symptoms of dementia. Am J Psychiatry 2005; 162:1996–2021.
95. Robinson L et al. Effectiveness and acceptability of non-pharmacological interventions to reduce wandering in dementia: a systematic review. Int J Geriatr Psychiatry 2007; 22:9–22.
96. Chung JC et al. Snoezelen for dementia. Cochrane Database Syst Rev 2002;CD003152.
97. McCarney R et al. Homeopathy for dementia. Cochrane Database Syst Rev 2003;CD003803.
98. Thorgrimsen L et al. Aroma therapy for dementia. Cochrane Database Syst Rev 2003;CD003150.
99. Ballard CG et al. Aromatherapy as a safe and effective treatment for the management of agitation in severe dementia: the results of a double-blind, placebo-controlled trial with Melissa. J Clin Psychiatry 2002; 63:553–558.
100. Nguyen QA et al. The use of aromatherapy to treat behavioural problems in dementia. Int J Geriatr Psychiatry 2008; 23:337–346.

Special groups

Further reading

European Medicines Agency. CHMP Assessment Report on conventional antipsychotics. 2008. http://www.emea.europa.eu
Medicines and Healthcare Products Regulatory Agency. PhVWP Assessment report. Antipsychotics and cerebrovascular accident. http://www.mhra.gov.uk. 2005.
Royal College of Psychiatrists. Atypical antipsychotics and BPSD. Prescribing update v4c. http://www.rcpsych.ac.uk/. 2004.

Covert administration of medicines within food and drink

In mental health settings, it is common for patients to refuse medication. In some cases, particularly in those with dementia or a learning disability, the patient may lack capacity to make an informed choice about whether medication will be beneficial to them or not. In these cases, the clinical team may consider whether it would be in the patient's best interests to conceal medication in food or drink. This practice is known as covert administration of medicines. Guidance from the Nursing and Midwifery Council[1,2], the Royal College of Psychiatrists[3], and the Mental Capacity Act[4] exists in order to protect patients from the unlawful and inappropriate administration of medication in this way.

Assessment of mental capacity[4,5]
The assessment of capacity is primarily a matter for doctors treating the patient[4,5]. It is important to make the assessment in relation to the particular treatment proposed. Capacity can vary over time and the assessment should be made at the time of the proposed treatment.

A patient is presumed to have the capacity to make treatment decisions unless he/she is unable to:

- understand information relevant to the treatment, its purpose and why it is being proposed (even when given in simple language)
- understand the principal benefits, risks, and alternatives
- understand the consequences of not receiving the proposed treatment
- retain the information long enough to make a decision
- weigh up the information and make a free choice.

Guidance on covert administration
The *routine* practice of administering medication within food or drink must be discouraged.

A distinction needs to be made between patients who have the capacity to give a valid refusal to medication (whose refusal should be respected, unless treatment is under the auspices of the Mental Health Act[6]), and those who lack this capacity. Among the latter, a further distinction can be made between those for whom no covert use is necessary (because they are unaware that they are receiving medication) and others who would be aware, if they were not deceived into thinking otherwise[2].

The covert administration of medication in patients with schizophrenia and other severe mental illnesses where patients can learn and understand that they will be required to take medication is generally unacceptable[7]. However, covert administration could be used to administer oral medication to a patient detained under the Mental Health Act and refusing treatment as long as they also lack capacity to give valid refusal.

There should be a clear expectation that the patient will benefit from covert administration, and that this will avoid significant harm (both mental or physical) to the patient or others. The treatment must be necessary to save the patient's life, to prevent deterioration in health or to ensure an improvement in physical or mental health[2].

The decision to administer medication covertly should not be made by a single individual but should involve discussion with the multidisciplinary team caring for the patient and the patient's relatives or informal carers. Any decisions should be carefully documented and each instance of covert administration recorded on the prescription chart[2,7]. The decision should be subject to regular review[2].

Special groups

Health professionals should be sure that their actions are in the best interests of the patient and are accountable for their decisions[2].

Summary of process
Covert administration of medication should be subject to the following safeguards:

- All efforts must be made to give medication openly in its normal form.
- A record of the examination of the patient's capacity must be made in the clinical notes, and evidence for incapacity documented.
- The proposed treatment plan and reasons for the plan should be discussed with the multidisciplinary team and the immediate relatives/carers or nominated representatives. Records of these discussions should be made in the clinical notes.
- A check should be made with the pharmacy to determine whether the properties of the medication are likely to be affected by crushing and/or being mixed with food or drink.
- The prescription card should be amended to describe how the medication is to be administered.
- The administration of medicines in this way should be reviewed regularly within care reviews.
- When the medication is administered in foodstuff, it is the responsibility of the dispensing nurse to ensure that the medication is taken. This can be facilitated by direct observation or by nominating another member of the clinical team to observe the patient taking the medication.

References

1. Nursing and Midwifery Council. Covert administration of medicines - disguising medicine in food and drink. 2007. http://www.nmc-uk.org/
2. Nursing and Midwifery Council. UKCC position statement on the covert administration of medicines - disguising medicine in food and drink. 2001. http://www.nmc-uk.org/
3. Royal College of Psychiatrists. College Statement on Covert Administration of Medicines. Psychiatr Bull 2004; 28:385–386.
4. Office of Public Sector Information. Mental Capacity Act 2005 – Chapter 9. 2005. http://www.opsi.gov.uk/
5. British Medical Association. Assessment of Mental Capacity: Guidance for Doctors and Lawyers. 2nd Edition. London: BMJ Books; 2004.
6. Department of Health. Code of Practice: Mental Health Act 1983 – 2008 revision. http://www.dh.gov.uk/. 2008.
7. Treloar A et al. Concealing medication in patients' food. Lancet 2001; 357:62–64.

Special groups

Parkinson's disease

Parkinson's disease is a progressive, degenerative neurological disorder characterised by resting tremor, cogwheel rigidity, bradykinesia, and postural instability. The prevalence of co-morbid psychiatric disorders is high. Approximately 25% will suffer from major depression at some point during the course of their illness, a further 25% from milder forms of depression, 25% from anxiety spectrum disorders, 25% from psychosis and up to 80% will develop dementia[1,2]. While depression and anxiety can occur at any time, psychosis, dementia, and also delirium are more prevalent in the later stages of the illness. Close co-operation between the psychiatrist and neurologist is required to optimise treatment for this group of patients.

Depression in Parkinson's disease
Depression in Parkinson's disease predicts greater cognitive decline, deterioration in functioning and progression of motor symptoms[3]; possibly reflecting more advanced and widespread neurodegeneration involving multiple neurotransmitter pathways[4]. Pre-existing dementia is an established risk factor for the development of depression.

Recommendations for treatment – depression in PD	
Step	Intervention
1	Exclude/treat organic causes such as hypothyroidism (the prevalence of which is higher in Parkinson's disease[3]).
2	**SSRIs** are considered to be first-line treatment. Some patients may experience a worsening of motor symptoms although the absolute risk is low[5,6]. Care must be taken when combining SSRIs with selegiline, as the risk of serotonin syndrome is increased[3]. TCAs are generally poorly tolerated because of their anticholinergic (can worsen cognitive problems; constipation) and alpha-blocking effects (can worsen symptoms of autonomic dysfunction). Note though that RCTs have shown low dose amitriptyline to be more effective than fluoxetine[7], and low dose amitriptyline and sertraline to be equally effective[8]. Nortipyline may be more effective than paroxetine[9].
3	Consider augmentation with dopamine agonists/releasers such as pramiprexole[10].
4	Consider **ECT**. Depression and motor symptoms generally respond well[3] but the risk of inducing delirium is high[11], particularly in patients with pre-existing cognitive impairment.
5	Follow the algorithm for treatment-resistant depression (see relevant section) from this point. Be aware of the increased propensity for side-effects and drug interactions in this patient group.

Psychosis in Parkinson's disease
Psychosis in Parkinson's disease is often characterised by visual hallucinations. Auditory hallucinations and delusions occur far less frequently[12], and usually in younger patients[13]. Psychosis and dementia frequently co-exist. Having one predicts the development of the other[14]. Sleep disorders are also an established risk factor for the development of psychosis[1].

Abnormalities in dopamine, serotonin, and acetylcholine neurotransmission have all been implicated, but the exact aetiology of Parkinson's disease psychosis is poorly understood. In the majority of patients, psychotic symptoms are thought to be secondary to dopaminergic medication rather than part of Parkinson's disease itself; psychosis secondary to medication may be determined at least in part, through polymorphisms of the ACE gene[15]. From the limited data available, anticholinergics and dopamine agonists seem to be associated with a higher risk of inducing psychosis than levodopa or COMT inhibitors[12,16]. Psychosis is a major contributor to caregiver distress and a risk factor for institutionalisation and early death[14].

Recommendations for treatment – psychosis in PD	
Step	Intervention
1	Exclude organic causes (delirium).
2	Optimise the environment to maximise orientation and minimise problems due to poor caregiver–patient interactions.
3	If the patient has insight and hallucinations are infrequent and not troubling, do not treat.
4	Consider reducing or stopping anticholinergics and dopamine agonists. Monitor for signs of motor deterioration. Be prepared to restart/increase the dose of these drugs again to achieve the best balance between psychosis and mobility.
5	Try an atypical antipsychotic. The efficacy of clozapine is supported by two placebo-controlled RCTs[17]. In contrast, there are two negative placebo-controlled trials each for quetiapine and olanzapine[17]. Low dose quetiapine is the best tolerated[18], although EPS[19] and stereotypical movements[20] can occur. It is therefore reasonable to try quetiapine before clozapine but the success rate may be low. Olanzapine[17], aripiprazole[21] and ziprasidone[22] probably all have greater adverse effects on motor function than quetiapine. Risperidone and typical antipsychotics should be avoided completely. Severe rebound psychosis has been described when antipsychotic drugs (quetiapine or clozapine) are discontinued[23]. Note that all antipsychotics may be even less effective in managing psychotic symptoms in patients with dementia, and such patients may be more prone to developing motor and cognitive side effects[24]. Antipsychotics have been associated with an increased risk of vascular events in the elderly. See section on antipsychotics and BPSD.
6	Consider a **cholinesterase inhibitor**, particularly if the patient has co-morbid dementia[25].
7	Try **clozapine**. Start at 6.25 mg – usual dose 25 mg/day[17,26]. Monitor as for clozapine. The elderly are more prone to develop serious blood dyscrasia. A case of aplastic anaemia has been reported[27].
8	Consider ECT[28]. Psychotic and motor symptoms usually respond well[29] but the risk of inducing delirium is high[11], particularly in patients with pre-existing cognitive impairment.

Dementia in Parkinson's disease

Cholinesterase inhibitors have been shown to improve cognition, delusions, and hallucinations in patients with Lewy body dementia (which has some similarities to Parkinson's disease). Motor function may deteriorate[30,31]. Improvements in cognitive functioning are modest[32,33]. A Cochrane review concluded that there was most evidence for rivastigmine; 15% of patients experience clinically meaningful improvements in cognition and activities of daily living[34].

References

1. Reich SG et al. Ten most commonly asked questions about the psychiatric aspects of Parkinson's disease. Neurologist 2003; 9:50–56.
2. Hely MA et al. The Sydney multicenter study of Parkinson's disease: the inevitability of dementia at 20 years. Mov Disord 2008; 23:837–844.
3. McDonald WM et al. Prevalence, etiology, and treatment of depression in Parkinson's disease. Biol Psychiatry 2003; 54:363–375.
4. Palhagen SE et al. Depressive illness in Parkinson's disease—indication of a more advanced and widespread neurodegenerative process? Acta Neurol Scand 2008; 117:295–304.
5. Gony M et al. Risk of serious extrapyramidal symptoms in patients with Parkinson's disease receiving antidepressant drugs: a pharmacoepidemiologic study comparing serotonin reuptake inhibitors and other antidepressant drugs. Clin Neuropharmacol 2003; 26:142–145.
6. Kulisevsky J et al. Motor changes during sertraline treatment in depressed patients with Parkinson's disease*. Eur J Neurol 2008; 15:953–959.
7. Serrano-Duenas M. A comparison between low doses of amitriptyline and low doses of fluoxetine used in the control of depression in patients suffering from Parkinson's disease (Spainish). Rev Neurol 2002; 35:1010–1014.
8. Antonini A et al. Randomized study of sertraline and low-dose amitriptyline in patients with Parkinson's disease and depression: effect on quality of life. Mov Disord 2006; 21:1119–1122.
9. Menza M et al. A controlled trial of antidepressants in patients with Parkinson disease and depression. Neurology 2008; 72:886–892.
10. Barone P et al. Pramipexole versus sertraline in the treatment of depression in Parkinson's disease: a national multicenter parallel-group randomized study. J Neurol 2006; 253:601–607.
11. Figiel GS et al. ECT-induced delirium in depressed patients with Parkinson's disease. J Neuropsychiatry Clin Neurosci 1991; 3:405–411.
12. Ismail MS et al. A reality test: How well do we understand psychosis in Parkinson's disease? J Neuropsychiatry Clin Neurosci 2004; 16:8–18.
13. Kiziltan G et al. Relationship between age and subtypes of psychotic symptoms in Parkinson's disease. J Neurol 2007; 254:448–452.
14. Factor SA et al. Longitudinal outcome of Parkinson's disease patients with psychosis. Neurology 2003; 60:1756–1761.
15. Lin JJ et al. Genetic polymorphism of the angiotensin converting enzyme and L-dopa-induced adverse effects in Parkinson's disease. J Neurol Sci 2007; 252:130–134.
16. Ives NJ et al. Dopamine agonist therapy in early Parkinson's disease: a systematic review of randomised controlled trials. Mov Disord 2004; 19 Suppl 9:S209.
17. Frieling H et al. Treating dopamimetic psychosis in Parkinson's disease: structured review and meta-analysis. Eur Neuropsychopharmacol 2007; 17:165–171.
18. Fernandez HH et al. Long-term outcome of quetiapine use for psychosis among Parkinsonian patients. Mov Disord 2003; 18:510–514.
19. Prueter C et al. Akathisia as a side effect of antipsychotic treatment with quetiapine in a patient with Parkinson's disease. Mov Disord 2003; 18:712–713.
20. Miwa H et al. Stereotyped behaviors or punding after quetiapine administration in Parkinson's disease. Parkinsonism Relat Disord 2004; 10:177–180.
21. Friedman JH et al. Open-label flexible-dose pilot study to evaluate the safety and tolerability of aripiprazole in patients with psychosis associated with Parkinson's disease. Mov Disord 2006; 21:2078–2081.
22. Schindehutte J et al. Treatment of drug-induced psychosis in Parkinson's disease with ziprasidone can induce severe dose-dependent off-periods and pathological laughing. Clin Neurol Neurosurg 2007; 109:188–191.
23. Fernandez HH et al. Rebound psychosis: effect of discontinuation of antipsychotics in Parkinson's disease. Mov Disord 2005; 20:104–105.
24. Prohorov T et al. The effect of quetiapine in psychotic Parkinsonian patients with and without dementia. An open-labeled study utilizing a structured interview. J Neurol 2006; 253:171–175.
25. Marti M et al. Dementia in Parkinson's disease. J Neurol 2007; 254 Suppl 1:41–48.
26. Merims D et al. Rater-blinded, prospective comparison: quetiapine versus clozapine for Parkinson's disease psychosis. Clin Neuropharmacol 2006; 29:331–337.
27. Ziegenbein M et al. Clozapine-induced aplastic anemia in a patient with Parkinson's disease. Can J Psychiatry 2003; 48:352.
28. Factor SA et al. Combined clozapine and electroconvulsive therapy for the treatment of drug-induced psychosis in Parkinson's disease. J Neuropsychiatry Clin Neurosci 1995; 7:304–307.
29. Martin BA. ECT for Parkinson's? CMAJ 2003; 168:1391–1392.
30. Richard IH et al. Rivastigmine-induced worsening of motor function and mood in a patient with Parkinson's disease. Mov Disord 2001; 16:33–34.
31. McKeith I et al. Efficacy of rivastigmine in dementia with Lewy bodies: a randomised, double-blind, placebo-controlled international study. Lancet 2000; 356:2031–2036.
32. Emre M et al. Rivastigmine for dementia associated with Parkinson's disease. N Engl J Med 2004; 351:2509–2518.
33. Aarsland D et al. Donepezil for cognitive impairment in Parkinson's disease: a randomised controlled study. J Neurol Neurosurg Psychiatry 2002; 72:708–712.
34. Maidment I et al. Cholinesterase inhibitors for Parkinson's disease dementia. Cochrane Database Syst Rev 2006;CD004747.

Further reading

Miyasaki JM et al. Practice Parameter: evaluation and treatment of depression, psychosis, and dementia in Parkinson disease (an evidence-based review): report of the Quality Standards Subcommittee of the American Academy of Neurology. Neurology 2006; 66:996–1002.
National Institute for Clinical Excellence. Dementia: Supporting people with dementia and their carers in health and social care. Clinical Guidance 42. http://www.nice.org.uk. 2006.

Special groups

Multiple sclerosis

Multiple sclerosis (MS) is a common cause of neurological disability affecting approximately 85 000 people in the UK, with the onset of the condition usually occurring between 20–50 years of age. Individuals with MS may experience a variety of psychiatric/neurological disorders such as depression, anxiety, pathological laughter and crying, mania and euphoria, psychosis/bipolar disorder, fatigue, and cognitive impairment. Psychiatric disorders may result from the psychological impact of MS diagnosis and prognosis, perceived lack of social support or unhelpful coping styles[1], increased stress[2], iatrogenic effects of treatments commonly used with MS[3], or damage to neuronal pathways[3]. According to some studies, shorter duration of illness is also implicated in risk of depression.

Depression in multiple sclerosis

In people with MS, depression is common with a point prevalence of 14–27%[4,5] and lifetime prevalence of up to 50%[5]. Suicide rates are 2–7.5 times higher than the general population[6]. Depression may be associated with fatigue and pain, though the relationship direction is unclear. Overlapping symptoms of depression and MS can complicate the diagnosis, therefore co-operation between neurologists and liaison psychiatrists should occur to ensure optimal treatment for individuals with MS.

The role of interferon-beta in the aetiology of MS depression is unclear; however recent reports suggest there is no evidence that depression occurs more frequently in people treated with interferon-beta[7,8]. Standard care for initiation of interferon-beta should include assessment for depression and for those with a past history of depressive illness, prophylactic treatment with an antidepressant[3].

Recommendations for treatment – depression in MS	
Step	Intervention
1	Screen for depression; can supplement with HADS/BDI[9]/CES-D[10]. Exclude and treat any organic causes. Consider iatrogenic effects of medications as a potential cause of depression. Ensure there is no past history of mania. People with mild depression could be considered for cognitive behaviour therapy or self-help[11]
2	SSRIs should be first line treatment[3,10,12] due to their benign side effect profile. Sertraline proved as effective as CBT in one trial[13], however paroxetine was not found to be more effective than placebo in another study[14] although the study was underpowered. Due to reduced tolerability of side effects in this patient group, medications should be titrated from an initial half dose. Many MS patients may be prescribed low dose TCAs for pain/bladder disturbance therefore SSRIs should be used with caution and patients should be observed for serotonin syndrome. For those with co-morbid pain consideration should be given to treating with an SNRI such as duloxetine or venlafaxine[15]. One RCT of desipramine showed it was more effective than placebo but tricyclics may be poorly tolerated[16]
3	If SSRIs are not tolerated or there is no response there are limited data that moclobemide is effective and well tolerated[15,17]. There are no published trials on venlafaxine, duloxetine and mirtazapine but these are used widely
4	ECT could be considered for people who are actively suicidal or severely depressed and at high risk, but it may trigger an exacerbation of MS symptoms[18], although some studies suggest that no neurological disturbance occurs[19]
5	CBT is the most appropriate psychological intervention with best efficacy in comparison to supportive therapy or usual care, and should be used in conjunction with medication for those who are moderately–severely depressed[12,13,20]

Special groups

Anxiety in multiple sclerosis

Anxiety affects many people with MS, with a point prevalence of 14–25%[21] and lifetime incidence of 35–37%[22]. Elevated rates in comparison with the general population are higher for generalized anxiety disorder, panic disorder, obsessive compulsive disorder[22], and social anxiety. Anxiety appears linked to perceived lack of support, increased pain, fatigue, sleep disturbance, depression, alcohol misuse, and suicidal ideas. As yet there are no published trials for the treatment of anxiety but SSRIs could be used and in non-responsive cases, venlafaxine might be an option.

Benzodiazepines may be used for acute and severe anxiety of less than 4 weeks' duration but should not be prescribed in the long term. Buspirone and beta-blockers could also be considered although as yet there is unproven efficacy in MS. Pregabalin is also licensed for anxiety and may be useful in this population group. People with MS may also respond to CBT. Generally treatment is as for non-MS anxiety disorders (see anxiety section, Chapter 4)

Pathological laughter and crying (PLC)

Up to 10% of individuals with MS experience PLC. It is more common in the advanced stages of the disease and is associated with cognitive impairment[22]. There have been a few open label trials recommending the use of small doses of TCAs, e.g. amitriptyline, or SSRIs, e.g. fluoxetine[21,23] in MS. Citalopram[24] or sertraline[25] have been investigated in people with post-stroke PLC with reasonable efficacy and rapid response and could also be useful.

Mania/euphoria/bipolar disorder

Incidence of bipolar disorder can be as high as 13% in the MS population[2] compared with 1–6% in the general population. Mania can be induced by drugs such as steroids or baclofen[26].

Anecdotal evidence suggests that patients presenting with mania/bipolar disorder should be treated with mood-stabilisers such as sodium valproate as these are better tolerated than lithium[27].

Lithium can cause diuresis and thus lead to increased difficulties with tolerance. Mania accompanied by psychosis could be treated with low-dose atypical antipsychotics such as risperidone, olanzapine[2], ziprasidone[28]. Patients requiring psychiatric treatment for steroid-induced mania with psychosis have been known to respond well to olanzapine[29], further case reports suggest risperidone is also useful. There have been no trials in this area.

Psychosis in multiple sclerosis

Psychosis occurs in 1.1% of the MS population and is relatively uncommon[28]. There have been few published trials in this area, but risperidone or clozapine have been recommended as useful because of their low risk of extrapyramidal symptoms[26].

Psychosis may rarely be the presentation of an MS relapse in which case steroids may be beneficial but would need to be given under close supervision.

Cognitive impairment

Cognitive impairment occurs in at least 40–65% of people with MS. Some of the iatrogenic effects of medications commonly prescribed can worsen cognition, e.g. tizanidine, diazepam, gabapentin[30]. Although there are no published trials, evidence from clinical case studies suggests that the treatment of sleep difficulties, depression, and fatigue can enhance cognitive function[30]. There have been two small, underpowered trials with donepezil for people with mild–moderate cognitive impairment with moderate efficacy[31,32] but as yet it is premature to recommend the use of acetylcholinesterase inhibitors within this group[33].

Fatigue

Fatigue is a common symptom in MS with up to 80% of people with MS affected[34]. The aetiology of fatigue is unclear but there have been suggestions that disruption of neuronal networks[35], depression or psychological reactions[26], sleep disturbances or medication may play a role in its development.

Pharmacological and non-pharmacological strategies[34]

Non-pharmacological strategies include reviewing history for any possible contributing factors, assessment and treatment of underlying depression if present, pacing activities and appropriate exercise. One trial suggests that CBT reduces fatigue scores[36].

Pharmacological strategies include the use of amantadine[37] or modafinil. NICE guidelines suggest no medicine should be used routinely, however amantadine could have a small benefit[38]. A Cochrane review of amantadine in people with MS suggests that the quality and outcomes of the amantadine trials are inconsistent and therefore efficacy remains unclear[37]. Modafinil has mixed results in clinical trials. Early studies[39,40] showed statistically significant improvements in fatigue, however these studies were subject to bias. A later randomised placebo-controlled double-blind study[41] found no improvement in fatigue compared with placebo. Further studies are required before any definitive answer can be provided.

Other pharmacological agents recommended for use in MS fatigue include pemoline or aspirin. A double-blind crossover study of aspirin compared with placebo favoured aspirin but further studies are required[42].

References

1. Ron MA. Do neurologists provide adequate care for depression in patients with multiple sclerosis? Nat Clin Pract Neurol 2006; 2:534–535.
2. Patten SB et al. Biopsychosocial correlates of lifetime major depression in a multiple sclerosis population. Mult Scler 2000; 6:115–120.
3. Servis ME. Psychiatric comorbidity in parkinson's disease, multiple sclerosis, and seizure disorder. Continuum 2006; 12:72–86.
4. Gottberg K et al. A population-based study of depressive symptoms in multiple sclerosis in Stockholm county: association with functioning and sense of coherence. J Neurol Neurosurg Psychiatry 2007; 78:60–65.
5. Patten SB et al. Major depression in multiple sclerosis: a population-based perspective. Neurology 2003; 61:1524–1527.
6. Sadovnick AD et al. Cause of death in patients attending multiple sclerosis clinics. Neurology 1991; 41:1193–1196.
7. Zephir H et al. Multiple sclerosis and depression: influence of interferon beta therapy. Mult Scler 2003; 9:284–288.
8. Patten SB et al. Anti-depressant use in association with interferon and glatiramer acetate treatment in multiple sclerosis. Mult Scler 2008; 14:406–411.
9. Moran PJ et al. The validity of Beck Depression Inventory and Hamilton Rating Scale for Depression items in the assessment of depression among patients with multiple sclerosis. J Behav Med 2005; 28:35–41.
10. Pandya R et al. Predictive value of the CES-D in detecting depression among candidates for disease-modifying multiple sclerosis treatment. Psychosomatics 2005; 46:131–134.
11. Rickards H. Depression in neurological disorders: Parkinson's disease, multiple sclerosis, and stroke. J Neurol Neurosurg Psychiatry 2005; 76 Suppl 1:i48–i52.
12. Siegert RJ et al. Depression in multiple sclerosis: a review. J Neurol Neurosurg Psychiatry 2005; 76:469–475.
13. Mohr DC et al. Comparative outcomes for individual cognitive-behavior therapy, supportive-expressive group psychotherapy, and sertraline for the treatment of depression in multiple sclerosis. J Consult Clin Psychol 2001; 69:942–949.
14. Ehde DM et al. Efficacy of paroxetine in treating major depressive disorder in persons with multiple sclerosis. Gen Hosp Psychiatry 2008; 30:40–48.
15. Hilty DM et al. Psychopharmacology for neurologists: principles, algorithms, and other resources. Continuum 2006; 12:33–46.
16. Barak Y et al. Treatment of depression in patients with multiple sclerosis. Neurologist 1998; 4:99–104.
17. Schiffer RB et al. Antidepressant pharmacotherapy of depression associated with multiple sclerosis. Am J Psychiatry 1990; 147:1493–1497.
18. Barak Y et al. Moclobemide treatment in multiple sclerosis patients with comorbid depression: an open-label safety trial. J Neuropsychiatry Clin Neurosci 1999; 11:271–273.
19. Then BF et al. Combined treatment with corticosteroids and moclobemide favors normalization of hypothalamo-pituitary-adrenal axis dysregulation in relapsing-remitting multiple sclerosis: a randomized, double blind trial. J Clin Endocrinol Metab 2001; 86:1610–1615.
20. Larcombe NA et al. An evaluation of cognitive-behaviour therapy for depression in patients with multiple sclerosis. Br J Psychiatry 1984; 145: 366–371.
21. Feinstein A et al. The effects of anxiety on psychiatric morbidity in patients with multiple sclerosis. Mult Scler 1999; 5:323–326.
22. Korostil M et al. Anxiety disorders and their clinical correlates in multiple sclerosis patients. Mult Scler 2007; 13:67–72.
23. Feinstein A et al. Prevalence and neurobehavioral correlates of pathological laughing and crying in multiple sclerosis. Arch Neurol 1997; 54: 1116–1121.
24. Andersen G et al. Citalopram for post-stroke pathological crying. Lancet 1993; 342:837–839.
25. Burns A et al. Sertraline in stroke-associated lability of mood. Int J Geriatr Psychiatry 1999; 14:681–685.
26. Jefferies K. The neuropsychiatry of multiple sclerosis. Adv Psychiatr Treat 2006; 12:214–220.

27. Stip E et al. Valproate in the treatment of mood disorder due to multiple sclerosis. Can J Psychiatry 1995; 40:219–220.
28. Davids E et al. Antipsychotic treatment of psychosis associated with multiple sclerosis. Prog Neuropsychopharmacol Biol Psychiatry 2004; 28: 743–744.
29. Budur K et al. Olanzapine for corticosteroid-induced mood disorders. Psychosomatics 2003; 44:353.
30. Pierson SH et al. Treatment of cognitive impairment in multiple sclerosis. Behav Neurol 2006; 17:53–67.
31. Krupp LB et al. Donepezil improved memory in multiple sclerosis in a randomized clinical trial. Neurology 2004; 63:1579–1585.
32. Greene YM et al. A 12-week, open trial of donepezil hydrochloride in patients with multiple sclerosis and associated cognitive impairments. J Clin Psychopharmacol 2000; 20:350–356.
33. Christodoulou C et al. Treatment of cognitive impairment in multiple sclerosis: is the use of acetylcholinesterase inhibitors a viable option? CNS Drugs 2008; 22:87–97.
34. Bakshi R. Fatigue associated with multiple sclerosis: diagnosis, impact and management. Mult Scler 2003; 9:219–227.
35. Sepulcre J et al. Fatigue in multiple sclerosis is associated with the disruption of frontal and parietal pathways. Mult Scler 2009; 15:337–344.
36. van KK et al. A randomized controlled trial of cognitive behavior therapy for multiple sclerosis fatigue. Psychosom Med 2008; 70:205–213.
37. Pucci E et al. Amantadine for fatigue in multiple sclerosis. Cochrane Database Syst Rev 2007;CD002818.
38. National Institute for Clinical Excellence. Management of multiple sclerosis in primary and secondary care. Clinical Guidance 8. 2003. http://www.nice.org.uk/
39. Rammohan KW et al. Efficacy and safety of modafinil (Provigil) for the treatment of fatigue in multiple sclerosis: a two centre phase 2 study. J Neurol Neurosurg Psychiatry 2002; 72:179–183.
40. Zifko UA et al. Modafinil in treatment of fatigue in multiple sclerosis. Results of an open-label study. J Neurol 2002; 249:983–987.
41. Stankoff B et al. Modafinil for fatigue in MS: A randomized placebo-controlled double-blind study. Neurology 2005; 64:1139–1143.
42. Wingerchuk DM et al. A randomized controlled crossover trial of aspirin for fatigue in multiple sclerosis. Neurology 2005; 64:1267–1269.

Special groups

Eating disorders

Prevalence rates in young females are 0.3% for anorexia nervosa and 1% for bulimia nervosa. In men the rate is about a 10th of that seen in women[1]. There are many similarities between the different types of eating disorders and patients often traverse diagnoses, which can complicate treatment[2].

Other psychiatric conditions (particularly anxiety, depression, and obsessive compulsive disorder) often coexist with eating disorders and this may in part explain the benefit seen with medication.

Anorexia nervosa carries considerable risk of mortality or serious physical morbidity. Patients may present with multiple physical conditions including amenorrhoea, muscle wasting, electrolyte abnormalities, cardiovascular complications, and osteoporosis. Patients who purge through vomiting are at high risk of loss of tooth enamel, gastro-oesophageal erosion, and dehydration[2]. Other modes of purging include laxative and diuretic misuse.

Any medication prescribed should be accompanied by close monitoring to check for possible adverse reactions.

Anorexia nervosa

General guidance

There are few controlled trials to guide treatment in anorexia nervosa. Prompt weight restoration, family therapy, and structured psychotherapy are the main choices of treatment[3,4]. The aim of (physical) treatment is to improve nutritional health through re-feeding with very limited evidence base for pharmacological treatment. Drugs may be used to treat co-morbid conditions[3], but have a limited role in weight restoration[5]. Olanzapine is the only drug shown conclusively to have any effect on weight restoration in anorexia nervosa[6,7].

Healthcare professionals should be aware of the risk of drugs that prolong the QTc interval. All patients with a diagnosis of anorexia nervosa should have an alert placed in their prescribing record concerning the risk of side effects. ECG monitoring should be undertaken if the prescription of medication that may compromise cardiac functioning is essential[3].

Physical aspects

VITAMINS AND MINERALS

Treatment with a multivitamin/multimineral supplement in oral form is recommended during both inpatient and outpatient weight restoration[3] (in the UK, Forceval or Sanatogen Gold one capsule daily may be used).

ELECTROLYTES

Electrolyte disturbances (e.g. hypokalaemia) may develop slowly over time and may be asymptomatic and resolve with re-feeding. Hypophosphataemia may also be precipitated by re-feeding. Rapid correction may be hazardous. Oral supplementation is therefore used to prevent serious sequelae rather than simply to restore normal levels. If supplements are used urea and electrolytes, HCO_3, Ca, P, and Mg need to be monitored and ECG needs to be performed[8].

OSTEOPOROSIS

Bone loss is a serious complication of anorexia with serious consequences. Hormonal treatment using oestrogen or dehydroepiandrosterone (DHEA) does not have a positive impact on bone density and oestrogen is not recommended in children and adolescence due to the risk of premature fusion of the bones[3].

Psychiatric aspects

ACUTE ILLNESS: ANTIDEPRESSANTS

A Cochrane review found no evidence from four placebo-controlled trials that antidepressants improved weight gain, eating disorder or associated psychopathology[9]. It has been suggested that neurochemical abnormalities in starvation may partially explain this non-response[9]. Co-prescribing nutritional supplementation (including tryptophan) with fluoxetine has not been shown to increase efficacy[10].

OTHER PSYCHOTROPIC DRUGS

Antipsychotic drugs (e.g. olanzapine), minor tranquilisers or antihistamines (e.g. promethazine) are often used to reduce the high levels of anxiety associated with anorexia nervosa but they are not usually recommended for the promotion of weight gain[3]. Case reports and retrospective studies have suggested that olanzapine may reduce agitation (and possibly improve weight gain)[11,12]. One RCT[7] showed that 87.5% of patients given olanzapine achieved weight restoration (55.6% placebo). Many other medications have been investigated in small placebo-controlled trials of varying quality and success, these include zinc[13], naltrexone[14], and cyproheptadine[15] amongst many others[5].

RELAPSE PREVENTION

There is evidence from one small trial that fluoxetine may be useful in improving outcome and preventing relapse of patients with anorexia nervosa after weight restoration[16]. Other studies have found no benefit[9,17].

CO-MORBID DISORDERS

Antidepressants are often used to treat co-morbid major depressive disorder and obsessive compulsive disorder. However, caution should be used as these conditions may resolve with weight gain alone[3].

Bulimia nervosa and binge eating disorder

Adults with bulimia nervosa and binge eating disorder (BED) may be offered a trial of an antidepressant. SSRIs (specifically fluoxetine[18-20]) are the drugs of first choice. The effective dose of fluoxetine is 60 mg daily[21]. Patients should be informed that this can reduce the frequency of binge eating and purging but long-term effects are unknown[3].

Antidepressant drugs may be used for the treatment of bulimia nervosa in adolescents but they are not licensed for this age group and there is no evidence for this practice. They should not be considered as a first-line treatment in adolescent bulimia nervosa[3].

There is some evidence that topiramate reduces frequency of binge-eating[22].

Other atypical eating disorders

There have been no studies of the use of drugs to treat atypical eating disorders other than anorexia nervosa and BED[3,23].

In the absence of evidence to guide the management of atypical eating disorders (also known as eating disorders not otherwise specified) other than binge eating disorder, it is recommended that the clinician considers following the guidance of the eating disorder that mostly resembles the individual patient's eating disorder[3].

Special groups

Summary of NICE guidance in eating disorders[3]

Anorexia nervosa
- Psychological interventions are the treatments of choice and should be accompanied by monitoring of the patient's physical state
- No particular medication is recommended. A range of drugs may be used in the treatment of co-morbid conditions

Bulimia nervosa
- An evidence based self-help programme or cognitive behaviour therapy for bulimia nervosa should be the first choice of treatment
- A trial of fluoxetine may be offered as an alternative or additional first step

Binge eating disorder
- An evidence based self-help programme of cognitive behavioural therapy for binge eating disorder should be the first choice of treatment
- A trial of an SSRI can be considered as an alternative or additional first step

References

1. Hoek HW et al. Review of the prevalence and incidence of eating disorders. Int J Eat Disord 2003; 34:383–396.
2. Steffen KJ et al. Emerging drugs for eating disorder treatment. Expert Opin Emerg Drugs 2006; 11:315–336.
3. National Institute for Clinical Excellence. Eating disorders: Core interventions in the treatment and management of anorexia nervosa, bulimia nervosa and related eating disorders. Clinical Guidance 9. http://www.nice.org.uk. 2004.
4. American Psychiatric Association. Treatment of patients with eating disorders, third edition. Am J Psychiatry 2006; 163:4–54.
5. Crow SJ et al. What potential role is there for medication treatment in anorexia nervosa? Int J Eat Disord 2009; 42:1–8.
6. Dunican KC et al. The role of olanzapine in the treatment of anorexia nervosa. Annal Pharmacotherapy 2007; 41:111–115.
7. Bissada H et al. Olanzapine in the treatment of low body weight and obsessive thinking in women with anorexia nervosa: a randomized, double-blind, placebo-controlled trial. Am J Psychiatry 2008; 165:1281–1288.
8. Connan F et al. Biochemical and endocrine complications. Eur Eat Disord Rev 2007; 8:144–157.
9. Claudino AM et al. Antidepressants for anorexia nervosa. Cochrane Database Syst Rev 2006;CD004365.
10. Barbarich NC et al. Use of nutritional supplements to increase the efficacy of fluoxetine in the treatment of anorexia nervosa. Int J Eat Disord 2004; 35:10–15.
11. Malina A et al. Olanzapine treatment of anorexia nervosa: a retrospective study. Int J Eat Disord 2003; 33:234–237.
12. La Via MC et al. Case reports of olanzapine treatment of anorexia nervosa. Int J Eat Disord 2000; 27:363–366.
13. Su JC et al. Zinc supplementation in the treatment of anorexia nervosa. Eat Weight Disord 2002; 7:20–22.
14. Marrazzi MA et al. Naltrexone use in the treatment of anorexia nervosa and bulimia nervosa. Int Clin Psychopharmacol 1995; 10:163–172.
15. Halmi KA et al. Anorexia nervosa. Treatment efficacy of cyproheptadine and amitriptyline. Arch Gen Psychiatry 1986; 43:177–181.
16. Kaye WH et al. Double-blind placebo-controlled administration of fluoxetine in restricting- and restricting-purging-type anorexia nervosa. Biol Psychiatry 2001; 49:644–652.
17. Walsh BT et al. Fluoxetine after weight restoration in anorexia nervosa: a randomized controlled trial. JAMA 2006; 295:2605–2612.
18. Fluoxetine Bulimia Nervosa Collaborative Study Group. Fluoxetine in the treatment of bulimia nervosa. A multicenter, placebo-controlled, double-blind trial. Arch Gen Psychiatry 1992; 49:139–147.
19. Goldstein DJ et al. Long-term fluoxetine treatment of bulimia nervosa. Fluoxetine Bulimia Nervosa Research Group. Br J Psychiatry 1995; 166:660–666.
20. Romano SJ et al. A placebo-controlled study of fluoxetine in continued treatment of bulimia nervosa after successful acute fluoxetine treatment. Am J Psychiatry 2002; 159:96–102.
21. Bacaltchuk J et al. Antidepressants versus placebo for people with bulimia nervosa. Cochrane Database Syst Rev 2003;CD003391.
22. Arbaizar B et al. Efficacy of topiramate in bulimia nervosa and binge-eating disorder: a systematic review. Gen Hosp Psychiatry 2008; 30:471–475.
23. Leombruni P et al. A 12 to 24 weeks pilot study of sertraline treatment in obese women binge eaters. Hum Psychopharmacol 2006; 21:181–188.

Special groups

Acutely disturbed or violent behaviour

Acute behavioural disturbance can occur in the context of psychiatric illness, physical illness, substance abuse, or personality disorder. Psychotic symptoms are common and the patient may be aggressive towards others secondary to persecutory delusions or auditory, visual or tactile hallucinations.

The clinical practice of rapid tranquillisation (RT) is used when appropriate psychological and behavioural approaches have failed to de-escalate acutely disturbed behaviour. It is, essentially, a treatment of last resort. RT is not underpinned by a strong evidence base. Patients who require RT are often too disturbed to give informed consent and therefore cannot participate in randomised controlled trials (RCTs). Recommendations are therefore based partly on research data, partly on theoretical considerations and partly on clinical experience.

Several studies supporting the efficacy of oral atypicals[2-8] have been published. The level of behavioural disturbance exhibited by the patients in these studies was moderate at most, and all subjects accepted oral treatment (this degree of compliance would be unusual in clinical practice). Note too that patients recruited to these studies received the atypical as antipsychotic monotherapy; the efficacy and safety of adding a second antipsychotic as 'PRN' has not been tested in formal RCTs.

Larger, placebo-controlled RCTs support the efficacy of IM olanzapine, ziprasidone, and aripiprazole[9]. When considered together these trials suggested that IM olanzapine is more effective than IM haloperidol which in turn is more effective than IM aripiprazole[1]. Again, the level of behavioural disturbance in these studies was moderate at most. Two small open studies support the effectiveness of IM ziprasidone and IM olanzapine in clinical emergencies (where disturbance was severe)[10,11].

Four large RCTs (the TREC studies[12-15]) have investigated the effectiveness of parenteral medication in 'real-life' acutely disturbed patients. Overall:

- IM midazolam 7.5–15 mg was more rapidly sedating than a combination of haloperidol 5–10 mg and promethazine 50 mg (TREC 1)[12]
- Olanzapine 10 mg was as effective as a combination of haloperidol 10 mg and promethazine 25–50 mg in the short term, but the effect did not last as long (TREC 4)[15]
- A combination of haloperidol 5–10 mg and promethazine 50 mg was more effective and better tolerated than haloperidol 5–10 mg alone (TREC 3)[14]
- A combination of haloperidol 10 mg and promethazine 25–50 mg was more effective than lorazepam 4 mg (TREC 2)[13].

Note that TREC 3[14] found IM haloperidol alone to be poorly tolerated; 6% of patients had an acute dystonic reaction. Acute EPS may adversely affect longer-term compliance[16]. In addition, the SPC for haloperidol requires a pre-treatment ECG[17,18] and recommends that concomitant antipsychotics are not prescribed. A small observational study supports the effectiveness of buccal midazolam in a PICU setting[19]. Lorazepam IM is an established treatment and TREC 2[13] supports its efficacy.

Plans for the management of individual patients should ideally be made in advance. The aim is to prevent disturbed behaviour and reduce risk of violence. Nursing interventions (de-escalation, time out), increased nursing levels, transfer of the patient to a psychiatric intensive care unit (PICU) and pharmacological management are options that may be employed. Care should be taken to avoid combinations and high cumulative doses of antipsychotic drugs. The monitoring of routine physical observations after RT is essential. Note that RT is often viewed as punitive by patients.

Special groups

The aims of RT are threefold:

1. To reduce suffering for the patient: psychological or physical (through self-harm or accidents)
2. To reduce risk of harm to others by maintaining a safe environment
3. To do no harm (by prescribing safe regimes and monitoring physical health).

Note: Despite the need for rapid and effective treatment, concomitant use of two or more antipsychotics (antipsychotic polypharmacy) should be avoided on the basis of risk associated with QT prolongation (common to almost all antipsychotics). This is a particularly important consideration in RT where the patient's physical state predisposes to cardiac arrhythmia.

In an emergency situation	
Step	**Intervention**
1	De-escalation, time out, placement, etc., as appropriate
2	Offer **oral** treatment **If the patient is prescribed a regular antipsychotic, lorazepam 1–2 mg or promethazine 25–50 mg** avoids the risks associated with combining antipsychotics Repeat after 45–60 min Monotherapy with **buccal midazolam, 10 – 20 mg may avoid the need for IM treatment.** Note that this preparation is unlicensed Go to step 3 if two doses fail or sooner if the patient is placing themselves or others at significant risk An oral antipsychotic is an option in patients not already taking a regular oral or depot antipsychotic • olanzapine 10 mg or • quetiapine 100–200 mg or • risperidone 1–2 mg or • haloperidol 5 mg Note that the SPC for **haloperidol** recommends; • **avoid concomitant antipsychotics** • **a pre-treatment ECG**
3	Consider **IM treatment** From this point on: Consider • The patient's legal status • Consulting a senior colleague Lorazepam 1–2 mg[ab] or Promethazine 50 mg[c] or Olanzapine 10 mg[d] or Aripiprazole 9.75 mg or Haloperidol 5 mg Repeat after 30–60 min if insufficient effect Have flumazenil to hand in case of benzodiazepine-induced respiratory depression. IM promethazine is a useful option in a benzodiazepine-tolerant patient IM olanzapine should NOT be combined with an IM benzodiazepine Less hypotension than olanzapine but possibly less effective[1] **Haloperidol should be the last drug considered** • The incidence of acute dystonia is high; ensure IM procyclidine is available • The SPC recommends a pre-treatment ECG
4	Consider **IV treatment** Diazepam 10 mg over at least 5 minutes[be] Repeat after 5–10 minutes if insufficient effect (up to 3 times) Have flumazenil to hand
5	**Seek expert advice** from the consultant or senior clinical pharmacist on call[f]

Notes

a. Mix lorazepam 1:1 with water for injections before injecting. Some centres use 2–4 mg.

b. Caution in the very young and elderly and those with pre-existing brain damage or impulse control problems, as disinhibition reactions are more likely[20].

c. Promethazine has a slow onset of action but is often an effective sedative. Dilution is not required before IM injection. May be repeated up to a maximum of 100 mg/day. Wait 1–2 hours after injection to assess response. Note that promethazine alone has been reported to cause NMS[21] although it is an extremely weak dopamine antagonist.

d. Recommended by NICE only for moderate behavioural disturbance.

e. Use Diazemuls to avoid injection site reactions. IV therapy may be used instead of IM when a very rapid effect is required. IV therapy also ensures near immediate delivery of the drug to its site of action and effectively avoids the danger of inadvertent accumulation of slowly absorbed IM doses. Note also that IV doses can be repeated after only 5–10 min if no effect is observed.

f. Options at this point are limited. IM amylobarbitone and paraldehyde have been used in the past but are used now only extremely rarely. ECT is probably a better option.

Rapid tranquillisation – physical monitoring

After any parenteral drug administration, monitor as follows:

Temperature

Pulse

Blood pressure

Respiratory rate

Every 5–10 min for 1 hour, and then half-hourly until patient is ambulatory. Patients who refuse to have their vital signs monitored or who remain too behaviourally disturbed to be approached should be observed for signs/symptoms of pyrexia, hypotension, oversedation, and general physical wellbeing.

If the patient is asleep or **unconscious**, the continuous use of pulse oximetry to measure oxygen saturation is desirable. A nurse should remain with the patient until ambulatory.

ECG and haematological monitoring are also strongly recommended when parenteral antipsychotics are given, especially when higher doses are used[22,23]. Hypokalaemia, stress and agitation place the patient at risk of cardiac arrhythmia[24] (see section on 'QT prolongation'). ECG monitoring is formally recommended for all patients who receive haloperidol.

Remedial measures in rapid tranquillisation

Problem	Remedial measures
Acute dystonia (including oculogyric crises)	Give **procyclidine** 5–10 mg IM or IV or **benzatropine** 1–2 mg IM
Reduced respiratory rate (<10/min) or oxygen saturation (<90%)	Give oxygen, raise legs, ensure patient is not lying face down Give **flumazenil** if benzodiazepine-induced respiratory depression suspected (see protocol) If induced by any other sedative agent: **transfer to a medical bed and ventilate mechanically**
Irregular or slow (<50/min) **pulse**	**Refer** to specialist medical care immediately
Fall in blood pressure (>30 mmHg orthostatic drop or <50 mmHg diastolic)	**Have patient lie flat**, tilt bed towards head. Monitor closely
Increased temperature	Check creatinine kinase urgently (risk of NMS and perhaps arrhythmia).

Guidelines for the use of flumazenil

Indication for use	If, after the administration of lorazepam or diazepam, respiratory rate falls below 10/min
Contra-indications	Patients with epilepsy who have been receiving long-term benzodiazepines
Caution	Dose should be carefully titrated in hepatic impairment
Dose and route of administration	*Initial:* 200 µg *intravenously* over 15 seconds – if required level of consciousness not achieved after 60 seconds, then, *Subsequent dose:* 100 µg over 10 seconds
Time before dose can be repeated	60 seconds
Maximum dose	1 mg in 24 hours (one initial dose and eight subsequent doses)
Side-effects	Patients may become agitated, anxious or fearful on awakening Seizures may occur in regular benzodiazepine users
Management	Side-effects usually subside
Monitoring • **What to monitor?** • **How often?**	Respiratory rate Continuously until respiratory rate returns to baseline level Flumazenil has a short half-life (much shorter than diazepam) and respiratory function may recover and then deteriorate again *Note: If respiratory rate does not return to normal or patient is not alert after initial doses given, assume that sedation is due to some other cause*

Guidelines for the use of Clopixol Acuphase (zuclopenthixol acetate)

Acuphase should be used only after an acutely psychotic patient has required *repeated* injections of short-acting antipsychotic drugs such as haloperidol or olanzapine, or sedative drugs such as lorazepam.

Acuphase should be given only when enough time has elapsed to assess the full response to previously injected drugs: allow 15 min after IV injections; 60 min after IM.

Acuphase is sometimes appropriately used in patients known to respond to it or in physically violent patients for whom repeated attempts at injection would be dangerous for all parties.

*Acuphase should **never** be administered:*
- in an attempt to 'hasten' the antipsychotic effect of other antipsychotic therapy
- for rapid tranquillisation (onset of effect is too slow)
- at the same time as other parenteral antipsychotics or benzodiazepines (may lead to oversedation which is difficult to reverse)
- as a 'test dose' for zuclopenthixol decanoate depot
- to a patient who is physically resistant (risk of intravasation and oil embolus).

*Acuphase should **never** be used for, or in, the following:*
- patients who accept oral medication
- patients who are neuroleptic naïve
- patients who are sensitive to EPS
- patients who are unconscious
- patients who are pregnant
- those with hepatic or renal impairment
- those with cardiac disease.

Onset and duration of action
Sedative effects usually begin to be seen 2 hours after injection and peak after 12 hours. The effects may last for up to 72 hours. Note: Acuphase has no place in rapid tranquillisation: *its action is not rapid.*

Dose
Acuphase should be given in a dose of 50–150 mg, up to a maximum of 400 mg over a 2-week period. This maximum duration ensures that a treatment plan is put in place. It does not indicate that there are known harmful effects from more prolonged administration, although such use should be very exceptional. There is no such thing as a 'course of Acuphase'. The patient should be assessed before each administration.

Injections should be spaced at least 24 hours apart.

Note: zuclopenthixol acetate is widely misused as a sort of 'chemical straitjacket'. In reality, it is a potentially toxic preparation with very little published information to support its use[25]. It is perhaps best reserved for those few patients who have a prior history of good response to Acuphase.

References

1. Citrome L. Comparison of intramuscular ziprasidone, olanzapine, or aripiprazole for agitation: a quantitative review of efficacy and safety. J Clin Psychiatry 2007; 68:1876–1885.
2. Lejeune J et al. Oral risperidone plus oral lorazepam versus standard care with intramuscular conventional neuroleptics in the initial phase of treating individuals with acute psychosis. Int Clin Psychopharmacol 2004; 19:259–269.
3. Currier GW et al. Acute treatment of psychotic agitation: a randomized comparison of oral treatment with risperidone and lorazepam versus intramuscular treatment with haloperidol and lorazepam. J Clin Psychiatry 2004; 65:386–394.
4. Yildiz A et al. Observational data on the antiagitation effect of risperidone tablets in emergency settings: a preliminary report. Int J Psychiatry Clin Pract 2003; 7:217–221.
5. Currier GW et al. Risperidone liquid concentrate and oral lorazepam versus intramuscular haloperidol and intramuscular lorazepam for treatment of psychotic agitation. J Clin Psychiatry 2001; 62:153–157.
6. Ganesan S et al. Effectiveness of quetiapine for the management of aggressive psychosis in the emergency psychiatric setting: a naturalistic uncontrolled trial. Int J Psychiatry Clin Pract 2005; 9:199–203.
7. Simpson JR, Jr. et al. Impact of orally disintegrating olanzapine on use of intramuscular antipsychotics, seclusion, and restraint in an acute inpatient psychiatric setting. J Clin Psychopharmacol 2006; 26:333–335.
8. Villari V et al. Oral risperidone, olanzapine and quetiapine versus haloperidol in psychotic agitation. Prog Neuropsychopharmacol Biol Psychiatry 2008; 32:405–413.
9. Andrezina R et al. Intramuscular aripiprazole for the treatment of acute agitation in patients with schizophrenia or schizoaffective disorder: a double-blind, placebo-controlled comparison with intramuscular haloperidol. Psychopharmacology 2006; 188:281–292.
10. San L et al. A naturalistic multicenter study of intramuscular olanzapine in the treatment of acutely agitated manic or schizophrenic patients. Eur Psychiatry 2006; 21:539–543.
11. Fulton JA et al. Intramuscular ziprasidone: an effective agent for sedation of the agitated ED patient. Am J Emerg Med 2006; 24:254–255.
12. TREC Collaborative Group. Rapid tranquillisation for agitated patients in emergency psychiatric rooms: a randomised trial of midazolam versus haloperidol plus promethazine. BMJ 2003; 327:708–713.
13. Alexander J et al. Rapid tranquillisation of violent or agitated patients in a psychiatric emergency setting. Pragmatic randomised trial of intramuscular lorazepam v. haloperidol plus promethazine. Br J Psychiatry 2004; 185:63–69.
14. Huf G et al. Rapid tranquillisation in psychiatric emergency settings in Brazil: pragmatic randomised controlled trial of intramuscular haloperidol versus intramuscular haloperidol plus promethazine. BMJ 2007; 335:869.
15. Raveendran NS et al. Rapid tranquillisation in psychiatric emergency settings in India: pragmatic randomised controlled trial of intramuscular olanzapine versus intramuscular haloperidol plus promethazine. BMJ 2007; 335:865.
16. van Harten PN et al. Acute dystonia induced by drug treatment. Br Med J 1999; 319:623–626.
17. Janssen-Cilag Ltd. Summary of Product Characteristics. Haldol Injection. 2009. http://emc.medicines.org.uk/.
18. MHRA. Pharmacovigilance Working Party. Public assessment report on neuroleptics and cardiac safety. http://www.mhra.gov.uk. 2008.
19. Taylor D et al. Buccal midazolam for rapid tranquillisation. Int J Psychiatry Clin Pract 2008; 12:309–311.
20. Paton C. Benzodiazepines and disinhibition: a review. Psychiatr Bull 2002; 26:460–462.
21. Chan-Tack KM. Neuroleptic malignant syndrome due to promethazine. South Med J 1999; 92:1017–1018.
22. Appleby L et al. Sudden unexplained death in psychiatric in-patients. Br J Psychiatry 2000; 176:405–406.
23. Yap YG et al. Risk of torsades de pointes with non-cardiac drugs. Doctors need to be aware that many drugs can cause QT prolongation. BMJ 2000; 320:1158–1159.
24. Taylor DM. Antipsychotics and QT prolongation. Acta Psychiatr Scand 2003; 107:85–95.
25. Gibson RC et al. Zuclopenthixol acetate for acute schizophrenia and similar serious mental illnesses. Cochrane Database Syst Rev 2004;CD000525.

Further reading

Currier GW et al. Orally versus intramuscularly administered antipsychotic drugs in psychiatric emergencies. J Psychiatr Pract 2006; 12:30–40.
Macpherson R et al. A growing evidence base for management guidelines: revisting… guidelines for the managment of acutely disturbed psychiatric patients. Adv Psychiatr Treat 2005; 11:404–415.
McAllister Williams RH et al. Rapid tranquillisation: time for a reappraisal of options for parenteral therapy. Br J Psychiatry 2002; 180:485–489.
National Institute for Clinical Excellence. Violence – The short-term management of disturbed/violent behaviour in in-patient psychiatric settings and emergency departments. Guideline No 25, 2005. www.nice.org.uk
Pratt JP et al. Establishing gold standard approaches to rapid tranquillisation: a review and discussion of the evidence on the safety and efficacy of medications currently used. J Psych Inten Care 2008; 4: 43–57.

Chronic behavioural disturbance (challenging behaviour) in learning disability (LD)

Behavioural disturbance is common in those with a learning disability; 16–50% exhibit aggression or a related challenging behaviour[1]. Those who are aggressive are more likely to be young, male, and have more severe cognitive impairment[2]. Up to a third of adults with LD who do not have a comorbid mental illness are prescribed psychotropic medication, mostly for the management of challenging behaviour[3].

It is often very difficult to determine the aetiology of behavioural disturbance. For example, stereotypical behaviour and irritability could be manifestations of a psychiatric illness or epilepsy (which is common in this patient group[4]). Some anticonvulsant drugs have marked behavioural side effects, most notably topiramate[5]. Stopping drugs such as benzodiazepines and SSRIs can also lead to problems (see Chapter 4).

The following may be useful prompts:

- Is there or could there be an underlying physical illness? (look for and treat)
- Could the behaviour be ictal in origin or a side effect of anticonvulsant drugs? (consider altering)
- Could environmental factors be contributing either as precipitants or reinforcants? (consider and alter if possible)
- Is there an underlying psychiatric illness? (consider and treat if applicable)

Antipsychotic drugs are frequently used to manage persistent aggression towards self or others; it is hoped that they will reduce arousal and treat any underlying psychotic symptoms. The NACHBID study[1] demonstrated that antipsychotics are probably no more effective than placebo for this indication (in patients who do not have a comorbid psychiatric illness); antipsychotics should therefore not be used routinely as a first-line treatment for the management of persistent aggression alone.

Also consider:

- Does the patient have a history of mood disturbance? (consider a trial of an antidepressant/mood-stabiliser)
- Is the disturbance cyclical? (consider a trial of a mood-stabiliser)
- Is the patient aggressive? (consider a trial of carbamazepine or a ß-blocker)
- Are there any signs of adrenergic overactivity such as tachycardia or tremor? (consider a trial of a ß-blocker)
- Is the patient impulsive? (consider a trial of an SSRI)
- Is the patient self-injurious? (consider a trial of an antipsychotic, SSRI or naltrexone)
- Could the behaviour be driven by psychosis? (consider a trial of an antipsychotic)

If medication is prescribed it should be as part of a co-ordinated multidisciplinary care plan. Efficacy against target symptoms should be monitored and particular attention paid to screening for side effects. Try, if possible, to avoid drugs with anticholinergic effects and the use of antipsychotics on a PRN basis.

Special groups

References

1. Tyrer P et al. Risperidone, haloperidol, and placebo in the treatment of aggressive challenging behaviour in patients with intellectual disability: a randomised controlled trial. Lancet 2008; 371:57–63.
2. Tyrer F et al. Physical aggression towards others in adults with learning disabilities: prevalence and associated factors. J Intellect Disabil Res 2006; 50: 295–304.
3. Deb S. Medication for behaviour problems associated with learning disabilities. Psychiatry 2006; 5:368–371.
4. Wilcox J et al. Epilepsy in people with learning disabilities. Psychiatry 2006; 5:372–377.
5. Coppola G et al. Topiramate in children and adolescents with epilepsy and mental retardation: a prospective study on behavior and cognitive effects. Epilepsy Behav 2008; 12:253–256.

Further reading

Bhaumik S, Branford D. The Frith Prescribing Guidelines in Adults with Learning Disability. London: Taylor & Francis; 2005.

Special groups

Self-injurious behaviour in learning disability

Repetitive or stereotypical acts that produce self-inflicted injury (self-injurious behaviour (SIB))[1–3]:

- occur in approximately 20% of adults with learning disability (up to 50% in those requiring institutional care)
- may at least partially be a response to life events in the same way that self-harm may be in people who do not have a learning disability[4]
- most commonly take the form of head-banging, banging other body parts, biting, scratching, pinching, gouging, hair-pulling and pica
- occur more frequently in males; younger adults; those with impairments in hearing, vision, mobility and communication; and those with a diagnosis of autism and epilepsy. As the IQ falls, the prevalence of SIB (and multiple behaviours) increases
- SIB is a major cause of distress to carers and a major cause of institutional care.

Aetiology[4–8]

SIB is best understood as being caused by a combination of organic and environmental factors. Organic factors include rare genetic syndromes (such as Lesch-Nyhan or Smith-Magenis syndrome), developmental brain damage, neurological disorders (such as epilepsy), physical illness, psychiatric illness and communication problems. SIB may be linked to the menstrual cycle in some women. Environmental factors include lack of stimulation/overstimulation, lack of/too much affection, rejection/lack of attention and adverse life events.

Some factors may predispose to SIB (e.g. genetic syndromes), others precipitate it (e.g. depression, dysphoria) and others perpetuate it (e.g. secondary changes in neuroregulatory systems).

The prevalence of mental illness is increased in those with learning disabilities, and non-specific and atypical presentations of mental illness increase in frequency as the IQ falls. Diagnosis often has to be made from observing behaviour rather than directly eliciting symptoms.

Non-drug treatments[9–11]

It is important to try to understand why the patient self-harms (e.g. self-stimulation, relief of dysphoria, attention, frustration, social escape through being removed from communal areas, material reward). Psychological/behavioural strategies for dealing with the behaviour can then be put in place. This should always be tried before resorting to drug treatment.

Successfully preventing one form of SIB may lead to the emergence of another form. Staff may perceive SIB to be due to different causes in the same patient and may react with fear, irritation, anger, disgust, or despair. Interventions based on individual belief systems will lead to inconsistent care. Effective management and support of staff is essential.

Special groups

Drug treatment options – SIB in learning disability	
Drug	*Rationale*
Antipsychotics[12-14]	• Supersensitivity of dopamine neurons in nigro-striatal pathways may predispose to SIB. D_1 blockers (such as thioxanthines) may be more effective than D_2 blockers. Atypical antipsychotics are poorly evaluated; one small naturalistic study found no benefit for atypicals as a group and weight gain was marked[15] • Dopamine is involved in reward mechanisms (blocking dopamine blocks reward) • Low-dose antipsychotics reduce stereotypies
Opiate antagonists[5,8]	• SIB leads to the release of endogenous opiates (endorphins), which may lead to a rewarding mood-state (positive reinforcement) • Naltrexone (an opiate antagonist) may decrease SIB acutely but is less effective in the long term (?opiate mechanisms are important in the early stages, but SIB is perpetuated via dopamine reward mechanisms)
Anticonvulsants[13]	• The prevalence of epilepsy is high in moderate/severe learning disabilities • Aggression (to others or self) can be related to seizure activity (pre-ictal, ictal or post-ictal). Note: anticonvulsant drugs may precipitate behavioural disturbance, most notably topiramate and vigabatrin • Rapid-cycling mood disorders and mixed affective states are more common in learning disabilities and may respond best to carbamazepine or valproate
Buspirone[16] Lithium[13,17] SSRIs[5,8] Venlafaxine[18]	• Drugs that increase 5HT neurotransmission have been shown to reduce SIB in some patients • These drugs may act by targeting the behaviour that precipitates SIB (e.g. fear, irritability, anxiety or depression) • Lithium is licensed for 'the control of aggressive behaviour or intentional self-harm'
Others[8,13,19]	• Other drugs may be useful in some circumstances (e.g. propranolol – probably through reducing anxiety), methylphenidate (when ADHD has been diagnosed), cyproterone (when severely problematic sexual behaviour contributes)

Most data originate from case reports and small open trials, often of heterogeneous patient groups.

Lithium is the only drug licensed for the treatment of SIB.

Prescribing and monitoring[13,20-22]
There is concern that antipsychotic drugs are prescribed excessively and inappropriately in the learning disability population and may cause undue harm. It is unclear if this patient population is more prone to side effects. It is therefore important to document:

- The rationale for treatment (including some measure of baseline target behaviours), potential risk/benefit and consent in the patient's notes. If the patient is unable to understand the nature, purpose and side-effects of treatment, a relative or carer should be consulted
- The impact of medication and any side-effects experienced, each time the patient is reviewed
- Drug interactions. These should always be considered (both kinetic and dynamic) before prescribing, particularly when anticonvulsant drugs are involved.

References

1. Schroeder SR et al. Self-injurious behavior: gene-brain-behavior relationships. Ment Retard Dev Disabil Res Rev 2001; 7:3–12.
2. Saloviita T. The structure and correlates of self-injurious behavior in an institutional setting. Res Dev Disabil 2000; 21:501–511.
3. Collacott RA et al. Epidemiology of self-injurious behaviour in adults with learning disabilities. Br J Psychiatry 1998; 173:428–432.
4. Lovell A. Learning disability against itself: the self-injury/self-harm conundrum. Br J Learning Disabil 2008; 36:109–121.
5. Mikhail AG et al. Self-injurious behavior in mental retardation. Curr Opin Psychiatry 2001; 14:457–462.
6. Moss S et al. Psychiatric symptoms in adults with learning disability and challenging behaviour. Br J Psychiatry 2000; 177:452–456.
7. Deb S. Self-injurious behaviour as part of genetic syndromes. Br J Psychiatry 1998; 172:385–388.
8. Clarke DJ. Psychopharmacology of severe self-injury associated with learning disabilities. Br J Psychiatry 1998; 172:389–394.
9. Xeniditis K et al. Management of people with challenging behaviour. Adv Psychiatr Treat 2001; 7:109–116.
10. Halliday S et al. Psychological interventions in self-injurious behaviour. Working with people with a learning disability. Br J Psychiatry 1998; 172:395–400.
11. Bromley J et al. Beliefs and emotional reactions of care staff working with people with challenging behaviour. J Intellect Disabil Res 1995; 39 (Pt 4):341–352.
12. Branford D. Antipsychotic drugs in learning disabilities (mental handicap). Pharm J 1997; 258:451–456.
13. Einfeld SL. Systematic management approach to pharmacotherapy for people with learning disability. Adv Psychiatr Treat 2001; 7:43–49.
14. Gagiano C et al. Short- and long-term efficacy and safety of risperidone in adults with disruptive behavior disorders. Psychopharmacology 2005; 179:629–636.
15. Ruedrich SL et al. Atypical antipsychotic medication improves aggression, but not self-injurious behaviour, in adults with intellectual disabilities. J Intellect Disabil Res 2008; 52:132–140.
16. Ratey JJ et al. Buspirone therapy for maladaptive behavior and anxiety in developmentally disabled persons. J Clin Psychiatry 1989; 50:382–384.
17. Craft M et al. Lithium in the treatment of aggression in mentally handicapped patients. A double-blind trial. Br J Psychiatry 1987; 150:685–689.
18. Carminati GG et al. Low-dose venlafaxine in three adolescents and young adults with autistic disorder improves self-injurious behavior and attention deficit/hyperactivity disorders (ADHD)-like symptoms. Prog Neuropsychopharmacol Biol Psychiatry 2006; 30:312–315.
19. Aman MG et al. Clinical effects of methylphenidate and thioridazine in intellectually subaverage children. J Am Acad Child Adolesc Psychiatry 1991; 30:246–256.
20. Janowsky DS et al. Minimally effective doses of conventional antipsychotic medications used to treat aggression, self-injurious and destructive behaviors in mentally retarded adults. J Clin Psychopharmacol 2005; 25:19–25.
21. Janowsky DS et al. Antipsychotic withdrawal-induced relapse predicts future relapses in institutionalized adults with severe intellectual disability. J Clin Psychopharmacol 2008; 28:401–405.
22. McGillivray JA et al. Pharmacological management of challenging behavior of individuals with intellectual disability. Res Dev Disabil 2004; 25:523–537.

Further reading

Bhaumik S, Branford D. The Frith Prescribing Guidelines in Adults with Learning Disability. London: Taylor & Francis; 2005.
Deb S, Clarke D, Unwin G. Using medication to manage behaviour problems among adults with a learning disability. www.ld-medication.bham.ac.uk. 2006
Read S. Self-injury and violence in people with severe learning disabilities. Br J Psychiatry 1998; 172:381–384.
Thompson CL et al. Behavioural symptoms among people with severe and profound intellectual disabilities: a 26-year follow-up study. Br J Psychiatry 2002; 181:67–71.

Psychotropics and surgery

There are few worthwhile studies of the effects of non-anaesthetic drugs on surgery and the anaesthetic process[1,2]. Practice is therefore largely based on theoretical considerations, case reports, clinical experience, and personal opinion. Any guidance given in this area is therefore somewhat speculative.

The decision as to whether or not to continue a drug during surgery and the perioperative period should take into account a number of interacting factors. Some general considerations include:

- Patients are at risk of aspirating their stomach contents during general anaesthesia. For this reason they are usually prevented from eating for at least 6 hours before surgery. However, clear fluids leave the stomach within 2 hours of ingestion and so fluids that enable a patient to take routine medication may be allowed up to 2 hours before surgery. A clear fluid is described as one through which newspaper print can be read[3].
- There are some interactions between drugs used during surgery and routine medication that requires concurrent administration to be avoided. This is usually managed by the anaesthetist through their choice of anaesthetic technique. Significant drug interactions between medicines used during surgery and psychotropics include:
  - enflurane may precipitate seizures in patients taking tricyclic antidepressants[4–6]
  - pethidine may precipitate fatal 'excitatory' reactions in patients taking MAOIs and may cause serotonin syndrome in patients taking SSRIs[4–7].
- Major procedures induce profound physiological changes, which include electrolyte disturbances and the release of cortisol and catacholamines.
- Postoperatively, surgical stress and some agents used in anaesthesia often lead to gastric or gastrointestinal stasis. Oral absorption is therefore likely to be compromised.

For the most part, psychotropic drugs should be continued during the perioperative period, assuming agreement of the anaesthetist concerned. The table overleaf provides some discussion of the merits or otherwise of continuing individual psychotropics during surgery. Note, however, that psychotropic and other drugs are frequently (accidentally and/or unthinkingly) withheld from preoperative patients simply because they are 'nil by mouth'[1]. Patients may be labelled 'nil by mouth' for several reasons, including unconsciousness, to rest the gut or postoperatively or as a result of the surgery itself. Patients may also develop an intolerance of oral medicines at any time during a stay in hospital, often because of nausea and vomiting. When one decides to continue a psychotropic, this needs to be explicitly outlined to appropriate medical and nursing staff.

For many patients undergoing surgery and recovery in a hospital there will be little or no opportunity to smoke, Abrupt cessation is likely to affect mental state and may also result in drug toxicity if psychotropics are continued (see section on 'Psychotropics and smoking').

Alternative routes and formulations may be sought. When changing the route or formulation, care should be taken to ensure the appropriate dose and frequency is prescribed as these may not be the same as for the oral route or previous formulation. Oral preparations may sometimes be administered via a nasogastric (NG), PEG or jejunostomy tube.

Risks associated with discontinuing psychotropics
- Relapse (especially if treatment ceased for more than a few days)[8]
- Worsening of condition. For example, abrupt cessation of lithium worsens outcome in BAD[9]
- Cessation of antidepressants may increase risk of suicide[10]
- Discontinuation symptoms. These may complicate diagnosis in the perioperative period
- Delirium. May be more common in those discontinuing antipsychotics[11] or antidepressants[6].

Risks associated with continuing psychotropics

- Potential for interactions, both pharmacokinetic and pharmacodynamic
- Increased likelihood of bleeding (e.g. with SSRIs)[12]
- Hypo/hypertension (depending on psychotropic)[13,14]
- Effects on core body temperature.

Psychotropics and surgery

Drug or drug group	Considerations	Safe in surgery?	Alternative formulations
Anticonvulsants[4,15]	• CNS depressant activity may reduce anaesthetic requirements • Drug level monitoring may be required	Probably, usually continued for people with epilepsy	Carbamazepine liquid or suppositories are available: 100 mg tablet = 125 mg suppository. Maximum by rectum 1 g daily in four divided doses. Phenytoin is available IV or liquid: IV dose = oral dose Sodium valproate is available IV or liquid: IV dose = oral dose. Before crushing tablets and mixing with water, confirm with either local guidelines or the drug company for stability information
Antidepressants – MAOIs[4,3,16–19]	• Dangerous, potentially fatal interaction with pethidine and dextromethorphan (serotonin syndrome or coma/ respiratory depression may occur) • Sympathomimetic agents may result in hypertensive crisis • MAO inhibition lasts for up to 2 weeks: early withdrawal is required • Switching to moclobemide 2 weeks before surgery allows continued treatment up until day of surgery (do not give moclobemide on the day of surgery)	Probably not, but careful selection of anaesthetic agents may reduce risks if continuation is essential	None

Psychotropics and surgery (Cont.)

Drug or drug group	Considerations	Safe in surgery?	Alternative formulations
Antidepressants – SSRIs[4,6,7,19–22]	• Danger of serotonin syndrome if administered with pethidine, pentazocine or tramadol • Occasional seizures reported • Cessation may result in withdrawal syndrome • Various interactions with drugs used in surgery • Venlafaxine may provoke opioid-induced rigidity • May increase bleeding time	Probably, but avoid other serotonergic agents	Liquid escitalopram, fluoxetine and paroxetine are available.
Antidepressants – tricyclics[4,6,14,19–21]	• α_1 blockade may lead to hypotension and interfere with effects of epinephrine/ norepinephrine • Danger of serotonin syndrome (clomipramine; amitriptyline) if administered with pethidine, pentazocine or tramadol • Many drugs prolong QT interval so arrhythmia more likely • Most drugs lower seizure threshold • May decrease core hypothermia • Sympathomimetic agents may give exaggerated response • Effects persist for several days after cessation so will need to be stopped some time before surgery	Unclear, but anaesthetic agents need to be carefully chosen Some authorities recommend slow discontinuation before surgery	Liquid amitriptyline is available. It is acidic and may interact with enteral feeds. Dosulepin (dothiepin) capsules can be opened and mixed with water before flushing well. This is preferred over crushing tablets
Antipsychotics[4,13,19,23–25]	• Some antipsychotics widely used in anaesthetic practice • Increased risk of arrhythmia with most drugs • α_1 blockade may lead to hypotension and interfere with effects of epinephrine/ norepinephrine • Most drugs lower seizure threshold • May enhance interoperative core hypothermia • Clozapine may delay recovery from anaesthesia • Gaseous anaesthetics may affect dopamine metabolism	Probably, usually continued to avoid relapse	Liquid preparations of some antipsychotics are available. Some 'specials' liquids can be made for NG delivery. Before crushing tablets and mixing with water, confirm with either local guidelines or the drug company for stability information

Special groups

430

Psychotropics and surgery (Cont.)

Drug or drug group	Considerations	Safe in surgery?	Alternative formulations
Benzodizepines[4,15]	• Reduced requirements for induction and maintenance anaesthetics • Many have prolonged action (days or weeks), so early withdrawal is necessary • Withdrawal symptoms possible	Probably; usually continued	Liquid, IM, IV and rectal diazepam are available (do not use IM route). Buccal liquid available for midazolam. Sublingual (use normal tablets), IM, IV and lorazepam are available
Lithium[4,16,3,19]	• Prolongs the action of both depolarising and non-depolarising muscle relaxants • Surgery-related electrolyte disturbance and reduced renal function may precipitate lithium toxicity. • Avoid dehydration and NSAIDs • Possible increased risk of arrhythmia	Probably safe in minor surgery but usually discontinued before major procedures and re-started once electrolytes normalise. Slow discontinuation is essential	The bioavailability of lithium varies between brands. Care is needed with equivalent doses of salts: lithium carbonate 200 mg = lithium citrate 509 mg. Liquid lithium citrate is available and is usually administered twice daily
Methadone[3,15]	• May reduce opiate requirements • Naloxone may induce withdrawal • Methadone prolongs QT interval • When using opiates, use only full agonists (avoid buprenorphine)	Probably, usually continued	IM dose = oral dose
Modafinil[26,27]	• Limited data suggest no interference with anaesthesia • Improves recovery after anaesthesia	Probably, data limited	None

References

1. Noble DW et al. Interrupting drug therapy in the perioperative period. Drug Saf 2002; 25:489–495.
2. Noble DW et al. Risks of interrupting drug treatment before surgery. BMJ 2000; 321:719–720.
3. Anon. Drugs in the peri-operative period: 1—Stopping or continuing drugs around surgery. Drug Ther Bull 1999; 37:62–64.
4. Smith MS et al. Perioperative management of drug therapy, clinical considerations. Drugs 1996; 51:238–259.
5. Chui PT et al. Medications to withhold or continue in the preoperative consultation. Curr Anaesth Crit Care 1998; 9:302–306.
6. Kudoh A et al. Antidepressant treatment for chronic depressed patients should not be discontinued prior to anesthesia. Can J Anaesth 2002; 49: 132–136.
7. Spivey KM et al. Perioperative seizures and fluvoxamine. Br J Anaesth 1993; 71:321.
8. De Baerdemaeker L et al. Anaesthesia for patients with mood disorders. Curr Opin Anaesthesiol 2005; 18:333–338.
9. Faedda GL et al. Outcome after rapid vs gradual discontinuation of lithium treatment in bipolar disorders. Arch Gen Psychiatry 1993; 50:448–455.
10. Yerevanian BI et al. Antidepressants and suicidal behaviour in unipolar depression. Acta Psychiatr Scand 2004; 110:452–458.
11. Copeland LA et al. Postoperative complications in the seriously mentally ill: a systematic review of the literature. Ann Surg 2008; 248:31–38.
12. Paton C et al. SSRIs and gastrointestinal bleeding. BMJ 2005; 331:529–530.
13. Kudoh A et al. Chronic treatment with antipsychotics enhances intraoperative core hypothermia. Anesthesia Analgesia 2004; 98:111–115.
14. Kudoh A et al. Chronic treatment with antidepressants decreases intraoperative core hypothermia. Anesthesia Analgesia 2003; 97:275–279.
15. Morrow JI et al. Essential drugs in the perioperative period. Curr Pract Surg 1990; 90:106–109.
16. Rahman MH et al. Medication in the peri-operative period. Pharm J 2004; 272:287–289.
17. Blom-Peters L et al. Monoamine oxidase inhibitors and anesthesia: an updated literature review. Acta Anaesthesiol Belg 1993; 44:57–60.
18. Hill S et al. MAOIs to RIMAs in anaesthesia – a literature review. Psychopharmacology 1992; 106 Suppl:S43–S45.
19. Huyse FJ et al. Psychotropic drugs and the perioperative period: a proposal for a guideline in elective surgery. Psychosomatics 2006; 47:8–22.
20. Chui PT et al. Medications to withhold or continue in the preoperative consultation. Curr Anaesth Crit Care 1998; 9:302–306.
21. Takakura K et al. Refractory hypotension during combined general and epidural anaesthesia in a patient on tricyclic antidepressants. Anaesth Intensive Care 2008; 34:111–114.
22. Roy S et al. Fentanyl-induced rigidity during emergence from general anesthesia potentiated by venlafexine. Can J Anaesth 2003; 50:32–35.
23. Doherty J et al. Implications for anaesthesia in a patient established on clozapine treatment. Int J Obstet Anesth 2006; 15:59–62.
24. Geeraerts T et al. Delayed recovery after short-duration, general anesthesia in a patient chronically treated with clozapine. Anesth Analg 2006; 103:1618.
25. Adachi YU et al. Isoflurane anesthesia inhibits clozapine- and risperidone-induced dopamine release and anesthesia-induced changes in dopamine metabolism was modified by fluoxetine in the rat striatum: An in vivo microdialysis study. Neurochem Intern 2008; 52:384–391.
26. Larijani GE et al. Modafinil improves recovery after general anesthesia. Anesth Analg 2004; 98:976–981.
27. Doyle A et al. Day case general anaesthesia in a patient with narcolepsy. Anaesthesia 2008; 63:880–882.

Special groups

432

Atrial fibrillation – using psychotropics

Atrial fibrillation (AF) is the most common cardiac arrhythmia which particularly affects older people but may occur in an important proportion of people under 40. Risk factors include obesity, diabetes, hypertension, long-standing aerobic exercise, and high alcohol consumption[1,2]. AF itself is not usually life-threatening but stasis of blood in the atria during fibrillation predisposes to clot formation and substantially increases the risk of stroke[3]. The use of aspirin (younger patients at lower risk of stroke) or warfarin (older patients or those with other risk factors) is therefore essential.

AF can be defined as 'lone' or paroxysmal (occurring infrequently and spontaneously reverting to sinus rhythm), persistent (repeated and prolonged (> one week) episodes usually, if temporarily, responsive to treatment) or permanent (unresponsive). Risk of stroke is increased in all three conditions[1].

Treatment may involve DC conversion, rhythm control (usually flecainide, propafenone or amiodarone) or rate control (with diltiazem, verapamil, or sotalol). With rhythm control the aim is to maintain sinus rhythm, although this is not always achieved. With rate control, atrial fibrillation is allowed to continue but ventricular response is controlled and ventricles are filled passively.

Atrial fibrillation is commonly encountered in psychiatry not least because of the high rates of obesity, diabetes, and alcohol misuse seen in mental health patients. When considering the use of psychotropics several factors need to be taken into account:

- Interactions between psychotropics and anticoagulant therapy
- Arrhythmogenicity of psychotropics prescribed (AF usually results from cardiovascular disease; drugs affecting cardiac ion channels may increase mortality in these patients, especially those with ischaemic disease[4,5])
- Effect on ventricular rate (some drugs induce reflex tachycardia via postural hypotension, others (clozapine, quetiapine) directly increase heart rate)
- Reported association between individual psychotropics and AF
- Risk of interaction with co-prescribed antiarrhythmics or rate-controlling drugs
- Whether AF is paroxysmal (aim to avoid precipitating AF), persistent (aim to avoid prolonging AF) or permanent (aim to avoid increasing ventricular rate).

Table   Recommendations – psychotropics in AF

Condition	Suggested drugs	Drugs to avoid
Schizophrenia/ schizoaffective disorder	In paroxysmal or persistent AF, **aripiprazole** may be an appropriate choice In permanent AF with rate control, drug choice is less crucial but probably best to avoid drugs with potent effects on the ECG (pimozide, sertindole, etc) and those which increase heart rate	AF reported with clozapine[6], olanzapine[7] and paliperidone[8]. Causation not established but avoid use in paroxysmal or persistent AF Avoid QT-prolonging drugs in ischaemic heart disease (see section on QT prolongation)
Bipolar disorder	Valproate Lithium	Mood-stabilisers appear not to affect risk of AF
Depression (note – untreated depression predicts recurrence of AF[9])	SSRIs (may be beneficial in paroxysmal AF[10]) but beware interaction with warfarin/aspirin Venlafaxine does not affect atrial conduction[11] and may cardiovert paroxysmal AF[12]	Avoid tricyclics in coronary disease[13] Tricyclics may also provoke AF[14,15]
Anxiety disorders (anxiety symptoms increase risk of AF[16])	Benzodiazepines SSRIs (see above)	Tricyclics (see above)
Alzheimer's disease	Acetylcholinesterase inhibitors (but beware bradycardic effects in patients with paroxysmal 'vagal' AF (paroxysmal AF provoked by low heart rate) Rivastigmine has least interaction potential Memantine	Avoid cholinesterase inhibitors in paroxysmal 'vagal' AF

References

1. National Institute for Clinical Excellence. Atrial fibrillation. The management of atrial fibrillation. Clinical Guidance 36. 2006. http://www.nice.org.uk.
2. Chen LY et al. Epidemiology of atrial fibrillation: a current perspective. Heart Rhythm 2007; 4:S1–S6.
3. Lakshminarayan K et al. Clinical epidemiology of atrial fibrillation and related cerebrovascular events in the United States. Neurologist 2008; 14: 143–150.
4. The Cardiac Arrhythmia Suppression Trial II Investigators. Effect of the antiarrhythmic agent moricizine on survival after myocardial infarction. N Engl J Med 1992; 327:227–233.
5. Epstein AE et al. Mortality following ventricular arrhythmia suppression by encainide, flecainide, and moricizine after myocardial infarction. The original design concept of the Cardiac Arrhythmia Suppression Trial (CAST). JAMA 1993; 270:2451–2455.
6. Low RA Jr et al. Clozapine induced atrial fibrillation. J Clin Psychopharmacol 1998; 18:170.
7. Waters BM et al. Olanzapine-associated new-onset atrial fibrillation. J Clin Psychopharmacol 2008; 28:354–355.
8. Schneider RA et al. Apparent seizure and atrial fibrillation associated with paliperidone. Am J Health Syst Pharm 2008; 65:2122–2125.
9. Lange HW et al. Depressive symptoms predict recurrence of atrial fibrillation after cardioversion. J Psychosom Res 2007; 63:509–513.
10. Shirayama T et al. Usefulness of paroxetine in depressed men with paroxysmal atrial fibrillation. Am J Cardiol 2006; 97:1749–1751.
11. Emul M et al. The influences of depression and venlafaxine use at therapeutic doses on atrial conduction. J Psychopharmacol 2008; 23:163–167.
12. Finch SJ et al. Cardioversion of persistent atrial arrhythmia after treatment with venlafaxine in successful management of major depression and post-traumatic stress disorder. Psychosomatics 2006; 47:533–536.
13. Taylor D. Antidepressant drugs and cardiovascular pathology: a clinical overview of effectiveness and safety. Acta Psychiatr Scand 2008; 118:434–442.
14. Moorehead CN et al. Imipramine-induced auricular fibrillation. Am J Psychiatry 1965; 122:216–217.
15. Rosen BH. Case report of auricular fibrillation following the use of imipramine (Tofranil). J Mt Sinai Hosp NY 1960; 27:609–611.
16. Eaker ED et al. Tension and anxiety and the prediction of the 10-year incidence of coronary heart disease, atrial fibrillation, and total mortality: the Framingham Offspring Study. Psychosom Med 2005; 67:692–696.

General principles of prescribing in HIV

Individuals with HIV/AIDS may experience symptoms of mental illness either as a direct consequence of (organic origin), a reaction to, or in addition to their underlying infection. In the first scenario, the focus of treatment should be the underlying infection. Where this is not feasible, or the presentation is not of organic origin, psychotropic medication will be the primary treatment.

When prescribing psychotropics, the following principles should be adhered to:

1. Start with a low dose and titrate according to tolerability and response.
2. Select the simplest dosing regime possible. (Remember that the patient's drug regime is likely to be complex already.)
3. Select an agent with the fewest side effects/interactions. Medical co-morbidity and potential drug interactions must be considered.
4. Ensure that management is conducted in close cooperation with the HIV physicians and the rest of the multidisciplinary team.

Although most psychotropic agents are thought to be safe in HIV-infected individuals, definitive data are lacking in many cases, and it has been suggested that this group may be more sensitive to higher doses, adverse side effects and interactions[1]. Patients with low CD4 counts and high viral loads are more likely to have exaggerated adverse reactions to psychotropic medications.

Psychosis
Atypicals are usually used first line. Risperidone is the most widely studied[2] and generally appears to be safe, although idiosyncratic interactions with ritonavir have been reported[3,4]. The use of clozapine is not routinely recommended, although it may be useful in low doses in patients with higher CD4 counts who are otherwise medically stable. Clozapine may also be helpful in the treatment of individuals with HIV-associated psychosis with drug-induced parkinsonism[5]. Although it is not known whether patients with HIV have a greater risk of agranulocytosis, extremely close monitoring of the WCC is recommended. Patients with HIV may be more susceptible to EPS[6], NMS[7], and TD[8].

Delirium
Organic causes should be identified and treated. Short-term symptomatic treatment may include low-dose atypicals such as risperidone[9], olanzapine[10], quetiapine[11], or ziprasidone[12]. The concomitant use of short courses of low-dose, short-acting benzodiazepines such as lorazepam may also be helpful.

Depression
Depression is common in individuals with HIV, and a recent study estimated the prevalence in this population to be as high as 84%[13]. Of note, depression may be a risk factor for HIV[14], and it has been further suggested that much of this depression is either unrecognised or insufficiently managed[15]. First-line agents include SSRIs, especially citalopram[16] (because it does not inhibit CYP2D6 or CYP3A4), with further treatment as per standard protocols. The risk of serotonin syndrome may be increased[17]. The use of TCAs may be appropriate in some cases, although side effects may limit efficacy and compliance[18]. MAOIs are not recommended in this population. There are limited data regarding other antidepressants, with some evidence suggesting that nefazodone[19]

(now withdrawn) may be helpful in treating depressive symptoms related to HIV infection. Other agents (bupropion[20], mirtazapine[21], reboxetine[22], and trazodone[23]) have been investigated, and although these agents were shown to reduce depressive symptoms, the high prevalence of side-effects limited their utility. Their routine use is therefore not recommended.

Bipolar affective disorder
Mania is a recognised presentation in HIV[24] and individuals with HIV may be more sensitive to the side effects of mood-stabilisers such as lithium[25], especially if they have neurocognitive dysfunction[24]. Conventional agents such as valproate, lamotrigine, and gabapentin may be used cautiously, but carbamazepine should be avoided because of important interactions with antiretroviral agents such as ritonavir[26], as well as the risk of neutropenia. In one case series lithium was shown to be poorly tolerated[27] and it may be advisable to limit its use to asymptomatic individuals with higher CD4 counts and to monitor closely these individuals.

Anxiety disorders
Benzodiazepines may have some utility in the acute treatment of anxiety in individuals with HIV, but caution should be exercised because of the potential for both misuse and multiple and, in rare cases, potentially serious interactions. SSRIs (remember interactions) and other antidepressants may be efficacious, and there is evidence that buspirone may be especially useful[28].

HIV neurocognitive disorders
Individuals with HIV may present with cognitive impairment at any time in the course of their illness; this may range from mild forgetfulness ('minor cognitive and motor disorder') to severe and debilitating dementia. The mainstay of treatment is combination antiretroviral therapy[29], with judicious, short-term use of an antipsychotic such as risperidone[30] if necessary. Treatment of these individuals is carried out primarily by HIV physicians, with liaison psychiatric input as required.

Important drug interactions
Although the majority of psychotropic agents are deemed safe for co-administration with antiretroviral agents, there are a number of clinically important interactions. These are shown in the following table. It should be noted that complete data are lacking, and that there is potential for other interactions not listed in the table. Although many of these interactions are not absolute contra-indications to co-prescribing, extreme caution is advised. As those receiving HIV treatment may be taking medication for many different medical indications, additional interactions cannot be excluded.

A number of psychotropic agents that are potent enzyme inducers are **contra-indicated** for use with antiretroviral agents of all classes, as they can compromise antiretroviral therapy; these include **carbamazepine, phenobarbital, phenytoin, primidone, and St John's Wort**. Enzyme inhibitors can cause severe exacerbation of side effects (e.g. SSRIs, benzodiazepines). Caution is advised when the patient is taking ritonavir and lopinavir/ritonavir, as these drugs are potent enzyme inducers that may compromise the efficacy of psychotropic drugs.

In the following table, interactions are both specific and illustrative, but not exhaustive: reported or sample interactions are outlined; many more interactions are possible. Check the latest literature *and* estimate risk of interaction from first principles (i.e. from understanding of CYP involvement).

Table Reported and suspected interactions of antiretrovirals and psychotropics[31–33] (see also individual SPCs)

Antiretroviral	Psychotropic	Clinical effect
Abacavir (negligible inhibitory effect on CYP3A4, none on CYP2C9 or CYP2D6)	Methadone	↓ Methadone levels
Amprenavir (CYP3A4 inhibitor)	Alprazolam, diazepam, midazolam, triazolam	↑ Sedation, confusion, respiratory depression
	Carbamazepine	↑ Carbamazepine effect; ↓ Amprenavir effect
	Clozapine	↑ Clozapine effect*
	Lamotrigine	↓ Lamotrigine levels*
	Methadone	↓ Methadone levels
	Phenobarbital, phenytoin	↓ Amprenavir effect
	Pimozide	↑ Cardiac arrhythmia
	Primidone	↓ Amprenavir effect
	St John's Wort	↓ Amprenavir effect
	Tricyclic Antidepressants	↑ Tricyclic levels
Delavirdine (inhibitor of CYP3A4, CYP2C9, CYP2C19)	Alprazolam, midazolam, triazolam	↑ Sedation, confusion, respiratory depression
	Carbamazepine	↓ Delavirdine effect
	Fluoxetine	↑ Delavirdine effect*
	Lamotrigine	↓ Lamotrigine levels*
	Phenobarbital, phenytoin	↓ Delavirdine effect
	Pimozide	↑ Cardiac arrhythmia
	Primidone	↓ Amprenavir effect
Efavirenz (inhibitor and inducer of CYP3A4)	Carbamazepine	↓ Carbamazepine effect; ↓ Efavirenz effect
	Fluoxetine	Possible serotonin syndrome
	Lamotrigine	↓ Lamotrigine levels*
	Methadone	↓ Methadone levels
	Phenobarbital	↓ Efavirenz effect
	Phenytoin	↓ Efavirenz effect; ↓ Phenytoin effect
	Pimozide	↑ Cardiac arrhythmia
	Primidone	↓ Efavirenz effect
	Sertraline	↓ Sertraline levels
	St John's Wort	↓ Efavirenz effect

Table Reported and suspected interactions of antiretrovirals and psychotropics[31-33] (see also individual SPCs) (Cont.)

Antiretroviral	Psychotropic	Clinical effect
Indinavir *(inhibitor of CYP3A4)*	Carbamazepine	↓ Indinavir effect
	Lamotrigine	↓ Lamotrigine levels*
	Midazolam	↑ Sedation, confusion, respiratory depression
	Phenobarbital, phenytoin	↓ Indinavir effect
	Pimozide	↑ Cardiac arrhythmia
	Primidone	↓ Efavirenz effect
	St John's Wort	↓ Indinavir effect; possible indinavir resistance
	Trazodone	↑ Sedation, confusion
	Venlafaxine	↓ Indinavir levels
Fosamprenavir *(inhibitor of CYP3A4)*	Carbamazepine	↓ Fosamprenavir levels
	Tricyclic Antidepressants	↑ Tricyclic levels
Lopinavir + Ritonavir *(inhibitor of CYP3A4, CYP2D6) (may induce glucuronidation)*	Bupropion	↑ Bupropion levels
	Buspirone	↑ Parkinsonism
	Carbamazepine	↓ Lopinavir/ritonavir effect
	Citalopram	↑ Citalopram levels*
	Clozapine	↓ Clozapine levels
	Desipramine	↑ Antimuscarinic effects*
	Fluoxetine	↑ Fluoxetine levels; possible serotonin syndrome
	Lamotrigine	↓ Lamotrigine levels*
	Midazolam, flurazepam, diazepam	↑ Sedation, confusion, respiratory depression
	Mirtazapine	↑ Mirtazapine levels*
	Methadone	↓ Methadone levels
	Olanzapine	↓ Olanzapine levels
	Phenobarbital, phenytoin	↓ Lopinavir/ritonavir effect
	Pimozide	↑ Cardiac arrhythmia
	Primidone Risperidone	↓ Lopinavir/ritonavir effect Reversible coma/↑ EPS
	St John's Wort	↓ Lopinavir/ritonavir effect
	Trazodone	↑ Trazodone levels*

Table Reported and suspected interactions of antiretrovirals and psychotropics[31-33] (see also individual SPCs) (Cont.)

Antiretroviral	Psychotropic	Clinical effect
Nelfinavir (inhibitor of CYP3A4, CYP1A2)	Bupropion	↑ Bupropion levels*
	Carbamazepine	↓ Nelfinavir effect
	Desipramine	↑ Antimuscarinic effects*
	Lamotrigine	↓ Lamotrigine levels*
	Methadone	↓ Methadone levels
	Midazolam, triazolam	↑ Sedation, confusion, respiratory depression
	Phenobarbital	↓ Nelfinavir effect
	Phenytoin	↓ Phenytoin effect
	Pimozide	↑ Cardiac arrhythmia
	Primidone	↓ Nelfinavir effect
	St John's Wort	↓ Nelfinavir effect
Nevirapine (CYP3A4, ? effect)	Methadone	↑ Methadone effect
	St John's Wort	↓ Nevirapine effect
Ritonavir (may inhibit and induce CYP3A4, inhibits CYP2D6, CYP2C9, CYP2C19)	Alprazolam, diazepam, midazolam, triazolam	↑ Sedation, confusion, respiratory depression
	Amitriptyline	↑ Antimuscarinic effects*
	Bupropion	↑ Bupropion levels
	Carbamazepine	↓ Ritonavir effect; ↑ carbamazepine levels
	Citalopram	↑ Citalopram levels*
	Clozapine	↓ Clozapine levels
	Desipramine	↑ Antimuscarinic effects*
	Disulphiram	↓ Disulphiram reaction
	Fluoxetine	↑ Fluoxetine levels; possible serotonin syndrome
	Lamotrigine	↓ Lamotrigine levels*
	Methadone	↓ Methadone levels
	Mirtazapine	↑ Mirtazapine levels*
	Olanzapine	↓ Olanzapine effect*
	Phenytoin	↑ Phenytoin effect
	Pimozide	↑ Cardiac arrhythmia
	Primidone	↓ Ritonavir effect
	Risperidone	↑ Risk of coma*
	St John's Wort	↓ Ritonavir effect
	Trazodone	↑ Trazodone levels*

Table Reported and suspected interactions of antiretrovirals and psychotropics[31–33] (see also individual SPCs) (Cont.)

Antiretroviral	Psychotropic	Clinical effect
Saquinavir (inhibits CYP3A4)	Carbamazepine	↓ Saquinavir effect
	Fluoxetine	Possible serotonin syndrome
	Lamotrigine	↑ Lamotrigine levels*
	Midazolam, triazolam	↑ Sedation, confusion, respiratory depression
	Phenobarbital, phenytoin	↓ Saquinavir effect
	Pimozide	↑ Cardiac arrhythmia
	Primidone	↓ Saquinavir effect
	St John's Wort	↓ Saquinavir effect
	Tricyclic Antidepressants	↑ Tricyclic levels
Tipranavir (induces and inhibits CYP3A4, may inhibit CYP1A2, CYP2C9, CYP2D6)	Desipramine	↑ Desipramine levels
	Methadone	↓ Methadone levels
	Trazodone	↑ Trazodone levels
Zidovudine (inhibits CYP3A4)	Methadone	↑ Zidovudine levels
	Valproic Acid	↑ Zidovudine levels

*Effects of interaction may be reduced/eliminated by reduction in psychotropic dose.
Note: all antiretrovirals are metabolised via CYP3A4; some also utilise additional enzymatic routes such as CYP2D6.

Psychotropic effects of HIV drugs

Psychosis, mania, agitation, and suicidal ideation have occasionally been associated with antiretroviral treatment (see following table), most commonly with efavirenz. The most common neuropsychiatric presentation is depression, although any of these conditions can appear de novo in HIV-positive individuals. There is, as yet, no conclusive evidence supporting an association between HIV infection and psychosis[34]. Psychosis is associated with efavirenz, zidovudine, nevirapine and, most recently, abacavir treatment[35]. In many of the reported cases, symptoms abated either when the putative offending agent was stopped or prophylactic agents were added to the medication regimen. It is possible that individuals with a prior history of psychiatric disorder may be at increased risk of neuropsychiatric side effects.

Although most reports suggest that these changes in mental state occur within a month of commencing antiretroviral therapy, the time frame can be highly variable, ranging from 2 days in the case of efavirenz[36] to 14 months[37] or even longer[38]. Treatment involves cessation of the putative offending agent and initiation of a suitable alternative. Inclusion of an appropriate prophylactic agent or agents can be useful, usually for a short period of time (1–3 months). It should be remembered that other drugs used to treat physical problems (apart from antiretrovirals) may also induce changes in mental state.

Table Psychotropic effects of antiretrovirals	
Diagnosis	**Implicated agent**
Depression	Abacavir[39] Amprenavir[40] Efavirenz[36,40,41] Enfuvirtide* Indinavir[42] Nevirapine[43] Ritonavir/lopinavir* Saquinavir* Stavudine* Zidovudine*
Mania	Didanosine[44] Efavirenz[45,46] Zidovudine[47–49]
Psychosis	Abacavir[35,39] Efavirenz[36,50–52] Nevirapine[43]
PTSD	Efavirenz[53]
Vivid dreams	Abacavir[54] Enfuvirtide* Entricitabine* Nevirapine[55] Efavirenz[56]
Suicidal ideation	Abacavir[39] Efavirenz[55,56]
Miscellaneous symptoms (anxiety, sleep disturbance, emotional lability, etc.)	Efavirenz[56,57] Ritonavir/lopinavir* Stavudine* Zalcitabine*

*Adverse effects reported in individual SPCs.

References

1. Ayuso JL. Use of psychotropic drugs in patients with HIV infection. Drugs 1994; 47:599–610.
2. Singh AN et al. Risperidone in HIV-related manic psychosis. Lancet 1994; 344:1029–1030.
3. Jover F et al. Reversible coma caused by risperidone-ritonavir interaction. Clin Neuropharmacol 2002; 25:251–253.
4. Kelly DV et al. Extrapyramidal symptoms with ritonavir/indinavir plus risperidone. Ann Pharmacother 2002; 36:827–830.
5. Lera G et al. Pilot study with clozapine in patients with HIV-associated psychosis and drug-induced parkinsonism. Mov Disord 1999; 14:128–131.
6. Hriso E et al. Extrapyramidal symptoms due to dopamine-blocking agents in patients with AIDS encephalopathy. Am J Psychiatry 1991; 148:1558–1561.
7. Horwath E et al. NMS and HIV. Psychiatr Serv 1999; 50:564.
8. Shedlack KJ et al. Rapidly progressive tardive dyskinesia in AIDS. Biol Psychiatry 1994; 35:147–148.
9. Sipahimalani A et al. Treatment of delirium with risperidone. Int J Geriatr Psychopharmacol 1997; 1:24–26.
10. Sipahimalani A et al. Olanzapine in the treatment of delirium. Psychosomatics 1998; 39:422–430.
11. Schwartz TL et al. Treatment of delirium with quetiapine. Prim Care Companion J Clin Psychiatry 2000; 2:10–12.
12. Leso L et al. Ziprasidone treatment of delirium. Psychosomatics 2002; 43:61–62.
13. Anon. Depression is common among AIDS patients. Psych consult often is necessary. AIDS Alert 2002; 17:153–154.

Special groups

441

14. McDermott BE et al. Diagnosis, health beliefs, and risk of HIV infection in psychiatric patients. Hosp Community Psychiatry 1994; 45:580–585.
15. Katz MH et al. Depression and use of mental health services among HIV-infected men. AIDS Care 1996; 8:433–442.
16. Currier MB et al. Citalopram treatment of major depressive disorder in Hispanic HIV and AIDS patients: a prospective study. Psychosomatics 2004; 45:210–216.
17. DeSilva KE et al. Serotonin syndrome in HIV-infected individuals receiving antiretroviral therapy and fluoxetine. AIDS 2001; 15:1281–1285.
18. Elliott AJ et al. Randomized, placebo-controlled trial of paroxetine versus imipramine in depressed HIV-positive outpatients. Am J Psychiatry 1998; 155:367–372.
19. Elliott AJ et al. Antidepressant efficacy in HIV-seropositive outpatients with major depressive disorder: an open trial of nefazodone. J Clin Psychiatry 1999; 60:226–231.
20. Currier MB et al. A prospective trial of sustained-release bupropion for depression in HIV-seropositive and AIDS patients. Psychosomatics 2003; 44:120–125.
21. Elliott AJ et al. Mirtazapine for depression in patients with human immunodeficiency virus. J Clin Psychopharmacol 2000; 20:265–267.
22. Carvalhal AS et al. An open trial of reboxetine in HIV-seropositive outpatients with major depressive disorder. J Clin Psychiatry 2003; 64:421–424.
23. De WS et al. Efficacy and safety of trazodone versus clorazepate in the treatment of HIV-positive subjects with adjustment disorders: a pilot study. J Int Med Res 1999; 27:223–232.
24. El-Mallakh RS. Mania in AIDS: clinical significance and theoretical considerations. Int J Psychiatry Med 1991; 21:383–391.
25. Tanquary J. Lithium neurotoxicity at therapeutic levels in an AIDS patient. J Nerv Ment Dis 1993; 181:518–519.
26. Berbel GA et al. Protease inhibitor-induced carbamazepine toxicity. Clin Neuropharmacol 2000; 23:216–218.
27. Parenti DM et al. Effect of lithium carbonate in HIV-infected patients with immune dysfunction. J Acquir Immune Defic Syndr 1988; 1:119–124.
28. Batki SL. Buspirone in drug users with AIDS or AIDS-related complex. J Clin Psychopharmacol 1990; 10:111S–115S.
29. Portegies P et al. Guidelines for the diagnosis and management of neurological complications of HIV infection. Eur J Neurol 2004; 11:297–304.
30. Belzie LR. Risperidone for AIDS-associated dementia: a case series. AIDS Patient Care STDS 1996; 10:246–249.
31. HIV InSite. Database of antiretroviral drug interactions. 2008. http://www.hivinsite.com/.
32. Anon. Toronto General Hospital Immunodeficiency Clinic. Drug Interaction Tables. 2009. http://www.tthhivclinic.com/.
33. Liverpool HIV Pharmacology Group. Drug Interaction Charts. 2008. http://www.hiv-druginteractions.org/.
34. Harris MJ et al. New-onset psychosis in HIV-infected patients. J Clin Psychiatry 1991; 52:369–376.
35. Foster R et al. Antiretroviral therapy-induced psychosis: case report and brief review of the literature. HIV Med 2003; 4:139–144.
36. de la Garza CL et al. Efavirenz-induced psychosis. AIDS 2001; 15:1911–1912.
37. Maxwell S et al. Manic syndrome associated with zidovudine treatment. JAMA 1988; 259:3406–3407.
38. Foster R. Personal Communication. 2005.
39. Colebunders R et al. Neuropsychiatric reaction induced by abacavir. Am J Med 2002; 113:616.
40. Lang JP et al. [Apropos of atypical melancholia with Sustiva (efavirenz)] (Article in French). Encephale 2001; 27:290–293.
41. Puzantian T. Central nervous system adverse effects with efavirenz: case report and review. Pharmacotherapy 2002; 22:930–933.
42. Harry TC et al. Indinavir use: associated reversible hair loss and mood disturbance. Int J STD AIDS 2000; 11:474–476.
43. Wise ME et al. Drug points: Neuropsychiatric complications of nevirapine treatment. BMJ 2002; 324:879.
44. Brouillette MJ et al. Didanosine-induced mania in HIV infection. Am J Psychiatry 1994; 151:1839–1840.
45. Blanch J et al. Manic syndrome associated with efavirenz overdose. Clin Infect Dis 2001; 33:270–271.
46. Shah MD et al. A manic episode associated with efavirenz therapy for HIV infection. AIDS 2003; 17:1713–1714.
47. O'Dowd MA et al. Manic syndrome associated with zidovudine (Letter). JAMA 1988; 260:3587.
48. Anon. Manic syndrome associated with zidovudine. JAMA 1988; 260:3587–3588.
49. Wright JM et al. Zidovudine-related mania. Med J Aust 1989; 150:339–341.
50. Sabato S et al. Efavirenz-induced catatonia. AIDS 2002; 16:1841–1842.
51. Poulsen HD et al. Efavirenz-induced psychosis leading to involuntary detention. AIDS 2003; 17:451–453.
52. Peyriere H et al. Management of sudden psychiatric disorders related to efavirenz. AIDS 2001; 15:1323–1324.
53. Moreno A et al. Recurrence of post-traumatic stress disorder symptoms after initiation of antiretrovirals including efavirenz: a report of two cases. HIV Med 2003; 4:302–304.
54. Foster R et al. More on abacavir-induced neuropsychiatric reactions. AIDS 2004; 18:2449.
55. Morlese JF et al. Nevirapine-induced neuropsychiatric complications, a class effect of non-nucleoside reverse transcriptase inhibitors? AIDS 2002; 16:1840–1841.
56. Lochet P et al. Long-term assessment of neuropsychiatric adverse reactions associated with efavirenz. HIV Med 2003; 4:62–66.
57. Foster R. Personal communication. 2008.

Drug treatment of borderline personality disorder

Borderline personality disorder (BPD) is common in psychiatric settings with up to 15% of inpatients meeting diagnostic criteria[1]. In BPD, co-morbid depression, anxiety spectrum disorders, and bipolar illness occur more frequently than would be expected by chance association alone. The suicide rate in BPD is similar to that seen in affective disorders and schizophrenia[2,3].

Although it is classified as a personality disorder, several 'symptoms' of BPD may intuitively be expected to respond to drug treatment. These include affective instability, transient stress-related psychotic symptoms, suicidal and self-harming behaviours, and impulsivity[4].

Drug treatments are often used during periods of crisis when 'symptoms' can be severe, distressing, and potentially life-threatening. By their very nature, these symptoms can be expected to wax and wane[2]. Drug therapy may then be required intermittently. It is generally easy to see when treatment is required, but much more difficult to decide when modest gains are worthwhile and whether or not continuation is likely to be necessary.

Management of crisis
NICE[5] recommends that during periods of crisis, time-limited treatment with a sedative drug may be helpful. Anticipated side-effect profile and potential toxicity in overdose should guide choice. For example, benzodiazepines (particularly short-acting drugs) can cause disinhibition in this group of patients[6], potentially compounding problems; sedative antipsychotics can cause EPS and/or considerable weight gain (see section on antipsychotics and weight gain), and tricyclic antidepressants are particularly toxic in overdose (see section on psychotropics in overdose). A sedative antihistamine such as promethazine is relatively well tolerated and may be a helpful short-term treatment when used as part of a co-ordinated care plan.

Medium to longer term treatment
Evidence supporting the effectiveness of pharmacological interventions in reducing the symptoms of borderline personality disorder is weak and prescribing in the medium to long term for patients who do not have co-morbid mental illness is discouraged by NICE[5]. Co-morbid mental illness should be treated in line with the relevant evidence-based guideline. Note however that a diagnosis of BPD predicts a poorer outcome from treatment of depression with antidepressants[7] and ECT[8]. Symptoms of OCD in BPD may be less responsive to clomipramine[9].

The majority of studies of drug treatment in BPD last for only 6 weeks and a large number of different outcome measures have been used, making it difficult to evaluate and compare studies. Not all RCTs report attrition data, but where this information is available, less than half of subjects tend to complete studies. Symptoms often improve in an unexpected way; for example depressive symptoms may improve with antipsychotics and psychotic symptoms with antidepressants. The placebo response rate in RCTs of BPD is uniformly high. Caution is required when evaluating uncontrolled studies or case reports.

Antipsychotics
Open studies have found benefit for a number of first- and second-generation antipsychotics over a wide range of symptoms. In contrast, placebo-controlled RCTs generally show only very modest benefits for active drug over placebo[10,11]. Open studies report reductions in aggression and self-harming behaviour with clozapine[12,13] and clozapine has been shown to have an anti-aggressive effect in people with schizophrenia[14]. Dysphoria and depression may develop during treatment with conventional antipsychotics[15,16].

Special groups

Antidepressants

Several open studies have found that SSRIs reduce impulsivity and aggression in BPD, but controlled studies show very modest benefits[17,18]. Tranylcypromine[19] and amitriptyline[20] have been shown not to be effective, and both may cause behavioural disinhibition. Reboxetine has also been reported to worsen symptoms[21].

Mood-stabilisers

Up to a half of people with BPD may also have a bipolar spectrum disorder[22] and mood-stabilisers are commonly prescribed. Open studies report benefit, but again the findings from RCTs are considerably more modest[23-25]. Lithium may reduce mood variation[26], anger, and suicidal ideation[27]; lithium is licensed for the control of aggressive behaviour or intentional self-harm[28]. Note that behavioural disinhibition has been reported with carbamazepine[29].

References

1. Winston AP. Recent developments in borderline personality disorder. Adv Psychiatr Treat 2000; 6:211–217.
2. Links PS et al. Prospective follow-up study of borderline personality disorder: prognosis, prediction of outcome, and Axis II comorbidity. Can J Psychiatry 2001; 62:265–270.
3. Paris J. Chronic suicidality among patients with borderline personality disorder. Psychiatr Serv 2002; 53:738–742.
4. American Psychiatric Association. Practice guideline for the treatment of patients with borderline personality disorder. Am J Psychiatry 2001; 158:1–52.
5. National Institute for Clinical Excellence. Borderline Personality Disorder: treatment and management. http://www.nice.org.uk. 2009
6. Gardner DL et al. Alprazolam-induced dyscontrol in borderline personality disorder. Am J Psychiatry 1985; 142:98–100.
7. Shea MT et al. Personality disorders and treatment outcome in the NIMH Treatment of Depression Collaborative Research Program. Am J Psychiatry 1990; 147:711–718.
8. DeBattista C et al. Is electroconvulsive therapy effective for the depressed patient with comorbid borderline personality disorder? J ECT 2001; 17:91–98.
9. Baer L et al. Effect of axis II diagnoses on treatment outcome with clomipramine in 55 patients with obsessive-compulsive disorder. Arch Gen Psychiatry 1992; 49:862–866.
10. Zanarini MC et al. Olanzapine treatment of female borderline personality disorder patients: a double-blind, placebo-controlled pilot study. J Clin Psychiatry 2001; 62:849–854.
11. Bogenschutz MP et al. Olanzapine versus placebo in the treatment of borderline personality disorder. J Clin Psychiatry 2004; 65:104–109.
12. Chengappa KN et al. Clozapine reduces severe self-mutilation and aggression in psychotic patients with borderline personality disorder. J Clin Psychiatry 1999; 60:477–484.
13. Benedetti F et al. Low-dose clozapine in acute and continuation treatment of severe borderline personality disorder. J Clin Psychiatry 1998; 59:103–107.
14. Volavka J et al. Heterogeneity of violence in schizophrenia and implications for long-term treatment. Int J Clin Pract 2008; 62:1237–1245.
15. Teicher MH et al. Open assessment of the safety and efficacy of thioridazine in the treatment of patients with borderline personality disorder. Psychopharmacol Bull 1989; 25:535–549.
16. Soloff PH et al. Efficacy of phenelzine and haloperidol in borderline personality disorder. Arch Gen Psychiatry 1993; 50:377–385.
17. Zanarini MC et al. A preliminary, randomized trial of fluoxetine, olanzapine, and the olanzapine-fluoxetine combination in women with borderline personality disorder. J Clin Psychiatry 2004; 65:903–907.
18. Rinne T et al. SSRI treatment of borderline personality disorder: a randomized, placebo-controlled clinical trial for female patients with borderline personality disorder. Am J Psychiatry 2002; 159:2048–2054.
19. Cowdry RW et al. Pharmacotherapy of borderline personality disorder. Alprazolam, carbamazepine, trifluoperazine, and tranylcypromine. Arch Gen Psychiatry 1988; 45:111–119.
20. Soloff PH et al. Paradoxical effects of amitriptyline on borderline patients. Am J Psychiatry 1986; 143:1603–1605.
21. Anghelescu I et al. Worsening of borderline symptoms under reboxetine treatment. J Neuropsychiatry Clin Neurosci 2005; 17:559–560.
22. Deltito J et al. Do patients with borderline personality disorder belong to the bipolar spectrum? J Affect Disord 2001; 67:221–228.
23. Tritt K et al. Lamotrigine treatment of aggression in female borderline-patients: a randomized, double-blind, placebo-controlled study. J Psychopharmacol 2005; 19:287–291.
24. Hollander E et al. A preliminary double-blind, placebo-controlled trial of divalproex sodium in borderline personality disorder. J Clin Psychiatry 2001; 62:199–203.
25. Frankenburg FR et al. Divalproex sodium treatment of women with borderline personality disorder and bipolar II disorder: a double-blind placebo-controlled pilot study. J Clin Psychiatry 2002; 63:442–446.
26. Rifkin A et al. Lithium carbonate in emotionally unstable character disorder. Arch Gen Psychiatry 1972; 27:519–523.
27. Links PS et al. Lithium therapy for borderline patients: preliminary findings. J Pers Disord 1990; 4:173–181.
28. Sanofi-Aventis. Summary of Product Characteristics. Priadel 200mg & 400mg prolonged release tablets. 2009. http://emc.medicines.org.uk/.
29. de la Fuente JM et al. A trial of carbamazepine in borderline personality disorder. Eur Neuropsychopharmacol 1994; 4:479–486.

Further reading

Binks CA et al. Pharmacological interventions for people with borderline personality disorder. Cochrane Database Syst Rev 2006;CD005653.
Lieb K et al. Borderline personality disorder. Lancet 2004; 364:453–461.

Special groups

Delirium

Delirium is a common neuropsychiatric condition that presents in medical and surgical settings and is known by various names including organic brain syndrome, intensive care psychosis, and acute confusional state[1].

Diagnostic criteria for delirium[2]

- Disturbance of *consciousness* (reduced clarity of awareness of the environment) with reduced ability to focus, sustain or shift attention
- A change in *cognition* (such as memory deficit, disorientation, language disturbance or perceptual disturbance) not better explained by a pre-existing or evolving dementia
- The disturbance develops over a *short period of time* (usually hours to days) and tends to fluctuate over the course of the day
- There is often evidence from the history, physical examination or laboratory findings that the disturbance is due to concomitant medications, a medical condition, substance intoxication or substance withdrawal.

Two distinct clinical subtypes of delirium are recognised[3,4]:

- Hyperactive delirium: characterised by increased motor activity with agitation, hallucinations and inappropriate behaviour
- Hypoactive delirium: characterised by reduced motor activity and lethargy and has a poorer prognosis.

Prevalence

Delirium occurs in 10% of hospitalised medical patients and a further 10–30% develop delirium after admission[3]. Postoperative delirium occurs in 15–53% of patients and in 70–87% of those in intensive care[5].

Risk factors

Delirium is almost invariably multifactorial and it is often inappropriate to isolate a single precipitant as the cause[3].

The most important risk factors have consistently emerged as[3,4]:

- Prior cognitive impairment
- Older age
- Severity of medical illness
- Psychoactive drug use
- Polypharmacy (>4 medications).

Outcome

Patients with delirium have an increased length of hospital stay, increased mortality and increased risk of long-term institutional placement[1,4]. Hospital mortality rates of patients with delirium range from 6% to 18% and are twice that of matched controls[4]. The one-year mortality rate associated with cases of delirium is 35–40%[5]. Up to 60% of individuals suffer persistent cognitive impairment and these patients are also three times more likely to develop dementia[1,4].

Management

Preventing delirium is the most effective strategy for reducing its frequency and complications[5]. Delirium is a medical emergency and the identification and treatment of the underlying cause should be the first aim of management[6].

Non-pharmacological or environmental support strategies should be instituted wherever possible, these include, co-ordinating nursing care, preventing sensory deprivation and disorientation, and maintaining competence[4,7]. Pharmacological treatment should be directed at the relief of specific symptoms of delirium.

The common errors in the pharmacological management of delirium are to use antipsychotic medications in excessive doses, give them too late, or overuse benzodiazepines[3].

General principles[3,4,8]

- Keep the use of sedatives and antipsychotics to a minimum.
- Use one drug at a time.
- Tailor doses according to age, body size and degree of agitation.
- Titrate doses to effect.
- Prescribe "as needed" or "prn" in the first instance.
- Review at least every 24 hours. Once an effective "as needed" or "prn" dose has been established, a regular dose should be prescribed.
- Increase scheduled doses if regular "as needed" doses are required after the initial 24 hour period.
- Maintain at an effective dose and discontinue 7–10 days after symptoms resolve.

Table Drugs used to treat delirium

Drug	Dose	Adverse effects	Notes
First-generation antipsychotics			
Haloperidol[1,4,5,7,9,10]	Oral 0.5–1 mg bd with additional doses every 4 hours as needed (peak effect: 4–6 h) IM 0.5–1 mg, observe for 30–60 minutes and repeat if necessary (peak effect: 20–40 minutes)	EPS can occur especially at doses above 3 mg Prolonged QT interval	Considered first line agent. No trial data has demonstrated superiority of other anti-psychotics to haloperidol, however care must be taken to monitor for extrapyramidal and cardiac side effects Baseline ECG recommended ? increased risk of stroke Avoid in withdrawal of alcohol or sedative hypnotics, anticholinergic toxicity, hepatic failure or neuroleptic malignant syndrome Avoid in Lewy Body Dementia Avoid intravenous use where possible. However in the medical ICU setting, IV is often used with close continuous ECG monitoring
Second-generation antipsychotics			
Amisulpride[7,8,11,12]	Oral 50–300 mg od Maximum of 800 mg od		Very limited evidence ? increased risk of stroke
Aripiprazole[7,8,11,12]	Oral 5–15 mg/day Maximum of 30 mg/day	Akathisia or worsening sleep cycle may be problematic	Very limited evidence ? increased risk of stroke
Olanzapine[13–15]	Oral 2.5–5 mg od Usual maximum 20 mg/day	EPS occur at a lower rate than haloperidol Sedation is the most common reported side effect	Increased risk of stroke among older patients with dementia The intramuscular preparation has not been assessed for the treatment of delirium

Table Drugs used to treat delirium (Cont.)

Drug	Dose	Adverse effects	Notes
Risperidone[15–20]	Oral 0.5 mg bd with additional doses every 4 hourly as needed Usual maximum 4 mg/day	The most common reported side effects are hypotension and EPS	Increased risk of stroke among older patients with dementia
Quetiapine[21,22]	Oral 12.5–25 mg bd This may be increased every 1–2 days to 100 mg daily if it is well tolerated	Sedation and postural hypotension are the most common reported side effects	? increased risk of stroke
Ziprasidone[23]	IM 10mg every 2 hourly Usual maximum 40mg/day		Very limited evidence. Not available in the UK ? increased risk of stroke
Benzodiazepines			
Lorazepam[1,4,5]	Oral/IM 0.25–1 mg every 2–4 hours as needed Usual maximum 3 mg in 24 hours IV use is usually reserved for emergencies	More likely than antipsychotics to cause respiratory depression, over sedation and paradoxical excitement	Considered second-line agent Used in alcohol or sedative hypnotic withdrawal, in Parkinson's disease and in neuroleptic malignant symptoms Associated with prolongation and worsening of delirium symptoms demonstrated in clinical trials
Diazepam[24]	Starting oral dose of 5–10 mg In the elderly a starting dose of 2 mg is recommended	Much longer half life in comparison with lorazepam so is preferred in the treatment of alcohol withdrawal Associated with prolongation and worsening of delirium symptoms demonstrated in clinical trials	Used in alcohol or sedative hypnotic withdrawal, Parkinson's disease and in neuroleptic malignant syndrome

Cholinesterase inhibitors		
Donepezil[25,26]	Oral 5 mg od	Reasonably well tolerated compared with placebo. Nausea and vomiting are the most common adverse effects reported	Very limited evidence. In the small studies where it has been used, clinical benefits have not been convincing
Rivastigmine[27]	Oral 3–9 mg od	As donepezil	Limited experience Usually used in chronic delirium as an adjunct to antipsychotics. Usually used in Lewy body dementia
Other drugs		
Melatonin[28,29]	Oral 2 mg od	Sedation is the most commonly reported adverse effect	Very limited experience, used mainly to correct altered sleep–wake cycle
Trazodone[3,5]	25–150 mg nocte	Over sedation is problematic	Limited experience – used only in uncontrolled studies
Sodium valproate[30]	Oral/IM 250 mg bd increased to plasma level of 50–100 mg/L	Contra-indicated in active liver disease	Some case reports of its use where antipsychotics and/or benzodiazepines are ineffective

References

1. van Zyl LT et al. Delirium concisely: condition is associated with increased morbidity, mortality, and length of hospitalization. Geriatrics 2006; 61:18–21.
2. American Psychiatric Association. Diagnostic and Statistical Manual of Mental Disorders, 4th edition. Washington DC: American Psychiatric Association; 1994.
3. Nayeem K et al. Delirium. Clin Med 2003; 3:412–415.
4. Potter J et al. The prevention, diagnosis and management of delirium in older people: concise guidelines. Clin Med 2006; 6:303–308.
5. Inouye SK. Delirium in older persons. N Engl J Med 2006; 354:1157–1165.
6. Burns A et al. Delirium. J Neurol Neurosurg Psychiatry 2004; 75:362–367.
7. Schwartz TL et al. The role of atypical antipsychotics in the treatment of delirium. Psychosomatics 2002; 43:171–174.
8. Seitz DP et al. Antipsychotics in the treatment of delirium: a systematic review. J Clin Psychiatry 2007; 68:11–21.
9. Fricchione GL et al. Postoperative delirium. Am J Psychiatry 2008; 165:803–812.
10. Lonergan E et al. Antipsychotics for delirium (review). Cochrane Database Syst Rev 2007;CD005594.
11. Boettger S et al. Atypical antipsychotics in the management of delirium: a review of the empirical literature. Palliat Support Care 2005; 3:227–237.
12. Leentjens AF et al. Delirium in elderly people: an update. Curr Opin Psychiatry 2005; 18:325–330.
13. Skrobik YK et al. Olanzapine vs haloperidol: treating delirium in a critical care setting. Intensive Care Med 2004; 30:444–449.
14. Sipahimalani A et al. Olanzapine in the treatment of delirium. Psychosomatics 1998; 39:422–430.
15. Duff G. Atypical antipsychotic drugs and stroke. http://www.mhra.gov.uk. 2004.
16. Bourgeois JA et al. Prolonged delirium managed with risperidone. Psychosomatics 2005; 46:90–91.
17. Gupta N et al. Effectiveness of risperidone in delirium. Can J Psychiatry 2005; 50:75.
18. Liu CY et al. Efficacy of risperidone in treating the hyperactive symptoms of delirium. Int Clin Psychopharmacol 2004; 19:165–168.
19. Horikawa N et al. Treatment for delirium with risperidone: results of a prospective open trial with 10 patients. Gen Hosp Psychiatry 2003; 25:289–292.
20. Han CS et al. A double-blind trial of risperidone and haloperidol for the treatment of delirium. Psychosomatics 2004; 45:297–301.
21. Torres R et al. Use of quetiapine in delirium: case reports. Psychosomatics 2001; 42:347–349.
22. Sasaki Y et al. A prospective, open-label, flexible-dose study of quetiapine in the treatment of delirium. J Clin Psychiatry 2003; 64:1316–1321.
23. Young CC et al. Intravenous ziprasidone for treatment of delirium in the intensive care unit. Anesthesiology 2004; 101:794–795.
24. Chan D et al. Delirium: making the diagnosis, improving the prognosis. Geriatrics 1999; 54:28–42.
25. Overshott R et al. Cholinesterase inhibitors for delirium. Cochrane Database Syst Rev 2008;CD005317.
26. Sampson EL et al. A randomized, double-blind, placebo-controlled trial of donepezil hydrochloride (Aricept) for reducing the incidence of postoperative delirium after elective total hip replacement. Int J Geriatr Psychiatry 2007; 22:343–349.
27. Dautzenberg PL et al. Adding rivastigmine to antipsychotics in the treatment of a chronic delirium. Age Ageing 2004; 33:516–517.
28. Hanania M et al. Melatonin for treatment and prevention of postoperative delirium. Anesth Analg 2002; 94:338–339, table.
29. Cronin AJ et al. Melatonin secretion after surgery. Lancet 2000; 356:1244–1245.
30. Bourgeois JA et al. Adjunctive valproic acid for delirium and/or agitation on a consultation-liaison service: a report of six cases. J Neuropsychiatry Clin Neurosci 2005; 17:232–238.

Special groups

450

Huntington's disease – pharmacological treatment

Huntington's disease (HD) is a genetic disease involving slow progressive degeneration of neurones in the basal ganglia and cerebral cortex. Neurones are damaged when the mutated Huntington protein gradually aggregates and interferes with normal metabolism and functioning. The mechanism is poorly understood[1] making it difficult to develop drugs that slow or stop progression. Therefore, only symptomatic treatment is used to improve quality of life. Choreiform movements occur in approximately 90% of patients, and between 23% and 73% develop depression or psychosis during the course of their illness[2]. Dementia is inevitable.

There is very little primary literature to guide practice in this area. A summary can be found below. Clinicians who treat patients with HD are encouraged to publish reports of both positive and negative outcomes to increase the primary literature base.

Symptoms	Treatment
Choreiform movements	Note that these are often more distressing for carers and healthcare professionals than they are for the patient and it should not be assumed that intervention is always in the patient's best interests. • Discontinue dopaminergic drugs such as piracetam, amantadine, and cabergoline[3]. Consider the contribution of psychotropic drugs with dopaminergic effects such as aripiprazole and venlafaxine. • The use of tetrabenazine is supported by RCTs[4,5] but up to 80% of patients experience dose-limiting symptoms[6] such as depression, anxiety, and insomnia. A diagnosis of pre-existing depression is not an absolute contra-indication though[6]. Studies suggest that clinical benefits can be observed rapidly and a multiple daily dosing regimen (TDS) may be needed[7]. • A small dose of a conventional antipsychotic such as haloperidol, fluphenazine[8], or sulpiride[6] is established clinical practice[9]. • Findings with second-generation antipsychotics are mixed. Two open studies of olanzapine 5 mg were negative[10,11] but a third using 30 mg showed improved motor function[12]. Case reports support the use of risperidone both at low[13] and higher dose[14,15]. Quetiapine may also be effective[16]. • A small, open-label study suggested levetiracetam may be effective in reducing chorea. Side effects included somnolence and dyskinesias[17]. • A large, double-blind trial found no benefit with riluzole in beneficial symptomatic effects or neuroprotection[18]. • The results of several small studies suggest that amantadine may help chorea at a dose of >400 mg/day. Possible side effects include agitation, confusion, and sleep disturbances[6]. • Valproic acid does not seem to be effective in treating chorea[6]. However, cortical myoclonus, a rare, but potentially disabling feature of adult Huntington's disease, was shown in several case reports to improve with valproic acid[6,19]. • Positive and negative data also exist for lamotrigine in the treatment of motor and mood symptoms in Huntington's disease[6,20].
Hypokinetic rigidity	• Treatment is similar to that of Parkinson's disease although response is often suboptimal. Anticholinergics and dopamine agonists are sometimes used. Note the potential to exacerbate choreiform movements and precipitate psychosis. • Muscle relaxants, such as diazepam can also be effective in treating rigidity and are usually well tolerated[3], although aspiration secondary to sedation is a potential risk.

(Cont.)	
Symptoms	*Treatment*
Psychosis	There are no RCTs to guide choice. Treatment is empirical. Note that antipsychotic drugs may exacerbate the underlying movement disorder. • Some evidence supports the efficacy of conventional antipsychotics, particularly haloperidol, when the HD is mild to moderate[9]. As HD progresses, typicals tend to be poorly tolerated due to dystonia and parkinsonism[9]. • Case reports support the efficacy of risperidone[14,15,21], quetiapine[22], and amisulpride[23] although EPS can be problematic with all of these drugs. A positive case report also exists for aripiprazole[24].
Depression	There are no RCTs to guide choice. Note that the suicide rate in patients with HD is 4–6 times higher than in the background population[9]. • Case reports support the efficacy of a wide range of antidepressants but TCAs are poorly tolerated (sedation, falls, and anticholinergic-induced cognitive impairment) and MAOIs can worsen choreiform movements. SSRIs are preferred[25,26]. • Reviews state that lithium is best avoided; clinical experience suggests that response is likely to be poor and that toxic effects may be particularly problematic[9] . There is no primary literature. • ECT seems to be relatively well tolerated in HD patients[9].
Dementia	Positive and negative case reports exist for the use of cholinesterase inhibitors in Huntington's disease patients. • Based on available evidence, the treatment of Huntington's disease with acetylcholinesterase inhibitors does not significantly alter cognitive decline, and has little impact on daily functionality of the Huntington disease patients. Therefore these drugs have no specific indication in the treatment of this disease[6]. • One small sample study concluded that donepezil was not an effective treatment for Huntington's disease[27]. • However, a 2-year follow-up of rivastigmine treatment showed positive results in slowing motor deterioration and possibly reducing cognitive impairment[28]. • Positive case reports also exist for memantine in preventing the progression of cognitive symptoms[29].

The above table represents a review of the literature rather than a guide to treatment. Readers are directed to the reports cited here for details of dosage, frequency, and monitoring.

References

1. Jankovic J . Huntington's disease http://www.bcm.edu. 2006
2. Petrikis P et al. Treatment of Huntington's disease with galantamine. Int Clin Psychopharmacol 2004; 19:49–50.
3. Bonelli RM et al. Huntington's disease: present treatments and future therapeutic modalities. Int Clin Psychopharmacol 2004; 19:51–62.
4. McLellan DL. et al. A double-blind trial of tetrabenazine, thiopropazate, and placebo in patients with chorea. Lancet 1974; 1:104–107.
5. Jankovic J. Treatment of hyperkinetic movement disorders with tetrabenazine: a double-blind crossover study. Ann Neurol 1982; 11:41–47.
6. Adam OR et al. Symptomatic treatment of Huntington disease. Neurotherapeutics 2008; 5:181–197.
7. Kenney C et al. Short-term effects of tetrabenazine on chorea associated with Huntington's disease. Mov Disord 2007; 22:10–13.
8. Bonelli RM et al. Pharmacological management of Huntington's disease: an evidence-based review. Curr Pharm Des 2006; 12:2701–2720.
9. Rosenblatt A et al. Neuropsychiatry of Huntington's disease and other basal ganglia disorders. Psychosomatics 2000; 41:24–30.
10. Squitieri F et al. Short-term effects of olanzapine in Huntington disease. Neuropsychiatry Neuropsychol Behav Neurol 2001; 14:69–72.
11. Paleacu D et al. Olanzapine in Huntington's disease. Acta Neurol Scand 2002; 105:441–444.
12. Bonelli RM et al. High-dose olanzapine in Huntington's disease. Int Clin Psychopharmacol 2002; 17:91–93.
13. Erdemoglu AK et al. Risperidone in chorea and psychosis of Huntington's disease. Eur J Neurol 2002; 9:182–183.
14. Dallocchio C et al. Effectiveness of risperidone in Huntington chorea patients. J Clin Psychopharmacol 1999; 19:101–103.
15. Duff K et al. Risperidone and the treatment of psychiatric, motor, and cognitive symptoms in Huntington's disease. Ann Clin Psychiatry 2008; 20:1–3.
16. Bonelli RM et al. Quetiapine in Huntington's disease: a first case report. J Neurol 2002; 249:1114–1115.

17. Zesiewicz TA et al. Open-label pilot study of levetiracetam (Keppra) for the treatment of chorea in Huntington's disease. Mov Disord 2006; 21: 1998–2001.
18. Landwehrmeyer GB et al. Riluzole in Huntington's disease: a 3-year, randomized controlled study. Ann Neurol 2007; 62:262–272.
19. Saft C et al. Dose-dependent improvement of myoclonic hyperkinesia due to Valproic acid in eight Huntington's disease patients: a case series. BMC Neurol 2006; 6:11.
20. Shen YC. Lamotrigine in motor and mood symptoms of Huntington's disease. World J Biol Psychiatry 2008; 9:147–149.
21. Madhusoodanan S et al. Use of risperidone in psychosis associated with Huntington's disease. Am J Geriatr Psychiatry 1998; 6:347–349.
22. Seitz DP et al. Quetiapine in the management of psychosis secondary to huntington's disease: a case report. Can J Psychiatry 2004; 49:413.
23. Saft C et al. Amisulpride in Huntington's disease. Psychiatr Prax 2005; 32:363–366.
24. Lin WC et al. Aripiprazole effects on psychosis and chorea in a patient with Huntington's disease. Am J Psychiatry 2008; 165:1207–1208.
25. De Marchi N et al. Fluoxetine in the treatment of Huntington's disease. Psychopharmacology 2001; 153:264–266.
26. Rosenblatt A, Ranen NG, Nance MA, Paulsen JS. A Physician's Guide to the Management of Huntington's Disease. 2nd ed. New York: Huntington's Disease Society of America; 1999.
27. Cubo E et al. Effect of donepezil on motor and cognitive function in Huntington disease. Neurology 2006; 67:1268–1271.
28. de TM et al. Two years' follow-up of rivastigmine treatment in Huntington disease. Clin Neuropharmacol 2007; 30:43–46.
29. Cankurtaran ES et al. Clinical experience with risperidone and memantine in the treatment of Huntington's disease. J Natl Med Assoc 2006; 98: 1353–1355.

Special groups

Velo-cardio-facial syndrome (VCFS)

Description of syndrome

Velo-cardio-facial syndrome, also known as DiGeorge or Shprintzen syndrome, is a congenital disorder caused by a microdeletion of chromosome 22 at band q11.2. It has an estimated incidence of 1 in 5000 births[1]. Although considerable phenotypic variability occurs, with over 180 clinical features described, it is characterised by:

Cardiac defects, Abnormal facies, Thymic hypoplasia, Cleft palate and Hypocalcaemia

These abnormalities have been collectively named **CATCH 22** (22 refers to chromosome 22)[2], a somewhat inappropriate name for a syndrome that can often be treated very effectively[3]. The typical facial features of patients with VCFS include a long face, prominent nose with bulbous tip and narrow orbital features[4].

Mental retardation and learning disabilities (including impairment in the development of language, reading, spelling and numeracy skills) are common. A high rate of psychiatric morbidity has also been identified in VCFS patients, with schizophrenia and bipolar disorder being most commonly reported[4].

There are currently limited data on the treatment of psychiatric disorders in VCFS with most of the evidence coming from a small number of anecdotal reports. The majority of patients do not require medication to treat the behavioural symptoms associated with the syndrome[3]. However, the range of psychiatric disorders seen in VCFS has been observed to respond to standard treatment protocols in both children and adults[1].

Adults

Neuropsychiatric symptoms in VCFS

A large study evaluating rates of psychiatric disorders in adult patients with VCFS reported that about 30% had a psychotic disorder; with 24% fulfilling DSM-IV criteria for schizophrenia and 12% had major depression without psychotic features[5]. Individuals with schizophrenia associated with VCFS were noted to have fewer negative symptoms and a relatively later age of onset (mean = 26 years) compared with control patients who did not have VCFS[6]. Results from genetic studies have estimated the prevalence of schizophrenia in VCFS patients as 22%, a much higher figure than the 0.5% prevalence of schizophrenia in the general population[7]. In fact, VCFS has been found to be the highest known risk factor for the development of schizophrenia[8].

Management of psychiatric symptoms

It has been suggested that neuropsychiatric symptoms of VCFS only partially respond to typical antipsychotics[4]. While the early introduction of clozapine is favoured[4], experience suggests that newer atypical antipsychotics are also effective in the treatment of VCFS-related schizophrenia[1]. Caution is required with most antipsychotics in VCFS because of the potential for cardiac toxicity (see section on QT changes).

The use of atypical antipsychotics in VCFS patients with general developmental disabilities has been investigated and studies have found them to be broadly effective against challenging behaviours such as self-injury and aggression[9,10]. In addition, they have been found to be better tolerated than typical antipsychotics in this population[11]. Most evidence supports the use of risperidone[9]. The frequency of use of clozapine in learning disabilities still lags behind its use in the general population, despite the higher prevalence of psychiatric disorders in these patients. Clozapine has been associated with marked improvements in psychosis and aggressive behaviours in learning disabled patients. However, although it showed no worsening of seizure control or provocation of seizures in one study, a reduction in seizure threshold is a well-established and potentially serious adverse effect of clozapine. Unlike the other antipsychotics that do not precipitate seizures in patients with intellectual disability who have no history of seizures, this is not the case with clozapine. Therefore special caution should be observed in this population[12].

Children
Neuropsychiatric symptoms
Children with VCFS have been reported to have high rates of bipolar II disorder (47%), attention deficit hyperactivity disorder (ADHD) (27%) and attention deficit disorder without hyperactivity (ADD) (13%). Data suggest that the inattentive subtype is the most common subtype of ADHD in children with VCFS. These children are less likely to be hyperactive or impulsive than children with idiopathic ADHD[13]. Some studies have also shown high rates of autism spectrum disorder, anxiety disorders, and emotional instability in children with VCFS[1].

Management of psychiatric symptoms
Concern has been raised over the theoretical risk of inducing psychosis in children with VCFS and comorbid ADHD by using the psychostimulant methylphenidate. This is of particular concern in older adolescents or young adults. However, standard treatment for ADHD is recommended following experience suggesting psychosis is not a significant clinical risk[1]. Low doses of methylphenidate (0.3 mg/kg) have been shown to be effective in controlling VCFS-related ADHD and were generally well tolerated[14].

References

1. Murphy KC. Annotation: velo-cardio-facial syndrome. J Child Psychol Psychiatry 2005; 46:563–571.
2. Buchanan LM et al. Velocardiofacial syndrome or DiGeorge's anomaly. Lancet 2001; 358:420.
3. Shprintzen RJ. Velo-cardio-facial syndrome: 30 Years of study. Dev Disabil Res Rev 2008; 14:3–10.
4. Gothelf D et al. Clinical characteristics of schizophrenia associated with velo-cardio-facial syndrome. Schizophr Res 1999; 35:105–112.
5. Murphy KC et al. High rates of schizophrenia in adults with velo-cardio-facial syndrome. Arch Gen Psychiatry 1999; 56:940–945.
6. Murphy KC et al. Velo-cardio-facial syndrome: a model for understanding the genetics and pathogenesis of schizophrenia. Br J Psychiatry 2001; 179:397–402.
7. Karayiorgou M et al. Schizophrenia susceptibility associated with interstitial deletions of chromosome 22q11. Proc Natl Acad Sci U S A 1995; 92:7612–7616.
8. Eliez S et al. Parental origin of the deletion 22q11.2 and brain development in velocardiofacial syndrome: a preliminary study. Arch Gen Psychiatry 2001; 58:64–68.
9. Aman MG et al. Atypical antipsychotics in persons with developmental disabilities. Ment Retard Dev Disabil Res Rev 1999; 5:253–263.
10. Williams H et al. Use of the atypical antipsychotics olanzapine and risperidone in adults with intellectual disability. J Intellect Disabil Res 2000; 44 (Pt 2):164–169.
11. Connor DF et al. A brief review of atypical antipsychotics in individuals with developmental disability. Ment Health Aspects Dev Disabil 1998; 1:93–101.
12. Gladston S et al. Clozapine treatment of psychosis associated with velo-cardio-facial syndrome: benefits and risks. J Intellect Disabil Res 2005; 49:567–570.
13. Antshel KM et al. Comparing ADHD in velocardiofacial syndrome to idiopathic ADHD: a preliminary study. J Atten Disord 2007; 11:64–73.
14. Gothelf D et al. Methylphenidate treatment for attention-deficit/hyperactivity disorder in children and adolescents with velocardiofacial syndrome: an open-label study. J Clin Psychiatry 2003; 64:1163–1169.

Summary of commonly reported physical side effects of psychotropics

All psychotropic medications in current use have physical side effects, most of which are rare, idiosyncratic and of variable clinical significance. When these effects are common and clinically relevant, such medications may require specific monitoring and intervention, such as the monitoring of plasma drug levels, although in general, appropriate physical and mental state examination will detect changes from baseline. On occasion it may be necessary to undertake additional investigations (imaging, electrophysiology, and laboratory). The effects of psychotropics on biochemical and haematological parameters are summarised elsewhere.

Although side-effects may arise at any time during treatment, they may be particularly common in the first few weeks of therapy, when doses are increased, on chronic, high doses, in patients with co-morbid medical and psychiatric disorders, in the elderly, and in association with polypharmacy. Most adverse effects may be predicted from the specific receptor profiles of each agent but in general the most common side effects of psychotropics are constitutional (dizziness, effects on body habitus), gastrointestinal (nausea, vomiting, altered bowel habit) and neurological (headache, movement disorders). Further details regarding individual drugs may be found in other sections.

The following table summarises the commonly reported physical side effects of those psychotropics in current use, with data compiled from various secondary sources. It should be noted that the data reflecting the actual frequency of these adverse effects are incomplete, and are based on information provided by pharmaceutical companies, clinical trials, case reports, and post-marketing surveillance. Thus the information provided below is intended as a general guide only, and will be subject to change. When in doubt, additional sources of information should be consulted. Note also that the following table is restricted to adverse effects reported to be common (usually occurring in more than 1% of patients). Less frequent associations are possible.

Table Commonly reported physical side effects of psychotropics[1-12]

System	Specific event	Associated psychotropic
Cardiovascular	Palpitations	Duloxetine; modafinil
	Tachycardia	Chlorpromazine; clozapine; flupentixol; fluphenazine; loxapine; molindone; olanzapine; paliperidone; perphenazine; pipotiazine; promazine; quetiapine; risperidone; zotepine
Constitutional	Decreased appetite	Atomoxetine; bupropion; dexamphetamine; donepezil; duloxetine; galantamine; isocarboxazid; methylphenidate; modafinil; naltrexone; phenelzine; rivastigmine; SSRIs; sulpiride; valproate; venlafaxine
	Dizziness	Aripiprazole; atomoxetine; benzodiazepines; buprenorphine; bupropion; buspirone; carbamazepine; chloral hydrate; chlorpromazine; clozapine; dexamphetamine; donepezil; fluphenazine; galantamine; haloperidol; isocarboxazid; lamotrigine; levomepromazine; lofexidine; memantine; maprotiline; meprobamate; methylphenidate; mianserin; moclobemide; olanzapine; pericyazine; perphenazine; phenelzine; pregabalin; prochlorperazine; reboxetine; risperidone; rivastigmine; quetiapine; SSRIs; sertindole; sulpiride; thioridazine; TCAs; tranylcypromine; trazodone; tryptophan; valproate; venlafaxine; zaleplon; zolpidem; zopiclone; zuclopenthixol
	Feeling cold	morphine; zotepine
	Feeling hot	tryptophan; zotepine
	Increased appetite	Isocarboxazid; maprotiline; mianserin; mirtazapine; phenelzine; pregabalin; TCAs
	Increased pain sensation	Olanzapine
	Weakness	Aripiprazole; benzodiazepines; isocarboxazid; maprotiline; meprobamate; methylphenidate; phenelzine; rivastigmine; TCAs; tranylcypromine; valproate; zotepine
	Weight gain	Amisulpride; benperidol; chlorpromazine; clozapine; flupentixol; fluphenazine; haloperidol; isocarboxazid; lithium; maprotiline; mianserin; mirtazapine; olanzapine; paliperidone; perphenazine; phenelzine; pimozide; pipotiazine; pregabalin; promazine; risperidone; quetiapine; thioridazine; tranylcypromine; TCAs; valproate; zotepine; zuclopenthixol
	Weight loss	Bupropion; dexamphetamine; donepezil; galantamine; rivastigmine

Special groups

Table Commonly reported physical side effects of psychotropics[1–12] (Cont.)

System	Specific event	Associated psychotropic
Ears	Tinnitus	Bupropion
Eyes	Blurred vision	Benperidol; buprenorphine; chlorpromazine; fluphenazine; haloperidol; isocarboxazid; lamotrigine; levomepromazine; maprotiline; meprobamate; methylphenidate; mianserin; molindone; perphenazine; phenelzine; pipotiazine; pregabalin; prochlorperazine; promazine; thioridazine; trazodone; TCAs; zotepine; zuclopenthixol
	Diplopia	Carbamazepine; lamotrigine; pregabalin
	Other visual disturbance (not specified)	Loxapine; morphine
	Pigmentary retinopathy	Thioridazine (high doses)
Gastrointestinal	Abdominal pain	Atomoxetine; bupropion; lamotrigine; methylphenidate; naloxone; naltrexone; quetiapine; risperidone; valproate
	Constipation	Amisulpride; aripiprazole; atomoxetine; benperidol; buprenorphine; bupropion; chlorpromazine; clozapine; fluphenazine; haloperidol; isocarboxazid; lamotrigine; loxapine; maprotiline; memantine; mianserin; mirtazapine; moclobemide; molindone; morphine; naltrexone; olanzapine; pericyazine; perphenazine; phenelzine; pregabalin; prochlorperazine; promazine; quetiapine; reboxetine; risperidone; SSRIs; sulpiride; thioridazine; tranylcypromine; trazodone; TCAs; trifluoperazine; valproate; venlafaxine; zotepine; zuclopenthixol
	Diarrhoea	Benperidol; carbamazepine; chloral hydrate; dexamphetamine; donepezil; duloxetine; galantamine; lithium; maprotiline; moclobemide; modafinil; naltrexone; pericyazine; prochlorperazine; rivastigmine; SSRIs; TCAs; tranylcypromine; valproate; venlafaxine
	Dry mouth	Atomoxetine; benperidol; benzodiazepines; bupropion; chlorpromazine; clozapine; dexamphetamine; duloxetine; fluphenazine; haloperidol; isocarboxazid; lofexidine; loxapine; maprotiline; mianserin; mirtazapine; moclobemide; molindone; morphine; olanzapine; pericyazine; perphenazine; phenelzine; pipotiazine; pregabalin; prochlorperazine; promazine; quetiapine; reboxetine; SSRIs; sulpiride; thioridazine; TCAs; tranylcypromine; trazodone; trifluoperazine; venlafaxine; zotepine; zuclopenthixol
	Dyspepsia	Atomoxetine; lamotrigine; olanzapine; quetiapine; rivastigmine; TCAs; valproate; zotepine
	Flatulence	Chloral hydrate; pregabalin
	Gastro-oesophageal reflux disease	Maprotiline Clozapine?

Table   Commonly reported physical side effects of psychotropics[1–12] (Cont.)

System	Specific event	Associated psychotropic
	Hypersalivation	Benzodiazepines; clozapine
	Nausea	Acamprosate; aripiprazole; atomoxetine; buprenorphine; bupropion; buspirone; carbamazepine; chloral hydrate; clomethiazole; clozapine; dexamphetamine; donepezil; duloxetine; galantamine; isocarboxazid; lamotrigine; lithium; meprobamate; methylphenidate; mianserin; moclobemide; modafinil; morphine; naloxone; naltrexone; phenelzine; pipotiazine; risperidone; rivastigmine; SSRIs; TCAs; tranylcypromine; trazodone; triclofos; tryptophan; valproate; venlafaxine
	Vomiting	Acamprosate; aripiprazole; atomoxetine; buprenorphine; donepezil; carbamazepine; clomethiazole; galantamine; lamotrigine; meprobamate; moclobemide; naltrexone; pregabalin; rivastigmine; sulpiride; trazodone; triclofos; tryptophan; valproate
Musculo-skeletal	Muscle cramp	Donepezil
	Myalgia	Bupropion
	Musculoskeletal pain	Naltrexone; tryptophan; venlafaxine
Nervous	Abnormal Coordination	Lamotrigine; meprobamate; pregabalin; trazodone
	Akathisia	Aripiprazole; chlorpromazine; fluphenazine; loxapine; molindone; pericyazine; perphenazine; pimozide; prochlorperazine; sulpiride; thioridazine; trifluoperazine
	Ataxia	Benzodiazepines; carbamazepine; haloperidol; lamotrigine; lithium; pregabalin; valproate; zaleplon; zolpidem; zopiclone
	Dysarthria	Benzodiazepines; lithium; pregabalin
	Dysgeusia	Chloral hydrate; maprotiline; TCAs
	Extrapyramidal side effects	Amisulpride; benperidol; chlorpromazine; flupentixol; fluphenazine; haloperidol; loxapine; molindone; pericyazine; perphenazine; pimozide; prochlorperazine; risperidone; sulpiride; thioridazine; trifluoperazine; zuclopenthixol
	Headache	Benperidol; bupropion; buspirone; carbamazepine; chloral hydrate; clomethiazole; clozapine; dexamphetamine; donepezil; duloxetine; galantamine; isocarboxazid; lamotrigine; maprotiline; memantine; meprobamate; methylphenidate; mianserin; modafinil; naloxone; naltrexone; paliperidone; pericyazine; prochlorperazine; risperidone; rivastigmine; SSRIs; sulpiride; TCAs; trazodone; triclofos; tryptophan; valproate; venlafaxine; zotepine

Table Commonly reported physical side effects of psychotropics[1–12] (Cont.)

System	Specific event	Associated psychotropic
	Movement disorder (unspecified)	Isocarboxazid; phenelzine
	Paraesthesia	Pregabalin; sertindole
	Parkinsonism	Benperidol; chlorpromazine; flupentixol; fluphenazine; haloperidol; loxapine; molindone; pericyazine; perphenazine; pimozide; prochlorperazine; thioridazine; trifluoperazine
	Tardive dyskinesia	Chlorpromazine; flupentixol; fluphenazine; haloperidol; loxapine; molindone; perphenazine; pimozide; promazine; thioridazine; trifluoperazine; zuclopenthixol
	Tremor	Bupropion; isocarboxazid; lamotrigine; lithium; methylphenidate; pericyazine; phenelzine; pregabalin; prochlorperazine; trazodone; valproate
	Unsteadiness	Carbamazepine
Renal and urinary	Urinary hesitation	Atomoxetine; reboxetine
	Urinary retention	Atomoxetine; buprenorphine; chlorpromazine; fluphenazine; haloperidol; loxapine; maprotiline; molindone; perphenazine; promazine; reboxetine; TCAs; trifluoperazine; zuclopenthixol
Reproductive and breast	Abnormal orgasm (men)	Atomoxetine; venlafaxine
	Abnormal orgasm (women)	Atomoxetine; duloxetine; SSRIs
	Decreased libido	Atomoxetine; duloxetine; maprotiline; pregabalin; SSRIs; TCAs
	Delayed ejaculation	SSRIs
	Ejaculation disorder (unspecified)	Venlafaxine
	Erectile dysfunction	Atomoxetine; pregabalin; SSRIs; venlafaxine
	Galactorrhoea	Amisulpride; chlorpromazine; flupentixol; fluphenazine; haloperidol; loxapine; moclobemide; molindone; perphenazine; pimozide; pipotiazine; sulpiride; thioridazine; trifluoperazine; zuclopenthixol
	Impotence	Atomoxetine; duloxetine; maprotiline; pipotiazine; reboxetine; sulpiride; TCAs; venlafaxine
	Menstrual cycle disorders	Atomoxetine; chlorpromazine; flupentixol; fluphenazine; loxapine; molindone; morphine; sulpiride
	Priapism	Chlorpromazine; fluphenazine; thioridazine; trifluoperazine; zuclopenthixol
	Sexual dysfunction (unspecified)	Chlorpromazine; fluphenazine; isocarboxazid; perphenazine; phenelzine; risperidone; thioridazine; tranylcypromine; trifluoperazine

Table Commonly reported physical side effects of psychotropics[1-12] (Cont.)

System	Specific event	Associated psychotropic
Respiratory	Nasal congestion	Clomethiazole
	Nasopharyngitis	Modafinil
	Rhinitis	Lamotrigine; modafinil
Skin and subcutaneous tissue	Decreased sweating	Chlorpromazine; fluphenazine; haloperidol; perphenazine; thioridazine; trifluoperazine
	Increased sweating	Atomoxetine; bupropion; clozapine; duloxetine; isocarboxazid; maprotiline; phenelzine; pipotiazine; reboxetine; rivastigmine; TCAs; venlafaxine; zotepine
	Pruritis	Acamprosate; maprotiline; nicotine; TCAs
	Rash	Bupropion; carbamazepine; lamotrigine; maprotiline; TCAs; trifluoperazine
	Urticaria	Carbamazepine
Vascular	Hypertension	Bupropion; haloperidol; modafinil; venlafaxine
	Hypotension	Chlorpromazine; clozapine; fluphenazine; haloperidol; loxapine; mirtazapine; molindone; perphenazine; pimozide; pipotiazine; promazine; reboxetine; thioridazine; trazodone; trifluoperazine; zotepine; zuclopenthixol
	Mild increase in blood pressure	Duloxetine
	Orthostatic hypotension	Aripiprazole; buprenorphine; isocarboxazid; lofexidine; olanzapine; pericyazine; phenelzine; prochlorperazine; promazine; quetiapine; sertindole; tranylcypromine
	Syncope	Chlorpromazine; fluphenazine; perphenazine; trazodone

References

1. ABPI. Medicines Compendium. Leatherhead: Datapharm Communications Ltd; 2008.
2. Balon R. Practical Management of the Side Effects of Psychotropic Drugs. New York: Marcel Dekker Ltd; 1999.
3. British Medical Association and Royal Pharmaceutical Society of Great Britain. British National Formulary. 57th edition. London: BMJ Group and RPS Publishing; 2009.
4. Buckley PF et al. Schizophrenia and Mood Disorders: The New Drug Therapies in Clinical Practice. London: Hodder Arnold; 2001.
5. Dubovsky SL. Clinical Guide to Psychotropic Medications. New York: WW Norton and Company; 2005.
6. Healy D. Psychiatric Drugs Explained. 3rd Edition. Oxford: Churchill Livingstone; 2002.
7. Kane JM et al. Adverse Effects of Psychotropics. New York: The Guilford Press; 1992.
8. Oyewumi LK et al. Managing Side Effects of Psychotropic Drugs: A Clinical Handbook for Healthcare Professionals. London (Ontario): ZZmazz Communications; 1998.
9. Pies RW et al. Handbook of Essential Psychopharmacology. 2nd Edition. Washington: American Psychiatric Press Inc; 2005.
10. Stahl SM. Essential Psychopharmacology: The Prescriber's Guide. 2nd edition. New York: Cambridge University Press; 2006.
11. Rosenbaum JF et al. Handbook of Psychiatric Drug Therapy. Fifth Edition. Philadelphia: Lippincott Williams and Wilkins; 2005.
12. Bazire S. Psychotropic Drug Directory 2009. Aberdeen: HealthComm UK Limited; 2009.

Special groups

Summary of commonly reported behavioural, cognitive, and psychiatric side effects of psychotropics

A number of psychotropics in current use have psychiatric, cognitive, and behavioural side effects that may limit their utility or may complicate diagnosis and management. While these effects are usually rare, they should be considered in patients with abnormal or complex presentations in which lack of clinical improvement is apparent, despite being on suitable treatment. It should be noted that ALL psychotropics may be associated with delirium, especially in susceptible populations (the elderly, polypharmacy, medical co-morbidity, individuals with co-morbid drug and alcohol use), on initial treatment and on increasing/high doses, especially when chronic. Many of the commonly prescribed psychotropics are also associated with sedation and fatigue.

The table below summarises the psychiatric, behavioural, and cognitive side effects of those psychotropics in current use, with data compiled from a variety of secondary sources. It should be noted that the reported frequencies of side effects vary widely and that there are currently no definitive data. Thus the information provided below is intended as a general guide only, and will be subject to change. When in doubt, additional sources of information should be consulted.

Table Commonly reported behavioural, cognitive, and psychiatric side effects of psychotropics[1–12]

Event	Associated psychotropic
Abnormal dreams	Donepezil; mirtazapine
Agitation	Amisulpride; atomoxetine; bupropion; flupentixol; moclobemide; pipotiazine; reboxetine; SSRIs; tranylcypromine; zotepine
Aggression	Atomoxetine
Anxiety	Amisulpride; atomoxetine; bupropion; maprotiline; moclobemide; modafinil; naltrexone; reboxetine; risperidone; TCAs; tranylcypromine; zotepine
Asthenia	Naloxone; naltrexone; venlafaxine
Depression	Benzodiazepines; donepezil; fluphenazine; galantamine; zotepine
Disorientation/ confusion	Benzodiazepines; carbamazepine; mirtazapine; pregabalin
Drowsiness/ fatigue	Atomoxetine; benzodiazepines; carbamazepine; donepezil; galantamine; isocarboxazid; lamotrigine; maprotiline; meprobamate; phenelzine; pregabalin; rivastigmine; TCAs; trazodone
Hallucinations	Buprenorphine
Impaired concentration	Pregabalin; sulpiride
Insomnia	Amisulpride; aripiprazole; atomoxetine; bupropion; dexamphetamine; donepezil; duloxetine; flupentixol; lamotrigine; methylphenidate; moclobemide; modafinil; pipotiazine; reboxetine; risperidone; SSRIs; tranylcypromine; venlafaxine; zotepine
Irritability	Atomoxetine; dexamphetamine; pregabalin

Table Commonly reported behavioural, cognitive, and psychiatric side effects of psychotropics[1-12] (Cont.)

Event	Associated psychotropic
Mania, euphoria, hypomania	Benzodiazepines; flupentixol; pregabalin
Memory impairment	Benzodiazepines; chlorpromazine; lithium; pregabalin; zaleplon; zolpidem; zopiclone
Nervousness	Benzodiazepines; buspirone; dexamphetamine; methylphenidate; modafinil; naloxone; naltrexone; TCAs; venlafaxine; zaleplon; zolpidem
Psychomotor restlessness	Buspirone; flupentixol; maprotiline; moclobemide; morphine; naloxone; pericyazine; pipotiazine; zaleplon; zolpidem
Sleep disorders (unspecified)	Isocarboxazid; naloxone; naltrexone; phenelzine; sulpiride
Sedation	Amisulpride; aripiprazole; atomoxetine; benperidol; benzodiazepines; buprenorphine; carbamazepine; chloral hydrate; chlorpromazine; clomethiazole; clozapine; duloxetine; flupentixol; fluphenazine; haloperidol; isocarboxazid; lamotrigine; levomepromazine; lofexidine; loxapine; maprotiline; meprobamate; mianserin; mirtazapine; morphine; olanzapine; paliperidone; pericyazine; perphenazine; phenelzine; pimozide; pregabalin; prochlorperazine; promazine; quetiapine; risperidone; SSRIs; sulpiride; thioridazine; tranylcypromine; trazodone; TCAs; triclofos; trifluoperazine; tryptophan; valproate; venlafaxine; zaleplon; zolpidem; zopiclone; zotepine; zuclopenthixol

References

1. ABPI. Medicines Compendium. Leatherhead: Datapharm Communications Ltd; 2008.
2. Balon R. Practical Management of the Side Effects of Psychotropic Drugs. New York: Marcel Dekker Ltd; 1999.
3. British Medical Association and Royal Pharmaceutical Society of Great Britain. British National Formulary. 57th edition. London: BMJ Group and RPS Publishing; 2009.
4. Brown TM et al. Psychiatric Side Effects of Prescription and Over-the-Counter Medications: Recognition and Management. Washington: American Psychiatric Press Inc; 1998.
5. Buckley PF et al. Schizophrenia and Mood Disorders: The New Drug Therapies in Clinical Practice. London: Hodder Arnold; 2001.
6. Dubovsky SL. Clinical Guide to Psychotropic Medications. New York: WW Norton and Company; 2005.
7. Healy D. Psychiatric Drugs Explained. 3rd Edition. Oxford: Churchill Livingstone; 2002.
8. Kane JM et al. Adverse Effects of Psychotropics. New York: The Guilford Press; 1992.
9. Oyewumi LK et al. Managing Side Effects of Psychotropic Drugs: A Clinical Handbook for Healthcare Professionals. London (Ontario): ZZmazz Communications; 1998.
10. Pies RW et al. Handbook of Essential Psychopharmacology. 2nd edition. Washington: American Psychiatric Press Inc; 2005.
11. Stahl SM. Essential Psychopharmacology: The Prescriber's Guide. 2nd edition. New York: Cambridge University Press; 2006.
12. Rosenbaum JF et al. Handbook of Psychiatric Drug Therapy. Fifth Edition. Philadelphia: Lippincott Williams and Wilkins; 2005.

chapter 8

Miscellaneous conditions and substances

Psychotropics in overdose

Suicide attempts and suicidal gestures are frequently encountered in psychiatric and general practice, and psychotropic drugs are often taken in overdose. This section gives brief details of the toxicity in overdose of commonly used psychotropics. It is intended to help guide drug choice in those thought to be at risk of suicide and to help identify symptoms of overdose. This section gives no information on the treatment of psychotropic overdose and readers are directed to specialist poisons units. In all cases of suspected overdose, urgent referral to acute medical facilities is, of course, strongly advised.

Table Psychotropics in overdose

Drug or drug group	Toxicity in overdose	Smallest dose likely to cause death	Signs and symptoms of overdose
Antidepressants			
Tricyclics[1–5] (not lofepramine)	High	Around 500 mg. Doses over 50 mg/kg usually fatal	Sedation, coma, tachycardia, arrhythmia (QRS, QT prolongation), hypotension, seizures
Lofepramine[4,6,7]	Low	Unclear. Fatality unlikely if lofepramine taken alone	Sedation, coma, tachycardia, hypotension
SSRIs[6–12]	Low	Unclear. Probably above 1–2 g. Fatality unlikely if SSRI taken alone	Vomiting, tremor, drowsiness, tachycardia, ST depression. Seizures and QT prolongation possible. Citalopram most toxic of SSRIs inoverdose (coma, seizures, arrhythmia)
Venlafaxine[13–16]	Moderate	Probably above 5 g, but seizures may occur after ingestion of 1 g	Vomiting, sedation, tachycardia, hypertension, seizures. Rarely QT prolongation, arrhythmia. Very rarely cardiac arrest
Duloxetine[17]	Unclear (probably low)	Unclear – no deaths from single overdose reported	Drowsiness, bradycardia, hypotension
Moclobemide[18,19]	Low	Unclear, but probably more than 8 g. Fatality unlikely if moclobemide taken alone	Vomiting, sedation, disorientation
Trazodone[20–24]	Low	Unclear but probably more than 10 g. Fatality unlikely in overdose of trazodone alone	Drowsiness, nausea, hypotension, dizziness. Rarely QT prolongation, arrhythmia
Reboxetine[13,25]	Low	Not known. Fatality unlikely in overdose of reboxetine alone	Sweating, tachycardia, changes in blood pressure
Mirtazapine[13,26–28]	Low	Unclear but probably more than 2.25 g. Fatality unlikely if mirtazapine taken alone	Sedation; even large overdose may be asymptomatic. Occasionally, tachycardia is seen
Bupropion[13,29–31]	Moderate	Around 4.5 g	Tachycardia, seizures, QRS prolongation, QT prolongation, arrhythmia

Table Psychotropics in overdose (Cont.)

Drug or drug group	Toxicity in overdose	Smallest dose likely to cause death	Signs and symptoms of overdose
Mianserin[32,33]	Low	Unclear but probably more than 1 g. Fatality unlikely if mianserin taken alone	Sedation, coma, hypertension, tachycardia, possible QT prolongation
MAOIs (not moclobemide)[1,2,4,34]	High	Phenelzine – 400 mg Tranylcypromine – 200 mg	Tremor, weakness, confusion, sweating, tachycardia, hypertension
Antipsychotics			
Phenothiazines[35–38]	High	Chlorpromazine 5–10 g	Sedation, coma, tachycardia, arrhythmia, pulmonary oedema, hypotension, QT prolongation, seizures, dystonia, NMS
Butyrophenones[37,39,40]	Moderate	Haloperidol – probably above 500 mg. Arrhythmia may occur at 300 mg	Sedation, coma, dystonia, NMS, QT prolongation, arrhythmia
Aripiprazole[41–44]	Unclear (probably low)	Unclear. Fatality unlikely when taken alone	Sedation, lethargy, GI disturbance, drooling
Amisulpride[45,45,46]	Moderate	Around 16 g	QT prolongation, arrhythmia
Clozapine[47,48]	Moderate	Around 2 g	Lethargy, coma, tachycardia, hypotension, hypersalivation, pneumonia, seizures
Olanzapine[47,49–51]	Moderate	Unclear. Probably more than 200 mg	Lethargy, confusion, myoclonus, myopathy, hypotension, tachycardia, delirium. Possibly QT prolongation
Risperidone[47]	Low	Unclear. Fatality rare in those taking risperidone alone	Lethargy, tachycardia, changes in blood pressure, QT prolongation
Quetiapine[47,52–57]	Low	Unclear. Probably more than 5 g. Fatalities rare	Lethargy, tachycardia, QT prolongation, respiratory distress, depression, hypotension, rhabdomyolysis, NMS
Ziprasidone[58–61]	Unclear (probably low)	Unclear. Fatality unlikely when taken alone	Drowsiness, lethargy. QT prolongation rarely reported
Mood-stabilisers			
Lithium[62–64]	Low (acute overdose)	Acute overdose does not normally result in fatality. Insidious, chronic toxicity is more dangerous	Nausea, diarrhoea, tremor, confusion, weakness, lethargy, seizures, coma, cardiovascular collapse, arrhythmia, heart block

Table Psychotropics in overdose (Cont.)

Drug or drug group	Toxicity in overdose	Smallest dose likely to cause death	Signs and symptoms of overdose
Carbamazepine[65,66]	Moderate	Around 20 g, but seizures may occur at around 5 g	Somnolence, coma, respiratory depression, ataxia, seizures, tachycardia, arrhythmia, electrolyte disturbance
Valproate[67–71]	Moderate	Unclear but probably more than 20 g. Doses over 400 mg/kg cause severe toxicity	Somnolence, coma, cerebral oedema, respiratory depression, blood dyscrasia, hypotension, hypothermia, seizures, electrolyte disturbance (hyper ammonaemia)
Lamotrigine[72–74]	Low	Unclear. No deaths from overdose reported	Drowsiness, vomiting, ataxia, tachycardia, dyskinesia
Others			
Benzodiazepines[75,76]	Low	Probably more than 100 mg diazepam equivalents. Fatality unusual if taken alone. Alprazolam is most toxic	Drowsiness, ataxia, nystagmus, respiratory dysarthria, depression, coma
Zopiclone[75,77,78]	Low	Unclear. Probably above 100 mg. Fatality rare in those taking zopiclone alone	Ataxia, nausea, diplopia, drowsiness, coma
Zolpidem[79,80]	Low	Unclear. Probably above 200 mg. Fatality rare in those taking zolpidem alone	Drowsiness, agitation, respiratory depression, tachycardia, coma
Methadone[81,82]	High	20–50 mg may be fatal in non-users. Co-ingestion of benzodiazepines increases toxicity	Drowsiness, nausea, hypotension, respiratory depression, coma, rhabdomyolysis
Modafinil[83]	Low	Unclear. Overdoses of >6 g have not caused death	Tachycardia, insomnia, agitation, anxiety, nausea

High = Less than 1 week's supply likely to cause serious toxicity or death
Moderate = 1–4 weeks' supply likely to cause serious toxicity or death
Low = Death or serious toxicity unlikely even if more than 1 month's supply taken

Miscellaneous

References

1. Crome P. Antidepressant overdosage. Drugs 1982; 23:431–461.
2. Henry JA. Epidemiology and relative toxicity of antidepressant drugs in overdose. Drug Saf 1997; 16:374–390.
3. Power BM, Hackett LP, Dusci LJ, Ilett KF. Antidepressant toxicity and the need for identification and concentration monitoring in overdose. Clin Pharmacokinet 1995; 29:154–171.
4. Cassidy S, Henry J. Fatal toxicity of antidepressant drugs in overdose. Br Med J 1987; 295:1021–1024.
5. Caksen H, Akbayram S, Odabas D, et al. Acute amitriptyline intoxication: an analysis of 44 children. Hum Exp Toxicol 2006; 25:107–110.
6. Henry JA, Alexander CA, Sener EK. Relative mortality from overdose of antidepressants. BMJ 1995; 310:221–224.
7. Cheeta S, Schifano F, Oyefeso A, Webb L, Ghodse AH. Antidepressant-related deaths and antidepressant prescriptions in England and Wales, 1998–2000. Br J Psychiatry 2004; 184:41–47.
8. Barbey JT, Roose SP. SSRI safety in overdose. J Clin Psychiatry 1998; 59 Suppl 15:42–48.
9. Luchini D, Morabito G, Centini F. Case report of a fatal intoxication by citalopram. Am J Forensic Med Pathol 2005; 26:352–354.
10. Jimmink A, Caminada K, Hunfeld NG, Touw DJ. Clinical toxicology of citalopram after acute intoxication with the sole drug or in combination with other drugs: overview of 26 cases. Ther Drug Monit 2008; 30:365–371.
11. Isbister GK, Friberg LE, Stokes B, Buckley NA, Lee C, Gunja N et al. Activated charcoal decreases the risk of QT prolongation after citalopram overdose. Ann Emerg Med 2007; 50:593–600.
12. Tarabar AF, Hoffman RS, Nelson L. Citalopram overdose: late presentation of torsades de pointes (TdP) with cardiac arrest. J Med Toxicol 2008; 4:101–105.
13. Buckley NA, Faunce TA. 'Atypical' antidepressants in overdose: clinical considerations with respect to safety. Drug Saf 2003; 26:539–551.
14. Whyte IM, Dawson AH, Buckley NA. Relative toxicity of venlafaxine and selective serotonin reuptake inhibitors in overdose compared to tricyclic antidepressants. QJM 2003; 96:369–374.
15. Howell C, Wilson AD, Waring WS. Cardiovascular toxicity due to venlafaxine poisoning in adults: a review of 235 consecutive cases. Br J Clin Pharmacol 2007; 64:192–197.
16. Hojer J, Hulting J, Salmonson H. Fatal cardiotoxicity induced by venlafaxine overdosage. Clin Toxicol (Phila) 2008; 46:336–337.
17. Menchetti M, Ferrari GB, Addolorata SM, Mercolini L, Petio C, Augusta RM. Non-fatal overdose of duloxetine in combination with other antidepressants and benzodiazepines. World J Biol Psychiatry 2008;1–5.
18. Hetzel W. Safety of moclobemide taken in overdose for attempted suicide. Psychopharmacology 1992; 106 Suppl:S127–S129.
19. Myrenfors PG, Eriksson T, Sandsted CS, Sjoberg G. Moclobemide overdose. J Intern Med 1993; 233:113–115.
20. Gamble DE, Peterson LG. Trazodone overdose: four years of experience from voluntary reports. J Clin Psychiatry 1986; 47:544–546.
21. Martinez MA, Ballesteros S, Sanchez dIT, Almarza E. Investigation of a fatality due to trazodone poisoning: case report and literature review. J Anal Toxicol 2005; 29:262–268.
22. Dattilo PB, Nordin C. Prolonged QT associated with an overdose of trazodone. J Clin Psychiatry 2007; 68:1309–1310.
23. Service JA, Waring WS. QT Prolongation and delayed atrioventricular conduction caused by acute ingestion of trazodone. Clin Toxicol (Phila) 2008; 46:71–73.
24. Wittebole X, Hantson P, Wallemacq P. Prolonged hypotension due to deliberate trazodone overdose in the presence of fluoxetine. Ann Clin Psychiatry 2007; 19:201–202.
25. Baldwin DS, Buis C, Carabel E. Tolerability and safety of reboxetine. Rev Contemp Pharmacother 2000; 11:321–330.
26. Montgomery SA. Safety of mirtazapine: a review. Int Clin Psychopharmacol 1995; 10 Suppl 4:37–45.
27. Bremner JD, Wingard P, Walshe TA. Safety of mirtazapine in overdose. J Clin Psychiatry 1998; 59:233–235.
28. LoVecchio F, Riley B, Pizon A, Brown M. Outcomes after isolated mirtazapine (Remeron) supratherapeutic ingestions. J Emerg Med 2008; 34:77–78.
29. Paris PA, Saucier JR. ECG conduction delays associated with massive bupropion overdose. J Toxicol Clin Toxicol 1998; 36:595–598.
30. Curry SC, Kashani JS, LoVecchio F, Holubek W. Intraventricular conduction delay after bupropion overdose. J Emerg Med 2005; 29:299–305.
31. Mercerolle M, Denooz R, Lachatre G, Charlier C. A fatal case of bupropion (Zyban) overdose. J Anal Toxicol 2008; 32:192–196.
32. Chand S, Crome P, Dawling S. One hundred cases of acute intoxication with mianserin hydrochloride. Pharmacopsychiatry 1981; 14:15–17.
33. Scherer D, von LK, Zitron E, et al. Inhibition of cardiac hERG potassium channels by tetracyclic antidepressant mianserin. Naunyn Schmiedebergs Arch Pharmacol 2008; 378:73–83.
34. Waring WS, Wallace WA. Acute myocarditis after massive phenelzine overdose. Eur J Clin Pharmacol 2007; 63:1007–1009.
35. Anon. Phenothiazines. POISINDEX® System [database on CD-ROM].Version 7.1. Greenwood Village, Colo: Thomson Micromedex; 2004.
36. Buckley NA, Whyte IM, Dawson AH. Cardiotoxicity more common in thioridazine overdose than with other neuroleptics. J Toxicol Clin Toxicol 1995; 33:199–204.
37. Haddad PM, Anderson IM. Antipsychotic-related QTc prolongation, torsade de pointes and sudden death. Drugs 2002; 62:1649–1671.
38. Li C, Gefter WB. Acute pulmonary edema induced by overdosage of phenothiazines. Chest 1992; 101:102–104.
39. Levine BS, Wu SC, Goldberger BA, Caplan YH. Two fatalities involving haloperidol. J Anal Toxicol 1991; 15:282–284.
40. Henderson RA, Lane S, Henry JA. Life-threatening ventricular arrhythmia (torsades de pointes) after haloperidol overdose. Hum Exp Toxicol 1991; 10:59–62.
41. Lofton AL, Klein-Schwartz W. Atypical experience: a case series of pediatric aripiprazole exposures. Clin Toxicol (Phila) 2005; 43:151–153.
42. Seifert SA, Schwartz MD, Thomas JD. Aripiprazole (abilify) overdose in a child. Clin Toxicol (Phila) 2005; 43:193–195.
43. Carstairs SD, Williams SR. Overdose of aripiprazole, a new type of antipsychotic. J Emerg Med 2005; 28:311–313.
44. Forrester MB. Aripiprazole exposures reported to Texas poison control centers during 2002–2004. J Toxicol Environ Health A 2006; 69:1719–1726.
45. Isbister GK, Murray L, John S, Hackett LP, Haider T, O'Mullane P et al. Amisulpride deliberate self-poisoning causing severe cardiac toxicity including QT prolongation and torsades de pointes. Med J Aust 2006; 184:354–356.
46. Ward DI. Two cases of amisulpride overdose: A cause for prolonged QT syndrome. Emerg Med Australas 2005; 17:274–276.
47. Trenton A, Currier G, Zwemer F. Fatalities associated with therapeutic use and overdose of atypical antipsychotics. CNS Drugs 2003; 17:307–324.
48. Flanagan RJ, Spencer EP, Morgan PE, Barnes TR, Dunk L. Suspected clozapine poisoning in the UK/Eire, 1992–2003. Forensic Sci Int 2005; 155:91–99.
49. Chue P, Singer P. A review of olanzapine-associated toxicity and fatality in overdose. J Psychiatry Neurosci 2003; 28:253–261.
50. Waring WS, Wrate J, Bateman DN. Olanzapine overdose is associated with acute muscle toxicity. Hum Exp Toxicol 2006; 25:735–740.
51. Morissette P, Hreiche R, Mallet L, Vo D, Knaus EE, Turgeon J. Olanzapine prolongs cardiac repolarization by blocking the rapid component of the delayed rectifier potassium current. J Psychopharmacol 2007; 21:735–741.
52. Smith RP, Puckett BN, Crawford J, Elliott RL. Quetiapine overdose and severe rhabdomyolysis. J Clin Psychopharmacol 2004; 24:343.
53. Langman LJ, Kaliciak HA, Carlyle S. Fatal overdoses associated with quetiapine. J Anal Toxicol 2004; 28:520–525.
54. Hunfeld NG, Westerman EM, Boswijk DJ, et al. Quetiapine in overdosage: a clinical and pharmacokinetic analysis of 14 cases. Ther Drug Monit 2006; 28:185–189.
55. Strachan PM, Benoff BA. Mental status change, myoclonus, electrocardiographic changes, and acute respiratory distress syndrome induced by quetiapine overdose. Pharmacotherapy 2006; 26:578–582.
56. Ngo A et al. Acute quetiapine overdose in adults: a 5-year retrospective case series. Ann Emerg Med 2008; 52:541–547.
57. Khan KH, Tham TC. Neuroleptic malignant syndrome induced by quetiapine overdose. Br J Hosp Med 2008; 69:171.
58. Gomez-Criado MS, Bernardo M, Florez T, Gutierrez JR, Gandia R, Ayani I. Ziprasidone overdose: cases recorded in the database of Pfizer-Spain and literature review. Pharmacotherapy 2005; 25:1660–1665.

59. Arbuck DM. 12,800-mg ziprasidone overdose without significant ECG changes. Gen Hosp Psychiatry 2005; 27:222–223.
60. Insa Gomez FJ, Gutierrez C, Jr. Ziprasidone overdose: cardiac safety. Actas Esp Psiquiatr 2005; 33:398–400.
61. Klein-Schwartz W, Lofton AL, Benson BE, Spiller HA, Crouch BI. Prospective observational multi-poison center study of ziprasidone exposures. Clin Toxicol (Phila) 2007; 45:782–786.
62. Tuohy K, Shemin D. Acute lithium intoxication. Dial Transplant 2003; 32:478–481.
63. Chen KP, Shen WW, Lu ML. Implication of serum concentration monitoring in patients with lithium intoxication. Psychiatry Clin Neurosci 2004; 58:25–29.
64. Serinken M, Karcioglu O, Korkmaz A. Rarely seen cardiotoxicity of lithium overdose: complete heart block. Int J Cardiol 2007.
65. Spiller HA. Management of carbamazepine overdose. Pediatr Emerg Care 2001; 17:452–456.
66. Schmidt S, Schmitz-Buhl M. Signs and symptoms of carbamazepine overdose. J Neurol 1995; 242:169–173.
67. Isbister GK, Balit CR, Whyte IM, Dawson A. Valproate overdose: a comparative cohort study of self poisonings. Br J Clin Pharmacol 2003; 55:398–404.
68. Spiller HA, Krenzelok EP, Klein-Schwartz W, et al. Multicenter case series of valproic acid ingestion: serum concentrations and toxicity. J Toxicol Clin Toxicol 2000; 38:755–760.
69. Sztajnkrycer MD. Valproic acid toxicity: overview and management. J Toxicol Clin Toxicol 2002; 40:789–801.
70. Eyer F, Felgenhauer N, Gempel K, Steimer W, Gerbitz KD, Zilker T. Acute valproate poisoning: pharmacokinetics, alteration in fatty acid metabolism, and changes during therapy. J Clin Psychopharmacol 2005; 25:376–380.
71. Robinson P, Abbott C. Severe hypothermia in association with sodium valproate overdose. N Z Med J 2005; 118:U1681.
72. Miller MA, Levsky ME. Choreiform dyskinesia following isolated lamotrigine overdose. J Child Neurol 2008; 23:243.
73. Reimers A, Reinholt G. Acute lamotrigine overdose in an adolescent. Ther Drug Monit 2007; 29:669–670.
74. Lofton AL, Klein-Schwartz W. Evaluation of lamotrigine toxicity reported to poison centers. Annal Pharmacotherapy 2004; 38:1811–1815.
75. Reith DM, Fountain J, McDowell R, Tilyard M. Comparison of the fatal toxicity index of zopiclone with benzodiazepines. J Toxicol Clin Toxicol 2003; 41:975–980.
76. Isbister GK, O'Regan L, Sibbritt D, Whyte IM. Alprazolam is relatively more toxic than other benzodiazepines in overdose. Br J Clin Pharmacol 2004; 58:88–95.
77. Pounder D, Davies J. Zopiclone poisoning. J Anal Toxicol 1996; 20:273–274.
78. Bramness JG, Arnestad M, Karinen R, Hilberg T. Fatal overdose of zopiclone in an elderly woman with bronchogenic carcinoma. J Forensic Sci 2001; 46:1247–1249.
79. Gock SB, Wong SH, Nuwayhid N et al. Acute zolpidem overdose –report of two cases. J Anal Toxicol 1999; 23:559–562.
80. Garnier R, Guerault E, Muzard D, Azoyan P, Chaumet-Riffaud AE, Efthymiou ML. Acute zolpidem poisoning--analysis of 344 cases. J Toxicol Clin Toxicol 1994; 32:391–404.
81. Gable RS. Comparison of acute lethal toxicity of commonly abused psychoactive substances. Addiction 2004; 99:686–696.
82. Caplehorn JR, Drummer OH. Fatal methadone toxicity: signs and circumstances, and the role of benzodiazepines. Aust N Z J Public Health 2002; 26:358–362.
83. Spiller HA et al. Toxicity from modafinil ingestion. Clin Toxicol (Phila) 2009; 47:153–156.

Further reading

Flanagan RJ. Fatal toxicity of drugs used in psychiatry. Hum Psychopharmacol 2008; 23:43–51.

Miscellaneous

Biochemical and haematological effects of psychotropics

Almost all psychotropics currently used in clinical practice have haematology or biochemistry-related adverse effects that may be detected using routine blood tests. While many of these changes are idiosyncratic and not clinically significant, others, such as the agranulocytosis associated with agents such as clozapine, will require regular monitoring of the full blood count. In general, where an agent has a high incidence of biochemical/haematological side effects or a rare but potentially fatal effect, regular monitoring is required as discussed in other sections.

For other agents, laboratory-related side effects are comparatively rare (prevalence usually less than 1%), are often reversible upon cessation of the putative offending agent and not always clinically significant although expert advice should be sought. It should further be noted that medical co-morbidity, polypharmacy and the effects of non-prescribed agents including substances of abuse and alcohol may also influence biochemical and haematological parameters. In some cases, where a clear temporal association between starting the agent and the onset of laboratory changes is unclear, then re-challenge with the agent in question may be considered. Where there is doubt as to the aetiology and significance of the effect, the appropriate source of expert advice should always be consulted.

The following tables summarise those agents with identified biochemical and haematological effects, with information compiled from various sources[1-11]. In many cases the evidence for these various effects is limited, with information obtained mostly from case reports, case series and information supplied by manufacturers. For further details about each individual agent, the reader is encouraged to consult the appropriate section of the Guidelines as well as other, expert sources, particularly product literature relating to individual drugs.

Miscellaneous

Table Summary of biochemical changes associated with psychotropics

Parameter	Reference range	Agents reported to raise levels	Agents reported to lower levels
Alanine transferase	0–45 IU/L (may be higher in males and obese subjects)	**Antipsychotics:** Benperidol, chlorpromazine, clozapine, haloperidol, olanzapine, quetiapine, zotepine **Antidepressants:** Duloxetine, mianserin, mirtazapine, moclobemide, monoamine oxidase inhibitors, SSRIs (especially paroxetine and sertraline); TCAs, trazodone, venlafaxine **Anxiolytics/hypnotics:** Barbiturates, benzodiazepines, chloral hydrate, chlormethiazole, promethazine **Miscellaneous agents:** Caffeine, dexamfetamine, disulfiram, opioids **Mood-stabilisers:** Carbamazepine, lamotrigine, valproate	Vigabatrin
Albumin	3.5–4.8 g/dL (gradually decreases after age 40)		Chronic use of amfetamine or cocaine. Microalbuminuria may be a feature of metabolic syndrome secondary to psychotropic use (especially phenothiazines, clozapine, olanzapine and possibly quetiapine) Plasma albumin may fall
Alkaline phosphatase	50–120 IU/L	Caffeine (excess/chronic use), carbamazepine, clozapine, disulfiram, duloxetine, galantamine, haloperidol, memantine, modafinil, nortriptyline, olanzapine, phenytoin, sertraline; also – associated agents that induce neuroleptic malignant syndrome	None known
Amylase	<300 IU/L	Clozapine, donepezil, methadone, olanzapine, opiates, pregabalin, rivastigmine, SSRIs (rarely), valproate	None known
Aspartate aminotransferase	10–50 IU/L (values slightly higher in males)	As for alanine transferase	Trifluoperazine

Table Summary of biochemical changes associated with psychotropics (Cont.)

Parameter	Reference range	Agents reported to raise levels	Agents reported to lower levels
Bicarbonate	22–30 mmol/l	None known	Agents associated with SIADH: all antidepressants, antipsychotics (clozapine, haloperidol, olanzapine, phenothiazines, pimozide, risperidone, quetiapine); carbamazepine
Bilirubin	3–20 μmol/l (total bilirubin)	Amitriptyline, benzodiazepines, carbamazepine, chlordiazepoxide, chlorpromazine, clomethiazole, disulfiram, imipramine, fluphenazine, meprobamate, phenothiazines, phenytoin, promethazine, trifluoperazine, valproate	None known
C-reactive protein	<10 μg/ml	Buprenorphine (rare)	None known
Calcium (corrected)	2.2–2.6 mmol/L	Lithium (rare)	Barbiturates Haloperidol
Carbohydrate-deficient transferrin	1.9–3.4 g/L	None known	None known
Chloride	98–107 mmol/L	None known	Medications associated with SIADH: all antidepressants, antipsychotics (clozapine, haloperidol, olanzapine, phenothiazines, pimozide, risperidone, quetiapine); carbamazepine
Cholesterol (total)	<5.2 mmol/L	Antipsychotic treatment, especially those implicated in the metabolic syndrome (phenothiazines, clozapine, olanzapine and possibly quetiapine). Rarely: aripiprazole, beta-blockers, disulfiram, memantine, mirtazapine, modafinil, phenytoin, rivastigmine, venlafaxine, zotepine	Ziprasidone

Table Summary of biochemical changes associated with psychotropics (Cont.)

Parameter	Reference range	Agents reported to raise levels	Agents reported to lower levels
Creatine kinase	<90 iu/L	Clozapine (when associated with seizures), donepezil, olanzapine; may also be also associated with agents causing neuroleptic malignant syndrome and SIADH; cocaine, dexamphetamine	None known
Creatinine	60–110 µmol/L	Clozapine, lithium, thioridazine, valproate, zotepine; medications associated with rhabdomyolysis (benzodiazepines, dexamphetamine, pregabalin, thioridazine); may also be also associated with agents causing neuroleptic malignant syndrome and SIADH	None known
Ferritin	Males: 40–340 µg/L; Females: 14–150 µg/L	None known	None known
Gamma-glutamyl transferase	<60 IU/L (higher levels may be found in males)	**Antidepressants:** mirtazapine, SSRIs (paroxetine and sertraline implicated); TCAs, trazodone, venlafaxine **Anticonvulsants/ mood-stabilisers:** carbamazepine, lamotrigine, phenytoin, phenobarbitone, valproate **Antipsychotics:** benperidol, chlorpromazine, clozapine, fluphenazine, haloperidol, olanzapine, quetiapine, zotepine **Miscellaneous:** barbiturates, clomethiazole, dexamphetamine, modafinil	None known
Glucose	Fasting: 2.8–6.0 mmol/L; Random <11.1 mmol/L	**Antidepressants:** MAOI, SSRI*, TCAs*; **Antipsychotics:** chlorpromazine, clozapine, olanzapine*, quetiapine, zotepine **Substances of abuse:** methadone, opioids **Other:** Beta-blockers*, bupropion, donepezil, galantamine, lithium *may also be associated with hypoglycaemia	Rarely with duloxetine, haloperidol, pregabalin, TCAs, zotepine. Medications associated with metabolic syndrome may result in raised or decreased glucose levels

Table Summary of biochemical changes associated with psychotropics (Cont.)

Parameter	Reference range	Agents reported to raise levels	Agents reported to lower levels
Glycated haemoglobin	3.5–5.5% (4–6% in diabetics)	All antipsychotics associated with hyperglycaemia (excluding amisulpride, and ziprasidone); galantamine, methadone, morphine, TCA	Lithium, MAOIs, SSRIs
Lactate dehydrogenase	90–200 U/L (levels rise gradually with age)	TCAs (especially imipramine), valproate; methadone, agents associated with neuroleptic malignant syndrome	None known
Lipoproteins: HDL	>1.2 mmol/L	Carbamazepine, phenobarbitone, phenytoin	Olanzapine, phenothiazines, valproate
Lipoproteins: LDL	<3.5 mmol/L	Beta-blockers, caffeine (controversial), chlorpromazine, clozapine, memantine, mirtazapine, modafinil, olanzapine, phenothiazines, quetiapine, risperidone, rivastigmine, venlafaxine, zotepine	None known
Phosphate	0.8–1.4 mmol/L	Acamprosate, carbamazepine, dexamphetamine; agents associated with neuroleptic malignant syndrome	None known
Potassium	3.5–5.0 mmol/L	Pregabalin	Haloperidol, lithium, mianserin, reboxetine, rivastigmine; alcohol, caffeine, cocaine
Prolactin	Normal <350 mU/L; Abnormal >600 mU/L;	Antidepressants (especially MAOIs and TCAs, venlafaxine also implicated); Antipsychotics e.g. amisulpride, haloperidol, pimozide, risperidone, sulpiride, zotepine (aripiprazole, clozapine, olanzapine, quetiapine and ziprasidone have minimal effects on prolactin levels)	None known
Protein (total)	60–80 g/L	None known	None known

Table	Summary of biochemical changes associated with psychotropics (Cont.)		
Parameter	Reference range	Agents reported to raise levels	Agents reported to lower levels
Sodium	135–145 mmol/L	None known	Benzodiazepines, carbamazepine, chlorpromazine, donepezil, duloxetine, haloperidol, lithium, memantine, mianserin, phenothiazines, reboxetine, rivastigmine, SSRIs (especially fluoxetine), tricyclic antidepressants (especially amitriptyline) **Note: The UK CSM advises that hyponatraemia should be considered in any patient on an antidepressant who develops confusion, convulsions or drowsiness.**
Thyroid-stimulating hormone	0.3–4.0 mU/L	Aripiprazole, carbamazepine, lithium, rivastigmine	Moclobemide
Thyroxine	Free: 9–26 pmol/L; total: 60–150 nmol/L	Dexamphetamine, moclobemide (rare)	Lithium (causes decreased T4 secretion); heroin, methadone (increase serum thyroxine-binding globulin); carbamazepine, phenytoin treatment. Rarely implicated: Aripiprazole, quetiapine and rivastigmine
Triglycerides	0.4–1.8 mmol/L	Beta-blockers, chlorpromazine, clozapine, memantine, mirtazapine, modafinil, olanzapine, quetiapine, phenothiazines, rivastigmine, valproate, venlafaxine, zotepine	Ziprasidone (controversial)
Tri-iodothyronine	Free 3.0–8.8 pmol/L; total 1.2–2.9 nmol/L	Heroin, methadone; moclobemide	Free T3: Valproate; total T3: carbamazepine, lithium
Urate (uric acid)	0.1–0.4 mmol/L	Rarely: zotepine, rivastigmine	None known
Urea	1.8–7.1 mmol/L (levels increase slightly after age 40)	Rarely with agents associated with anticonvulsant hypersensitivity syndrome and rhabdomyolysis	None known

Table Summary of haematological changes associated with psychotropics

Parameter	Reference range	Agents reported to raise levels	Agents reported to lower levels
Activated partial thromboplastin time	25–39 seconds	Bupropion*, phenothiazines (especially chlorpromazine) *may raise or lower levels	Modafinil (rare)
Basophils	0.0–0.10 x 10^9/L	TCAs (especially desipramine)	None known
Eosinophils	0.04–0.45 x 10^9/L	Amitriptyline, beta-blockers, carbamazepine, chloral hydrate, chlorpromazine, clonazepam, clozapine, donepezil, fluphenazine, haloperidol, imipramine, meprobamate, modafinil, nortriptyline, olanzapine, promethazine, quetiapine, SSRIs, tryptophan, valproate, zotepine	None known
Erythrocytes	Males: 4.5– 6.0 x 10^{12}/L; Females: 3.8–5.2 x 10^{12}/L	None known	Carbamazepine, chlordiazepoxide, chlorpromazine, donepezil, meprobamate, phenytoin, trifluoperazine
Erythrocyte sedimentation rate	<20 mm/hour; (Note: levels increase with age and are slightly higher in females)	Buprenorphine, clozapine, dexamphetamine, levomepromazine, maprotiline, SSRIs, zotepine	None known
Haemoglobin	Male 14–18 g/dL; Female 12–16 g/dL	None known	Aripiprazole, barbiturates, bupropion, carbamazepine, chlordiazepoxide, chlorpromazine, donepezil, duloxetine, galantamine, MAOIs, memantine, meprobamate, mianserin, phenytoin, promethazine, rivastigmine, trifluoperazine, zotepine
Lymphocytes	1.0–4.8 x 10^9/L	Opioids, valproate	Chloral hydrate, lithium

Parameter	Normal range		
Mean cell haemoglobin	27–37 pg. Note: Levels are slightly higher in males and may be raised in the elderly	Medications associated with megaloblastic anaemia, e.g. all anticonvulsants	None known
Mean cell haemoglobin concentration	300–350 g/L		
Mean cell volume	80–100 fL		
Monocytes	0.21–0.92 x 10^9/L	Haloperidol	None known
Neutrophils	2–9 x 10^9/L (may be lower in people of African descent due to benign ethnic neutropenia)	Bupropion, carbamazepine*, citalopram, chlorpromazine, clozapine*, duloxetine, fluphenazine, haloperidol, lithium, olanzapine, quetiapine, risperidone, rivastigmine, trazodone, venlafaxine, zotepine *rare, usually associated with leucopoenia	**Agents associated with agranulocytosis:** amitriptyline, amoxapine, aripiprazole, barbiturates, carbamazepine, chlordiazepoxide, chlorpromazine, clomipramine, clozapine†, diazepam, fluphenazine, haloperidol, imipramine, meprobamate, mianserin, mirtazapine, nortriptyline, olanzapine, promethazine, tranylcypromine, valproate †Note that in rare cases clozapine has been associated with a 'morning pseudo–neutropenia' with lower levels of circulating neutrophil levels. As neutrophil counts may show circadian rhythms, repeating the FBC at a later time of day may be instructive **Agents associated with leucopoenia:** amitriptyline, amoxapine, bupropion, carbamazepine, chlorpromazine, citalopram, clomipramine, clonazepam, clozapine, duloxetine, fluphenazine, galantamine, haloperidol, lamotrigine, lorazepam, MAOIs, memantine, meprobamate, mianserin, mirtazapine, modafinil, nefazodone, olanzapine, oxazepam, pregabalin, promethazine, quetiapine, risperidone, tranylcypromine, valproate, venlafaxine, zotepine **Agents associated with neutropenia:** trazodone, valproate

Table Summary of haematological changes associated with psychotropics (Cont.)

Parameter	Reference range	Agents reported to raise levels	Agents reported to lower levels
Packed cell volume	Adult males: 42–52%; Adult females: 35–47% (levels slightly lower in pregnant versus non-pregnant women)	None known	None known
Platelets	150–400 x10⁹/L	Lithium	Amitriptyline, barbiturates, bupropion, carbamazepine, clomipramine, chlordiazepoxide, chlorpromazine, clonazepam, clozapine, diazepam, donepezil, duloxetine, fluphenazine, imipramine, lamotrigine, MAOIs, meprobamate, mirtazapine, olanzapine, promethazine, risperidone, rivastigmine, sertraline, tranylcypromine, trazodone, trifluoperazine, valproate, zotepine, cocaine, methadone **Agents associated with impaired platelet aggregation:** chlordiazepoxide, citalopram, diazepam, fluoxetine, fluvoxamine, paroxetine, sertraline
Prothrombin time/inter-national normalised ratio	10–13 seconds	Fluoxetine, fluvoxamine, disulfiram, bupropion	Barbiturates, carbamazepine, phenytoin
Red cell distribution width	11.5–14.5%	Agents associated with anaemia e.g.: Carbamazepine, chlordiazepoxide, citalopram, clonazepam, diazepam, lamotrigine, mirtazapine, nefazodone, sertraline, tranylcypromine, trazodone, valproate, venlafaxine	None known
Reticulocyte count	0.5–1.5%	None known	Carbamazepine, chlordiazepoxide, chlorpromazine, meprobamate, phenytoin, trifluoperazine

References

1. Balon R et al. Hematologic side effects of psychotropic drugs. Psychosomatics 1986; 27:119–117.
2. Bazire S. Psychotropic Drug Directory: the Professional's Pocket Handbook and Aide Memoire. Malta: Gutenberg Press; 2009.
3. British Medical Association and Royal Pharmaceutical Society of Great Britain. *British National Formulary*. 57th edition. London: BMJ Group and RPS Publishing; 2009.
4. Aronson JK. Meyler's Side Effects of Drugs: The International Encyclopedia of Adverse Drug Reactions and Interactions. 15th Edition. Amsterdam: Elsevier Science; 2006.
5. Foster R. Clinical Laboratory Investigation and Psychiatry. *A Practical Handbook*. New York: Informa; 2008.
6. Jacobs DS, De Mott WR, oxley DK. Laboratory Test Handbook. 5th Edition. Hudson, Cleveland: Lexi-Comp Inc; 2001.
7. Livingstone C et al. The role of clinical biochemistry in psychiatry. Clin Biochem 2004; 6:59–65.
8. Oyesanmi O et al. Hematologic side effects of psychotropics. Psychosomatics 1999; 40:414–421.
9. Stubner S et al. Blood dyscrasias induced by psychotropic drugs. Pharmacopsychiatry 2004; 37 Suppl 1:S70–S78.
10. Sweetman SC. *Martindale: The Complete Drug Reference 35*. [Online]. London: Pharmaceutical Press; 2008. http://www.medicinescomplete.com.
11. Wu AHB. *Tietz Clinical Guide to Laboratory Tests. 4th Edition*. Philadelphia, Pennsylvania: WB Saunders and Company; 2006.

Miscellaneous

Prescribing drugs outside their licensed indications

A Product Licence is granted when regulatory authorities are satisfied that the drug in question has proven efficacy in the treatment of a specified disorder, along with an acceptable side-effect profile, relative to the severity of the disorder being treated and other available treatments.

The decision of a manufacturer to seek a Product Licence for a given indication is essentially a commercial one; potential sales are balanced against the cost of conducting the necessary clinical trials. It therefore follows that drugs may be effective outside their licensed indications for different disease states, age ranges, doses, and durations. The absence of a formal Product Licence or labelling may simply reflect the absence of controlled trials supporting the drug's efficacy in these areas. Importantly, however, it is possible that trials have been conducted but given negative results.

The application of common sense is important here. Prescribing a drug within its licence does not guarantee that the patient will come to no harm. Likewise, prescribing outside a licence does not mean that the risk–benefit ratio is automatically adverse. Prescribing outside a licence, usually called 'off-label', does confer extra responsibilities on prescribers, who will be expected to be able to show that they acted in accordance with a respected body of medical opinion (the Bolam test)[1] and that their action was capable of withstanding logical analysis (the Bolitho test)[2].

The psychopharmacology special interest group at the Royal College of Psychiatrists has published a consensus statement on the use of licensed medicines for unlicensed uses[3]. They note that unlicensed use is common in general adult psychiatry with cross-sectional studies showing that up to 50% of patients are prescribed at least one drug outside the terms of its licence. They also note that the prevalence of this type of prescribing is likely to be higher in patients under the age of 18 or over 65, in those with a learning disability, in women who are pregnant or lactating and in those patients who are cared for in forensic psychiatry settings. The main recommendations in the consensus statement are summarised below.

Before prescribing 'off-label':

1. Exclude licensed alternatives (e.g. they have proved ineffective or poorly tolerated).
2. Ensure familiarity with the evidence base for the intended unlicensed use. If unsure, seek advice.
3. Consider and document the potential risks and benefits of the proposed treatment. Share this risk assessment with the patient, and carers if applicable. Document the discussion and the patient's consent or lack of capacity to consent.
4. If prescribing responsibility is to be shared with primary care, ensure that the risk assessment and consent issues are shared with the GP.
5. Monitor for efficacy and side-effects.
6. Consider publishing the case to add to the body of knowledge.

The more experimental the unlicensed use is, the more important it is to adhere to the above guidance.

Examples of acceptable use of drugs outside their Product Licences

The table below gives examples of common unlicensed uses of drugs in psychiatric practice. These examples would all fulfil the Bolam and Bolitho criteria in principle. An exhaustive list of unlicensed uses is impossible to prepare as:

- The evidence base is constantly changing.

- The expertise and experience of prescribers varies. A strategy may be justified in the hands of a specialist in psychopharmacology based in a tertiary referral centre but be much more difficult to justify if initiated by someone with a special interest in psychotherapy who rarely prescribes.

Note that some drugs do not have a UK licence for any indication. Two commonly prescribed examples in psychiatric practice are immediate-release formulations of melatonin (used to treat insomnia in children and adolescents) and pirenzepine (used to treat clozapine-induced hypersalivation). Awareness of the evidence base and documentation of potential benefits, side effects and patient consent are especially important here.

Drug/drug group	Unlicensed use(s)	Further information
Second-generation antipsychotics	Psychotic illness other than schizophrenia	Licensed indications vary markedly, and in most cases are unlikely to reflect real differences in efficacy between drugs
Cyproheptadine	Akathisia	Some evidence to support efficacy in this distressing and difficult to treat side-effect of antipsychotics
Fluoxetine	Maintenance treatment of depression	Few prescribers are likely to be aware that this is not a licensed indication
Lamotrigine	Bipolar depression	RCTs demonstrate benefit
Melatonin (Circadin)	Insomnia in children	Licence covers adults >55 years only. Probably preferable to unlicensed formulations of melatonin
Methylphenidate	ADHD in children under 6 ADHD in people over 18	Established clinical practice Supported by evidence base
Naltrexone	Self-injurious behaviour in people with learning disabilities Maintenance of abstinence from alcohol	Limited evidence base Acceptable in specialist hands
Sodium valproate	Treatment and prophylaxis of bipolar disorder	Established clinical practice

References

1.   Bolam v Friern Barnet Hospital Management Committee. WLR 1957; 1:582.
2.   Bolitho v City and Hackney Health Authority. WLR 1997; 3:1151.
3.   Baldwin DS. Royal College of Psychiatrists' Special Interest Group in Psychopharmacology. The use of licensed medicines for unlicensed applications in psychiatric practice. http://www.rcpsych.ac.uk/. 2006.

Further reading

Frank B et al. Psychotropic medications and informed consent: a review. Ann Clin Psychiatry 2008; 20:87–95.
General Medical Council. Good Practice in Prescribing Medicines (2008). http://www.gmc-uk. Org. 2008.

Miscellaneous

Observations on the placebo effect in mental illness

Target symptoms improve, to varying degrees, in approximately a third of patients given a placebo[1]. Side effects also occur; the so-called nocebo effect. Although pharmacologically inert, placebo can cause direct physiological effects, at least in the short term, that are consistent with the effects of active drugs; this has been demonstrated in neuroimaging studies[2,3]. The following considerations apply when interpreting the results of placebo-controlled studies. Although the references for each point are drawn from the depression literature, the same principles apply to the treatment of other disorders. The relative importance of each point will vary depending on the disorder that is being treated.

- Placebo is not the same as no care: patients who maintain contact with services have a better outcome than those who receive no care[4].
- The placebo response is greater in mild illness[5].
- The higher the placebo response rate, the more difficult it is to power studies to show treatment effects. Where the placebo response rate exceeds 40%, studies have to recruit very large numbers of patients to be adequately powered to show differences between treatments[6].
- It is difficult to separate placebo effects from spontaneous remission. The higher the spontaneous remission rate, the more difficult it is to power studies to show treatment effects[4].
- Patients who enter RCTs generally do so when acutely unwell. Symptoms are likely to improve in the majority, irrespective of the intervention. This is so-called 'regression to the mean'[7].
- The placebo response rate in published studies is increasing over time[8]. This may be because of increasing numbers of mildly ill patients being recruited into trials because of clinicians' reluctance to risk severely ill patients being randomised into placebo arms.
- 'Breaking the blind' may influence outcome. The resultant 'expectancy effect' may explain why active placebos are more effective than inert placebos[9,10]. That is, if patients and observers note adverse effects, the placebo effect is enhanced.
- Overt administration of placebo is more effective than covert administration.
- Not all placebos are the same. Patients perceive two brightly coloured tablets to be more effective than one small white one. Capsules, injections and branding also increase expectations of efficacy[1]. This may partly explain different placebo response rates in studies of similar design.
- Most psychotropic drugs have side effects such as sedation that may improve scores on rating scales without actually treating the target illness.
- Placebo response may be short-lived: studies are usually too short to pick up placebo relapsers[11].
- Statistical significance and clinical significance are not the same thing: a study may report on a highly statistically significant difference in efficacy between active drug and placebo, but the magnitude of the difference may be too small to be clinically meaningful.
- Publication bias remains a problem[12–14]. Many negative studies are never published. Underpowered positive studies often are.
- Placebo response increases according to expectancy. For example, placebo response is greater in studies randomising 2:1 active: placebo than in those randomising 1:1 (chance of receiving active is greater).
- Note that other effects may operate: 'wish bias' probably exaggerates the efficacy of new drugs compared with established agents[15].

References

1. Rajagopal S. The placebo effect. Psychiatr Bull 2006; 30:185–188.
2. Scott DJ et al. Placebo and nocebo effects are defined by opposite opioid and dopaminergic responses. Arch Gen Psychiatry 2008; 65:220–231.
3. Mayberg HS et al. The functional neuroanatomy of the placebo effect. Am J Psychiatry 2002; 159:728–737.
4. Andrews G. Placebo response in depression: bane of research, boon to therapy. Br J Psychiatry 2001; 178:192–194.
5. Khan A et al. Severity of depression and response to antidepressants and placebo: an analysis of the Food and Drug Administration database. J Clin Psychopharmacol 2002; 22:40–45.
6. Thase ME. Studying new antidepressants: if there were a light at the end of the tunnel, could we see it? J Clin Psychiatry 2002; 63 Suppl 2:24–28.
7. McDonald CJ et al. How much of the placebo 'effect' is really statistical regression? Stat Med 1983; 2:417–427.
8. Walsh BT et al. Placebo response in studies of major depression: variable, substantial, and growing. JAMA 2002; 287: 1840–1847.
9. Kirsch I et al. The Emperor's new drugs: An analysis of antidepressant medication data submitted to the US Food and Drug Administration. Prevention and Treatment 2002; 5:10–23.
10. Moncrieff J et al. Active placebos versus antidepressants for depression. Cochrane Database Syst Rev 2004;CD003012.
11. Ross DC et al. A typological model for estimation of drug and placebo effects in depression. J Clin Psychopharmacol 2002; 22:414–418.
12. Lexchin J et al. Pharmaceutical industry sponsorship and research outcome and quality: systematic review. BMJ 2003; 326: 1167–1170.
13. Melander H et al. Evidence b(i)ased medicine – selective reporting from studies sponsored by pharmaceutical industry: review of studies in new drug applications. BMJ 2003; 326:1171–1173.
14. Werneke U et al. How effective is St John's wort? The evidence revisited. J Clin Psychiatry 2004; 65:611–617.
15. Barbui C et al. "Wish bias" in antidepressant drug trials? J Clin Psychopharmacol 2004; 24:126–130.

Further reading

Diederich NJ et al. The placebo treatments in neurosciences: New insights from clinical and neuroimaging studies. Neurology 2008; 71:677–684.

Miscellaneous

Drug interactions with alcohol

Drug interactions with alcohol are complex. Many patient-related and drug-related factors need to be considered. It can be difficult to predict accurately outcomes as a number of processes may occur simultaneously.

Pharmacokinetic interactions[1,2]

Alcohol (ethanol) is absorbed from the GI tract and distributed in body water. The volume of distribution is smaller in women and the elderly where plasma levels of alcohol will be higher for a given 'dose' of alcohol than in males. Approximately 10% of ingested alcohol is subjected to first-pass metabolism by alcohol dehydrogenase (ADH). A small proportion of alcohol is metabolised by ADH in the stomach. The remainder is metabolised in the liver by ADH and CYP2E1; women have less capacity to metabolise via ADH than men. CYP2E1 plays a minor role in occasional drinkers but is an important metabolic route in chronic, heavy drinkers. CYP1A2, CYP3A4 and many other CYP enzymes also play a minor role[3,4].

CYP2E1 and ADH convert alcohol to acetaldehyde which is the toxic substance responsible for the unpleasant symptoms of the 'antabuse reaction' (e.g. flushing, headache, nausea, malaise). Acetaldehyde is then further metabolised by aldehyde dehydrogenase to acetic acid and then to carbon dioxide and water.

All of the major enzymes involved in the metabolism of alcohol exhibit genetic polymorphism. For example, forty percent of people of Asian origin are poor metabolisers via ADH. Chronic consumption of alcohol induces CYP2E1 and CYP3A4. The effects of alcohol on other hepatic metabolising enzymes have been poorly studied.

Metabolism of alcohol

Interactions are difficult to predict in alcohol misusers because two opposing processes may be at work: competition for enzymatic sites during periods of intoxication (increasing drug plasma levels) and enzyme induction prevailing (reducing plasma levels) during periods of sobriety. In chronic drinkers, particularly those who binge drink, serum levels of prescribed drugs may reach toxic levels during periods of intoxication with alcohol and then be sub-therapeutic when the patient is sober. This makes it very difficult to optimise treatment of physical or mental illness.

Interactions of uncertain aetiology include increased blood alcohol concentrations in people who take verapamil and decreased metabolism of methylphenidate in people who consume alcohol.

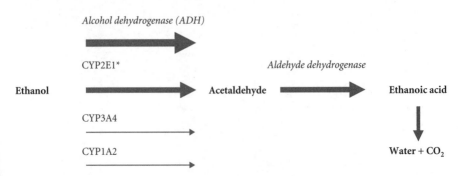

Alcohol dehydrogenase (ADH)

CYP2E1*

Aldehyde dehydrogenase

Ethanol → Acetaldehyde → Ethanoic acid

CYP3A4

CYP1A2

Water + CO$_2$

*Minor route in occasional drinkers; major route in misusers.

Table	Co-administration of alcohol and substrates for CYP2E1 and CYP3A4	
	CYP2E1	**CYP3A4**
Substrates for enzyme (note: this is not an exhaustive list)	• Paracetamol • Isoniazid • Phenobarbitone	• Benzodiazepines • Carbamazepine • Clozapine • Donepezil • Galantamine • Mirtazapine • Risperidone • Sildenafil • Tricyclics • Valproate • Venlafaxine • "Z" hypnotics
Effects in an intoxicated patient	Competition between alcohol and drug leading to reduced rates of metabolism of both compounds. Increased plasma levels may lead to toxicity	Competition between alcohol and drug leading to reduced rates of metabolism of both compounds. Increased plasma levels may lead to toxicity
Effects in a chronic, sober drinker	Activity of CYP2E1 is increased up 10 fold. Increased metabolism of drugs potentially leading to therapeutic failure	Increased rate of drug metabolism potentially leading to therapeutic failure

Table	Drugs that inhibit alcohol dehydrogenase and aldehyde dehydrogenase	
Enzyme	**Inhibited by:**	**Potential consequences:**
Alcohol dehydrogenase	• Aspirin • H_2 antagonists	Reduced metabolism of alcohol resulting in higher plasma levels for longer periods of time
Aldehyde dehydrogenase	• Chlorpropamide • Disulfiram • Griseofulvin • Isoniazid • Isosorbide dinitrate • Metronidazole • Nitrofurantoin • Sulphamethoxazole • Tolbutamide	Reduced ability to metabolise acetaldehyde leading to 'Antabuse' type reaction: facial flushing, headache, tachycardia, nausea and vomiting, arrhythmias and hypotension

Pharmacodynamic interactions[1,2,5]

Alcohol enhances inhibitory neurotransmission at $GABA_a$ receptors and reduces excitatory neurotransmission at glutamate NMDA receptors. It also increases dopamine release in the mesolimbic pathway and may have some effects on serotonin and opiate pathways. Alcohol alone would therefore be expected to cause sedation, amnesia, ataxia and give rise to feelings of pleasure (or worsen psychotic symptoms in vulnerable individuals).

Note that heavy alcohol consumption can lead to hypoglycaemia in people with type 2 diabetes who take oral hypoglycaemics, and can also increase blood pressure. Alcohol can cause or worsen psychotic symptoms by increasing dopamine release in mesolimbic pathways. The effect of antipsychotic drugs may be competitively antagonised, rendering them less effective.

Electrolyte disturbances secondary to alcohol-related dehydration can be exacerbated by other drugs that cause electrolyte disturbances such as diuretics.

Note that:
- **In the presence of pharmacokinetic interactions, pharmacodynamic interactions will be more marked.** For example, in a chronic heavy drinker who is sober, enzyme induction will increase the metabolism of diazepam which may lead to increased levels of anxiety (treatment failure). If the same patient becomes intoxicated with alcohol, the metabolism of diazepam will

(Cont.)

Table Pharmacodynamic interactions with alcohol

Effect of alcohol	Effect exacerbated by	Potential consequences
Sedation	Other sedative drugs e.g.: • Antihistamines • Antipsychotics • Baclofen • Benzodiazepines • Lofexidine • Opiates • Tizanidine • Tricyclics • Z-hypnotics	Increased CNS depression ranging from increased propensity to be involved in accidents through to respiratory depression and death
Amnesia	Other amnesic drugs e.g.: • Barbiturates • Benzodiazepines • Z-hypnotics	Increased amnesic effects ranging from mild memory loss to total amnesia
Ataxia	• ACE inhibitors • ß-blockers • Ca channel blockers • Nitrates Adrenergic alpha receptor antagonists e.g. • Clozapine • Risperidone • Tricyclics	Increased unsteadiness and falls

Table   Psychotropic drugs: choice in patients who continue to drink

	Safest choice	*Best avoided*
Antipsychotics	**Sulpiride and amisulpride** (non-sedative and renally excreted)	**Very sedative antipsychotics** such as chlorpromazine and clozapine
Antidepressants	**SSRI** Potent inhibitors of CYP3A4 (fluoxetine, paroxetine) may decrease alcohol metabolism in chronic drinkers	**TCAs**, because impairment of metabolism by alcohol (while intoxicated) can lead to profound hypotension, seizures, arrhythmias and coma Cardiac effects can be exacerbated by electrolyte disturbances Combinations of TCAs and alcohol profoundly impair psychomotor skills **MAOIs** as can cause profound hypotension. Also potential interaction with tyramine-containing drinks which can lead to hypertensive crisis
Mood-stabilisers	**Valproate** **Carbamazepine** Note: higher plasma levels achieved during periods of alcohol intoxication may be poorly tolerated	**Lithium**, because it has a narrow therapeutic index and alcohol-related dehydration and electrolyte disturbance can precipitate lithium toxicity

be greatly reduced as it will have to compete with alcohol for the metabolic capacity of CYP3A4. Plasma levels of alcohol and diazepam will rise (toxicity). As both alcohol and diazepam are sedative (via $GABA_a$ affinity), loss of consciousness and respiratory depression may occur.

NB. Be aware of the possibility of hepatic failure or reduced hepatic function in chronic alcohol misusers. See section on 'hepatic impairment'. Also note risk of hepatic toxicity with some recommended drugs (e.g. valproate).

References

1. Weathermon R et al. Alcohol and medication interactions. Alcohol Res Health 1999; 23:40–54.
2. Tanaka E. Toxicological interactions involving psychiatric drugs and alcohol: an update. J Clin Pharm Ther 2003; 28:81–95.
3. Salmela KS et al. Respective roles of human cytochrome P-4502E1, 1A2, and 3A4 in the hepatic microsomal ethanol oxidizing system. Alcohol Clin Exp Res 1998; 22:2125–2132.
4. Hamitouche S et al. Ethanol oxidation into acetaldehyde by 16 recombinant human cytochrome P450 isoforms: role of CYP2C isoforms in human liver microsomes. Toxicol Lett 2006; 167:221–230.
5. Stahl SM, Muntner N. Essential Psychopharmacology: Neuroscientific Basis and Practical Applications. 2nd ed. Cambridge: Cambridge University Press; 2000.

Further reading

British National Formulary. 2008. No.56. Appendix 1: Drug interactions. British Medical Association and Royal Pharmaceutical Society of Great Britain. www.bnf.org.uk/bnf
Stockley's Drug Interactions (Online). 2008. http://www.medicinescomplete.com

Miscellaneous

Nicotine

The most common method of consuming nicotine is by smoking cigarettes. One-quarter of the general population, 40–50% of those with depression and up to 90% of those with schizophrenia smoke[1]. Nicotine causes peripheral vasoconstriction, tachycardia, and increased blood pressure[2]. Smokers are at increased risk of developing cardiovascular disease. As well as nicotine, cigarettes also contain tar (a complex mixture of organic molecules, many carcinogenic), a cause of cancers of the respiratory tract, chronic bronchitis and emphysema[3].

Nicotine is highly addictive; an effect which may be at least partially genetically determined[4]. People with mental illness are 2–3 times more likely than the general population to develop and maintain a nicotine addiction[1]. Chronic smoking contributes to the increased morbidity and mortality from respiratory and cardiovascular disease that is seen in this patient group. Nicotine also has psychotropic effects. Smoking can affect the metabolism (and therefore the efficacy and toxicity) of drugs prescribed to treat psychiatric illness[5]. See section on 'smoking and psychotropics'. Nicotine use may be a gateway to experimenting with other psychoactive substances.

Psychotropic effects
Nicotine is highly lipid-soluble and rapidly enters the brain after inhalation. Nicotine receptors are found on dopaminergic cell bodies and stimulation of these receptors leads to dopamine release[1]. Dopamine release in the limbic system is associated with pleasure: dopamine is the brain's 'reward' neurotransmitter. Nicotine may be used by people with mental health problems as a form of 'self-medication' (e.g. to alleviate the negative symptoms of schizophrenia or antipsychotic-induced EPS or for its anxiolytic effect[6]). Drugs that increase the release of dopamine reduce the craving for nicotine. They may also worsen psychotic illness (see under smoking cessation below).

Nicotine improves concentration and vigilance[1]. It also enhances the effects of glutamate, acetylcholine, and serotonin[6].

Schizophrenia
Up to 90% of people with schizophrenia regularly smoke cigarettes[1] and this increased tendency to smoke predates the onset of psychiatric symptoms[7]. Possible explanations are as follows: smoking causes dopamine release, leading to feelings of well-being and a reduction in negative symptoms[6]; to alleviate some of the side-effects of antipsychotics such as drowsiness and EPS[1] and cognitive slowing[8]; as a means of structuring the day (a behavioural filler); or as a means of alleviating the deficit in auditory gaiting that is found in schizophrenia[9]. Nicotine may also improve working memory and attentional deficits[10–12]. Nicotinic receptor agonists may have beneficial effects on neurocognition[13,14], although none are yet licensed for this purpose; note though that cholinergic drugs may exacerbate nicotine dependence[15]. A SPECT study has shown that the greater the occupancy of striatal D_2 receptors by antipsychotic drugs, the more likely the patient is to smoke[16]. This may partly explain the clinical observation that smoking cessation may be more achievable when clozapine (a weak dopamine antagonist) is prescribed in place of a conventional antipsychotic. It has been suggested that people with schizophrenia find it particularly difficult to tolerate nicotine withdrawal symptoms[5].

Depression and anxiety
In 'normal' individuals a moderate consumption of nicotine is associated with pleasure and a decrease in anxiety and feelings of anger[17]. The mechanism of this anxiolytic effect is not understood. People who suffer from anxiety and/or depression are more likely to smoke and find it more difficult to stop[17,18]. This is compounded by the fact that nicotine withdrawal can precipitate or exacerbate depression in those with a history of the illness[17]. Patients with depression are at

increased risk of cardiovascular disease. By directly causing tachycardia and hypertension[2], nicotine may, in theory, exacerbate this problem. More importantly, smoking is a well-known independent risk factor for cardiovascular disease.

Movement disorders and Parkinson's disease

By increasing dopaminergic neurotransmission, nicotine provides a protective effect against both drug-induced EPS and idiopathic Parkinson's disease. Smokers are less likely to suffer from antipsychotic-induced movement disorders than non-smokers[1] and use anticholinergics less often[5]. Parkinson's disease occurs less frequently in smokers than in non-smokers and the onset of clinical symptoms is delayed[1,19]. This may reflect the inverse association between Parkinson's disease and sensation-seeking behavioural traits, rather than a direct effect of nicotine[20].

Drug interactions

Polycyclic hydrocarbons in cigarette smoke are known to stimulate the hepatic microsomal enzyme system, particularly P4501A2[6], the enzyme responsible for the metabolism of many psychotropic drugs. Smoking can lower the blood levels of some drugs by up to 50%[6]. This can affect both efficacy and side effects and needs to be taken into account when making clinical decisions. The drugs most likely to be affected are: clozapine[21], fluphenazine, haloperidol, chlorpromazine, olanzapine, many tricyclic antidepressants, mirtazapine, fluvoxamine and propranolol. See section on 'smoking and psychotropics'.

Withdrawal symptoms[5]

Withdrawal symptoms occur within 12–14 hours of stopping smoking and include depressed mood, insomnia, anxiety, restlessness, irritability, difficulty in concentrating, and increased appetite. Nicotine withdrawal can be confused with depression, anxiety, sleep disorders, and mania. Withdrawal can also exacerbate the symptoms of schizophrenia.

Smoking cessation

In July 2007 a new law was introduced in England that made virtually all enclosed public places and workplaces smokefree[22]. In order to achieve this, NICE recommends a range of interventions from opportunistic advice to pharmacotherapy and behavioural support[23].

People with mental health problems generally have low motivation to stop smoking and may find withdrawal intolerable[10], factors which predict a lower success rate with smoking cessation interventions. Nicotine replacement in the form of patches, microtabs, gum, lozenges, sprays and inhalers, should be used first line[24]. Some preparations are also licensed to support smoking reduction. Full details can be found in the *BNF*. Bupropion/amfebutamone (a noradrenaline (norepinephrine) and dopamine reuptake inhibitor) has been shown to be effective in people with schizophrenia[25,26], particularly when combined with NRT[25,27]. Noradrenergic antidepressants such as nortriptyline[28,29] and venlafaxine[30] may also be effective, but SSRIs are not[29].

Bupropion should be avoided in those at risk of seizures (including those who take epileptogenic drugs). Varenicline, a selective nicotine receptor partial agonist, is perhaps the most effective treatment available[31], but may also be associated with the highest risks; treatment-emergent suicidal thoughts and behaviour have been reported. Note that NRT, bupropion and varenicline should be used alongside behavioural counselling and/or group therapy, the success rate of pharmacotherapy alone is likely to be low. Clinicians should be aware of the possible emergence of depression in patients who attempt to stop smoking.

References

1. Goff DC et al. Cigarette smoking in schizophrenia: relationship to psychopathology and medication side effects. Am J Psychiatry 1992; 149:1189–1194.
2. Benowitz NL et al. Cardiovascular effects of nasal and transdermal nicotine and cigarette smoking. Hypertension 2002; 39: 1107–1112.
3. Anderson JE et al. Treating tobacco use and dependence: an evidence-based clinical practice guideline for tobacco cessation. Chest 2002; 121:932–941.
4. Berrettini W. Nicotine addiction. Am J Psychiatry 2008; 165:1089–1092.
5. Ziedonis DM et al. Schizophrenia and nicotine use: report of a pilot smoking cessation program and review of neurobiological and clinical issues. Schizophr Bull 1997; 23:247–254.
6. Lyon ER. A review of the effects of nicotine on schizophrenia and antipsychotic medications. Psychiatr Serv 1999; 50:1346–1350.
7. Weiser M et al. Higher rates of cigarette smoking in male adolescents before the onset of schizophrenia: a historical-prospective cohort study. Am J Psychiatry 2004; 161:1219–1223.
8. Harris JG et al. Effects of nicotine on cognitive deficits in schizophrenia. Neuropsychopharmacology 2004; 29:1378–1385.
9. McEvoy JP et al. Smoking and therapeutic response to clozapine in patients with schizophrenia. Biol Psychiatry 1999; 46:125–129.
10. Jacobsen LK et al. Nicotine effects on brain function and functional connectivity in schizophrenia. Biol Psychiatry 2004; 55:850–858.
11. Sacco KA et al. Effects of cigarette smoking on spatial working memory and attentional deficits in schizophrenia: involvement of nicotinic receptor mechanisms. Arch Gen Psychiatry 2005; 62:649–659.
12. Smith RC et al. Effects of nicotine nasal spray on cognitive function in schizophrenia. Neuropsychopharmacology 2006; 31:637–643.
13. Olincy A et al. Proof-of-concept trial of an alpha7 nicotinic agonist in schizophrenia. Arch Gen Psychiatry 2006; 63:630–638.
14. Lieberman JA et al. Cholinergic agonists as novel treatments for schizophrenia: the promise of rational drug development for psychiatry. Am J Psychiatry 2008; 165:931–936.
15. Kelly DL et al. Lack of beneficial galantamine effect for smoking behavior: a double-blind randomized trial in people with schizophrenia. Schizophr Res 2008; 103:161–168.
16. de Haan L et al. Occupancy of dopamine D2 receptors by antipsychotic drugs is related to nicotine addiction in young patients with schizophrenia. Psychopharmacology 2006; 183:500–505.
17. Glassman AH. Cigarette smoking: implications for psychiatric illness. Am J Psychiatry 1993; 150:546–553.
18. Wilhelm K et al. Clinical aspects of nicotine dependence and depression. Med Today 2004; 5:40–47.
19. Scott WK et al. Family-based case-control study of cigarette smoking and Parkinson disease. Neurology 2005; 64:442–447.
20. Evans AH et al. Relationship between impulsive sensation seeking traits, smoking, alcohol and caffeine intake, and Parkinson's disease. J Neurol Neurosurg Psychiatry 2006; 77:317–321.
21. Derenne JL et al. Clozapine toxicity associated with smoking cessation: case report. Am J Ther 2005; 12:469–471.
22. Office of Public Sector Information. Statutory Instrument 2006 No. 3368. The Smoke-free (Premises and Enforcement) Regulations 2006. http://www opsi gov uk
23. National Institute for Clinical Excellence. Brief interventions and referral for smoking cessation in primary care and other settings. Public Health Guidance PH1. 2006. http://www.nice.org.uk/
24. Stead LF et al. Nicotine replacement therapy for smoking cessation. Cochrane Database Syst Rev 2008;CD000146.
25. George TP et al. A placebo controlled trial of bupropion for smoking cessation in schizophrenia. Biol Psychiatry 2002; 52:53–61.
26. Evins AE et al. A double-blind placebo-controlled trial of bupropion sustained-release for smoking cessation in schizophrenia. J Clin Psychopharmacol 2005; 25:218–225.
27. Evins AE et al. A 12-week double-blind, placebo-controlled study of bupropion sr added to high-dose dual nicotine replacement therapy for smoking cessation or reduction in schizophrenia. J Clin Psychopharmacol 2007; 27:380–386.
28. Wagena EJ et al. Should nortriptyline be used as a first-line aid to help smokers quit? Results from a systematic review and meta-analysis. Addiction 2005; 100:317–326.
29. Hughes JR et al. Antidepressants for smoking cessation. Cochrane Database Syst Rev 2007;CD000031.
30. Cinciripini PM et al. Combined effects of venlafaxine, nicotine replacement, and brief counseling on smoking cessation. Exp Clin Psychopharmacol 2005; 13:282–292.
31. Cahill K et al. Nicotine receptor partial agonists for smoking cessation. Cochrane Database Syst Rev 2008;CD006103.

Further reading

Aguilar MC et al. Nicotine dependence and symptoms in schizophrenia: naturalistic study of complex interactions. Br J Psychiatry 2005; 186:215–221.
Campion J et al. Review of smoking cessation treatments for people with mental illness. Adv Psychiatr Treat 2008; 14:208–216.

Miscellaneous

Smoking and psychotropic drugs

Tobacco smoke contains polycyclic aromatic hydrocarbons that induce (increase the activity of) certain hepatic enzymes (CYP1A2 in particular)[1]. For some drugs used in psychiatry smoking significantly reduces drug plasma levels and higher doses are required than in non-smokers.

When smokers quit, enzyme activity reduces over a week or so. (Nicotine replacement has no effect on this process.) Plasma levels of affected drugs will then rise, sometimes substantially. Dose reduction will usually be necessary. If smoking is restarted, enzyme activity increases, plasma levels fall and dose increases are then required. The process is complicated and effects are difficult to predict. Of course, few people manage to give up smoking completely, so additional complexity is introduced by intermittent smoking and repeated attempts at stopping completely. Close monitoring of plasma levels (where useful), clinical progress and adverse effect severity are essential.

The table on the following pages gives details of psychotropic drugs known to be affected by smoking status.

Table Smoking and psychotropic drugs

Drug	Effect of smoking	Action to be taken on stopping smoking	Action to be taken on restarting
Benzodiazapines[2,3]	Plasma levels reduced by 0–50% (depends on drug and smoking status)	Monitor closely. Consider reducing dose by up to 25% over one week	Monitor closely. Consider restarting 'normal' smoking dose
Carbamazepine[2]	Unclear, but smoking may reduce carbamazepine plasma levels to a small extent	Monitor for changes in severity of adverse effects	Monitor plasma levels
Chlorpromazine[2-4]	Plasma levels reduced. Varied estimates of exact effect	Monitor closely, consider dose reduction	Monitor closely, consider restarting previous smoking dose
Clozapine[5-7]	Reduces plasma levels by up to 50% Plasma level reduction may be greater in those receiving valproate	Take plasma level before stopping. On stopping, reduce dose gradually (over a week) until around 75% of original dose reached (i.e. reduce by 25%). Repeat plasma level one week after stopping. Consider further dose reductions	Take plasma level before restarting. Increase dose to previous smoking dose over one week. Repeat plasma level
Duloxetine[8]	Plasma levels may be reduced by up to 50%	Monitor closely. Dose may need to be reduced	Consider re-introducing previous smoking dose
Fluphenazine[9]	Reduces plasma levels by up to 50%	On stopping, reduce dose by 25%. Monitor carefully over following 4–8 weeks. Consider further dose reductions	On restarting, increase dose to previous smoking dose

Fluvoxamine[10]	Plasma levels decreased by around a third	Monitor closely. Dose may need to be reduced	Dose may need to be increased to previous level
Haloperidol[11,12]	Reduces plasma levels by around 20%	Reduce dose by around 10%. Monitor carefully. Consider further dose reductions	On restarting, increase dose to previous smoking dose
Mirtazapine[13]	Unclear, but effect probably minimal	Monitor	Monitor
Olanzapine[14-16]	Reduces plasma levels by up to 50%	Take plasma level before stopping. On stopping, reduce dose by 25%. After one week, repeat plasma level. Consider further dose reductions	Take plasma level before restarting. Increase dose to previous smoking dose over one week. Repeat plasma level
Tricyclic antidepressants[2,3]	Plasma levels reduced by 25–50%	Monitor closely. Consider reducing dose by 10–25% over one week. Consider further dose reductions	Monitor closely. Consider restarting previous smoking dose
Zuclopentixol[17,18]	Unclear, but effect probably minimal	Monitor	Monitor

References

1. Kroon LA. Drug interactions with smoking. Am J Health Syst Pharm 2007; 64:1917–1921.
2. Desai HD et al. Smoking in patients receiving psychotropic medications: a pharmacokinetic perspective. CNS Drugs 2001; 15: 469–494.
3. Miller LG. Recent developments in the study of the effects of cigarette smoking on clinical pharmacokinetics and clinical pharmacodynamics. Clin Pharmacokinet 1989; 17:90–108.
4. Goff DC et al. Cigarette smoking in schizophrenia: relationship to psychopathology and medication side effects. Am J Psychiatry 1992; 149:1189–1194.
5. Haring C et al. Influence of patient-related variables on clozapine plasma levels. Am J Psychiatry 1990; 147:1471–1475.
6. Haring C et al. Dose-related plasma levels of clozapine: influence of smoking behaviour, sex and age. Psychopharmacology 1989; 99 Suppl:S38–S40.
7. Diaz FJ et al. Estimating the size of the effects of co-medications on plasma clozapine concentrations using a model that controls for clozapine doses and confounding variables. Pharmacopsychiatry 2008; 41:81–91.
8. Fric M et al. The influence of smoking on the serum level of duloxetine. Pharmacopsychiatry 2008; 41:151–155.
9. Ereshefsky L et al. Effects of smoking on fluphenazine clearance in psychiatric inpatients. Biol Psychiatry 1985; 20:329–332.
10. Spigset O et al. Effect of cigarette smoking on fluvoxamine pharmacokinetics in humans. Clin Pharmacol Ther 1995; 58: 399–403.
11. Jann MW et al. Effects of smoking on haloperidol and reduced haloperidol plasma concentrations and haloperidol clearance. Psychopharmacology 1986; 90:468–470.
12. Shimoda K et al. Lower plasma levels of haloperidol in smoking than in nonsmoking schizophrenic patients. Ther Drug Monit 1999; 21:293–296.
13. Grasmader K et al. Population pharmacokinetic analysis of mirtazapine. Eur J Clin Pharmacol 2004; 60:473–480.
14. Carrillo JA. Role of the smoking-induced cytochrome P450 (CYP)1A2 and polymorphic CYP2D6 in steady-state concentration of olanzapine. J Clin Psychopharmacol 2003; 23:119–127.
15. Gex-Fabry M et al. Therapeutic drug monitoring of olanzapine: the combined effect of age, gender, smoking, and comedication. Ther Drug Monit 2003; 25:46–53.
16. Bigos KL et al. Sex, race, and smoking impact olanzapine exposure. J Clin Pharmacol 2008; 48:157–165.
17. Jann MW et al. Clinical pharmacokinetics of the depot antipsychotics. Clin Pharmacokinet 1985; 10:315–333.
18. Jorgensen A et al. Zuclopenthixol decanoate in schizophrenia: serum levels and clinical state. Psychopharmacology 1985; 87: 364–367.

Caffeine

Caffeine is probably the most popular psychoactive substance in the world. Mean daily consumption in the UK is 350–620 mg[1]. A quarter of the general population and half of those with psychiatric illness regularly consume over 500 mg caffeine/day[2]. Consumption of caffeine can increase both systolic and diastolic BP by up to 10 mmHg; an effect that lasts up to 4 hours[3]. Caffeine has de novo psychotropic effects, may worsen existing psychiatric illness, and interact with psychotropic drugs. Caffeine can also enhance the reinforcing effects of nicotine and possibly other drugs of abuse[4].

Table Caffeine content of drinks

Brewed coffee	100 mg/cup
Red Bull	80 mg/can (other energy drinks may contain substantially more)
Instant coffee	60 mg/cup
Tea	45 mg/cup
Soft drinks	25–50 mg/can

Chocolate also contains caffeine. Martindale lists over 600 medicines that contain caffeine[5]. Most are available without prescription and are marketed as analgesics or appetite suppressants.

Pharmacokinetics
Caffeine is rapidly absorbed after oral administration and has a half-life of 2.5–4.5 hours. It is metabolised by CYP1A2, a hepatic cytochrome enzyme that exhibits genetic polymorphism. Oestrogens, cimetidine, fluvoxamine, and disulfiram can all inhibit caffeine metabolism. Metabolic pathways also become saturated at higher doses[6]. These factors may partially account for the large inter-individual differences that are seen in the ability to tolerate caffeine[7].

Psychotropic effects
Caffeine is associated with CNS stimulation and increased catecholamine release[8]. Low-to-moderate doses are associated with favourable subjective effects such as elation and peacefulness[2]. Doses of >600 mg/day invariably produce anxiety, insomnia, psychomotor agitation, excitement, rambling speech (and sometimes delirium and psychosis)[9]. In sensitive people, these effects are produced by much lower doses. Caffeine has been shown to influence central dopamine binding[10] and at high doses, it can inhibit benzodiazepine-receptor binding[8,9]. Tolerance develops to the effects of caffeine and an established withdrawal syndrome exists (headache, depressed mood, anxiety, fatigue, irritability, nausea, dysphoria, and craving)[11].

Caffeine intoxication (caffeinism)
The DSM-IV[12] defines caffeinism as the recent consumption of caffeine, usually in excess of 250 mg accompanied by five or more of the following: restlessness, nervousness, excitement, insomnia, flushed face, diuresis, GI disturbance, muscle twitching, rambling flow of thought and speech, tachycardia or cardiac arrhythmia, periods of inexhaustibility, and psychomotor agitation, when these symptoms cause significant distress or impairment in social, occupational or other important areas

of functioning and are not due to a general medical condition or better accounted for by another mental disorder (e.g. an anxiety disorder).

Schizophrenia

Patients with schizophrenia often consume large amounts of caffeine-containing drinks[1] and they are twice as likely as controls to consume >200 mg caffeine/day[13]. This may be to relieve dry mouth (as a side effect of antipsychotic drugs), for the stimulant effects of caffeine (to relieve dysphoria/sedation/negative symptoms) or simply because coffee/tea drinking structures the day or relieves boredom. Excessive caffeine consumption is of concern because caffeine increases the release of catecholamines and so may theoretically precipitate or worsen psychosis. Kruger[8] found that large doses of caffeine can worsen psychotic symptoms (in particular elation and conceptual disorganisation) and result in the prescription of larger doses of antipsychotic drugs. The removal of caffeine from the diets of chronically disturbed (challenging behaviour) patients, may lead to decreased levels of hostility, irritability and suspiciousness[14] although this may not hold true in less disturbed populations[15].

Caffeine can also interfere with the effectiveness of drug treatment. Clozapine plasma levels can be raised by up to 60%[16], presumably through competitive inhibition of CYP1A2. Other drugs metabolised by this enzyme, such as olanzapine, imipramine and clomipramine, may be similarly affected. Large doses of caffeine taken in combination with serotonergic antidepressants may increase the risk of developing serotonin syndrome[17]. The potential effects of caffeine on the metabolism of other drugs, as well as the potential to induce a caffeine-withdrawal syndrome, should always be considered before substituting caffeine-free drinks.

Mood disorders

Caffeine may elevate mood through increasing noradrenaline release (norepinephrine)[18]. The practice of self-medication with caffeine to improve mood is common in the general population. Excessive consumption of caffeine may precipitate mania[19,20]. Depressed patients may be more sensitive to the anxiogenic effects of caffeine[21]. MAOIs can be expected to enhance the effects of caffeine.

Caffeine can increase cortisol secretion (gives a false positive in the dexamethasone-suppression test)[22], increase seizure length during ECT[23] and increase the clearance of lithium by promoting diuresis[24]. Caffeine toxicity can be precipitated by drugs that inhibit CYP1A2. Fluvoxamine, for example, can decrease clearance of caffeine by 80%[25].

Anxiety disorders

Caffeine increases vigilance, decreases reaction times, increases sleep latency and worsens subjective estimates of sleep quality, effects that may be more marked in poor metabolisers. It can also precipitate or worsen generalised anxiety and panic attacks[26]; vulnerability to these effects may be mediated through adenosine $A2_a$ receptor gene polymorphism[4]. These effects are so marked that caffeine intoxication should always be considered when patients complain of anxiety symptoms or insomnia. Symptoms may diminish considerably or even abate completely if caffeine is avoided[27]. High doses of caffeine can reduce the efficacy of benzodiazepines (by reducing receptor binding[8,9]).

Summary

Caffeine

- is present in high quantities in coffee and some soft drinks
- can increase systolic and diastolic BP by up to 10 mmHg
- may worsen psychosis and anxiety
- can increase plasma clozapine levels
- may induce intoxication which is characterised by psychomotor agitation and rambling speech
- may be associated with toxicity when co-administered with CYP1A2 inhibitors such as fluvoxamine
- can enhance the reinforcing effects of nicotine and possibly other drugs of abuse.

References

1. Rihs M et al. Caffeine consumption in hospitalized psychiatric patients. Eur Arch Psychiatry Clin Neurosci 1996; 246:83–92.
2. Clementz GL et al. Psychotropic effects of caffeine. Am Fam Physician 1988; 37:167–172.
3. Mort JR et al. Timing of blood pressure measurement related to caffeine consumption. Ann Pharmacother 2008; 42:105–110.
4. Cauli O et al. Caffeine and the dopaminergic system. Behav Pharmacol 2005; 16:63–77.
5. Sweetman SC. Martindale: The Complete Drug Reference 35. [Online]. London: Pharmaceutical Press; 2008. http://www.medicinescomplete.com.
6. Kaplan GB et al. Dose-dependent pharmacokinetics and psychomotor effects of caffeine in humans. J Clin Pharmacol 1997; 37:693–703.
7. Butler MA et al. Determination of CYP1A2 and NAT2 phenotypes in human populations by analysis of caffeine urinary metabolites. Pharmacogenetics 1992; 2:116–127.
8. Kruger A. Chronic psychiatric patients' use of caffeine: pharmacological effects and mechanisms. Psychol Rep 1996; 78:915–923.
9. Sawynok J. Pharmacological rationale for the clinical use of caffeine. Drugs 1995; 49:37–50.
10. Kaasinen V et al. Dopaminergic effects of caffeine in the human striatum and thalamus. Neuroreport 2004; 15:281–285.
11. Silverman K et al. Withdrawal syndrome after the double-blind cessation of caffeine consumption. N Engl J Med 1992; 327:1109–1114.
12. American Psychiatric Association. Diagnostic and Statistical Manual of Mental Disorders, 4th edition. Washington DC: American Psychiatric Association; 1994.
13. Gurpegui M et al. Fewer but heavier caffeine consumers in schizophrenia: a case-control study. Schizophr Res 2006; 86:276–283.
14. De Freitas B et al. Effects of caffeine in chronic psychiatric patients. Am J Psychiatry 1979; 136:1337–1338.
15. Koczapski A et al. Effects of caffeine on behavior of schizophrenic inpatients. Schizophr Bull 1989; 15:339–344.
16. Carrillo JA et al. Effects of caffeine withdrawal from the diet on the metabolism of clozapine in schizophrenic patients. J Clin Psychopharmacol 1998; 18:311–316.
17. Shioda K et al. Possible serotonin syndrome arising from an interaction between caffeine and serotonergic antidepressants. Hum Psychopharmacol 2004; 19:353–354.
18. Achor MB et al. Diet aids, mania, and affective illness. Am J Psychiatry 1981; 138:392.
19. Ogawa N et al. Secondary mania caused by caffeine. Gen Hosp Psychiatry 2003; 25:138–139.
20. Machado-Vieira R et al. Mania associated with an energy drink: the possible role of caffeine, taurine, and inositol. Can J Psychiatry 2001; 46:454–455.
21. Lee MA et al. Anxiogenic effects of caffeine on panic and depressed patients. Am J Psychiatry 1988; 145:632–635.
22. Uhde TW et al. Caffeine-induced escape from dexamethasone suppression. Arch Gen Psychiatry 1985; 42:737–738.
23. Cantu TG et al. Caffeine in electroconvulsive therapy. DICP 1991; 25:1079–1080.
24. Mester R et al. Caffeine withdrawal increases lithium blood levels. Biol Psychiatry 1995; 37:348–350.
25. Stockleys Drug Interactions. [Online]. http://www.medicinescomplete.com . 2008.
26. Bruce MS. The anxiogenic effects of caffeine. Postgrad Med J 1990; 66 Suppl 2:S18–S24.
27. Bruce MS et al. Caffeine abstention in the management of anxiety disorders. Psychol Med 1989; 19:211–214.

Further reading

Caffeine: In AHFS Drug Information. American Society of Health Care Pharmacists. http://www.medicinescomplete.com
Paton C, Beer D. Caffeine: the forgotten variable. Int J Psychiatry Clin Pract 2002; 5:231–236.

Miscellaneous

Complementary therapies

A large proportion of the population currently use or have recently used complementary therapies (CTs)[1,2]. As health professionals are rarely consulted before purchase, a diagnosis is often not made and efficacy and side effects are not monitored. The majority of those who use CTs are also taking conventional medicines[2] and many people use more than one CT simultaneously. Many do not tell their doctor. The public associate natural products with safety and may be unwilling to report possible side effects[3]. Herbal medicines, in particular, can be toxic as they contain pharmacologically active substances[4]. Many conventional drugs prescribed today were originally derived from plants. These include medicines as diverse as aspirin, digoxin, and the vinca alkaloids used in cancer chemotherapy. Herbal medicines such as St John's Wort, *Gingko biloba*, and valerian are increasingly used as self-medication for psychiatric and neurodegenerative illnesses[5–7]. Few CTs have been subject to randomised, controlled trials, so efficacy is largely unproven. For some, Cochrane Reviews exist. These include the use of kava to treat anxiety[8] (some evidence of efficacy; although a more recent review disputes this conclusion[9]), Chinese herbal medicine as an adjunct to antipsychotics in schizophrenia (promising, more evidence required)[10], aromatherapy for behavioural problems in dementia (insufficient evidence, but worth further study)[11], and hypnosis for schizophrenia (insufficient evidence, but worth further study)[12]. Several complementary therapies are thought to be worthy of further study in the adjunctive management of substance misuse[13]. There is some preliminary, limited support for aromatherapy as an adjunct to conventional treatments in a range of psychiatric conditions[14].

There is little systematic monitoring of side effects caused by CTs, so safety is largely unknown. There are an increasing number of published case reports of significant drug–herb interactions[15]; these include ginko and aspirin or warfarin leading to increased bleeding, ginko and trazodone leading to coma, and ginseng and phenelzine leading to mania. Drug interactions with St John's Wort are outlined in the section 'Drug Interactions with Antidepressants'. Some herbs are known to be very toxic[16,17].

Whatever the perceived 'evidence base' for the use of complementary therapies, the feelings of autonomy engendered by taking control of one's own illness and treatment can result in important psychological benefits irrespective of any direct therapeutic benefits of the CT; the placebo effect is likely to be important here. (See section: 'Observation on the placebo effect in mental illness'.) There are many different complementary therapies, the most popular being homeopathy and herbal medicine with its branches of Bach's flower remedies, and Chinese and Ayurvedic medicine. Non-drug therapies such as acupuncture and osteopathy are also popular. Aromatherapy is usually considered to be a non-pharmacological treatment but this may not be the case[18]. To master one CT can take years of study; therefore, to ensure safe and effective treatment, referral to a qualified practitioner is recommended. Be aware, nonetheless, that scientific support for most complementary medicine is minimal and 'qualification' to practice may entail little in the way of regulation. The majority of doctors and pharmacists have no qualifications or specific training in CTs. The following table gives a brief introduction. Further reading is strongly recommended.

References

1. Barnes J, Anderson LL, Phillipson JD. *Herbal Medicines: A Guide for Healthcare Professionals*. 2nd ed. London: Pharmaceutical Press; 2002.
2. Astin JA. Why patients use alternative medicine: results of a national study. JAMA 1998; 279:1548–1553.
3. Barnes J et al. Different standards for reporting ADRs to herbal remedies and conventional OTC medicines: face-to-face interviews with 515 users of herbal remedies. Br J Clin Pharmacol 1998; 45:496–500.
4. Pies R. Adverse neuropsychiatric reactions to herbal and over-the-counter "antidepressants". J Clin Psychiatry 2000; 61:815–820.
5. Werneke U et al. Complementary medicines in psychiatry: review of effectiveness and safety. Br J Psychiatry 2006; 188:109–121.
6. van der WG et al. Complementary and alternative medicine in the treatment of anxiety and depression. Curr Opin Psychiatry 2008; 21:37–42.
7. Andreescu C et al. Complementary and alternative medicine in the treatment of bipolar disorder—a review of the evidence. J Affect Disord 2008; 110:16–26.
8. Pittler MH et al. Kava extract for treating anxiety. Cochrane Database Syst Rev 2003;CD003383.
9. Connor KM et al. Kava in generalized anxiety disorder: three placebo-controlled trials. Int Clin Psychopharmacol 2006; 21:249–253.
10. Rathbone J et al. Chinese herbal medicine for schizophrenia: Cochrane systematic review of randomised trials. Br J Psychiatry 2007; 190:379–384.
11. Thorgrimsen L et al. Aroma therapy for dementia. Cochrane Database Syst Rev 2003;CD003150.
12. Izquierdo de SA et al. Hypnosis for schizophrenia. Cochrane Database Syst Rev 2007;CD004160.
13. Dean AJ. Natural and complementary therapies for substance use disorders. Curr Opin Psychiatry 2005; 18:271–276.
14. Perry N et al. Aromatherapy in the management of psychiatric disorders: clinical and neuropharmacological perspectives. CNS Drugs 2006; 20:257–280.
15. Hu Z et al. Herb–drug interactions: a literature review. Drugs 2005; 65:1239–1282.
16. Ernst E. Serious psychiatric and neurological adverse effects of herbal medicines – a systematic review. Acta Psychiatr Scand 2003; 108:83–91.
17. De Smet PA. Health risks of herbal remedies: an update. Clin Pharmacol Ther 2004; 76:1–17.
18. Nguyen QA et al. The use of aromatherapy to treat behavioural problems in dementia. Int J Geriatr Psychiatry 2008; 23:337–346.
19. NHS Centre for Reviews and Dissemination. Homeopathy. Effect Health Care Bull 2002; 7:1–12.
20. Fulder S. *The Handbook of Complementary Medicine*, 2nd edition. London: Hodder and Stoughton; 1989.

Further reading

Complementary and alternative medicine specialist library. http://www.library.nhs.uk/cam/
Barnes J et al. Herbal medicines. http://www.medicinescomplete.com

Miscellaneous

Table An introduction to complementary therapies

Health beliefs	Homeopathy[11,12,19]	Herbal medicine (phytotherapy)[16,17]	Aromatherapy[20]
	• Treatment is selected according to the individual characteristics of the patient (hair colour and personality are as important as symptoms) • Treatment stimulates the body to restore health (there is no scientifically plausible theory to support this claim) • Like is treated with like (e.g. substances that cause a fever, treat a fever) • The more diluted the preparation, the more potent it is thought to be • Very potent preparations are unlikely to contain even one molecule of active substance	• Treatment is selected according to the individual characteristics of the patient (as with homeopathy) • Herbs are believed to stimulate the body's natural defences and enhance the elimination of toxins by increasing diuresis, defecation, bile flow and sweating • Attention to diet is important • The whole plant is used, not the specific active ingredient (this is believed to reduce side effects) • Active ingredients vary with the source of the herb (standardisation is contrary to the philosophy of herbal medicine) • Herbalists believe that if the correct treatment is chosen, treatment will be completely free of side effects	• Treatment is selected according to the individual characteristics of the patient (as with homeopathy and herbal medicine) • Illness is believed to be the result of imbalance in mental, emotional and physical processes, and aromatherapy is believed to promote balance • Purified oils are not used (the many natural constituents are believed to protect against adverse effects: similar to the beliefs held by herbalists) • There is no standard dose • Individual oils may be used for several unrelated indications
Used for	• A wide range of indications (except those outlined below) • May be taken with conventional treatments • Over 2000 remedies and many dilutions are available	• Everything except as outlined below • May be taken with conventional treatments but many significant interactions are possible (some have been reported) • Advertised in the lay press for a wide range of indications	• Everything except as outlined below • May be used as an adjunct to conventional treatments • Usually administered by massage onto the skin, which is known to relieve pain and tension, increase circulation and aid relaxation

Contra-indications	• Infection • Organ failure • Vitamin/mineral/hormone deficiency	• Use in pregnancy and lactation (many herbs are abortifacient) • Evening primrose oil should not be used in epilepsy	• Use in pregnancy (jasmine, peppermint, rose and rosemary may stimulate uterine contractions) • Rosemary should be avoided in epilepsy and hypertension
Side effects and other information	• None known or anticipated • Said to be inactivated by aromatherapy and strong smells (e.g. coffee, peppermint, toothpaste) • Said to be inactivated by handling • Healing follows the law of cure: symptoms disappear down the body in the reverse order to which they appeared, move from vital to less vital organs and ultimately appear as a rash (which is a sign of cure)	• Herbal remedies are occasionally adulterated (with conventional medicines such as steroids or toxic substances such as lead) • Many side effects can be anticipated (e.g. kelp and thyrotoxicosis, St John's wort and serotonin syndrome) • Overuse, adulteration, variation in plant constituents and misidentification of plants are common causes of toxicity. Some Chinese herbs are toxic	• Skin sensitivity • Significant systemic absorption can occur during massage • Ingestion can cause liver/kidney toxicity • All aromatherapy products should be stored in dark containers away from heat to avoid oxidation

Enhancing medication adherence

Recommendations made in clinical guidelines regarding the use of medicines are based on evidence from clinical trials supplemented by clinicians' opinions of the balance between the potential benefits and potential risks of treatment. In clinical practice however, a range of patient-related factors such as insight, health beliefs, and the perceived efficacy and tolerability of treatment influence whether medication is taken, and if so, for how long.

The patient and prescriber should agree jointly on the goals of treatment and how these can be reached. Sticking to this mutually agreed plan is termed concordance or adherence; non-adherence indicates that the treatment plan should be renegotiated, and not that the patient is at fault.

How common is non-adherence?
Approximately 50% of people do not take their medication as prescribed; this proportion is similar across chronic physical and mental disorders[1].

There is some **variation in adherence** rates both **over time** and **across settings**. For example, ten days after discharge from hospital, up to 25% of patients with schizophrenia are partially or non-adherent and this figure rises to 50% at one year and 75% by 2 years[2]. In some mental healthcare settings the rate of non-adherence may be up to 90%[3].

Not surprisingly, non-adherence is known to be more common when the patient disagrees with the need for treatment, the medication regimen is complex, or the patient perceives the side effects of treatment to be unacceptable[4,5]. Adherence may also therefore be **medication specific,** where some medicines are taken regularly, others intermittently and others not at all. Notably, half of those who stop treatment don't tell their doctor.

Why don't people take medication?
Non-adherence can be intentional (sometimes termed "intelligent" non-adherence) or unintentional or a mixture of both. Most non-adherence is intentional. Individual influences include:

- Illness-related factors such as denial of illness, specific symptoms such as grandiose or persecutory thoughts/delusions, or the impact of illness on lifestyle (e.g. cognitive deficits, disorganisation).
- Treatment-related factors such as the drug being perceived not to be effective or the side effects intolerable; akathisia, weight gain, and sexual dysfunction feature prominently here
- Clinician-related factors such as not feeling listened to or consulted, perceiving the clinician as authoritative or dismissive, being given a poor explanation of treatment or having infrequent contact
- Patient-related factors such as personal beliefs about illness, denial of illness/or lack of insight, perception of illness severity, being young and male, having co-morbid personality disorder(s), and/or substance misuse, personal beliefs about treatment such as concerns about dependency, concerns about long-term side-effects, a lack of knowledge about treatment, misunderstanding instructions, or simply forgetting
- Environmental and cultural factors such as the family's beliefs about illness and treatment, religious beliefs and peer pressure.

NICE (2008)[6] recommend that, as long as the patient has capacity to consent, their right not to take medication should be respected. If the prescriber considers that this decision may have an adverse effect, the reasons for the patient's decision and the prescriber's concerns should be recorded.

Assessing attitudes to medication?

A number of rating scales and checklists are available that help to guide and structure discussion around attitudes to medication. The most widely used is the Drug Attitude Inventory (DAI)[7], which consists of a mix of positive and negative statements about medication; 30 statements in its full form and 10 in its abbreviated form. It is designed to be completed by the patient who simply agrees or disagrees with each statement. The total score is an indicator of the patient's overall perception of the balance between the benefits and harms associated with taking medication, and therefore likely adherence. Attitudes to medication as measured using the DAI have been shown to be a useful predictor of compliance over time[8]. Other available checklists include the Rating of Medication Influences scale (ROMI)[9] and the Beliefs about Medicines Questionnaire[10].

How can you assess adherence?

It is very difficult to be certain about whether or not a patient is taking prescribed medicines. Clinicians are known to overestimate adherence rates and patients may not openly acknowledge that they are not taking all or any of their medication. NICE recommends that the patient should be asked in a non-judgemental way if they have missed any doses over a specific time period such as the previous week[6].

It is also important to ask the patient about perceived effectiveness and side effects. More intrusive methods include checks that prescriptions have been collected, asking to see the patient's medication (pill counts), and asking family or carers. For some antipsychotics such as clozapine, olanzapine, and risperidone, blood tests can be useful to directly assess plasma levels. It is important to note that plasma levels of these drugs achieved with a fixed dose vary somewhat and it is not possible to accurately determine partial non-adherence (i.e. total non-adherence will be readily revealed but partial and full adherence may be difficult to tell apart). See Chapter 1 on 'plasma level monitoring'.

Strategies for improving adherence

NICE has reviewed the evidence for adherence over a range of health conditions[6]. They conclude that no specific intervention can be recommended for all patients but, in general, **adherence is maximised if**

- the patient is offered information about medicines before the decision is taken to prescribe
- this information is actively discussed, taking into account the patient's understanding and beliefs about diagnosis and treatment
- the information includes the name of the medicine, how it works, the likely benefits and side effects, and how long it should be continued
- the patient is given the opportunity to be involved in making decisions about prescribed medicines
- at each contact, the patient is asked if they have any concerns about their medicines, and any identified concerns are addressed.

NICE further recommends that any intervention that is used to increase adherence should be tailored to overcome the specific difficulties experienced or reported by a patient.

It is essential that the **patient's perspective is understood and respected and a treatment plan agreed jointly.** The following strategies may help to achieve this:

- explore aspirations for the future and how medication could help, e.g. staying out of hospital or not getting into trouble with the police
- help the patient and carer understand their experiences in a culturally sensitive way that recognises the place of medication in recovery
- work with the patient to elicit and explore the positive and negative things about taking/not taking medication
- talk through past experiences of medication and exploring which medicines were helpful and less helpful from the patient's perspective
- listen to and acknowledge the concerns of patients and their carers about the use of medication and address any false beliefs
- work collaboratively with the patient to find a medication that the patient perceives to be helpful
- systematically monitor the effectiveness and side effects of medication so that the patient feels listened to and respected
- manage side effects when they occur. Consider dosage reduction, change of medication, alteration of the timing of doses, or additional medication for side-effects.

Overcoming **practical difficulties** can also help. Potentially useful strategies include:

- ensuring the patient knows how to obtain medication and is able to do this
- keeping medication regimens as simple as possible[11]
- using reminders and prompts, including telephone follow-up or mobile phone text messaging
- maximising engagement with services by introducing patients to their community team before discharge from hospital[12]
- providing support, encouragement, and regular planned follow up.

The need to consider multiple strategies tailored to the needs of individual patients is also the conclusion of a Cochrane review that examined medication adherence over a wide range of medical conditions[1]. Almost all of the interventions that were effective in improving adherence in long-term care were complex, and even the most effective interventions did not lead to large improvements in adherence and treatment outcomes. Haynes et al[1] emphasized that there is no evidence that low adherence can be 'cured'; efforts to improve adherence must be maintained for as long as treatment is needed.

'Compliance therapy' for schizophrenia

After early promise in improving insight, adherence, attitudes towards medication and rehospitalisation rates in an inpatient sample[13,14], further studies of compliance therapy have failed to replicate this finding. Compliance therapy has been shown to have no advantage over non-specific counselling in either inpatients[8] or outpatients[15], or those who have been clinically unstable in the last year[16].

Compliance aids

Compliance aids that contain compartments that accommodate up to four doses of multiple medicines each day may be helpful in patients who are clearly motivated to take medication but find this difficult due to disorganisation or cognitive deficits. It should be noted that only 10% of non-compliant patients say that they forgot to take medication[11] and that compliance aids are not a substitute for lack of insight or lack of motivation to take medication. Some medicines are unstable when removed from blister packaging and placed in a compliance aid; these include oro-dispersible formulations, which are often prescribed for non-adherent patients. In addition, compliance aids are labour-intensive (expensive) to fill and it can be difficult to change prescriptions at short notice.

Depot antipsychotics

Depot antipsychotics avoid covert non-adherence; if the patient defaults from treatment, it will be immediately apparent. NICE recommends that depots are an option in patients who are known to be non-adherent to oral treatment and/or those who prefer this method of administration[17].

Depots are likely to be underused, for example a recent US study found that depot preparations were prescribed for less than 1 in 5 patients with a recent episode of non-adherence[18].

Paying patients to take their medication

There is evidence from controlled trials across a number of disease areas supporting the potential of financial incentives to enhance medication adherence. Paying people to take their medication is extremely controversial, though some clinicians have found this strategy to be successful in high-risk patients with psychotic illness[19].

References

1. Haynes RB, Ackloo E, Sahota N, McDonald HP, Yao X. Interventions for enhancing medication adherence. Cochrane Database Syst Rev 2008;CD000011.
2. Leucht S, Heres S. Epidemiology, clinical consequences, and psychosocial treatment of nonadherence in schizophrenia. J Clin Psychiatry 2006; 67 Suppl 5:3–8.
3. Cramer JA, Rosenheck R. Compliance with medication regimens for mental and physical disorders. Psychiatr Serv 1998; 49:196–201.
4. Valenstein M, Copeland LA, Owen R, Blow FC, Visnic S. Adherence assessments and the use of depot antipsychotics in patients with schizophrenia. J Clin Psychiatry 2001; 62:545–551.
5. Mitchell AJ, Selmes T. Why don't patients take their medicine? reasons and solutions in psychiatry. Adv Psychiatr Treat 2007; 13:336–346.
6. National Institute for Clinical Excellence. Medicines concordance and adherence: involving adults and carers in decisions about prescribed medicines. Draft for Consultation; 2008. http://www nice org uk
7. Hogan TP, Awad AG, Eastwood R. A self-report scale predictive of drug compliance in schizophrenics: reliability and discriminative validity. Psychol Med 1983; 13:177–183.
8. O'Donnell C, Donohoe G, Sharkey L et al. Compliance therapy: a randomised controlled trial in schizophrenia. BMJ 2003; 327:834.
9. Weiden P, Rapkin B, Mott T et al. Rating of medication influences (ROMI) scale in schizophrenia. Schizophr Bull 1994; 20:297–310.
10. Horne R, Weinman J, Hankins M. The beliefs about medicines questionnaire: The development and evaluation of a new method for assessing the cognitive representation of medication. Psychol Health 1999; 14:1–24.
11. Perkins DO. Predictors of noncompliance in patients with schizophrenia. J Clin Psychiatry 2002; 63:1121–1128.
12. Nose M, Barbui C, Gray R, Tansella M. Clinical interventions for treatment non-adherence in psychosis: meta-analysis. Br J Psychiatry 2003; 183: 197–206.
13. Kemp R, Hayward P, Applewhaite G, Everitt B, David A. Compliance therapy in psychotic patients: randomised controlled trial. BMJ 1996; 312:345–349.
14. Kemp R, Kirov G, Everitt B, Hayward P, David A. Randomised controlled trial of compliance therapy. 18-month follow-up. Br J Psychiatry 1998; 172:413–419.
15. Byerly MJ, Fisher R, Carmody T, Rush AJ. A trial of compliance therapy in outpatients with schizophrenia or schizoaffective disorder. J Clin Psychiatry 2005; 66:997–1001.
16. Gray R, Leese M, Bindman J et al. Adherence therapy for people with schizophrenia. European multicentre randomised controlled trial. Br J Psychiatry 2006; 189:508–514.
17. National Institute for Clinical Excellence. Guidance on the use of newer (atypical) antipsychotic drugs for the treatment of schizophrenia. Health Technology Appraisal No. 43. 2002. http://www nice org uk
18. West JC, Marcus SC, Wilk J, Countis LM, Regier DA, Olfson M. Use of depot antipsychotic medications for medication nonadherence in schizophrenia. Schizophr Bull 2008; 34:995–1001.
19. Claassen D, Fakhoury WK, Ford R, Priebe S. Money for medication: financial incentives to improve medication adherence in assertive outreach. Psychiatr Bull 2007; 31:4–7.

Driving and psychotropic drugs

No one should drive if their performance is compromised by illness, prescribed medicines, alcohol, or other drugs. Everyone has a duty to drive reasonably and all drivers are legally responsible for accidents they cause[1].

Many factors have been shown to affect driving performance. These include age, personality, physical and mental state, and being under the influence of alcohol, prescribed medicines, street drugs, or over-the-counter medicines[2]. Studying the effects of any of these factors in isolation is extremely difficult. Some studies have assessed the effect of medication on tests such as response time and attention[3], but these tests do not directly measure ability or inability to drive.

It has been estimated that up to 10% of people killed or injured in road traffic accidents (RTAs) are taking psychotropic medication[4]. Patients with personality disorders and alcoholism have the highest rates of motoring offences and are more likely to be involved in accidents[4]. People whose driving ability may be impaired through their illness or prescribed medication should inform their insurance company. Failure to do so is considered to be 'withholding a material fact' and may render the insurance policy void.

Table Psychotropics and driving

Drug	Effect
Alcohol	Alcohol causes sedation and impaired coordination, vision, attention, and information-processing. Alcohol-dependent drivers are twice as likely to be involved in traffic accidents and offences than licensed drivers as a whole[4], and a third of all fatal RTAs involve alcohol-dependent drivers[4]. Young drivers who use alcohol in combination with illicit drugs are particularly high risk[5,6]
Anticonvulsants	Initial, dose-related side effects may affect driving ability (e.g. blurred vision, ataxia, and sedation). There are strict rules regarding epilepsy and driving
Antidepressants	People who are prescribed an antidepressant have an increased risk of being involved in a RTA; TCAs may not be associated with greater risks than SSRIs, suggesting that depression itself may make a major contribution[7]
Antipsychotics	Sedation and EPS can impair coordination and response time[2]. A high proportion of patients treated with antipsychotics may have an impaired ability to drive[8,9]. One study found patients with schizophrenia taking atypical antipsychotics or clozapine performed better in tests of skills related to car-driving ability than patients with schizophrenia taking typical antipsychotics[10]. Clinical assessment is required

Table	Psychotropics and driving (Cont.)
Drug	*Effect*
Hypnotics and anxiolytics	Benzodiazepines cause sedation and impaired attention, information processing, memory and motor coordination, and along with opiates are the drugs most frequently implicated in RTAs. The impairment is dose-related and greater with longer half-life drugs. When used as anxiolytics and hypnotics[11,12], benzodiazepines are associated with an increased risk of RTAs. One study found that zopiclone dramatically increased the risk of RTAs[11]. Another suggests middle-of-the-night administration of zolpidem can negatively affect driving ability[13]
Lithium	Lithium may impair visual adaptation to the dark[2] but the implications for driving safety are unknown. Elderly people who take lithium may be at increased risk of being involved in an injurious motor vehicle crash[14]
Methylphenidate	One small study found that methylphenidate improved driving perform-ance in adults with ADHD[15], again suggesting that illness may make a bigger contribution to fitness to drive than the specific pharmacology of the treatment

Effects of mental illness

Severe mental disorder is a prescribed disability for the purposes of the Road Traffic Act (1988). Regulations define mental disorder as including mental illness, arrested or incomplete development of the mind, psychopathic disorder, or severe impairment of intelligence or social functioning. The licence restrictions that apply to each disorder can be found in the following table. Note that licence restrictions may also apply to people with diabetes, particularly if treated with insulin or if there are established micro- or macro-vascular complications.

Effects of psychiatric medicines

The Road Traffic Act does not differentiate between illicit and prescribed drugs. Therefore any person who drives in a public place while unfit due to any drug is liable to prosecution. Many psychotropics can impair alertness, concentration, and driving performance. Drugs that block H_1, α_1-adrenergic or cholinergic receptors may be particularly problematic. Effects are particularly marked at the start of treatment and after increasing the dose. It is important to stop driving during this time if adversely affected. The use of alcohol will further increase any impairment. Many antipsychotic and antidepressant drugs lower the seizure threshold. The DVLA advises this is taken into consideration when prescribing for a driver. Further information about the effects of psychotropic drugs on driving can be found in the previous table.

Drug-induced sedation

Many psychotropic drugs are sedative. The more sedative a drug is, the more likely it is to impair driving ability. Other medicines, either prescribed or bought over the counter, may also be sedative and/or affect driving ability (e.g. antihistamines[4]). One study found that 89% of patients taking other psychotropic drugs in addition to antidepressants failed a battery of 'fitness to drive' tests[16]. Since the degree of sedation any individual will experience is very difficult to predict, patients prescribed sedative drugs should be advised not to drive if they feel sedated.

DVLA – duty of the driver

It is the duty of the licence holder or licence applicant to notify the DVLA of any medical condition which may affect safe driving. A list of relevant medical conditions can be found in the DVLA 'At a glance' guide (www.dvla.gov.uk).

DVLA – duty of the prescriber

Make sure the patient understands that their condition may impair their ability to drive. If the patient is incapable of understanding, notify the DVLA immediately. Explain to the patient that they have a legal duty to inform the DVLA.

Note: The DVLA guidance specifies that patients under S17 of the MHA must be able to satisfy the standards of fitness for their respective conditions and be free from any effects of medication which would affect driving adversely, before resuming driving. Very few patients will fulfil these criteria.

GMC guidelines for prescribers (www.dvla.gov.uk)

- Patients who disagree with the diagnosis or the effect of the condition on their ability to drive should seek a second opinion and refrain from driving until this has been obtained.
- If the patient continues to drive while unfit, you should make every reasonable effect to persuade them to stop. This may include telling their next of kin if they agree you may do so.
- If they continue to drive, inform the DVLA. Tell the patient you are going to do this and write to the patient to confirm you have done so.

Table Summary of DVLA regulations

Diagnosis	Group 1 Entitlement (cars and motorcycles)		Group 2 Entitlement (heavy goods or public service vehicles)	
	Notify DVLA?	Notes	Notify DVLA?	Notes
Uncomplicated anxiety or depression (without significant memory or concentration problems, agitation, behavioural disturbance or suicidal thoughts)	No	Consider effects of medication (see before).	No	Very minor short-lived illnesses need not be notified to DVLA. Consider effects of medication (see before)
Severe anxiety states or depressive illnesses (with significant memory or concentration problems, agitation, behavioural disturbance or suicidal thoughts)	Yes	Driving should cease pending the outcome of medical enquiry. A period of stability will be required before driving can be resumed	Yes	Licence revoked for minimum of 6 months. Driving usually permitted if illness long-standing but controlled on medication that does not impair driving

Table Summary of DVLA regulations (Cont.)

Diagnosis	Group 1 Entitlement (cars and motorcycles)		Group 2 Entitlement (heavy goods or public service vehicles)	
	Notify DVLA?	Notes	Notify DVLA?	Notes
Acute psychotic disorders of any type	Yes	Driving must cease during the acute episode. Relicensing can be considered (hypomania/mania following an isolated episode only) when all of the following conditions can be satisfied: a) has remained well and stable for at least 3 months b) is compliant with treatment c) has regained insight (hypomania/mania only) d) is free from adverse effects of medication which would impair driving e) subject to a favourable specialist report. Drivers with a history of instability or poor compliance will require a longer period off driving	Yes	Licence revoked for at least 3 years. Driving will only be permitted again if medication is minimal and does not interfere with driving ability and there is no significant likelihood of relapse

Hypomania/mania	Yes	See Acute psychotic disorders of any type. Repeated changes of mood: when there have been four or more episodes of mood swing in the last 12 months, at least 6 months' stability is required	Yes	As above
Chronic schizophrenia and other chronic psychoses	Yes	See Acute psychotic disorders of any type. Continuing symptoms even with limited insight do not necessarily preclude driving. Symptoms should be unlikely to cause significant concentration problems, memory impairment or distraction whilst driving	Yes	As above
Dementia or any organic brain syndrome	Yes	Patient should inform DVLA (see guidance overleaf). Decision regarding fitness to drive subject reports. In early dementia, licence may be issued based on medical subject to annual review	Yes	Licence revoked

Table Summary of DVLA regulations (Cont.)

Diagnosis	Group 1 Entitlement (cars and motorcycles)		Group 2 Entitlement (heavy goods or public service vehicles)	
	Notify DVLA?	Notes	Notify DVLA?	Notes
Learning disability	Yes	Severe LD – licence application will be refused. Mild LD – must be declared by patient on licence application form. Provisional licence may be issued: liaise with DVLA	Yes	Only persons with minor degrees of learning disability will be considered for a licence. When the condition is stable and there are no medical or psychiatric complications
Developmental disorders inc. Asperger's syndrome and ADHD	Yes	Diagnosis not in itself a bar to licensing. Factors such as impulsivity, lack of awareness of the impact of own behaviour on self or others need to be considered	Yes	Continuing minor symptomatology may be compatible with licensing cases considered individually
Behaviour disorders (e.g. violent behaviour)	Yes	Licence revoked. If behaviour is seriously disturbed. Licence reissued only after behaviour has been satisfactorily controlled. Medical report required	Yes	If behaviour is seriously disturbed, licence refused/revoked. Restoration of licence possible if psychiatric reports confirm stability
Alcohol misuse 'Persistent misuse of alcohol confirmed by medical enquiry'	Yes	Licence refused/revoked for confirmed, persistent alcohol misuse until minimum of 6 months' controlled drinking or abstinence attained	Yes	Same as Group 1 except 1 year's controlled drinking or abstinence required

Alcohol dependency	Yes	Licence refused/revoked until a 1-year period free from alcohol problems attained. Abstinence usually required. Medical reports required. Additional restrictions if seizures occur	Yes	Licence not granted if there is a history of alcohol dependency in the past 3 years. Additional restrictions if seizures occur. Medical reports required
Alcohol-related disorders (e.g. neuropsychiatric impairment or psychosis)	Yes	Patient should inform DVLA. Medical reports required. Licence usually refused/revoked until satisfactory recovery	Yes	Licence refused/revoked
Drug misuse and dependency NB: Benzodiazepines prescribed above BNF limits for any reason constitute misuse/dependency for DVLA purposes	Yes	Licence revoked until drug-free period shown below is attained. Assessment and urine screen arranged by DVLA may be required. If persistent use or dependency; **6-month drug-free period** for cannabis, amfetamines, ecstasy and other psychoactive substances. If persistent use or dependency; **1-year drug-free period** for heroin, morphine, methadone (there are exceptions for those on a supervised maintenance programme), cocaine and benzodiazepines. Additional restrictions if seizures occur	Yes	Licence revocation until drug-free period attained. Assessment and urine screen arranged by DVLA **will normally** be required. If persistent use of dependency; **1-year drug-free period** for cannabis, amfetamines, ecstasy and other psychoactive substances. If persistent use of dependency; **3-year drug-free period** for heroin, morphine, methadone, cocaine and benzodiazepines. Additional restrictions if seizures occur

Full information can be found at: www.dvla-gov.uk. On the left hand side of the page, click on "medical rules" then on the "At a Glance Guide".

References

1. Annas GJ. Doctors, drugs, and driving – tort liability for patient-caused accidents. N Engl J Med 2008; 359:521–525.
2. Metzner JL et al. Impairment in driving and psychiatric illness. J Neuropsychiatry Clin Neurosci 1993; 5:211–220.
3. Ray WA et al. Medications and the older driver. Clin Geriatr Med 1993; 9:413–438.
4. Noyes R, Jr. Motor vehicle accidents related to psychiatric impairment. Psychosomatics 1985; 26:569–566, 579.
5. Biecheler MB et al. SAM survey on "drugs and fatal accidents": search of substances consumed and comparison between drivers involved under the influence of alcohol or cannabis. Traffic Inj Prev 2008; 9:11–21.
6. Oyefeso A et al. Fatal injuries while under the influence of psychoactive drugs: a cross-sectional exploratory study in England. BMC Public Health 2006; 6:148.
7. Bramness JG et al. Minor increase in risk of road traffic accidents after prescriptions of antidepressants: a study of population registry data in Norway. J Clin Psychiatry 2008; 69:1099–1103.
8. Grabe HJ et al. The influence of clozapine and typical neuroleptics on information processing of the central nervous system under clinical conditions in schizophrenic disorders: implications for fitness to drive. Neuropsychobiology 1999; 40:196–201.
9. Wylie KR et al. Effects of depot neuroleptics on driving performance in chronic schizophrenic patients. J Neurol Neurosurg Psychiatry 1993; 56:910–913.
10. Brunnauer A et al. The impact of antipsychotics on psychomotor performance with regards to car driving skills. J Clin Psychopharmacol 2004; 24:155–160.
11. Barbone F et al. Association of road-traffic accidents with benzodiazepine use. Lancet 1998; 352:1331–1336.
12. Engeland A et al. Risk of road traffic accidents associated with the prescription of drugs: a registry-based cohort study. Ann Epidemiol 2007; 17:597–602.
13. Verster JC et al. Residual effects of middle-of-the-night administration of zaleplon and zolpidem on driving ability, memory functions, and psychomotor performance. J Clin Psychopharmacol 2002; 22:576–583.
14. Etminan M et al. Use of lithium and the risk of injurious motor vehicle crash in elderly adults: case-control study nested within a cohort. BMJ 2004; 328:558–559.
15. Verster JC et al. Methylphenidate significantly improves driving performance of adults with attention-deficit hyperactivity disorder: a randomized crossover trial. J Psychopharmacol 2008; 22:230–237.
16. Grabe HJ et al. The influence of polypharmacological antidepressive treatment on central nervous information processing of depressed patients: implications for fitness to drive. Neuropsychobiology 1998; 37:200–204.

Further reading

Driver and Vehicle Licensing Agency. For medical practitioners: at a glance guide to the current medical standards of fitness to drive. www.dvla.gov.uk

Miscellaneous

Use of antibiotics in psychiatry

Antibiotics are possibly the most frequently prescribed non-psychotropics in psychiatric institutions. Their use in psychiatry is often complicated by a number of factors: the absence of in-house specialist microbiologist advice; lack of experience or knowledge of modern antibiotic therapy; and restrictions on possible routes of administration because nursing staff are unlikely to hold necessary certification.

The following table sets out broad guidelines for the use of antibiotics in some commonly encountered conditions. In using this table, some general guidance should be noted:

- Take samples for microbiological examination before starting treatment.
- Start with oral therapy unless patient is very unwell or if condition requires a parenteral-only agent.
- Consult microbiology (where available) sooner rather than later – certainly if treatment has had no effect after 48 hours, ideally before starting treatment.
- Always check allergy status before giving any antibiotic. Check casenotes, the prescription chart and ask the patient.
- Be aware of the risk of antibiotic-associated colitis. Consult microbiology if this is suspected.

Table Use of antibiotics in psychiatry		
Infection/ condition	*First-line treatment*	*Second-line treatment*
Ears – e.g. otitis externa, otitis media	Consult microbiologist if otitis media suspected Chloramphenicol 0.5% drops, four times daily	Neomycin or polymyxin drops
Fungal infections	**Mouth/pharynx -** Nystatin suspension (100 000 iu/ml), 1 ml four times daily **Skin –** Clotrimazole 1% cream three times daily **Systemic or resistant skin infection –** fluconazole 50 mg daily for 7–14 days **Nail –** terbinafine 250mg daily (see BNF for duration)	Fluconazole Fluconazole Consult microbiology Consult microbiology
Gastro-enteritis	Not usually indicated – consult microbiology	
Pelvic inflammatory disease	Collect high vaginal swab; if *Neisseria gonococcus* excluded: Metronidazole 400 mg three times daily for seven days plus doxycycline 100 mg twice daily for 2 weeks. Give after food	Consult microbiology
Respiratory tract infections	Amoxycillin 250 mg three times daily or Erythromycin 500 mg three times daily	Co-amoxiclav 375 mg three times daily or Clarithromycin 250 mg twice daily
Throat infection	Usually has viral cause. Consult microbiology; if *Streptococcus* confirmed: Phenoxymethylpenicillin 250 mg four times daily or cefadroxil 500 mg twice daily or erythromycin 500 mg three times daily	Consult microbiology
Tuberculosis	Consult microbiology	
Urinary tract infections	Trimethoprim 200 mg twice daily or amoxycillin 250 mg three times daily	Nalidixic acid 1 g four times daily or co-amoxiclav 375 mg three times daily or ciprofloxacin 250 mg twice daily
Vaginal candidiosis	Oral fluconazole 150 mg as a single dose or clotrimazole 500 mg vaginal pessary	Consult microbiology
Wounds, ulcers, pressure sores	Do not use topical agents If cellulitis present – consult microbiology	

Index